# Fundamentals of Immunohematology

Theory and Technique

# Fundamentals of Immunohematology

## Theory and Technique

### 2nd edition

**Mary Louise Turgeon, Ed. D., MT(ASCP), CLS(NCA)**

Associate Director of Medical Education,
Robert Packer Hospital/Guthrie Healthcare System
Sayre, Pennsylvania
Research Assistant Professor
State University of New York
Health Science Center, College of Medicine
Syracuse, New York

**Williams & Wilkins**

BALTIMORE • PHILADELPHIA • HONG KONG
LONDON • MUNICH • SYDNEY • TOKYO

A WAVERLY COMPANY

1995

*Executive Editor:* Donna Balado
*Developmental Editor:* Lisa Stead
*Production Coordinator:* Marette D. Magargle
*Project Editor:* Robert D. Magee
*Cover:* Professors P.M. Motta and S. Correr, Science Source/Photo Researchers.

Copyright © 1995
Williams & Wilkins
Rose Tree Corporate Center
1400 North Providence Road, Building II, Suite 5025
Media, PA 19063-2043

Accurate indications, adverse reactions, and dosage schedules for drugs are provided in this book, but it is possible they may change. The reader is urged to review the package information data of the manufacturers of the medications mentioned.

*Printed in the United States of America*

**Library of Congress Cataloging-in-Publication Data**
Turgeon, Mary Louise.
    Fundamentals of immunohematology : theory and technique / Mary
Louise Turgeon. — 2nd ed.
       p.         cm.
    Includes bibliographical references and index.
    ISBN 0-683-08490-9
    1. Blood banks.   2. Immunohematology.   3. Blood—Transfusion.
I. Title.
    [DNLM:   1. Blood Groups—immunology.   2. Blood Grouping and
Crossmatching—methods.   3. Blood Transfusion—methods.   WH 420
T936f   1995]
RM172.T84   1995
615′.39—dc20
DNLM/DLC
for Library of Congress                                        94-29199
                                                 CIP

94 95 96 97 98
1 2 3 4 5 6 7 8 9 10

Dedicated to the memory of my husband, Don, who always supported my professional and personal goals.

# Preface

*Fundamentals of Immunohematology* has been written to meet the needs of undergraduate clinical laboratory science students, educators, and blood bank personnel for a book that encompasses the concepts, clinical practices, and techniques associated with modern transfusion therapy. Students, educators, and practitioners in other allied health disciplines, nursing, and medicine can also use the book as a primary blood banking-transfusion therapy reference.

The purpose of this book is to integrate the basic foundations of immunohematology and blood banking with the technical aspects of the discipline and clinical real-world problems. In the first two chapters, important safety and quality assurance information is presented. Subsequent chapters progress from theoretical concepts to technical issues of importance such as pretransfusion testing, blood components and synthetic blood substitutes, transfusion reactions, and blood-borne infectious diseases. The book concludes with two chapters on bench procedures and a new chapter on transplantation.

The second edition has been extensively revised to reflect contemporary theoretical information as well as current technical rules and regulations. Several chapters have been divided and developed into full chapters. In addition, a new chapter on transplantation has been added.

The pedagogy of the first edition has been retained in this edition. Specific chapter objectives have been condensed where appropriate and retained at the beginning of each chapter. Licensure type questions have been edited to reflect the new style of national examinations.

M.L. TURGEON
Waverly, New York

# Acknowledgments

My objective in writing *Fundamentals of Immunohematology* was to integrate the basic theory and current information in blood banking with real-world applications. This book has provided me with the opportunity to share with others my perspectives and experience as a practitioner and educator.

I would like to thank the staff at Lea & Febiger for their assistance in the production of this book. I would also like to thank the peer reviewers of the manuscript: Jay Wilborne, Teresa S. Nadder, Sandra Rothenberger, and Dixie Stone.

Since the publication of the first edition of this book, two significant individuals are no longer here to support my efforts. I will always affectionately remember the important roles that my husband, Don Turgeon, and my first editor, Christian "Kit" Febiger Spahr, played in sharing my dream to write.

# Contents

# Basic Foundations

# Part I

# Safety and Quality Assurance in the Blood Bank

At the conclusion of this chapter, the reader should be able to:

- Describe the role of the medical technologist or medical technician in providing quality patient care.
- List several functions of blood bank technicians and technologists.
- Explain the purpose and contents of a safety manual.
- Define the term *universal precautions* and discuss several protective techniques in the prevention of disease transmission.
- Describe four important safety practices.
- Name two types of hazardous waste and describe the appropriate management and control of these wastes.
- Name the essential components of a quality assurance program.
- Describe the major techniques for accomplishing quality in the blood bank and identify the daily quality assurance practices in the blood bank.

## Chapter Outline

## AN OVERVIEW OF IMMUNOHEMATOLOGY

Immunohematology is one of the specialized branches of medical science. Efforts to save human lives by transfusing blood have been recorded for several centuries. Although most of the blood used for early transfusions was of animal origin, in 1492 an unsuccessful attempt was recorded to transfuse Pope Innocent VII intravenously with the blood from three human donors. Because of the many disastrous consequences resulting from blood transfusions, transfusions were forbidden from 1667 until 1829, when James Blundell of England successfully transfused human blood to women suffering from postpartum hemorrhage.

Blood transfusions continued to produce unpredictable results, and were used only as a last resort, until Landsteiner's historic discovery of the ABO groups in 1900. This landmark event initiated the era of scientifically based transfusion therapy and was the foundation of immunohematology as a science. World War II ushered in the modern age of blood banking and transfusion therapy. More than 14 million units of whole blood are collected for use in the United States annually.

Medical technologists (clinical laboratory scientists) and technicians (clinical laboratory technicians) in the blood bank render a major service to the patient. To provide excellence in patient care through accurate, efficient, and cost-effective testing, the blood bank technologist or technician must be familiar with the *theory* and *practice* of a wide variety of procedures.

Functions of a modern blood bank include:

1. Recruiting blood donors
2. Collecting and storing whole blood or components from volunteer, paid, or autologous donors
3. Typing, screening, and preparing patient and donor blood for transfusion
4. Detecting and identifying unexpected antibodies in potential blood recipients or pregnant women
5. Establishing a database of HIV positive or questionable donors
6. Processing and dispensing blood components
7. Performing paternity testing
8. Conducting tissue typing prior to organ transplantation and participating in the processing of human materials, as in bone banking

## SAFETY IN THE BLOOD BANK

All blood banks and transfusion services need programs to minimize risks to the health and safety of employees, donors, volunteers, and patients. Suitable physical arrangements and appropriate equipment need to be available to maintain safe operations. In addition, all personnel need to be educationally qualified and properly trained.

The recognition and rapid increase in the number of patients identified with human immunodeficiency virus (HIV-1) has generated new policies from the Centers for Disease Control and Prevention (CDC) and mandated regulations by the Occupational Safety and Health Administration (OSHA). Compliance with the OSHA Bloodborne Pathogens Standard and the Occupational Exposure Standard is required in order to provide a safe work environment. OSHA mandates that the employer:

1. Educate and train all health care workers in universal precautions and in prevention of blood-borne infections
2. Provide proper equipment and supplies (for example, gloves)
3. Monitor compliance with the protective biosafety policies.

According to the CDC concept of universal precautions, all human blood and other body fluids are treated as potentially infectious for HIV-1, hepatitis B virus (HBV), or other blood-borne microorganisms that can cause disease in humans.

### Universal Blood and Body Fluid Precautions

In 1987 the CDC introduced the concept of *universal blood and body fluid precautions,* or *universal precautions,* in order to prevent parenteral, mucous membrane, and nonintact skin exposures of health care workers to blood-borne pathogens. The practice of universal precautions requires that blood and certain body fluids of *all* patients be treated as potentially infectious for HIV, hepatitis B virus (HBV), and other blood-borne pathogens. This approach to infection control eliminates the need for separate isolation procedures for patients known to be, or suspected of being, infectious. The application of universal precautions also eliminates the need for warning labels on specimens.

### Occupational Transmission of HBV and HIV

Blood bank personnel should be aware that HBV and HIV are totally different diseases, caused by totally unrelated viruses (see Chapter 13 for a full discussion of each of these viruses). The most feared hazard—the transmission of HIV through occupational exposure—is among the least likely to occur if proper safety practices are followed.

Exposure to HIV is uncommon, but cases of occupational transmission to health care personnel with no other known high-risk factors have been documented. As of December 1993, the CDC had received documented reports of 40 health care workers in the United States who have occupationally acquired HIV infection, as well as 83 *possible* cases of occupationally acquired HIV infection. Clinical laboratory personnel and nurses accounted for 15 and 13, respectively, of the documented cases. Laboratory personnel accounted for 14 of the possible cases of occupationally acquired HIV infection.

**Table 1-1. Potentially Infectious Materials**

Specific human fluids
- Amniotic fluid
- Blood
- Cerebrospinal fluid
- Pleural fluid
- Saliva (in dental procedures)
- Semen
- Synovial fluid
- Vaginal secretions

Other materials
- Any body fluid that is visibly contaminated with blood.
- All body fluids, in situations where it is difficult or impossible to differentiate among body fluids
- Unfixed tissue or organs (other than intact skin) from a human (living or dead)
- HIV-containing cell or tissue culture
- Organ cultures or HIV-containing culture medium

Occupational exposure is defined as a percutaneous injury (for example, a needle stick or cut with a sharp object). Other sources of exposure can include contact of mucous membranes or nonintact skin with infected blood, tissues, or blood-stained body fluid to which universal precautions apply, or contact with concentrated virus. Among health care personnel with documented occupationally acquired HIV infection, 84% had percutaneous exposure.

Although HIV is an unlikely work-related hazard, it cannot be ignored. At the present time, HIV, the virus that causes AIDS, is considered to be fatal. However, the transmission of HBV, which can also be fatal, is more probable. OSHA estimates that occupational exposures account for 5900 to 7400 cases of HBV infection annually.

Blood is the single most important source of HIV, HBV, and other blood-borne pathogens (Table 1-1) in the occupational setting. HBV can be present in extraordinarily high concentrations in blood, but HIV is usually found in lower concentrations. HBV may be stable in dried blood and blood products at 25°C for up to 7 days. HIV retains infectivity for more than 3 days in dried specimens at room temperature and for more than a week in an aqueous environment at room temperature. The likelihood of infection after exposure to blood infected with HBV or HIV depends on a variety of factors, including:

1. The concentration of HBV or HIV. Viral concentration is higher for HBV than for HIV.
2. The duration of the contact.
3. The presence of skin lesions or abrasions on the hands or exposed skin of the health care worker.
4. The immune status of the health care worker for HBV.

HBV and HIV may be *directly* transmitted by:

1. Percutaneous (parenteral) inoculation of blood, plasma, serum, or certain other body fluids due to accidental needlesticks, etc.
2. Contamination of the skin with blood or certain body fluids without overt puncture because of scratches, abrasions, burns, or exudative skin lesions.
3. Accidental exposure of mucous membranes (oral, nasal, or conjunctival) to infected blood or certain body fluids as the result of splashes or spattering.
4. Centrifuge accidents, or the improper removal of rubber stoppers from test tubes, can produce droplets. If these *aerosol* (introducing substances in droplet form into the air) products are infectious and come in direct contact with mucous membranes or nonintact skin, direct transmission of virus can result.

HBV and HIV may be *indirectly* transmitted. Viral transmission can result from contact with inanimate objects, such as work surfaces or equipment contaminated with infected blood or certain body fluids. If the virus is transferred to the skin or mucous membranes by hand contact, it can produce viral exposure.

## Protective Techniques for Infection Control

Universal precautions are intended to supplement rather than replace recommendations for routine infection control, such as handwashing. Infection control efforts for HIV, HBV, and other blood-borne pathogens must focus on prevention of exposure to blood. It is possible to be vaccinated against HBV, which is a wise preventive measure. The risk of nosocomial transmission of HBV, HIV, and other blood-borne pathogens can be minimized if blood bank personnel are aware of, and adhere to, essential safety guidelines.

### Selection and Use of Gloves

Gloves for medical use are either sterile surgical or nonsterile examination gloves made of vinyl or latex. There are no reported differences in barrier effectiveness between intact latex and intact vinyl gloves. Tactile differences have been observed between the two types of gloves, with latex gloves providing more tactile sensitivity; however, either type is usually satisfactory for phlebotomy and as a protective barrier when performing technical procedures. Rubber household gloves may be used for cleaning procedures.

The general guidelines related to the selection and use of gloves include:

1. Use sterile gloves for procedures involving contact with normally sterile areas of the body, or during procedures where sterility has been established and must be maintained. Use nonsterile examination gloves for procedures that do not require the use of sterile gloves.
2. Wear gloves when processing blood specimens, reagents, or blood products. Gloves should be changed frequently—and immediately if the gloves become visibility contaminated with blood or certain body fluids, or if physical damage occurs.
3. Do not wash or disinfect latex or vinyl gloves for reuse. Washing with detergents may cause increased penetra-

tion of liquids through undetected holes in the gloves. Rubber gloves can be decontaminated and reused, but disinfectants may cause deterioration. Rubber gloves should be discarded if they have punctures, tears, or evidence of deterioration, or if they peel, crack, or become discolored.

### Gloves as a Barrier Protection for Phlebotomy

Properly fitting vinyl or latex gloves do not interfere with the proper collection of samples from patients (see Chapter 2) or donors. The use of gloves reduces the incidence of blood contamination of hands during phlebotomy, but they cannot prevent skin punctures due to accidental needlesticks or other sharp objects. The likelihood of hand contamination with HIV, HBV, or other blood-borne pathogens depends on a variety of factors, including the following:

1. The skill, technique, and experience of the phlebotomist.
2. The number of phlebotomies performed. The cumulative risk of blood exposure increases for phlebotomists who perform more procedures.
3. The circumstances under which the specimen is being obtained. In emergency situations contact may be more likely.
4. The prevalence of either HBV or HIV in the patient or donor population.

As a result of the CDC modifications published in June 1988, some institutions have relaxed recommendations for using gloves for phlebotomy procedures by skilled phlebotomists in settings where the prevalence of blood-borne pathogens is known to be very low (for example, volunteer blood donation centers). Institutions or organizations that choose to modify the policy of requiring gloves for all phlebotomies must periodically reevaluate their policy and must provide gloves to all personnel who wish to use them for phlebotomy. Guidelines for the use of gloves during phlebotomy procedures include:

1. Gloves must be used by phlebotomists who have cuts, scratches, or other breaks in their skin. The presence of skin lesions will increase the likelihood of infection subsequent to skin exposure.
2. Gloves should be worn when the phlebotomist judges that hand contamination may occur (for example, when performing phlebotomy on an uncooperative patient).
3. Gloves must be worn when performing finger or heel sticks on infants and children.
4. Gloves must be worn when receiving phlebotomy training.
5. Gloves should be changed between each patient contact.

### Gloves as a Barrier Protection During Testing

Gloves should be worn when:

1. Handling blood, serum, plasma, or certain body fluids.
2. Handling blood or potentially infectious blood products, such as antisera of human origin and reagent red blood cells.
3. Testing serum, plasma, or red blood cells.
4. Using items potentially contaminated with blood or certain body fluids, such as specimen containers, laboratory instruments, and counter tops.

Care must be taken to avoid indirect contamination of work surfaces or objects in the work area. Gloves should be properly removed or covered with an uncontaminated glove or paper towel before answering the telephone, handling laboratory equipment, or touching door knobs.

### Facial Barrier Protection and Occlusive Bandages

Facial barrier protection should be used if there is a potential for splashing or spraying of blood or certain body fluids. Masks or other facial protection should be worn if mucous membrane contact with blood or certain body fluids is anticipated. All disruptions of exposed skin should be covered with a water-impermeable occlusive bandage. This includes defects on the arms, face, and neck. Blood should never be forced into an evacuated tube by exerting pressure on the syringe plunger. This practice may cause the rubber tube stopper to pop off and spray blood onto nonintact skin.

### Laboratory Coats or Gowns as Barrier Protection

A color-coded, two-lab-coat system (or equivalent system) should be used whenever laboratory personnel are working with potentially infectious specimens. The garment worn in the lab must be changed or covered with an uncontaminated coat when leaving the immediate work area. Garments should be changed immediately if grossly contaminated with blood or body fluids, to prevent seepage through to street clothes or skin. Contaminated coats or gowns should be placed in an appropriately designated biohazard bag for laundering. Disposable plastic aprons are recommended if there is a significant possibility that blood or certain body fluids may be splashed. Aprons should be discarded in a biohazard container.

## Important Safety Practices

### Handwashing

Frequent handwashing is an important safety precaution. It should be performed after contact with patients and laboratory specimens. Hands should be washed with soap and water:

**Table 1-2. Preparation of Diluted Household Bleach**

| Vol. of Bleach | Vol. of H₂O | Ratio | % Sodium Hyopchlorite |
|---|---|---|---|
| 1 mL | 9 mL | 1:10 | 0.5 |

1. After completing lab work and before leaving the laboratory.
2. After removing gloves.
3. Before eating, drinking, applying makeup, changing contact lenses, or using the lavatory.
4. Before all activities that involve hand contact with mucous membranes or breaks in the skin.
5. Immediately after accidental skin contact with blood, body fluids, or tissues. If the contact occurs through breaks in gloves, the gloves should be removed immediately and the hands thoroughly washed. If accidental contamination occurs to an exposed area of the skin, or because of a break in gloves, wash first with a liquid soap, rinse well with water, and apply a 1:10 dilution of bleach or 50% isopropyl or ethyl alcohol. Leave the bleach or alcohol on the skin for at least 1 minute before final washing with liquid soap and water.

## Decontamination of Work Surfaces, Equipment, and Spills

All work surfaces should be cleaned and sanitized at the beginning and end of each shift with a 1:10 dilution of household bleach (Table 1-2) or other approved disinfectant. Instruments, such as scissors used to cut donor blood segments or centrifuge carriages, should be sanitized daily with a dilute solution of bleach. Diluted household bleach prepared *daily* inactivates HBV in 10 minutes and HIV in 2 minutes. Disposable materials contaminated with blood must be placed in containers marked **Biohazard** and properly discarded.

All blood spills should be treated as *potentially* hazardous. In the event of a blood spill, this procedure for cleaning up the spill should be used:

1. Wear gloves and a lab coat.
2. Absorb the blood with disposable towels. (Bleach solutions are less effective in the presence of high concentrations of protein). Remove as much liquid blood or serum as possible before decontamination.
3. Using a diluted bleach solution, clean the spill site of all visible blood.
4. Wipe down the spill site with paper towels soaked with diluted bleach.
5. Place all disposable materials used for decontamination in a biohazard container.

## Needle Precautions

The Occupational Safety and Health Administration (OSHA) estimates that approximately six hundred thousand to one million needlestick injuries, the majority of which are unreported, occur in the United States each year. To prevent needlestick injuries, needles should *never* be recapped, separated from syringes, or otherwise manipulated by hand. Used needles should be placed intact into specifically designated red, puncture-proof, biohazard containers. The same criteria should be applied to used scalpel blades and any other sharp devices that may be contaminated with blood. The container should be located as close as possible to the work area. Phlebotomists should carry red, puncture-resistant containers in their collection trays. Needles should not project from the top of the container. To discard the containers, close and place them in a biohazard waste container. An accidental needlestick must be reported to the blood bank supervisor or other designated individual.

## Other Safety Precautions

A variety of other safety practices should be followed to reduce the risk of inadvertent contamination with blood or certain body fluids. These practices include:

1. All devices in contact with blood that are capable of transmitting infection to the donor or recipient must be sterile and nonreusable.
2. Food and drinks should not be consumed in work areas or stored in the same area as specimens. Containers, refrigerators, or freezers used for specimens should be marked as containing a biohazard.
3. Specimens needing centrifugation should be capped and placed in a centrifuge with a sealed dome.
4. Slowly and carefully open rubber-stoppered test tubes with a 2 × 2 gauze square placed over the stopper to minimize aerosol production.
5. Use safety bulbs for pipetting. Pipetting *by mouth* of any clinical material must be strictly forbidden.

## Hazardous Waste Management and Control

The control of infectious, chemical, and radioactive waste is regulated by a variety of government agencies, including the Occupational Safety and Health Administration (OSHA) and the Food and Drug Administration (FDA). Legislation and regulations that affect laboratories include the Resource Recovery and Conservation Act (RCRA), the Toxic Substances Control Act (TOSCA), clean air and water laws, right-to-know laws, and Toxic Waste and Hazardous Substance Communications (HAZCOM). Blood banks should implement applicable federal, state, and local laws that pertain to hazardous material and waste management.

### Infectious Waste

Infectious waste, such as contaminated gauze squares and test tubes, must be discarded into biohazard containers. These containers should:

1. Be conspicuously marked **Biohazard** and bear the universal biohazard symbol.
2. Be of the universal color—red, or red-and-black.
3. Be rigid, leakproof, and puncture-resistant (cardboard boxes lined with a leakproof plastic bag are available).
4. Be used for blood and certain body fluids* and disposable materials contaminated with them.

If the primary infectious waste containers are red plastic bags, they should be kept in secondary metal or plastic cans. Extreme care should be taken not to contaminate the exterior of these bags. If they do become contaminated on the outside, the entire bag must be placed into another red plastic bag. Secondary plastic or metal cans should be decontaminated regularly—and immediately after any grossly visible contamination—with an agent such as a 1 : 10 solution of household bleach.

Terminal disposal of infectious waste should be by incineration, however, an alternate method of terminal sterilization is autoclaving. If incineration is not done in the health care facility, or by an outside contractor, all contaminated disposables should be autoclaved prior to leaving the facility for disposal with routine waste.

### Chemical Hazards

OSHA recommends that all chemically hazardous material be properly labeled with the contents and hazardous severity of the material, and should bear a hazard symbol. Excellent guidelines for chemical hazards can be found in the National Fire Prevention Association's document NFPA 704.

Recent government regulations require that all employees who handle hazardous material and waste must be *trained* to use and handle these materials. Chemical-hazard education sessions must be presented to new employees and conducted annually for all employees.

### Safety Documents

Each laboratory *must* have an up-to-date safety manual. This manual should contain a comprehensive listing of approved policies, acceptable practices, and precautions, including universal blood and body fluid precautions. Specific regulations that conform to current state and federal requirements (such as OSHA regulations) must be included in the manual. Other sources of mandatory and voluntary standards include the Joint Commission on Accreditation of Healthcare Organizations (JCAHO), the College of American Pathologists (CAP), the Centers for

Disease Control and Prevention (CDC), and the American Association of Blood Banks (AABB) guidelines.

### Compliance with Universal Precautions

A clear policy on institutionally required universal precautions is needed. For usual blood bank activities, personal protective equipment consists of gloves and a laboratory coat or gown. Other equipment, such as masks, would normally not be needed.

Compliance with the enforcement of universal precautions also requires relevant training programs. The former OSHA categories of risk classifications for all routine and reasonably anticipated job-related tasks and personal protective equipment are useful in planning staff training programs.

Risk classification is divided into three categories:

**Category I.** Tasks that involve exposure to blood, body fluids, or tissues. All procedures or job-related tasks that involve an inherent potential for mucous membrane or skin contact with blood, body fluids, or tissues, or a potential for spills or splashes of them, are Category I tasks.

**Category II.** Tasks that involve no exposure to blood, body fluids, or tissues, but employment may require performing *unplanned* Category I tasks. The normal work responsibilities involve no exposure to blood, body fluids, or tissues, but exposure or potential exposure *may* be required as a condition of employment.

**Category III.** Tasks that involve *no* exposure to blood, body fluids, or tissues, and Category I tasks are *not* a condition of employment. Normal work responsibilities involve no exposure to blood, body fluids, or tissues. A person in this category does not perform, and is not expected to perform, tasks that can lead to potential exposure. Activities such as answering the telephone, or the use of shared bathroom facilities with workers in other categories, are not considered to be a risk.

In addition, Public Health Service (PHS) Biosafety Levels 1, 2, and 3 describe the relative risk that may be encountered in a work area (Table 1-3). Biosafety Level

**Table 1-3. Summary of Minimum Biosafety Level 2 Precautions**

- Decontaminate bench tops daily
- Use biosafety cabinet to contain aerosols, or wear gloves, gown, goggles, and mask
- Use gowns and gloves routinely
- No mouth pipetting
- Transport specimens properly
- Dispose of infectious waste properly
- No eating, drinking, smoking, or application of cosmetics or contact lenses in work areas
- Conduct high-risk activities in restricted areas
- Practice needle precautions
- Report accidental exposure to suspected or actual hazardous material immediately

---

* Some local health codes currently permit blood and body fluids to be disposed of by pouring them down the sink into the sanitary sewage system. If this disposal method is used, care must be taken to prevent splashing. Water should not be running into the sink, and facial protection and a plastic apron should be worn in addition to gloves and a laboratory coat. Sinks used for hazardous waste disposal should not be used for handwashing.

1 is the least threatening. The PHS biosafety levels of risk that may be encountered in a work area are:

**Level 1.** Work that involves agents of no known, or minimal, potential hazard to laboratory personnel and the environment.

**Level 2.** Work that involves agents of moderate potential hazard to personnel and the environment. *Note:* Most work with blood requires Biosafety Level 2 precautions (Table 1-3). Exceptions may be appropriate if no open specimens will be encountered.

**Level 3.** Work that involves indigenous or exotic agents that may cause serious or potentially lethal disease as a result of exposure by inhalation.

### Prophylaxis, Medical Followup and Records of Accidental Exposure

Vaccination against hepatitis B virus (HBV) and compliance with universal precautions is the best prophylaxis against blood-borne pathogens. Health care workers are urged to be vaccinated against HBV. If an individual has not been vaccinated, Hepatitis B immune globulin (HBIG) is usually given—concurrently with hepatitis B vaccine—postexposure to penetrating injuries. If administered in accordance with the manufacturer's directions, both products are considered safe and have proven free of any risk of infection with HBV or HIV.

If a known or suspected parenteral exposure takes place, a technician or technologist may request followup monitoring for HBV or HIV antibodies. This monitoring and followup counseling must be provided free of charge. If either voluntary informed consent—or in some states, disclosure, which bypasses consent requirements—is obtained, the source of the potentially infectious material and the health care worker should be tested immediately. The worker should also be tested at intervals after exposure. An injury report must also be filed after parenteral exposure.

### Compliance with Chemical Hazard Precautions

Legislation—such as state right-to-know laws, and OSHA document 29 CFR 1910—which sets the standards for chemical hazard communication (HAZCOM), determines the types of documents that must be on file in a laboratory. For example, a yearly physical inventory of all hazardous chemicals must be performed, and material safety data sheets (MSDS) should be available in each department of use. Each institution should also have at least one centralized area where all MSDS are stored.

## QUALITY ASSURANCE IN THE BLOOD BANK

Quality assurance is employed in the blood bank to support error-free performance in the delivery of the highest level of patient care. A systematic approach to quality en-

sures that patients will receive safe blood products and related transfusion services promptly and at a reasonable cost. Important factors in a comprehensive quality assurance program include:

1. Qualified personnel
2. An approved blood bank policies-and-procedures manual that is reviewed annually by the medical director
3. Correct blood collection and storage
4. Established quality assurance techniques
5. Accuracy in communications and records
6. Recognition and resolution of problems

### Qualified Personnel

One of the most important functions of a quality assurance program in the blood bank is the maintenance of high personnel standards. Assessment of these standards should include:

1. Evaluation of entry-level and continuing competency
2. Maintaining competency

### Evaluation of Competency

The entry-level examination competencies of all certified persons in blood banking must be validated. Validation should take the form of both external certification and formal education, plus new-employee orientation to the work environment.

At the beginning of employment, and periodically throughout the year, an employee's written job description should be reviewed. This document is important to an employee because it describes the employer's expectations. A job description includes the duties and responsibilities of a position and measurable standards of performance for each task described, as well as position title, hours worked, major functions and responsibilities of the position, qualifications for the position, the employees' immediate supervisor, and the departments with whom the employee frequently works and communicates. Staff members are required to document that they have read the manuals that apply to their tasks.

The formal annual performance evaluation, as well as periodic informal sessions, should focus on the job description as a tool to opening communication and promoting professional growth. Action plans for the correction of deficiencies need to be developed, with specific activities and timelines noted. Evaluations are maintained to document performance.

### Maintaining Competency

Participation in continuing education activities is essential to maintaining competency. If specific areas of performance need strengthening, continuing education can become a tool for corrective action.

For most staff, continuing education keeps them

abreast of new knowledge and practices in the field, as well as maintaining their job interest and motivation. It is important for individuals to share information gained after attendance at a continuing education activity. Forms of continuing education include antibody and journal clubs, self-instruction, professional meetings, writing for publication, and workshop presentations for peers. A person's job description should specify that continuing education is an expected professional activity, and it should be recognized and rewarded with positive comments on performance evaluations and appropriate merit-pay increases.

## Blood Bank Policies, Procedures, and Records

### Policies

Laboratory policies should be included in a reference manual that is available to all hospital personnel. This manual must contain all approved policies, including safety rules. The manual may refer to appropriate sections of the current *Standards* or *Technical Manual* published by the American Association of Blood Banks. Transfusion practices (such as the length of time a unit of crossmatched blood will be reserved for a patient) should be *clearly* stated in this document. The manual should be reviewed periodically by all blood bank personnel, and *must* be reviewed annually by the medical director.

### Procedures and Procedures Manuals

The procedures manual must be a complete document of current techniques and approved policies that is available at all times in the immediate work area of blood bank personnel. It is extremely important for all blood bank personnel periodically to review this manual. The manual should comply with the National Commission for Clinical Laboratory Standards (NCCLS) format standards for a procedures manual (Table 1-4). The procedural format

### Table 1-4. Written Procedural Protocol*

Procedure Name
Name of the test method
Principle and purpose of the test
Specimen collection and storage
Quality control
Reagents, equipment, and supplies
Procedural protocol
Expected or normal (reference) values
Procedural Notes:
   Sources of error
   Limitations
   Clinical applications
References

* Source: ''Summary of NCCLS Approved Guideline GP2-A2,'' *Clinical Laboratory Technical Procedural Manual*, 2nd ed. Villanova, PA: National Committee for Clinical Laboratory Standards, 1992

found in Chapters 14 and 15 of this text follows these guidelines.

Alternative techniques can be included with each procedure, if more than one technique is acceptable. New pages must be dated and initialed when inserted into the manual. Pages that have been removed must be retained for 5 years, with the date of removal from the manual and the reason for removal indicated. It may be necessary, for legal reasons, to identify the reason a particular procedure was followed.

### Record Keeping and Retention

Each blood bank and transfusion service must have a system of record keeping, manual or computerized. Policies and procedures related to the system must be established, written, and followed. Confidentiality of donor and patient records must be assured.

The actual results of each test must be recorded immediately, and the final interpretation must be recorded upon completion of testing. There must be a means to identify persons performing each significant step in collection, processing, compatibility testing, and distribution of blood or blood components.

If a computer system is used, records must be complete, retrievable in a reasonable period of time, and protected from accidental or malicious modification or destruction. A display system must be available before final recording of data. If the computer system is not available, an alternate system must be available. A computer system must document: program development, if done internally; installation of the system; validation of functionality and data integrity; training of personnel; and policies and procedures for system maintenance and operations. System modifications must be authorized and documented. In addition, all changes in operations or software must be documented, both in complete technical detail and in language understandable to the users.

The length of retention of blood bank records varies (Table 1-5). Some records must be stored for a minimum of 5 years; other records need to be stored indefinitely.

### Identification Errors

Strict adherence to proper blood collection and storage (discussed in Chapter 2) is *critical* to the safety and accuracy of blood transfusion. Identification is a major potential source of error. The most common cause of transfusion accidents (for example, hemolytic transfusion reactions) is inaccurate identification of the patient, the patient's blood specimen, or the donor unit; this is followed by clerical inaccuracies. The most detailed quality assurance program for reagents or equipment is no safeguard against an incorrectly labeled specimen or inaccurately identified patient.

Errors can be made from the time the unit of blood is collected until it is administered to a recipient. Whenever possible, two people should check the identification at all

**Table 1-5. Record Keeping and Retention**

| Category | Type of Information |
|---|---|
| *Indefinite Retention* | |
| Donors and Donor Blood | Medical history, physical examination, consent, and interpretations of tests for infectious disease markers for each donation, including hemapheresis. |
| | Blood and components received from outside sources, including numeric and alphanumeric identification of blood unit, and identification of the collecting facility. Information from an intermediate facility may be used if the intermediate facility retains the unit number and identification of the collecting facility. |
| | Information to identify facilities that carry out any part of the preparation of blood components and the function performed. |
| | Final disposition of each unit of blood or component. |
| | Names, signatures, and initials or identification code, and inclusive dates of employment of those authorized to sign or initial or review reports and records. |
| | Notification to donors of permanent deferral. |
| Patients | Notification to recipients of potential exposure to disease transmissible by blood. This must include patient notification (Look-Back) to identify recipients of blood or components from donors who are subsequently found to have infection with HIV or HTLV-I/II and to have these recipients informed of the risk of infection. |
| *Retention for 5 Years (Minimum)** | |
| Donors and Donor Blood | ABO group and Rh type. |
| | Blood typing difficulty. |
| | Severe adverse transfusion reaction. |
| | Hemapheresis procedure clinical record. |
| | Blood component inspection prior to issue. |
| Patients | ABO group and Rh type. |
| | Blood typing difficulty. |
| | Detection of clinically significant unexpected antibodies. |
| | Severe adverse reactions to transfusion. |
| | Interpretation of compatibility testing. |
| | Therapeutic procedures including phlebotomy, hemapheresis and outpatient transfusion. |
| Other Records | All superceded procedures, manuals, and publications including safety records. |
| | Temperature of storage and results of inspection of blood and component units. |
| | Control testing of components, reagents, and equipment and proficiency testing surveys (including dates, tests performed, observed results, interpretations, identification of personnel carrying out the tests, and any appropriate corrective actions. |
| *Indefinite Retention* | |
| Deferral Records | Records of persons who have been placed on permanent deferral or surveillance. |
| *Required Deferral Period* | Records of prospective donors who have been temporarily deferred for the protection of the potential recipient. |

Source: Adapted from *Standards for Blood Banks and Transfusion Services,* 15th ed. 1993, pp. 39–41.
* Or as required by applicable state and federal laws

stages involved in collection, pretransfusion testing, and administering blood or blood products in order to minimize this risk. The growing use of computerized bar code identification will continue to be an asset.

## Established Quality Assurance Techniques

### Daily Practices

Each procedure must have an established protocol to ensure the quality of the results. To support a quality control program, documentation of results is essential. Factors such as day-to-day variability, reagent variability, and differences between technologists need to be closely monitored. The daily testing of reagents and monitoring of refrigerators, freezers, and waterbaths (discussed in detail on pages 13–17) undergird the accuracy and safety of

blood banking practice. If reagent control results are not acceptable, the source of error must be identified before patient test results can be considered valid.

### Peer Review

Many voluntary or mandatory accrediting agencies—such as the American Association of Blood Banks (AABB), College of American Pathologists (CAP), Joint Commission on Accreditation of Healthcare Organizations (JCAHO), and state and federal regulatory agencies—have requirements or laws that are designed to ensure the safety of blood transfusion and related activities. It is important not only to satisfy various inspection and accreditation requirements but also to embrace the spirit and the letter of the law.

Peer review of transfusion practices related to blood and blood derivatives is required by the JCAHO, the *Code*

**Table 1-6. General Functions of the Transfusion Committee**

- Establish policies for blood utilization
- Develop criteria for, and audit, transfusion practices
- Monitor transfusion reactions, including posttransfusion infections
- Evaluate improvement in problem areas
- Assess safety, adequacy, and methods of blood procurement
- Develop and promote continuing medical education related to transfusion practices
- Review transfusion service written policies and procedures annually to ensure compliance with accepted standards
- Report to the hospital Quality Assurance Committee and recommend corrective action when indicated

*of Federal Regulations* that qualifies hospitals to receive Medicare reimbursement, and most states, for Medicaid or comparable reimbursement. The standards of the JCAHO require that the medical staff conduct a review of blood usage at least quarterly. Peer review is also required for voluntary accreditation of the blood bank/transfusion service by both the CAP and the AABB. The hospital transfusion committee usually performs the peer review function and has been delegated to make recommendations (Table 1-6) concerning policies governing transfusion practices.

In addition to the medical director of the blood bank, all medical departments that routinely order blood should have representation on the committee: surgery, anesthesiology, internal medicine, obstetrics, pediatrics, and high-blood-use subspecialties such as hemodialysis, oncology, hematology, and neonatology. Nonphysician members should include a blood bank technologist, hospital administrator, nurse, and health information technology librarian.

Although the blood bank medical director may make most of the day-to-day policy decisions, it is appropriate for the committee to review issues affecting the entire hospital staff. Blood usage review includes the following:

1. Review ordering practices for blood and blood products.
2. Review the use of all categories of blood and blood components.
3. Evaluate all confirmed transfusion reactions.
4. Monitor indicator data for appropriate blood utilization.
5. Evaluate blood use problems.
6. Take actions to resolve problems.
7. Assess the actions and document improvement.
8. Review the adequacy of transfusion services to meet the needs of patients.
9. Develop or approve policies and procedures relating to the distribution, handling, use, and administration of blood and blood components.
10. Communicate relevant information to the organization-wide quality assessment program.

Encouraging appropriate blood use (Table 1-7) is the basic task of the transfusion committee. The committee can base recommendations on review of retrospective blood bank records or retrospective and concurrent review of patients' charts.

### Continual Quality Improvement

The JCAHO has described a 10-step model for hospital quality assessment of blood use. These steps are:

1. Assign responsibility
2. Delineate the scope of blood use

**Table 1-7. Guidelines for Appropriate Blood Use**

| Blood Product | Purpose |
|---|---|
| Whole blood | To restore blood volume and oxygen-carrying capacity |
| Packed red blood cells | To restore oxygen-carrying capacity |
| Leukocyte-poor packed red blood cells | To minimize exposure of patient to donor leukocytes |
| Washed red blood cells | To remove plasma proteins |
| Neocyte-enriched red blood cells | To prolong the time between transfusions in chronically transfusion-dependent patients (e.g., sickle cell anemia or thalassemia) |
| Frozen/deglycerolized red blood cells | Prevention of nonhemolytic febrile transfusion reactions, plasma allergies, or exposure to cytomegalovirus; autologous transfusion |
| Irradiated red blood cells | To inactivate the replicative machinery of the donor leukocyte |
| Granulocytes concentrates | To elevate the leukocyte count in patients with neutropenia or granulocyte dysfunction who are suffering from, or at risk of, a life-threatening infection |
| Platelet concentrates | To replace platelets in patients who are bleeding or at a high risk of bleeding |
| Single-donor plasma | To treat hypovolemic shock or severe burns |
| Fresh frozen plasma | To replace plasma proteins and all coagulation factors except platelets in patients who are bleeding, or at risk of bleeding |
| Cryoprecipitate | Treatment of patients with von Willebrand's disease, hemophilia A (Factor VIII deficiency), or hypofibrinogenemia who are bleeding, or at risk of bleeding |
| Factor VIII concentrate | Treatment of patients with hemophilia A who are bleeding, or at risk of bleeding |
| Prothrombin complex | Treatment of patients with a deficiency of factors II, VII, IX, or X, who are bleeding or at risk of bleeding |
| Albumin (5%) | To increase blood volume while maintaining colloidal oncotic pressure |

3. Identify the important aspects of blood use
4. Identify indicators (audit criteria)
5. Establish thresholds for indicators
6. Monitor indicator activity
7. Evaluate blood use and problems
8. Take actions to resolve problems
9. Assess the actions and document improvement
10. Communicate relevant information to the organization-wide quality assessment program

Recently the JCAHO has defined an "agenda for change." This philosophy places blood transfusion review into a reorganized program with emphasis on continual quality improvement. Some aspects of transfusion functions can be performed by hospital-based groups other than the transfusion committee.

Participation in proficiency testing programs ensures maintenance of consistently high standards. In addition to monitoring quality through a paper trail or computer tracking, participation in external specimen quality control programs contributes to overall patient quality. In order to monitor ongoing performance, proficiency samples should not receive special handling by the laboratory. Testing should include weekend, evening, and night shift personnel.

## Donor Collection and Processing

Monitoring quality also includes donor collection and processing activities (Chapter 2). Review of the interview, physical examination, and other donor screening procedures (such as determination of hemoglobin/hematocrit) can be performed as a quality assurance monitoring step. Scales used to determine the weight of whole blood (Table 1-8) need to be monitored either daily or on the day of use.

Other categories to be monitored include donor reactions, infectious disease testing, labeling, component processing and storage, and transportation. The number, type, and severity of reactions before, during, and after phlebotomy must be recorded and evaluated. Testing for infectious diseases must include adequate quality measures in test performance, as well as an effective system to locate and quarantine all blood units (and their components) that are found to be positive during the processing of a donor unit. A system for monitoring compliance with labeling requirements is essential. Quality assurance related to blood components includes documentation of in vitro assays to validate the effective collection of specific elements or coagulation factors. Donor selection, blood volume, accuracy of scales, and anticoagulant volumes apply to component preparation as well as to whole-blood collection and processing. Specific requirements for the collection and storage of blood components are described in Chapters 2 and 10.

## Accuracy in Communications and Records

Blood bank personnel have frequent contact with physicians, nurses, hospital support staff, and donors. In many cases, the events requiring verbal communication are situations of high stress. It is critical that excellent communication skills be developed in order to interact effectively with coworkers (as well as others) in order to deliver high-quality patient care.

It is equally important, in reporting results, to be alert for clerical errors, particularly transcription errors. Clerical errors must be guarded against when:

1. Reporting results (grouping, typing, crossmatching)
2. Maintaining pre- and post-transfusion records
3. Releasing and transferring blood and blood components

## Recognition and Resolution of Problems

A *problem* can be described as a "critical incident," or it can be any deviation from the standard operating procedures of the blood bank. To resolve a critical incident, good communication and thorough analysis of the problem—with interconnected causes and overlapping factors such as inadequate training or knowledge, quality of materials or reagents, or improper procedures—may need to be considered. The incident (loss of a thawed unit of plasma, a donor reaction, a clerical error) should be thoroughly documented.

Ongoing assessment of the operation of a blood bank requires objective appraisal of important aspects of patient care and followup correction of identified problems. No one wants to make a mistake in the blood bank, but in the day-to-day operation of a blood bank, errors, near misses, and inefficient practices and problems can develop. It is essential to detect problems and resolve them appropriately.

## DAILY QUALITY ASSURANCE PRACTICES

To monitor and ensure the highest quality of patient care, some factors in the blood bank should be evaluated periodically; others are an integral part of the daily operation. Reagents and equipment are critical components in the accuracy of daily testing.

**Table 1-8. Weight of Whole Blood**

Problem: Determine the minimum weight of a 450 (±45) mL unit of whole blood.
- One milliliter of blood weighs no less than 1.053 grams (gms) (hemoglobin 12.5 g/dL).
- One unit of whole blood = 405 mL × 1.053 g/dL = 426 gms, plus the weight of the container and its anticoagulant.*
- Determine the weight of the container and its anticoagulant by weighing at least 10 containers from the lot in use.

* A practical maximum total weight is 522 gms.

## Quality Control of Reagents

Commercial reagent antisera and reagent red blood cells are licensed for clinical use only after they meet or exceed minimum criteria for specificity and potency as described by the FDA. Manufacturer's directions must be followed exactly. To guard against the loss of potency or specificity, the following additional practices should be followed:

1. Store all antisera at 2° C to 6° C when not in use.
2. Freeze all rare antisera for extended storage. It is best to divide antisera into aliquots to avoid repeated thawing and refreezing. Thaw at 37° C and mix thoroughly before use.

### Daily Quality Control of Antisera

The manufacturer's directions must be strictly followed. Because reagent antisera or red blood cells may deteriorate or become contaminated with other antisera, blood, or microorganisms, each blood bank must confirm that *each* reagent, on *each* day of use, is correctly reactive.

Positive and negative controls must be used for each reagent tested. The red blood cells selected as positive controls in the test system should be weakly reactive to provide accurate indication of antisera potency. This is best accomplished by choosing reagent red blood cells that are heterozygous for the antigen being tested. The following reagents should be tested daily: anti-A, anti-B, anti-A,B, anti-D, anti-D control, and antihuman globulin (AHG).

For routine daily quality control testing of AHG reagent, it is sufficient to use D positive red blood cells sensitized with anti-D. The anti-D reagent should be diluted to coat, but not agglutinate, D positive cells and produce no more than a 2+ reaction with AHG. Evaluation for anticomplementary activity is considered unnecessary, because AHG reagent that has lost potency due to improper storage demonstrates comparable loss of both anti-IgG and anticomplement activity.

Antisera that are infrequently used should be tested in parallel with an actual test. This requires simultaneous testing of both positive and negative control red blood cells.

### Daily Quality Control of Reagent Red Blood Cells

Reagent red blood cells used for determination of ABO grouping, and IgG-sensitized red blood cells used as a control for antiglobulin testing, may be prepared locally, provided there is adequate documentation that they are satisfactory for the intended use. Reverse grouping red blood cells (such as $A_1$, $A_2$, and B cells—and red blood cells being screened for the detection of clinically significant antibodies and Coombs control cells—should be tested on each day of use with both a positive and a negative control. Reverse grouping cells should be tested with anti-A and anti-B antisera. If a discrepancy is observed, the reagent red blood cells and antisera should be tested independently with cells or antisera of known reactivity.

It is particularly important visually to inspect each vial of screening red blood cells for hemolysis. If the supernatant fluid is hemoglobin-tinged and a single wash removes the color, these cells can be used on the day of processing as a freshly prepared saline suspension. Some technologists prefer to use a saline suspension of washed reagent red blood cells, especially if there is a problem in antibody identification. Screening cells can be examined with a weak saline-reactive antibody and a weak AHG antibody. It is impractical to perform testing on each vial of antibody identification panel red blood cells.

### Monitoring Serum-to-Cell Ratios

Pasteur-type pipettes are used in most blood banks to deliver serum in antibody screening and identification, and in compatibility testing. These pipettes vary considerably in the size of the drop delivered, according to the diameter of the orifice and the angle the pipette is held at the time the drop is delivered. The ratio of serum to cells affects the sensitivity of antibody detection. The average drop size and volume delivered by the pipettes in use as transfer pipettes and red cell droppers in a specific blood bank should be determined. Once the average delivery volume has been determined, the directions for antibody detection and compatibility testing should designate volumes that are near the optimal 80:1 serum-to-cell ratio.

In addition, when reagent red blood cell or antisera manufacturers are changed, the delivery volume should be checked. An appropriate adjustment should be made in the number of drops of serum that are added from the disposable pipettes in use.

### Daily Reagent Control Records

Records of daily quality control testing must be maintained. The form must include the reactions, the commercial source and lot identification numbers of the reagent tested, date of testing, and the initials of the person conducting the test (Fig. 1-1).

## Quality Control of Equipment

All instruments and equipment used in the laboratory must be properly maintained and monitored to ensure accurate testing. Continual monitoring of the temperatures of waterbaths, refrigerators, and freezers is important to the maintenance of reagent quality and test performance.

Equipment such as centrifuges, automatic cell washers, Rh view boxes (if used), and equipment (refrigerators, freezers, waterbaths) should be cleaned and checked for accuracy on a regular schedule. A preventive maintenance schedule should be followed on all pieces of equipment.

REAGENT CONFIDENCE RECORD

+ = POSITIVE
N = NEGATIVE

Reagent - Antisera Control

| CELLS | Anti A | Anti B | Anti A,B | Anti D | Rh-hr. control | AHG | Saline |
|---|---|---|---|---|---|---|---|
| A₁ | 1 | 4 | 7 | 10 | 12 | 13 | |
| A₂ | 2 | 5 | 8 | | | | |
| B | 3 | 6 | 9 | 11 | | 14 | |
| dilute ccc | | | | | | | 15 |

| | IS 37° | AHG | CCC |
|---|---|---|---|
| Searchcyte I | | | |
| Searchcyte II | | | |
| dilute Anti-D | 16 | | |
| Saline | 17 | | |

INTERPRETATION

| REAGENT | LOT NO. | EXP. DATE |
|---|---|---|
| Anti-A | | |
| Anti-B | | |
| Anti-A,B | | |
| Anti-D | | |
| Rh-hr. Control | | |
| Albumin | | |
| Reverse Cyte | | |
| Search Cyte | | |
| Coombs Control Cells | | |
| A₂ Cells | | |
| Anti-human Serum | | |

EQUIPMENT CONTROL

| | INCUBATOR TEMP (°C) | | | REFRIG. (°C) | | |
|---|---|---|---|---|---|---|
| I.D. | 37±1 Bath | 37±1 Block | 45-50 Rh Box | 1-6 Top Shelf | 1-6 Bottom Shelf | -20 to -35 Freezer | 22-25 Rm.Tp. | 56±1 |
| Temp. | | | | | | |

Date _____

Technician _____

**Figure 1-1.** Reagent confidence record

Failure to monitor equipment regularly can produce inaccurate test results and lead to expensive repairs.

### Centrifuges

The purpose of centrifugation in serologic testing is to enhance in vitro red blood cell antigen-antibody reactions. Centrifugation should pack the red blood cells into a well-defined cell button; tighter packing is undesirable because nonagglutinated red blood cells cannot be easily resuspended.

Quality control procedures for centrifuges and serofuges need to be addressed. Timing needs to be checked periodically with a stopwatch; speed should be checked with a tachometer at least every 6 months.

In the case of automated cell washers, the dual function of washing red blood cells and enhancing agglutination reactions is desired. In this situation, the supernatant fluid should be clear after centrifugation and produce a well-defined cell button. Some automated cell washing systems also add AHG reagent to each tube.

To ensure that a centrifuge is working efficiently, the operator's manual should describe initial quality control checks and calibration procedures, both following repairs and annually. With automated cell washers, a number of factors must be checked. Procedures include the following:

1. Testing to ensure that an equal volume of saline is being dispensed into each tube.
2. Checking that the total volume of saline added to each tube is less than 80% of the total volume of the tube, to eliminate the possibility of cross-contamination. Forceful overfilling of test tubes with saline can produce foaming of serum protein. Underfilling of test tubes produces inadequate washing, and residual protein can neutralize AHG antisera.
3. Verification that the time and speed of centrifugation are correct.
4. Examination of red blood cell buttons to be sure that each is correctly resuspended between washings, so that they can be washed properly and packed properly on the final decant cycle.
5. Inspection to see that the addition of AHG is proper, if this step is part of the cell washer's function.

### Waterbaths and Heat Blocks

Waterbaths and heat blocks are usually maintained at 37° C in the blood bank for the detection of warm reactive antibodies and thawing blood components (such as fresh frozen plasma) (30° C–37° C). The temperature of incubators should be monitored periodically by properly attaching a standard thermometer. The temperature of each piece of equipment needs to be checked and recorded on each day of use (refer to Fig. 1-1).

The temperature can vary in the wells of a multi-well heat block, but it is impractical to check the temperature of each well with a thermometer. A quick method of observing the temperature is to use cholesteric liquid crystals, which change color as the temperature changes (green at 37° C and blue at 37.5° C). A few crystals can be placed in a test tube in each well for 60 seconds and observed immediately.

### Refrigerators and Freezers

Written procedures must be readily available on how to maintain blood and components within permissible temperatures. They should include instructions to be followed in the event of a power failure.

Blood bank refrigerators and freezers must have a fan for circulating air, to ensure a constant temperature throughout, and must be equipped with an audible alarm system and a temperature-recording device. In addition, refrigerators and freezers must be connected to an emergency power system. Temperature checks must be performed and recorded daily. Alarms must be periodically tested.

Refrigerator and freezer compartments in which blood, blood components, or derivatives are stored may also be used for the storage of donor samples, patient samples, or blood bank reagents.

Refrigerators, freezers, and platelet incubators need to have the temperature monitored at least every 4 hours. If storage of certain components is in an open area, the ambient temperature must be recorded at least every 4 hours. If red blood cells are stored in liquid nitrogen, a gas phase temperature below $-120°$ C must be maintained.

The alarm must be set to activate at a temperature that will allow for proper action before the blood or components reach an undesirable temperature. Alarms must signal in an area that has adequate coverage to ensure that immediate corrective action can be taken. An alarm system in liquid nitrogen freezers must be activated when an unsafe level of contained liquid nitrogen is approached.

### Rh Viewing Boxes

When Rh testing is performed on a slide or plate, the lighted viewing box facilitates reading of the test and provides sufficient heat so that the temperature of the anti-D antisera and red blood cells is approximately 37° C. Therefore, the glass surface of the viewing box must remain between 45° C and 50° C. A thermometer should be properly attached to the glass surface of the box and the temperature checked routinely before use. When a test is conducted, the slide should be placed in the middle part of the heated surface to avoid possible cold spots.

### Platelet Incubators

Various types of incubators are available for platelet storage. These incubators rotate platelet concentrates to prevent platelet aggregation. The speed (rpms) should be checked periodically according to the manufacturer's directions.

In addition, a system must be in operation to monitor the temperature (20° C to 24° C) continuously and to record the temperature at least every 4 hours. If platelet concentrates stand in an open storage area, the ambient temperature should be recorded at least every 4 hours.

## CHAPTER SUMMARY

### Chapter Review

The medical technicians (MLTs/CLTs) and medical technologists (MTs/CLSs) working in the blood bank render a major service to patients. Personnel working in this area have diverse functions. Some of these functions include recruiting blood donors, collecting and processing donor blood, performing pretransfusion compatibility testing, and identifying unexpected antibodies that have been formed as the result of pregnancy or prior transfusion.

### Safety in the Blood Bank

Implementing universal precautions eliminates the need for specific warning labels. All blood, and certain body fluid specimens, should be treated as infectious and capable of transmitting disease.

Safety issues for patients, as well as employee protection, are a major concern for blood banks. Blood bank personnel must comply with the latest safety practices. The proper techniques to guard against infectious contamination, as well as against exposure to chemical hazards, is mandatory.

### Quality Assurance in the Blood Bank

Quality assurance is a method of ensuring error-free performance. Any system should encompass the categories of personnel, policies and procedures, and techniques. Techniques for accomplishing quality include daily practices, peer review, external quality control programs, accuracy in communications and records, and the recognition and resolution of problems.

### Daily Quality Assurance Practices

Daily practices must include the monitoring of antisera and reagent red cells. Equipment (for example, centrifuges and alarms) must be periodically tested for accuracy. Records of all of these procedures must be maintained.

## REVIEW QUESTIONS

1. Which of the following is *not* a function of a blood bank?
   A. Recruiting and collecting homologous blood donors

   B. Typing, screening, and preparing blood for transfusion
   C. Directly administering blood or blood components to patients
   D. Detecting and identifying antibodies in potential recipients

2. Universal blood and body fluid precautions mandate:
   A. Immunization against hepatitis B
   B. Immunization against tuberculosis
   C. Wearing gloves when handling specimens contaminated with blood
   D. Wearing masks for routine testing

3–7. Match the following precautions. (Use an answer only once).
   3. Food and drinks
   4. Needles
   5. Work surfaces
   6. Specimens
   7. Contaminated gauze squares

   A. Should be disinfected with diluted bleach
   B. Should be disposed of in biohazard bags
   C. Should *not* be in the same area as specimens
   D. Should *not* be recapped
   E. Should be treated as potentially hazardous

8. The purpose of quality assurance in blood banking is:
   A. To regulate inventory management
   B. To guarantee error-free performance
   C. To regulate personnel standards
   D. To monitor hospital budget practices

9. Which activity is helpful in maintaining competency as a continuing education activity?
   A. Antibody and journal clubs
   B. Professional meetings
   C. Writing for publication
   D. All of the above

10. A daily practice (or practices) that constitutes part of a quality assurance program includes:
   A. Daily monitoring of reagents
   B. Daily monitoring of refrigerators
   C. Daily monitoring of centrifuges
   D. Both A and B

11. Clerical errors must be guarded against when:
   A. Reporting results
   B. Maintaining pre- and post-transfusion records
   C. Releasing blood or components
   D. All of the above

12. Commonly used blood bank antisera should be routinely stored at _____° C when not in use.
   A. 2 to 6
   B. 0 to 2
   C. −10 to 0
   D. −20 to −10

13. Reagent antisera and reagent erythrocytes should be tested on each day of use with:
    A. A positive control
    B. A negative control
    C. Either a positive or negative control
    D. Both A and B

14. Heat blocks or waterbaths should be maintained at _____° C.
    A. 37
    B. 25
    C. 15
    D. 2

15. The glass surface of an Rh viewbox should be _____° C.
    A. Between 45 and 50
    B. Between 26 and 39
    C. Between 16 and 25
    D. Between 0 and 15.

**Bibliography**

Albertson, D.: Final OSHA regs mandate HIV, HBV protection. MLO, 24(2):17–18, 1992.

Alpert, L.I.: OSHA: New Player in the Battle Against AIDS. Med. Lab. Obs., 22(4):49–52, 1990.

Alpert, L.I.: Prevention of device-mediated bloodborne infections. Med. Lab Obs., 24(11):43–46, 1992.

Baer, D.M.: Bleach Stability. Med. Lab. Obs., 22(4):9, 1990.

Baron, E.J., and Finegold, S.M.: Baily and Scott's diagnostic microbiology, 9th ed., St. Louis: C.V. Mosby, 1994.

Brown, J.W.: Biosafety in the Laboratory. Testrends, 5(1):1–3, 1991.

Campbell, J.A.: Appropriateness of blood product ordering: Quality assurance techniques. Lab. Med., 20(1):15–18, 1989.

Clark, J.A. and Wilkes, N.C.: Computer-assisted implementation of maximum surgical blood order schedule. Lab. Med., 20(1):40–44, 1989.

Deutsch, C.E., and Malley, C.B.: Safety standards and laboratory procedures for exposure to chemicals. Laboratory Medicine, 23(7):482–484, July 1992.

Fahey, B.J. and Henderson, D.K.: Minimizing risks for occupational blood-borne infections. JAMA, 264(9):1189–1190, September 5, 1990.

Ferdinand, M.: OSHA's bloodborne pathogens standard: Enforcement, compliance and comment. J. Healthcare Materials Management, 11(8):12, 14, 16, September 1993.

Kuriyan, M.: Surgical blood use analysis: A microcomputer program. Lab. Med., 20(5):324–326, 1989.

McCullough, J.: The nation's changing blood supply system. JAMA, 269(17):2239–2245, May 5, 1993.

Miller, L.E.: Recommended concentrations of bleach. Lab. Med., 21(2):116, 1990.

Moses, B. et al.: Evaluation of the appropriateness of blood and blood product transfusion using preset criteria. JAMA, 263(1):95, 1990.

Perry, S., Ryan, J., and Polan, H.J.: Needlestick injury associated with venipuncture. JAMA, 276(1):54, 1992.

Schwartlander, B. et al.: Guidelines for designing rapid assessment surveys of HIV seroprevalence among hospitalized patients. Public Health Rep., 109(1):53–59, January–February, 1994.

Turgeon, M.L.: Clinical hematology, 2nd ed., Boston: Little, Brown, 1992.

U.S. Dept. of Health and Human Services, Update: Universal precautions for prevention of transmission of human immunodeficiency virus, hepatitis B virus, and other bloodborne pathogens in health care settings. MMWR, 37(24), June 1988.

U.S. Dept. of Health and Human Services. AIDS and human immunodeficiency virus infection in the United States: 1988 updates. MMWR, 38(S-4), May 12, 1989.

U.S. Dept. of Health and Human Services. Guidelines for prevention of transmission of human immunodeficiency virus and hepatitis B virus to health care and public safety workers. MMWR, 38(S-6):4, 5, 9, 11, June 23, 1989.

U.S. Dept. of Health and Human Services. HIV/AIDS Surveillance Report, Dec, 1993 Vol. 5, No. 4 Centers for Disease Control and Prevention, Atlanta.

U.S. Dept. of Health and Human Services. Regulations for implementing the clinical laboratory improvement amendments of 1988: A summary. MMWR, 41(RR-2), February 28, 1992.

U.S. Dept. of Health and Human Services. Surveillance for occupationally acquired HIV infection—United States, 1981–1992. MMWR, 41(43), October 30, 1992.

U.S. Dept. of Labor, Occupational Safety and Health Administration. Occupational exposure to bloodborne pathogens: Part 1910 to title 29 of the Code of Federal Regulations, 64175–64182, Fed. Reg., 56(235), December 6, 1991.

Voldish, K.: The "Dirty Dozen"—12 common violations of OSHA's bloodborne pathogens standard. Lab. Med., 24(5):305–306, 1993.

Wong, E.S. et al.: Are universal precautions effective in reducing the number of occupational exposures among health care workers? JAMA 265(9)1123–1128, March 6, 1991.

# Blood Collection, Storage, Processing, and Issue

At the conclusion of this chapter, the reader should be able to:

- Discuss the proper procedure for collecting blood from patients, including the possible problems that may be encountered and their resolution.
- Describe the medical history and physical criteria that would exclude an allogeneic donor.
- Delineate the proper steps in the preparation of a donor venipuncture site and the collection of blood.
- Explain the possible donor reactions and the appropriate initial first aid procedure for each.
- Define the term *autologous donation* and compare the four forms of autologous donation-transfusion.
- State the only generally accepted criterion for autologous donation.
- Briefly explain the process and purposes of hemapheresis.
- Describe the possible donor reactions that may be encountered in normal and in hemapheresis donors and explain the appropriate first aid procedures for each.
- Name the commonly used anticoagulants for donated blood and their respective approved maximum storage time.
- State at least three changes that occur in stored, anticoagulated blood.
- Define the term *storage lesion.*
- State the appropriate methods of storage of blood and blood components, including recipient and integral samples.
- List the tests that must be conducted on a unit of allogeneic blood.
- Describe the relevant information that should be checked before a unit of blood is issued from the blood bank and list the acceptable conditions for the reissue of blood.

The collection of blood from patients and donors is one
of the important functions of a blood bank. This chapter
discusses the techniques for collecting pretransfusion venous blood specimens and information related to the processing, storage, and dispensing of blood are discussed.

## PATIENT BLOOD SPECIMEN COLLECTION

A properly collected blood specimen is essential to the
accuracy and safety of blood transfusion. Strict adherence
to the rules of specimen collection is critical, because identification errors involving either the patient or the specimen are *major* potential sources of error.

### Blood Collection Equipment

Although disposable plastic syringes may be used in special
cases, evacuated blood-collecting tubes are the most widely
used system for collecting venous blood samples. This system (Figure 2-1A) consists of a collection needle, a holder,

**A**

**B**

**Figure 2-1.** Evacuated tube system. A. The end of the double-
pointed needle is partially inserted into the rubber stopper. B. After
the opposite end of the needle successfully enters the blood vessel, the evacuated tube is gently pushed until the partially inserted
needle fully pierces the rubber stopper. This allows the blood to
enter the evacuated tube.

and an evacuated glass tube containing enough vacuum to draw a specific amount of blood.

The collecting needle is a double-pointed needle. The longer end is for insertion into the patient's vein and the shorter end pierces the rubber stopper of the collection tube (Figure 2-1B). Sterile needles are used with a standard holder. Various needle sizes are available. In addition to length, needles are identified by gauge size. The higher the gauge number, the smaller the inner diameter (bore). These double-pointed needles are either single-sample or multiple-sample types. The multiple-sample type has a rubber sleeve on the short end of the needle that punctures the rubber stopper. The rubber sleeve prevents blood from leaving the system when more than one evacuated tube is needed for testing. The specially designed needle holder is used to secure the needle. This holder can be washed and reused.

Evacuated tubes are intended for one-time use. Using the evacuated tubes with the double-pointed collection needles make possible a closed sterile system for specimen collection. This preserves the quality of the specimen during transport prior to testing and protects the patient from infection.

Evacuated tubes come in various sizes (mL), including pediatric sizes, with color-coded stoppers. The stopper color denotes the type of anticoagulant; for example, lavender denotes EDTA and red indicates no anticoagulant. Two types of tubes—red-stoppered and lavender-stoppered—are used in routine blood banking. Because the red-stoppered tube contains no anticoagulant, venous blood will clot normally and produce the straw-colored fluid, *serum*. The lavender-stoppered tube, containing anticoagulant, allows whole blood to be separated into *plasma,* a straw-colored fluid, and its cellular components: erythrocytes, leukocytes, and platelets. *EDTA,* ($K_3$ *EDTA*), tripotassium ethylenediamine tetra-acetate, removes ionized calcium ($Ca^{++}$) through a process referred to as *chelation.* This process forms an insoluble salt of calcium that prevents blood coagulation.

## Blood Collection Techniques

### General Protocol

1. All medical personnel should introduce themselves pleasantly to the patient and briefly explain the phlebotomy procedure in easy-to-understand terms.
2. Patient identification is the *critical* first step in blood collection. Both asking the patient his/her name and checking the patient's hospital identification band, which *must* be physically attached to the patient, are necessary. In cases where patients are unable to give their name or where identification is attached to the bed or missing, nursing personnel should be asked to physically identify the patient. Verbal identification of

a patient should be noted on the test requisition. Many blood banks utilize a numbered blood bank bracelet and requisition system (Figure 2-2) in order to positively identify blood bank patients. This is particularly critical in emergency or outpatient situations when hospital identification bands may not be available.
3. Forms requesting whole blood or components, and forms accompanying blood samples from the recipient, must contain sufficient information for positive identification of the recipient. The first and last name and identification number of the patient are required. Optional information can include: sex, date of birth, clinical diagnosis, previous transfusion or pregnancy history, and attending physician's name. Incomplete or illegible forms must not be accepted. The appropriate equipment is then assembled.
4. All specimens should be properly labeled *immediately after* the specimen is drawn and *before* leaving the recipient's bedside. The label must state the recipient's first and last name, identification number, date, and name or initials of the phlebotomist. The specimen label and request form must agree.

## Venous Blood Collection (Phlebotomy)

### Supplies and Equipment

1. Test requisition.
2. Tourniquet.
3. 70% alcohol, and gauze square or alcohol wipes.
4. Sterile disposable needles (vacutainer or syringe type).
5. Evacuated blood tubes and a needle holder or a syringe (in special cases).
6. Spirits of ammonia breakable capsule (emergency use only).
7. Adhesive plastic strips or spots.
8. Disposable gloves.

### Initiation of the Procedure

1. Identify the patient.
2. Assemble all necessary equipment at the patient's bedside.
3. Wash your hands.
4. If a needle and syringe are to be used, firmly secure the hub of the needle with the shield in place on the syringe. If an evacuated tube is to be used, screw the short end of the needle on the needle holder. The plastic shield is to remain on the needle until *immediately* prior to performing the venipuncture. The evacuated tube is placed into the holder and gently pushed until the top of the stopper reaches the guideline on the holder. *Note:* Do not push the tube all the way into the holder or a loss of vacuum will result.

***Selection of an Appropriate Site.*** *Note:* Venous blood should not be drawn near an intravenous infusion (IV).

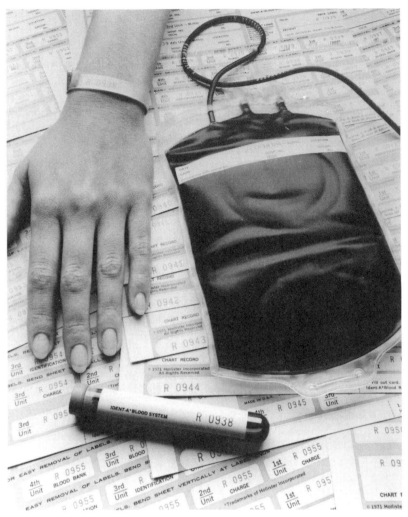

**Figure 2-2.** Blood bank identification system. A numbered patient identification system, such as the Ident-A-Blood Recipient System by Hollister Incorporated, Libertyville, IL, adds an additional safety precaution for correct identification of the patient, patient blood specimen, unit of blood, and related requisitions and reports. With this system, the patient receives a separate numbered bracelet at the time when the blood specimen is drawn. The number also appears on the blood specimen, any blood or blood components, the patient's chart, and related requisitions.

It is preferable to draw the sample from the opposite arm, if possible, or from below the infusion site. If possible, the IV should be shut off for 2 to 3 minutes before the sample is drawn. Note on the test requisition whether the sample was drawn from below an IV site and record the type of solution being administered. Obtaining a blood specimen from an IV line should be avoided because it increases the risk of mixing the fluid with the blood sample.

1. Visually inspect both arms. Choose the arm that has not been repeatedly used for previous venipunctures and one that is free of bruises, abrasions, or sites of infection. In the arm, three veins can be used for venipuncture: the cephalic, basilic, and median cubital veins (Figure 2-3).
2. Applying the tourniquet. Two general types of tourniquets are available. One type is a flat or rounded rubber

tube and the other is a strap with velcro ends for simple adjustment to the arm.

A. If a rubber tourniquet is used, slide the tourniquet under the arm a few inches above the expected venipuncture site. Evenly adjust both ends of the tourniquet (Figure 2-4A).
B. Grasp both ends of the tourniquet a few inches above the patient's arm. Pull up on the ends to create tension in the tourniquet. Cross the right side of the tourniquet over the left side. With the index finger of the right hand, create a small loop in the right side of the tourniquet while continuing to hold the tension in the tourniquet (Figure 2-4B).
C. Slip this small loop under the left side of the tourniquet. The resulting application will allow easy removal of the tourniquet with one hand,

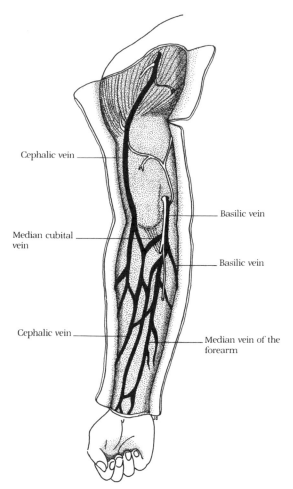

**Figure 2-3.** Veins of the arm. In the arm, the two most common veins used for venipuncture are the cephalic and median cubital. Illustration from Turgeon, M.L.: Clinical Hematology: Theory and Procedures. Boston, Little, Brown and Company, 2nd Ed., 1993, p. 19.

Cephalic vein

Median cubital vein

Cephalic vein

Basilic vein

Basilic vein

Median vein of the forearm

after the needle has been inserted into the vein (Figure 2-4C).

3. Ask the patient to make a fist (sometimes a roll of gauze is placed in the patient's hand). This usually makes the veins more prominent. With the index finger, palpate (feel) for an appropriate vein (Figure 2-4D). It is important to feel the vein, which has a resilient feeling compared to the surrounding tissues.

Large veins are not always a good choice because they have a tendency to roll as you attempt to venipuncture. Superficial and small veins should also be avoided. The ideal site is generally near, or slightly below, the bend in the arm (Figure 2-4E). If no appropriate veins are found in one arm, examine the other arm by applying the tourniquet and palpating the arm. Do not leave the tourniquet on for more than 2 minutes. Veins in other areas—wrists, hands, or feet—can be used as venipuncture sites; however, only experienced phlebotomists should use these sites.

### Preparation of the Venipuncture Site

1. After an appropriate site has been chosen, release the tourniquet.
2. Using a cotton ball saturated with 70% alcohol, or an alcohol pad saturated with 70% alcohol, cleanse the skin in the area of the venipuncture site. Using a circular motion, cleanse the area from the center outward. Do not go back over an area once it has been cleansed.
3. Allow the site to dry.

### Performing the Venipuncture

The appropriate steps in the venipuncture are shown in Figure 2-5A–E. *Note:* It is preferable to avoid touching the cleansed venipuncture site. In unusual situations, it may be allowable to touch the area with an alcohol-wiped finger to reestablish the location of the vein.

1. Put on disposable gloves.
2. Reapply the tourniquet and have the patient make a fist.
3. Use one hand to hold the evacuated tube or syringe. Use one or more fingers of the other hand to secure the skin area of the forearm below the intended venipuncture site. This will tighten the skin and secure the vein. Position the patient's arm in a slightly downward position.
4. Hold the needle with attached syringe or tube about 1 to 2 inches below, and in a straight line with, the intended venipuncture site. Position the blood-drawing unit at about a 20° angle. The bevel of the needle should be in an *upward* position.
5. Gently and smoothly insert the needle through the skin and into the vein. If a vacuum tube is used, one hand should steady the needle holder unit while the other hand pushes the tube to the end of the plastic holder. It is important to hold the needle still during the collection process to avoid interrupting the flow of blood. Multiple samples can be drawn by attaching each additional tube as soon as the tube attached to the needle holder has filled. If a syringe is used, one hand should steady the barrel of the syringe while the other hand slowly pulls the plunger backwards.

### Termination of the Procedure

1. The tourniquet may be released as soon as the blood begins to flow into the evacuated tube or syringe, or immediately before the final amount of blood is drawn.
2. Ask the patient to open the hand.
3. After the desired amount of blood is drawn, place a gauze pad over the venipuncture site.
4. Withdraw the blood-collection unit with one hand

**Figure 2-4A–E.** Venipuncture technique. To perform a venipuncture **A,** Adjust both ends of the tourniquet evenly. **B** and **C,** When applying the tourniquet place tension on the tourniquet, cross one side over the other, and slip a small loop under one side of the tourniquet. A properly applied tourniquet can be removed with one hand by simply pulling on one end of it. **D,** With the index finger, palpate the site for a suitable vein. **E,** The ideal site for venipuncture is usually near or slightly below the bend of the elbow. (Illustration from Turgeon, M.L.: Clinical Hematology: Theory and Procedures. Boston, Little, Brown and Company, 2nd Ed., 1993, p. 20.)

and *immediately* press down on the gauze pad with the other hand.

5. If possible, have the patient elevate the entire arm and press on the gauze pad with the opposite hand. If the patient is unable to do this, apply pressure until bleeding ceases.

6. Place a nonallergenic adhesive spot or strip over the venipuncture site. *Note:* Failure to apply sufficient pressure to the venipuncture site could result in a *hematoma* (a collection of blood under the skin that produces a bruise).

7. Remove the evacuated tube from the holder. Dispose of the needle immediately into a puncture-proof container.

8. Mix tubes with anticoagulant by inverting the tubes several times. If a syringe was used, carefully remove the needle with an appropriate instrument *before* dispensing the blood into a test tube. Never manipulate a needle with your fingers! Discard the used needle in an appropriate biohazard container.

9. Label all tubes.

10. Clean up supplies from the work area. Remove gloves

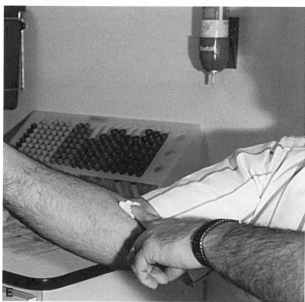

**Figure 2-5.** Phlebotomy procedure. A. Establishing the patient or donor's identity. B. The gloved forefinger of the phlebotomist's left hand locates the appropriate venipuncture site. C. The site is prepared with an alcohol sterile wipe and gauze square. D. The needle is gently inserted into the patient's vein. E. After the appropriate evacuated tubes are filled, the procedure is terminated by covering the venipuncture site with a square of sterile gauze and applying pressure.

25

and wash hands before leaving the patient's room. Place gloves and other contaminated supplies in a bio-hazard bag. Have outpatients wait for a few minutes after the venipuncture is complete to be sure they don't feel dizzy or nauseated.

### Phlebotomy Problems

Occasionally, a phlebotomist may experience an unsuc-cessful venipuncture. A venipuncture should not be at-tempted more than twice. If two attempts are unsuccessful, notify the blood bank supervisor or find someone who can assist you. Problems encountered in phlebotomy can include the following:

1. Refusal by the patient to have blood drawn. The proce-dure for solving this problem is to excuse yourself pol-itely from the patient's room. Note the refusal on the requisition and notify the blood bank supervisor.
2. Difficulty in obtaining a specimen because the bore of the needle is against the wall of the vein. Pulling back slightly on the needle may solve this problem.
3. Movement of the vein. To guard against this problem, always have firm pressure on the arm below the in-tended venipuncture site. The needle can be moved around slightly to attempt to reach the vein, but *exces-sive* probing around in the tissues must be avoided. Care must be exercised in moving the needle around because a hematoma can form if both sides of the vessel wall are pierced.
4. Sudden movement by the patient or phlebotomist that causes the needle to come out of the arm prematurely. Always anticipate the possibility of this situation. Quick action is needed! Immediately remove the tour-niquet and place a gauze pad on the venipuncture site. Apply pressure until bleeding has stopped to prevent the formation of a hematoma. It is a good practice to have gauze pads at hand whenever a venipuncture is being performed.
5. Blood clots form in anticoagulated tubes. In the phle-botomy procedure, red-top (plain) evacuated tubes should be drawn *first*. Promptly after terminating the venipuncture procedure, a tube containing EDTA anti-coagulant should be gently inverted at least 6 times to mix the specimen.
6. Fainting or illness subsequent to venipuncture. The first-aid procedures of the laboratory should be prac-ticed in this event. It is very important to prevent injury to the patient.

## DONOR BLOOD COLLECTION

Although most donor blood is furnished by large regional collection agencies, many hospital blood banks maintain active donor facilities for the collection of blood from au-tologous or emergency donors, or for the collection of special products. In this section, information related to the collection and processing of allogeneic, hemapheresis, and autologous donors is presented.

### Allogeneic Donors

The process of collecting blood from volunteer blood do-nors consists of three stages:

1. Registering and interviewing prospective donors to de-termine if they are appropriate candidates
2. Conducting a brief physical examination
3. Collecting a unit of blood or blood component

### Registering and Interviewing the Donor

Basic information from the donor includes:

1. Date of donation
2. Name: Last, first and middle initial
3. Address: Residence and/or business
4. Telephone: Residence and/or business
5. Sex
6. Age and/or date of birth
   Acceptable donors must be at least 17 years old. Collec-tion of blood from minors requires written consent obtained in accordance with applicable law. An elderly person may donate at the discretion of the blood bank physician.
7. Signed consent allowing the blood bank to take and use blood from the prospective donor.

On the day of blood donation, the prospective donor's medical history needs to be evaluated confidentially to determine that the donation will not be detrimental to the donor or potential recipient. Oral interviews are aimed at identifying donors who are at high risk of transmitting disease. Direct questions regarding at-risk behaviors (Table 2-1), especially sexual habits, are considerations. One of the important adjuncts in ensuring a safe blood supply in the volunteer donor system is reliance on the donor's integrity and good intentions when answering the predo-nation medical history.

A form similar to Figure 2-6 is the basic guideline for the medical history interview. This record must be kept

**Table 2-1. At-Risk Behaviors**

| At-Risk Behavior | Signs and Symptoms |
|---|---|
| Parenteral drug abuse | Inspect both arms for signs of repeated needle injections |
| Alcohol abuse | Intoxication or signs and symptoms (such as jaundice) of alcohol abuse |
| Sexually transmitted diseases | History of syphilis or gonorrhea, treatment for syphilis or gonorrhea, or reactive screening test for syphilis in the absence of a confirmatory test shall be cause for deferral for 12 months after completion of therapy |

DONOR REGISTRATION – BLOOD BANK

| DONOR'S NAME | ADDRESS (Street, City, State & Zip Code) | | HOME PHONE | DATE |
|---|---|---|---|---|
| DONOR'S BLOOD TYPE | SEX ☐ MALE ☐ FEMALE | I.D. INITIALS | | DATE OF BIRTH |
| DONOR'S EMPLOYER & ADDRESS | | | | BUSINESS PHONE |

PLEASE ANSWER YES OR NO TO QUESTIONS BELOW

| | | | | | |
|---|---|---|---|---|---|
| Ever had Yellow Jaundice, Liver Disease, Hepatitis or a Positive Blood Test for Hepatitis? | ☐ YES ☐ NO | Ever Had Heart Disease, Chest Pain, or Shortness of Breath? | | ☐ YES | ☐ NO |
| Ever Taken Self–Injected Drugs? | ☐ YES ☐ NO | Ever Had Convulsions, Seizures, or Fainting Spells? | | ☐ YES | ☐ NO |
| Received Blood Transfusions, Blood Injections, or Tattoos in Past Six Months? | ☐ YES ☐ NO | Ever Had a Blood Disease or Cancer? | | ☐ YES | ☐ NO |
| Been Exposed to Anyone With Yellow Jaundice, Hepatitis or a Kidney Machine in past Six Months? | ☐ YES ☐ NO | Had any Vaccinations or Immunizations in the Past Year? | | ☐ YES | ☐ NO |
| Ever Had Malaria? | ☐ YES ☐ NO | Do You Have Any Acute Respiratory Disease or Trouble Breathing? | | ☐ YES | ☐ NO |
| Ever Been Outside the U.S. in Past Three Years? | ☐ YES ☐ NO | Had Any Dental Work in the Past Three Days? | | ☐ YES | ☐ NO |
| Ever Had Any Serious Illness? | ☐ YES ☐ NO | Been Exposed to Anyone With AIDS? | | ☐ YES | ☐ NO |
| Been Hospitalized in Past Six Months? | ☐ YES ☐ NO | Been to Haiti or Zaire? | | ☐ YES | ☐ NO |
| Are You Feeling Well Today? | ☐ YES ☐ NO | Pregnant in the Past Six Months? | | ☐ YES | ☐ NO |
| Taken Any Medications in Past Month? | ☐ YES ☐ NO | Had Sweats, Unexplained Fever or Weight Loss, Lumps in Neck, Arm Pits or Groin, Discolored Areas of Skin or Mouth, Persistent Cough, or Diarrhea? | | ☐ YES | ☐ NO |
| Ever Been Deferred as a Blood Donor or Had Problems Donating Blood? | ☐ YES ☐ NO | | | | |

*The information I have given for this form is correct. I understand the information that has been given to me today about the spread of the AIDS virus through donated blood and plasma. If I am at risk for spreading the AIDS virus, I agree not to donate blood and plasma for transfusion to another person.*

▶ DONOR'S SIGNATURE                    DATE

FOR BLOOD BANK USE

| PACK Q.C. | BLOOD DONATION WT. | LOT. No. | WHOLE BLOOD NO. | COMMENTS: |
|---|---|---|---|---|
| DONOR WEIGHT | TEMP. | B.P. | PULSE | |
| ARMS ☐ SATISFACTORY ☐ UNSATISFACTORY | | SKIN DISEASE ☐ YES ☐ NO | | |
| PHLEB ☐ SATISFACTORY ☐ UNSATISFACTORY | | REACTION ☐ SLIGHT ☐ MODERATE ☐ SEVERE | | |
| Hb ☐ SATISFACTORY ☐ UNSATISFACTORY | Hct. | TIME DONATION Completed | | |

**Figure 2-6.** Donor form.

for at least 5 years or as required by local law, whichever is longer. Factors of importance include previous donations, previous deferral, surgery, illnesses, pregnancy, immunization, hepatitis, malaria, and other infectious diseases.

*Previous Donations.* The donation interval should be at least 8 weeks, except for reasonable qualifying circumstances. A program may be established to allow collection of blood components from a single donor for an individual patient—upon request of the recipient's physician and with the approval of the blood bank physician and the informed consent of the donor. The donor must meet all donor requirements except for frequency of donation. Whole-blood donation must be deferred for at least 48 hours after hemapheresis.

*Previous Deferral.* It is important to determine if a donor has been previously rejected as a blood donor and the reason for the deferral. This information should be considered when evaluating the donor's current eligibility.

Donor deferral registries (DDRs) are an important adjunct to screening procedures; they alert blood banks to attempted future donations from unacceptable donors (if the person returns to give blood and the original reason for rejection is no longer detectable). Records for permanent donor deferral must be maintained indefinitely.

*Surgery.* In cases of uncomplicated surgery, a donor is only disqualified until healing is complete and full activity has been resumed. A donor receiving blood or blood components should be deferred for 12 months (see Hepatitis).

*Illnesses.* Potential donors with diseases of the heart, liver, or lungs, or individuals with a history of cancer, or those with an abnormal bleeding tendency should be excluded subject to evaluation by a physician. Prospective donors who have had cancer—with the exception of those who have had minor skin cancer or cervical cancer in situ—must be evaluated by a qualified physician before being accepted as a blood donor. Donors who have had leukemia or lymphoma must be permanently deferred. A previous history of tuberculosis that has been successfully treated and is no longer active need not disqualify a donor. Questionable conditions—for example, an unexplained weight loss of 10 pounds (4.5 kg) or more—might suggest that a potential donor is not in good health. The donor should be referred to a qualified physician for further evaluation.

*Pregnancy.* If a woman knows she is pregnant, she should be excluded from donating. Ordinarily, a prospective donor shall be excluded for 6 weeks following the conclusion of her pregnancy. An exception can be made if a mother's blood is needed for an exchange transfusion of her infant. Note that pregnancy is not a contraindication for autologous donation.

*Medication.* In general, medications taken by a donor are not harmful to a recipient. Most donors taking medications, prescription and nonprescription, are acceptable blood donors; deferral of a donor because of drugs is based on the nature of the disease. Checking a list of permitted drugs (Table 2-2) or getting approval on an individual basis should be standard procedure. Ingestion of aspirin-containing medication within 3 days precludes use of a donor as the sole source of platelet preparations for a recipient.

*Immunization.* Persons recently immunized with toxoids and killed viral, bacterial, and rickettsial vaccines are acceptable, if they are symptom free and afebrile. Included in this group of immunizations are those for anthrax, cholera, diphtheria, influenza, paratyphoid, pertussis, plague, polio (injection, Salk), Rocky Mountain spotted fever, tetanus, typhoid, and typhus. It has been reported that up to 5% of donors who recently received influenza vaccination before blood donation will have false positive-screening enzyme-linked immunosorbent assays (ELISAs) for antibodies to human T-cell lymphotrophic virus type 1 (HTLV-1).

After smallpox vaccination, a donor is acceptable when the scab has fallen off, or 2 weeks after an immune reaction.

A donor who has received an attenuated live virus vaccine such as polio (oral), measles (rubeola), mumps, or yellow fever, is deferred for 2 weeks after the last immunization. In the case of German measles (rubella) vaccine, deferral is for 4 weeks after the last injection. If rabies vaccination has been given following a bite by a rabid animal, the donor must be deferred for 1 year after the bite.

Prospective donors shall be deferred for 12 months after receiving hepatitis B immune globulin (HBIG). Administration of immune serum globulin does not require that a donor be deferred. In addition, recipients of hepatitis B vaccine are acceptable donors if they are not disqualified for other reasons.

**Table 2-2. Drugs That May Be Permitted in a Prospective Blood Donor**

- Blood-pressure medications (if the donor is free of side effects and any cardiovascular symptoms
- Bronchodilators and decongestants (nonprescription)
- Hypnotics used at bedtime
- Isoniazid, if no evidence of active tuberculosis exists
- Oral hypoglycemic agents, if diabetes is well controlled without evidence of vascular complications
- Tetracyclines and other antibiotics for acne (Isoretinoin disqualifies a donor for 30 days)
- Topical steroid preparations applied to skin lesion not at the venipuncture site
- Tranquilizers (a physician should evaluate to exclude antipsychotic medications)
- Other medications: oral contraceptives, mild analgesics, vitamins, hormones or weight-reduction pills (marijuana may be permitted if the donor is not under the influence of the drug)

*Infectious Diseases.* A donor must be free from infectious diseases known to be transmissible by blood, as determined by the usual examinations and a medical history. Deferral of donors relates both to donations of whole blood and blood components.

HEPATITIS. Recipients of blood, or human blood components, or derivatives known to be possible sources of hepatitis are excluded for 12 months. Persons with a history of tattoo or having had close contact with an individual with viral hepatitis must be deferred for 12 months. Other reasons for donor deferral are listed in Table 2-3.

ACQUIRED IMMUNODEFICIENCY SYNDROME (AIDS). All donors must be given educational materials informing them of the high-risk behaviors associated with human immunodeficiency virus (HIV) infection and the signs and symptoms of the resultant diseases that characterize AIDS. Persons at risk for AIDS should refrain from donating blood for transfusion and should be provided with an opportunity to indicate in confidence that their blood, if collected, is not suitable for transfusion. A confidential, self-administered questionnaire that describes high-risk behaviors and requires the donor to designate their blood for either laboratory purposes or for transfusions is an effective way of implementing HIV screening.

MALARIA. Permanent residents of nonendemic countries who have been in an area where malaria is considered endemic may be accepted 6 months after their return to a nonendemic area, if they have been free of unexplained febrile illnesses and have not taken antimalarial drugs.

Donors who have a history of malaria, or were previously resident in an endemic area, should be deferred for 3 years after becoming asymptomatic or after leaving the endemic area. If donors have taken antimalarial prophylaxis and been in an endemic area, deferral should be for 3 years after cessation of therapy *and* after departure from the area, if they remain asymptomatic in the interim. Donations for plasma, plasma components, or derivatives lacking intact RBCs are exempted from the previous restrictions.

Physical Examination

The pre-donation physical examination should include:

1. Assessment of general appearance and health
2. Measurement of weight
3. Evaluation of temperature
4. Measurement of pulse and blood pressure
5. Quantitation of hemoglobin or microhematocrit (packed cell volume)

*General Appearance.* The prospective donor should appear to be in good health. Skin at the venipuncture site must be free of lesions. Evidence of repeated venipunctures (suggestive of narcotic use) excludes a donor. Alcoholic intoxication also excludes a donor.

**Table 2-3. Deferral of Donors Related to Infectious Diseases**

Hepatitis Related

*Indefinite deferral:*
1. History of viral hepatitis after the 11th birthday
2. History of hepatitis B
3. History of a confirmed positive test for hepatitis B surface antigen (HBsAg)
4. History of a repeatedly reactive test for antibody to hepatitis B core antigen (anti-HBc) on more than one occasion
5. Demonstrate an alanine aminotransferase (ALT) blood level that is more than 2× the highest acceptable value on one occasion, or above (but less than twice) the highest acceptable value for suitable donor blood on more than one occasion
6. Present or past clinical or laboratory evidence of infections with hepatitis C virus (HCV)
7. Donation of the only unit of blood or blood component transfused to a patient who developed transfusion-associated hepatitis. This patient must have received no other blood component or derivative known to transmit these infections and have no other probable source of infection.
8. History or evidence of intravenous drug abuse. Evidence of repeated parenteral drug use or other obvious stigmata of parental drug use permanently excludes a donor.

*12-month deferral:*
1. History of receiving a tattoo within the preceding 12 months
2. Mucous membrane exposure to blood within the preceding 12 months
3. Nonsterile skin penetration with instruments or equipment contaminated with blood or body fluids within the preceding 12 months (potential donors who have undergone ear piercing, depilitation, or acupuncture under questionable conditions should be considered in this category)
4. Close contact with a person who had viral hepatitis within the preceding 12 months
5. History of receiving hepatitis B immune globulin (HBIG) prophylaxis

Other Viral Causes

*Indefinite deferral:*
1. Present, or past, clinical or laboratory evidence of infections with human T-cell lymphotrophic virus types 1 and 2 (HTLV-I/II) or human immunodeficiency virus (HIV)
2. Excluded from donation by current FDA recommendations for the prevention of HIV transmission by blood and blood components
3. Donation of the only unit of blood or blood component transfused to a patient who developed transfusion-associated human immunodeficiency virus (HIV) or HTLV-I/II (this patient must have received no other blood component or derivative known to transmit these infections and have no other probable source of infection)
4. A history of injections with human pituitary growth hormone (pit-hGH) given between 1958 and 1986. This preparation may have contained the virus causing Creutzfeld-Jakob disease (CJD), which may be transmissible by transfusion. Deferral is not necessary if recombinant growth hormone has been received.

Bacterial Causes

*Indefinite deferral:*
1. History of babesiosis
2. History of Chagas' disease

*12-month deferral:*
1. History of syphilis or gonorrhea, treatment for syphilis or gonorrhea, or a reactive screening test for syphilis in the absence of a confirmatory test shall be cause for deferral for 12 months after completion of therapy

*Measurement of Weight.* Unexplained weight loss of a significant degree (more than 10 lb) shall be a reason for exclusion. Donors who weigh 110 lb (59 kg) or more may ordinarily donate 525 mL of blood, including samples. Donors weighing less than 110 lb may donate blood, but proportionately less.

*Anticoagulant Restrictions.* Packed red blood cells may be used for transfusion if 300–404 mL of blood has been collected into an anticoagulant volume calculated for 450 mL ± 45 mL and the unit is identified as a "low volume unit." The label should read "Low Volume Unit: _____ mL Red Blood Cells." If less than 300 mL of blood is collected, it may be used for transfusion if collected in a proportionately reduced volume of anticoagulant. (The excess anticoagulant must be reduced proportionately by expressing the excess into an integrally attached satellite bag and sealing the tubing, and the volume of blood must be accurately measured.) Other blood components shall not be made from low-volume units.

Example: Calculation of amount of anticoagulant to remove for drawing donors weighing less than 50 kg (110 lb):

1. $\dfrac{\text{Donor's weight in kg}}{50} \times 450 \text{ mL}$

   = Volume of blood to draw (approx. 12% of blood volume)

2. $\dfrac{\text{Answer from above}}{100} \times 14$

   = Amount of anticoagulant (CPDA = 1)

3. $63 - \text{(last answer)}$

   = Amount of anticoagulant to remove from a 450 mL bag

*Evaluation of Temperature.* A donor's temperature must not exceed 37.5° C. Care should be taken to remove the thermometer before obtaining a blood sample for hemoglobin/hematocrit testing.

*Measurement of Pulse and Blood Pressure.* Measurement of a donor's pulse must reveal no pathologic cardiac irregularities and should be between 50 and 100 beats per minute. If the prospective donor is an athlete with high exercise tolerance, a lower pulse rate may be acceptable.

In determination of blood pressure, the systolic pressure should be no higher than 180 mm Hg and the diastolic no higher than 100 mm Hg. Donors with values above these readings may be accepted only after evaluation by a qualified physician.

## Quantitation of Microhematocrit (Packed Cell Volume) or Hemoglobin

The donor's predonation hemoglobin should be no less than 12.5 g/dL (microhematocrit-packed cell volume

38%). In the case of autologous donors, the hemoglobin should be no less than 11.0 g/dL and the minimum microhematocrit 33%.

***Capillary Blood Collection.*** Several types of microcollection tubes are available for use in capillary blood collection. These small tubes may be heparinized or plain. Capillary blood collection is performed using a sterile, disposable lancet. These lancets should be properly discarded in a puncture-proof container after a single use.

### SUPPLIES AND EQUIPMENT

1. Alcohol (70%) and gauze squares or alcohol wipes
2. Sterile, small gauze squares
3. Sterile, disposable blood lancets
4. Microhematocrit tubes
5. Disposable gloves

### SELECTION OF AN APPROPRIATE SITE

1. The fingertip (usually of the third or fourth finger) is an appropriate site for the collection of small quantities of blood (Fig. 2-7). The earlobe may also be used as a site of last resort in adults. *Do not* puncture the skin through previous sites that may be infected.

2. The site of blood collection must be warm to ensure free flow of blood; otherwise, the blood sample will not be truly representative of the blood in the vascular system. If necessary, massage the finger several times or place a warm cloth on the area for a few minutes to increase blood circulation to the site.

### PREPARATION OF THE SITE

1. Put on a pair of disposable gloves and hold the area to be punctured with the thumb and index finger of one hand.
2. Wipe the area with 70% alcohol and allow to air dry.
3. Wipe the area with a dry gauze square or cotton ball. If the area is not dry, the blood will not form a rounded drop and will be difficult to collect.

### PUNCTURING THE SKIN

1. A disposable, sterile lancet is used *once* and must be properly discarded in a puncture-proof container.
2. Hold the area securely and puncture once with a firm motion. The lancet should puncture across the creases of the fingerprint—not with the grooves. If the finger is the chosen site, the area to be punctured should be

**Figure 2-7.** Collection of capillary blood. The areas of the fingertip designated by arrows are the preferred sites for collection of capillary blood from the finger. Illustration from Turgeon, M.L.: Clinical Hematology: Theory and Procedures. Boston, Little, Brown and Company, 2nd Ed., 1993, p. 22.

in the portion of the finger that is rich in capillaries, not the fleshy part.

3. The first drop of blood should be wiped away; it is not a true sample because it is mixed with extracellular (tissue) fluid and possibly alcohol.

4. Subsequent drops are obtained by *gently* applying pressure to the area. A good capillary puncture should require *no* forcing or hard squeezing of the site. If the site is squeezed too hard, extracellular fluid will mix with the blood and produce inaccurate test results.

COLLECTING THE SAMPLE

1. Filling a microhematocrit tube is accomplished by allowing free-flowing blood to enter the tube by capillary action. The tube must be held horizontally to avoid introducing air bubbles or breaks in the column of blood.

2. The site should be wiped frequently with a plain gauze square in order to prevent the accumulation of platelets, which will slow down or stop the blood flow.

TERMINATION OF THE PROCEDURE

1. Wipe the area with 70% alcohol on a gauze square or alcohol wipe.

2. Place a clean gauze square on the site and apply pressure. If the patient is unable to apply pressure to the site, hold the gauze square until the bleeding has stopped.

3. Label all specimens.

4. Place the used lancet in a puncture-proof container.

***Copper Sulfate Method.*** This is an alternate method that is based on specific gravity. A solution of copper sulfate, with a specific gravity of 1.053 (equivalent to 12.5 g/dL of hemoglobin), is used. Twenty-five tests can be performed in a 30 mL container of solution; the solution should be changed daily.

After collecting a capillary blood sample in an anticoagulated tube, one drop of blood is allowed to fall gently from the tube at a height of about 1 cm above the surface of the solution. Observe the droplet. An acceptable drop of blood will sink in the copper sulfate solution within 15 seconds. An unacceptable specimen will either remain suspended or will sink slightly and then rise to the top of the solution.

Although falsely acceptable results are rare, falsely unacceptable (low) results are common. In these cases, it is best to use a secondary method (usually the microhematocrit method) to verify the donor's ineligibility.

## Informing the Donor of Test Results

Blood donors must be provided with five categories of information:

1. Education related to the risks of infectious disease. This information must stress the importance of withdrawing as a blood donor if the blood is not suitable for transfusion.

2. Knowledge related to informed consent for the withdrawal of blood or blood components; this must be documented. Also, the process of phlebotomy must be explained.

3. A confidential opportunity to exclude their blood from being transfused, even if it is already drawn.

4. Post-phlebotomy care and possible adverse reactions.

5. The medical director of the facility collecting the blood shall be responsible for a mechanism to notify donors of any clinically significant abnormalities detected during the predonation evaluation, or during laboratory testing of the unit of blood or blood components.

## Collection of Blood from the Donor

In the collection of a donor unit or blood components, sterility must be maintained by using aseptic methods and sterile, pyrogen-free equipment and solutions. To maintain aseptic conditions, use a closed system and perform a single venipuncture. If more than one venipuncture is needed, another set and container must be used.

*Labeling* of a unit of blood, a blood component, bone marrow, or peripheral blood progenitor cells is as important as any other step in the processing of blood. The original label, and any added portions, shall be attached firmly to the container and be in clear, eye-readable type—which also may be machine-readable. A label from a single facility must comply with the AABB requirements for labeling at collection or preparation, labeling prior to issue (Table 2-4), and labeling of blood components (Table 2-5). These requirements apply to blood, blood components, bone marrow, and peripheral blood progenitor cells. Handwritten additions or changes shall be legible and in permanent, moisture-proof ink.

A numeric or alphanumeric labeling system must be used that will make it possible to trace any unit of blood or component from the donor source to final disposition. This system can be used to recheck records applying to the specific unit, including an investigation of any reported adverse reactions. The original identification number shall not be obscured, altered, or removed by subsequent facilities. Other facilities may assign and affix a local identification number to the unit, but the label must clearly identify the original facility. No more than two identifications may be visible on a blood or component container: those of the original collecting facility and the transfusing (or intermediate) shipping facility. It may be necessary to remove or obliterate identifications assigned by intermediate facilities. This does not preclude the use of a patient identification number.

Before labeling is completed, records must be reviewed to ensure that blood, and all components, from unsuitable donors will be quarantined and not issued for transfusion.

**Table 2-4. Label Requirements**

### Labeling at Collection or Preparation

| Category | Comments |
|---|---|
| 1. Name of product | Examples: whole blood, component, intended component, bone marrow, peripheral blood progenitor cells |
| 2. Numbering system | Numeric or alphanumeric identification |
| 3. Name of anticoagulant | Exceptions: components prepared by hemapheresis and for frozen, deglycerolized, rejuvenated or washed red blood cells |
| 4. Approximate amount of product collected from the donor | Examples: blood, bone marrow, or progenitor cells |
| 5. Approximate volume in the container | Examples: platelets, low-volume red blood cells, fresh frozen plasma, pooled components, components prepared by hemapheresis, bone marrow, and peripheral blood progenitor cells |
| 6. Sedimenting agent | Note: if applicable |
| 7. Intended recipient | Required for bone marrow and peripheral blood progenitor cells |

### Final Container Labeling Prior to Issue

| Category | Comments |
|---|---|
| 1. Temperature of storage | |
| 2. Expiration date | Time of expiration, if appropriate |
| 3. Identification of facility preparing final component | Exception: blood components |
| 4. ABO group and Rh type | Rh type not required for cryoprecipitated AHF |
| 5. Interpretation of unexpected antibody test | Interpretation needed only if test is positive/interpretation not required for frozen, deglycerolized, rejuvenated, or washed red blood cells |
| 6. Instructions to transfusionist | See circular of information for the use of human blood and blood components; Properly identify intended recipient; This product may transmit infectious agents; Caution: Federal law prohibits dispensing without a prescription |
| 7. Type of donor | Examples: volunteer donor, paid donor, or autologous donor if applicable |

Source: Adapted from American Association of Blood Bank *Standards,* 15th edition, Sections B 6.2, 6.3, and 6.4, 1993, pp. 13–15.

## *Supplies and Equipment*

1. Anticoagulated collection bag or other specialized equipment
2. Phlebotomy site preparation solutions:
   A. Scrub solution: 0.7% aqueous scrub solution of iodophor compound (for example, PVP-iodine or polymer-iodine complex; this is available in prepackaged single-use form).
   B. Prep solution: 10% PVP-iodine (this is available in prepackaged single-use form). *Note:* For donors sensitive to iodine (tincture or PVP) another method (e.g., Exidine scrub) should be designated by the medical director of the blood bank.
3. Sterile applicator swabs (optional)
4. Sterile gauze squares and adhesive tape
5. A pair of hemostat clamps and a tube stripper
6. Disposable gloves
7. Metal clips and hand sealer, if heat sealer is not used
8. Emergency supplies (spirits of ammonia, emesis basin, etc.)

## *Venipuncture Technique*

PREPARATION OF THE SITE. After selection of an appropriate vein (as discussed earlier), an area at least 1.5 inches in all directions from the intended venipuncture site needs to be prepared. The initial scrub, as well as subsequent applications, should be from the intended site outward in a ring. The method involves these steps:

1. Scrub the area for 30 seconds with 0.7% aqueous scrub solution of iodophor compound. Although excess foam must be removed, the arm need not be dry before the next step.
2. Apply prep solution and let stand for 30 seconds. This solution contains only 1% free iodine and need not be removed before completing the venipuncture. This

**Table 2-5  Label Requirements**

| Special Requirements for Component Labels | |
|---|---|
| Category | Comments |
| 1. Final container labeling prior to issue | Must comply with the requirements listed above for final container labels, including the name of the pooled component, final volume of the pooled component, name of the facility preparing the pooled component, unique numbering system |
| 2. Specific unit information on the label or tag | Required information: Number of units in the pool, ABO group and Rh type of units in the pool (exception-Rh type is not required for pooled cryoprecipitated AHF) |

Source: Adapted from American Association of Blood Bank *Standards,* 15th edition, Sections B 6.2, 6.3, and 6.4, 1993, pp. 13–15.

solution has the advantage of having less odor and staining properties than tincture of iodine, and seldom causes skin reactions even in iodine-sensitive individuals.

3. Cover the area with a dry sterile gauze, if venipuncture is not done immediately. Do not repalpate the vein at the intended venipuncture site.

THE PHLEBOTOMY PROCEDURE

1. Inspect the anticoagulant donor bag for leaks. Be sure that the anticoagulant solution is clear. Open the seal in the tubing at the point of connection to the bag.

2. Position the bag below the level of the donor-arm balance system, making sure that the counterbalance is level and adjusted for the amount of blood to be drawn. A loose knot should be made in the tubing if metal clips and a hand sealer are not used. If a vacuum-assist device is used, follow the manufacturer's instructions.

3. Reapply the tourniquet or blood-pressure cuff (inflated to 40–60 mm Hg) and have the donor open and close the hand until the selected vein is again prominent.

4. Apply the hemostat clamp to the tubing, uncover the sterile needle, and perform the venipuncture immediately. A clean venipuncture will guarantee a full, clot-free unit.

5. Open the hemostat and check that the blood flow is adequate. Carefully tape the tubing to hold the needle in place and cover the venipuncture site with a sterile gauze pad. Have the donor squeeze a rubber ball or other soft object every 10 to 12 seconds during collection.

6. Keep the donor under observation throughout the phlebotomy. A person should never be left unattended during, or immediately after, donation.

7. Mix the unit of blood periodically (every 30 seconds). Time limits for collecting a unit are not fixed, so long as the blood flow is continuous. However, units requiring more than 8 minutes may not be suitable for preparation of platelet concentrates, fresh frozen plasma, or cryoprecipitate. A unit containing 450–495 mL should weigh 425–520 g plus the weight of the container with its anticoagulant.

8. Additional samples may be obtained by disconnecting an in-line coupler, or by tightening the preformed knot, hemostating the end toward the needle and the opposite side, and cutting the tubing on the needle side of the knot. Additional blood may be collected for laboratory tests, provided containers are properly labeled before (or at the time of) collection. These additional tubes must accompany the blood container and be reidentified with the blood container after filling.

9. Deflate and remove the tourniquet. Hold a sterile gauze square lightly over the venipuncture site and remove the needle from the donor's arm. Apply pressure on the gauze. Have the donor raise the arm (elbow straight) and hold the gauze firmly over the phlebotomy site with the opposite hand.

10. Strip the donor tubing as completely as possible. Invert the donor unit and allow the line to refill, then strip again. Seal the tubing attached to bag into segments suitable for subsequent tests with either a heat sealer or metal clips. It must be possible to separate segments from the container without breaking the sterility of the container. Reinspect the bag for defects.

POSTPHLEBOTOMY CARE

1. Check the donor's arm. After bleeding has stopped, apply a bandage.

2. Have the donor remain reclining for a few minutes under close observation by staff. When the donor appears to be in satisfactory condition, allow the donor to sit upright. Remain with the donor as the donor assumes an upright position and walks to an observation area.

GENERAL TIPS. Have the donor drink something before leaving the donor site, increase fluids for the next few hours, and refrain from smoking for 30 minutes. Instruct the donor to raise the arm and apply pressure if bleeding from the venipuncture site occurs. If a donor feels faint or dizzy, instruct the donor to lie or sit down with the head between the knees.

If any symptoms persist, the donor should return to the blood bank or see a physician. Donors may resume normal activities after a half hour if feeling well, and may remove the bandage after a few hours.

***Donor Reactions.*** The blood bank physician must provide written instructions for handling donor reactions. These must include a procedure for obtaining emergency medical help. In all cases, be sure that the donor feels stable before discharge from the area.

GENERAL PROCEDURES

1. Remove the tourniquet and withdraw the needle immediately at the first sign of a reaction.

2. If possible, move the donor to a private area

3. Call the blood bank physician if recovery is not prompt

Donor reactions may include:

1. Fainting
2. Nausea and vomiting
3. Hyperventilation
4. Development of a hematoma

FAINTING. The symptoms of fainting include general weakness, sweating, dizziness, pallor, and loss of consciousness. The skin may feel cool; blood pressure drops. Pulse rate falls in fainting—as compared to cardiogenic or hypovolemic shock, in which the pulse rate rises. Convulsions, with the involuntary passage of feces or urine, are rare.

First aid procedures for fainting are:

1. Place the donor on the back and raise the feet above the level of the head.
2. Loosen tight clothing.
3. Be sure that an adequate airway exists.
4. Apply cold compresses to the forehead or back of the neck.
5. Administer aromatic spirits of ammonia by inhalation. (Smell the broken capsule cautiously to test for strength.) The donor should respond by coughing, which elevates the blood pressure.
6. Check the pulse, blood pressure, and respirations periodically.

NAUSEA AND VOMITING. If a patient feels nauseated:

1. Instruct the patient to breathe slowly and deeply.
2. Apply a cold compress to the patient's forehead, and turn the head to one side.
3. Provide an emesis basin and clean towels.
4. If the patient vomits, give water and mouthwash to cleanse the mouth.

HYPERVENTILATION. The early symptoms of hyperventilation may include twitching or muscular spasms. Nervousness may cause a donor to hyperventilate, which leads to faint muscular twitching or tetanic spasms of the hand or face. In many cases, diverting the donor's attention with conversation can interrupt the hyperventilation pattern. If symptoms are apparent, have the donor breathe into a paper bag.

HEMATOMA. At the first sign of swelling in the venipuncture site, remove the tourniquet, and remove the needle from the donor's arm. Place several sterile gauze pads over the hematoma and apply firm pressure for 7–10 minutes with the donor's arm held above heart level. Apply ice to the area for 5 minutes, if desired.

If an arterial puncture is suspected, immediately withdraw the needle and apply firm pressure for 10 minutes. Check for the presence of a radial pulse. If the pulse is not palpable, call the blood bank physician.

**Hemapheresis Donors**

Introduction

Hemapheresis is a unique type of blood donation. In this type of donation, whole blood is withdrawn from either a healthy donor or patient. After removal, separation, and retention of the desired cellular elements or plasma, the remaining products are recombined and returned to the donor or patient. The process of hemapheresis may be performed using an intermittent-flow instrument that requires only a single venipuncture, or with continuous-flow equipment that usually requires two venipunctures, one

for removal of whole blood and the other for the return of the undesired components. With automated equipment, citrate solution is added in a measured quantity to the whole blood as it enters the primary tubing. All personnel involved in performing hemapheresis procedures should be thoroughly familiar with current regulations and qualified by training or experience to perform the procedure.

The harvested components (see Chapter 11) of hemapheresis from healthy donors are valuable to a wide variety of patients, particularly those who require multiple transfusions of platelets. Therapeutic hemapheresis is directly beneficial to patients with specific disorders, such as Waldenstrom's macroglobulinemia, myasthenia gravis, Goodpasture syndrome, and Guillain-Barré syndrome. In therapeutic circumstances, hemapheresis is directed at removing a plasma component—or it may be used to remove excessive numbers of platelets or leukocytes (therapeutic cytapheresis).

In the early 1960s, Judson, an engineer employed by International Business Machines (IBM), spearheaded the initial efforts to design an automated instrument that would selectively remove cells from the extracorporeal circulation. Judson was interested in cytodepletion because he wanted to help his son, who was suffering from acute leukemia, avoid the toxic side effects of chemotherapy. It was hoped that maintenance of a low circulating leukocyte count would avert organ damage. In 1964, it was demonstrated that lowering the leukocyte count of leukemia patients would not reduce organ damage. Although depletion of leukocytes through cytapheresis was not advantageous to leukemia patients, components provided by hemapheresis therapy have proven beneficial to patients suffering from the toxic side effects of chemotherapy, as well as patients having neutropenic and thrombocytopenic symptoms.

Donor Guidelines

Informed consent must be obtained from the donor. If the frequency of donation does not exceed donation every 8 weeks, donors of components prepared by cytapheresis must meet the same requirements as donors of whole blood. Plateletpheresis or leukapheresis of donors who do not meet the usual requirements shall be performed only when the harvested cells are expected to be of particular value to an intended recipient, and only when a physician has certified in writing that the donor's health permits hemapheresis.

General criteria for donation include the following:

1. At least 48 hours should elapse between successive donations.
2. The amount of plasma collected should not exceed the amount approved by the FDA for the instrument being used.
3. A donor should not undergo hemapheresis more than two times in a week or 24 times in a year, except in

unusual circumstances as determined by a blood bank physician.

4. A donor must be tested appropriately to detect a developing cytopenia. Abnormal results shall be reviewed by a blood bank physician to determine suitability for continued donation.
5. If a cytapheresis donor donates a unit of whole blood, or if it becomes impossible to return the donor's red cells during plateletpheresis or leukapheresis, at least 8 weeks should elapse before a subsequent cytapheresis procedure, unless the harvested cells are expected to be of special value to a recipient and the physician supervising the procedure certifies in writing that the donor's health permits hemapheresis.
6. Extracorporeal blood volume should not exceed 15% of the donor's estimated blood volume.
7. Drugs to facilitate leukapheresis shall not be used for donors whose medical history suggests that such drugs may exacerbate previous or intercurrent disease. There must be a written policy indicating the maximal cumulative dose of any sedimenting agent that will be administered to a donor within a given time interval. The physician in charge is responsible for appropriate guidelines in such circumstances.

## Assessment of Donors

Hemapheresis donors must have the routine measurement of hemoglobin and/or hematocrit prior to donation. In addition, it is desirable to evaluate the platelet count, the leukocyte count and a leukocyte differential.

If plateletpheresis is performed more frequently than every 8 weeks, the donor must have a platelet count above $150 \times 10^9$/L or be deferred from donating platelets. A platelet count is not required prior to the first procedure or if the interval between plateletpheresis sessions is at least 8 weeks. The result of a platelet count may be used to qualify a donor for the next procedure. In addition, donors who are the sole source of platelets and who have taken aspirin or aspirin-containing medications within 3 days of donation must be deferred.

## Plasmapheresis

*Plasmapheresis* is a term used to describe the removal of plasma with or without replacement of the lost fluid with a physiologic solution such as normal saline. If donors undergo plasmapheresis no more frequently than once every 8 weeks, the standards that apply to whole-blood donation apply to the selection and care of the donor. If plasma is donated more frequently than once every 8 weeks, the FDA requirements and recommendations must be followed. Plasmapheresis of donors who do not meet the usual requirements shall be done only when the plasma is of unusual therapeutic value and only when a physician

who is aware of the health status of the donor has certified in writing that the donor's health permits plasmapheresis.

As in other hemapheresis procedures, informed consent from the donor is required. A qualified, licensed physician knowledgeable in all aspects of plasmapheresis must be responsible for all areas of plasmapheresis. Donors must be closely observed during the procedure and immediate assistance must be available if an adverse donor reaction occurs. If an adverse reaction occurs, the supervising physician should advise the donor regarding personal medical care and should make available such medical records as may be required.

Phlebotomists must be fully trained in the recognition and prevention of all potential procedural hazards. The system used in performing phlebotomy and processing the blood must be designed to ensure safe reinfusion of the autologous red blood cells. All administration and transfer sets inserted in the blood containers used for plasmapheresis shall be sterile, pyrogen-free, nontoxic, and compatible with the contents under normal conditions of use. Plasmapheresis shall be done aseptically under conditions that avoid possible air embolism. Only 0.9% sodium chloride injection USP shall be used as a red blood cell diluent. Before the blood container has been separated from the donor for processing, it shall bear two separate independent means of identification that will enable both the donor and the phlebotomist to determine with certainty that the contents are those of the donor.

All the available red blood cells from the phlebotomy should be returned to the donor before collecting a second unit of blood, or within 2 hours of the phlebotomy. The amount of whole blood, not including anticoagulant, withdrawn for processing from a donor during a manual plasmapheresis procedure shall not exceed 500 mL at one time or 1000 mL during the entire session or within a 48-hour period unless the donor's weight is or exceeds 80 kg (176 lb), in which case the amount of whole blood withdrawn at one time shall not exceed 600 mL of 1200 mL during the entire plasmapheresis session or within a 48-hour period. When plasmapheresis is performed by an automated procedure, the amount of plasma collected should not exceed the amount approved by the FDA for that specific instrument.

## Donor Reactions to Hemapheresis

Although they are infrequent, unusual reactions may be observed in hemapheresis donors. The negative consequences of component donation can include procedural reactions, vascular complications, or reactions specific to the type of component (such as leukapheresis). Procedural reactions can include a reaction to the citrate anticoagulant, hypovolemia, hypervolemia, hemolysis, chilling, and allergic or anaphylactic reactions. Vascular complications can involve development of sclerosis or thrombosis. Reactions subsequent to leukapheresis can encompass a state of hypervolemia, edema, skin manifestations, or reactions to steroids. Immediate hypersensitivity reactions have been occasionally observed in healthy plateletpheresis donors. This type of anaphylactic reaction due to basophil histamine release during an automated plateletpheresis procedure is believed to be caused by sensitization to the ethylene oxide gas used to sterilize the disposable plastic equipment used in the procedure.

If a donor reaction occurs, first-aid procedures should be instituted. These procedures should be approved by the medical director of the blood bank. If symptoms (such as shortness of breath) or other severe reactions occur, the pheresis procedure should be stopped and the blood bank physician should be notified. Examples of donor reactions and the immediate steps that should be taken include the following:

1. Chills should be treated by covering the donor with a blanket and connecting a blood warmer to the blood return channel.
2. Bleeding from the infusion site may occur in heparinized donors. If this occurs, the needle should be removed and light pressure applied. If applying pressure does not control the bleeding, cold and pressure should be applied concurrently.
3. Paresthesia and muscle cramping related to the binding of calcium by citrate anticoagulant should be treated by slowly reinfusing the donor's blood and delaying the next centrifugation cycle until symptoms disappear.
4. Heparin or protamine sensitivity may produce epistaxis or unusual bleeding, chills, urticaria, or symptoms of anaphylactic shock. The infusion should be disconnected immediately and emergency treatment (such as the administration of steroids or epinephrine) instituted.
5. Chest pain, shortness of breath, shock, pallor, sweating, and syncope can be symptoms of an air embolism. Immediately place the donor on the left side, administer oxygen, and obtain emergency care.

## Immediate and Chronic Effects of Hemapheresis

The immediate effects of hemapheresis donation may be demonstrated by changes in the donor's hemoglobin and hematocrit, platelet count, or leukocyte count, depending upon the harvested components and the type of equipment. Postdonation changes are generally considered to be acceptable with approved equipment. The platelet count in thrombocytapheresis donors decreases about 30% postdonation and may require up to 72 hours to return to normal. Immediate slight-to-moderate decreases in the blood lymphocyte count and plasma immunoglobin concentrations are without known adverse effects.

Automated hemapheresis has made it possible selectively to remove large quantities of cellular elements or plasma proteins. As a result, the concentration of these substances in the donor's circulation can fall below normal. Plateletpheresis may remove $2.0 \times 10^9$ to $3.0 \times 10^9$ leukocytes per procedure from the circulation of a normal donor. This represents a loss of approximately four times more mononuclear cells than from a typical, single-unit donation; during leukapheresis approximately eight times the number of mononuclear cells are lost. Mononuclear cell depletion produces significant decreases in both the absolute number and the percentage of CD4 lymphocytes. The normal ratio of CD4:CD8 cells is also altered.

The quantities of components, such as lymphocytes and immunoglobulins, that can be removed without causing significant immediate or long-term consequence is unknown, but frequent and sustained nonlymphocyte-sparing plateletpheresis is associated with changes in laboratory findings related to the immune system. Body defense mechanisms can become defective when plasma IgG levels are less than 200 mg/dL or when the circulating lymphocyte count is less than $1.0 \times 10^9$/L.

The chronic effects of hemapheresis donation have been studied less extensively than the immediate effects. Frequent donors have been found to exhibit a small but statistically significant decrease both in their absolute lymphocyte count and percentage of T lymphocytes, and in their IgM levels compared to controls. Current FDA standards for whole-blood donation allow an estimated loss of 6 to $8 \times 10^9$/L mononuclear cells per year. Intensive lymphocytapheresis for the treatment of rheumatoid arthritis demonstrates that lymphocyte depletion and immunosuppression are feasible with current technology. A concern exists that depletion of lymphocytes during routine cytapheresis may lead to immunosuppressive and associated infections, malignancy, or autoimmune disease.

## Donor Records and Testing

A written protocol of all procedures shall be maintained. This shall include criteria for, and dosage of, any ancillary agents used, and instruction for the prevention and treatment of donor reactions. A data sheet must be kept for each procedure and the following information recorded: identity of the donor, anticoagulants given, duration of procedure, volume of component, drugs used, and reactions that occurred and how they were treated.

Testing of donor blood must be identical to the testing that would have been performed for whole blood if the component to be prepared is intended for transfusion. For a cytapheresis donor dedicated to the support of a specific patient, testing required to prevent disease transmission must be performed prior to transfusion of the first component and at least every 10 days thereafter.

Testing of the plasmapheresis donor's blood must be identical to the testing that would have been performed for whole blood if the component to be prepared is intended for transfusion.

## Therapeutic Phlebotomy

### Plasmapheresis, Plasma Exchange, and Cytapheresis

If patients have disorders (e.g., immunoglobulin disorder or polycythemia vera), it is sometimes beneficial to remove certain components, such as plasma, or specific cells, or a portion of the total blood volume, from the patient. In these cases, the attending physician must order the procedure in writing, but the blood bank physician must decide whether to accept the responsibility for bleeding the patient. Informed consent must be obtained from the donor-patient and it must be documented.

A written procedure describing the method used, including (if applicable) the operation of hemapheresis equipment, must be included in the blood bank procedure manual. Records of therapeutic procedures must include patient identification, diagnosis, type of therapeutic procedure performed, method used, extracorporeal blood volume, nature and volume of the component removed, nature and volume of replacement fluids, any occurrence of adverse reactions, and medications administered. Provisions for emergency care are the same as those described on pages 33 and 34 for allogeneic donors.

The decision to transfuse such blood must be made by the medical director of the blood bank, in conjunction with the attending physician of the prospective recipient. Any units resulting from therapeutic phlebotomy that are to be used for allogeneic transfusion shall be labeled to indicate the patient's disease or condition.

### History of Autologous Transfusion

Autologous blood transfusion is not a new procedure. The first recorded use of autologous transfusion dates to 1818, when John Blundell utilized blood salvage to treat patients with severe postpartum hemorrhage. Despite Blundell's innovative therapy and reasonable rate of success, only five of the ten patients survived. Little serious attention was given to autotransfusion. Sporadic reports do appear in the medical literature throughout the remainder of the 19th century.

The direction of autotransfusion changed dramatically in 1915 with the development of the first sodium citrate anticoagulant. This made it possible to store blood in vitro. In 1921, the first documented autologous predeposit collection was performed. Autologous transfusion became standard practice in the 1920s and early 1930s. However, with the introduction of organized blood banks in 1937 at Cook County Hospital, Chicago, and catalyzed by World War II, homologous donation and transfusion emerged as the standard of practice, and interest in autologous transfusion diminished.

The modern period of autologous transfusion began in the 1960s. Renewed interest in autologous transfusion, in the form of intraoperative salvage, gained momentum as posttransfusion hepatitis became an issue of concern. The phenomenal growth in autologous predeposit programs has been fueled by anxiety about transfusion-associated AIDS. Although it is out of proportion to the actual risk, this concern has spurred public demand for a safe blood supply, and it is widely accepted that autologous blood is the safest blood available. Autologous blood now accounts for about 4.6% of donated blood. However, the nonutilization rate is very high (44% in 1989).

### Types of Autologous Donations

Autologous (self-donation) and directed blood donation have gained in popularity since preoperative patients and their physicians have become more concerned about the risk of transmitting blood-borne infectious diseases such as AIDS in allogeneic blood. The two major categories of autologous (perioperative) donation are:

1. Predeposit
2. Autotransfusion

***Predeposit.*** *Predeposit* refers to the removal and storage of blood or blood components from a donor-patient. One or more units of blood are collected before an elective surgical procedure, for reinfusion during or after the procedure. This form of autologous transfusion is important in blood banking and is discussed in more detail later in this section.

***Autotransfusion***

CATEGORIES. Autotransfusion can be divided into the following categories:

1. Intraoperative autotransfusion
2. Hemodilution
3. Postoperative autotransfusion

Blood may be collected in a variety of ways from the donor-patient intraoperatively, by intraoperative autotransfusion from the operative site or from an extracorporeal circuit.

In *isovolemic hemodilution,* whole blood is collected before a surgical procedure and simultaneously replaced with a comparable volume of crystalloid or colloid solution. Hemodilution was first developed by cardiac surgeons, with the primary purpose being a decrease in blood viscosity. The decrease in viscosity reduces stress on the heart and increases the microcirculation. Blood collected during hemodilution can be saved and retransfused as fresh, whole blood. Beneficial results from hemodilution have been achieved in cardiovascular surgery, vascular surgery, spinal surgery for scoliosis, and total hip replacements.

Under postoperative and posttraumatic situations, shed blood may be collected from body cavities, joint spaces, and other closed operative or traumatic sites. *Postoperative autotransfusion* utilizes shed mediastinal blood, blood from the chest, or blood from other sterile operative sites. The blood is sterile and defibrinogenated, and will not clot.

**Table 2-6. Potential Benefits of Predeposit Autologous Donation**

1. Potentially extends the available homologous blood supply, either by not using available homologous blood, or if was not used by the autologous donor and meets acceptable standards
2. Often decreases overall health care costs, if only minimal pre-transfusion testing is performed
3. Provides peace of mind to surgical candidates with anxiety about contracting infectious diseases such as AIDS
4. No risk of alloimmunization to erythrocyte, leukocyte, platelet, or plasma protein antigens
5. No transfusion-related reactions (hemolytic, febrile, allergic or graft-versus-host)
6. Supplies compatible blood for persons with rare RBC antibodies or blood types when compatible blood may not be available
7. Stimulates erythropoiesis

Collection and processing of blood utilizes the same devices as those for intraoperative autotransfusion. The blood is retransfused following open heart surgery and traumatic hemothorax.

## Advantages and Disadvantages of Predeposit Autologous Donation

The autologous predeposit of blood has many benefits (Table 2-6) including individual benefits such as elimination of sensitization to cellular blood components and allergic reactions, as well as nonexposure to infectious diseases such as hepatitis and AIDS. The societal benefits of autologous transfusion include reduction of demand on the homologous blood supply and potential reduction of cost associated with compatibility testing.

Some of the disadvantages of autologous predeposit include the fact that it is not possible for medically indicated transfusion, nor available to meet unanticipated needs. The most common adverse effects (Table 2-7) of autologous blood donation are anemia and hypovolemia. This situation can be minimized by adhering to the AABB guidelines and recommended phlebotomy schedules. Other adverse reactions are not unlike those seen in homologous donors.

## Special Requirements of Autologous Transfusion

There must be a physician responsible for the autologous blood recovery program. This person shall oversee compliance with the American Association of Blood Banks *Stan-*

**Table 2-7. Potential Problems of Predeposit Autologous Transfusion**

1. Presurgical anemia
2. Presurgical hypovolemia
3. Clerical identification errors
4. Oudating of liquid stored blood
5. Homologous blood transfused instead of autologous
6. Patient-donor unable to donate (poor veins, or a preexisting medical condition that precludes donation)
7. Inadequate length of time to collect suitable number of units

*dards,* the establishment of written policy and procedures, and their periodic review.

Blood collected under the circumstances of autotransfusion may not be transfused to other patients. The methods of collection and reinfusion shall be safe, aseptic, and ensure accurate identification of all blood and components collected. Equipment must be pyrogen-free and should include a filter capsule of retaining potentially harmful particles and precluding an air embolism.

A complete written protocol of all autologous collection procedures should be maintained, including selection of anticoagulants and solutions used for processing and labeling of collected blood or components. Procedures for the prevention and treatment of adverse reactions are also needed. A total quality-management program encompassing quality control and quality assurance is needed. This program should include written procedures, criteria for acceptable results, and records of results. In addition, issues related to safety of blood and components collected for the recipient need to be included.

## Criteria for Autologous Donation

Preoperative autologous donation procedures require the consent of the donor-patient's physician and the blood bank physician, as well as the donor's informed consent (Figure 2-8). Because of the special circumstances surrounding autologous transfusion, rigid criteria for donor selection are not applicable. Suitable guidelines need to be established by the blood bank medical director. These guidelines must be retained in the blood bank procedures manual. Individual deviations from the guidelines require approval by the blood bank physician, usually in consultation with the donor-patient's physician. Appropriate guidelines for autologous donors include collection of an amount of blood that complies with established donor weight provisions. Diseases and conditions that usually preclude blood donation do not exclude autologous blood donation. If a patient's status is stable enough to allow elective surgery, the patient can usually donate several units of blood. Pregnant women may donate safely. In some cases, patients with cardiac history must be approved as donors by a cardiologist. Preexisting medical conditions (e.g., active asthma or chronic obstructive pulmonary disease) usually exclude the person as a donor-patient. Preoperative donation of autologous blood should not be undertaken when the donor-patient has, or is being treated for, bacteremia, or has a significant bacterial infection that can be associated with bacteremia. Donors with a history of seizures should also be excluded.

No age limits have been established for autologous donation. Children between the ages of 8 and 18 years have successfully predeposited autologous blood. Younger children have also been autologous donors. However, the volume collected must comply with the donor weight and ratio of anticoagulant guidelines. Hemoglobin levels

---

Blood Bank and Transfusion Service
Statement of Consent for Autologous Donation and Transfusion

I consent to the withdrawal of my own blood by authorized members of the staff of the Blood Bank for autologous transfusion purposes. The purpose, nature, and advantages of autologous transfusion, the risks involved, and the possibility of complications have been explained to me by _____, M.D. I understand that:

1. The procedure for donating my own blood is identical to routine blood donation. Each unit (approximately one pint) is collected by placing a needle into a vein in my arm; blood flows into a sterile plastic bag containing an anticoagulant. After the procedure, the needle is removed, and pressure and a bandage are applied to my arm to prevent bleeding. Each unit is labeled and stored for my own use during my subsequent hospitalization.

2. I will be asked to take oral iron supplements to replenish the iron lost with each donated unit.

3. A mild anemia or decrease in my blood volume may be a temporary result after frequent blood donation for autologous transfusion. Symptoms of anemia may include feeling faint, lightheaded, or weak. Because of these possible symptoms, I understand I should refrain from strenuous athletic events or hazardous occupation during the period of time I am donating blood.

4. While every effort will be made to transfuse me with only my own units of blood, there may be occasional situations where additional blood products are required, or where my own blood is no longer available. I will accept homologous (other donors') blood if my physician deems it necessary.

I further consent to such additional procedures related to autologous transfusion as may be necessary or desirable.

Should I not require transfusion of the blood withdrawn from me, I consent to the use or disposal of my blood in any manner deemed appropriate by the Blood Bank Medical Director.

Donor Signature _____ Date_____

Hospital Unit Number _____ or S.S. #_____

Witness _____ Date_____

---

**Figure 2-8.** Autologous donor's consent form.

should be no less than 11 g/dL (or microhematocrit–packed cell volume no less than 33%). Although the frequency of phlebotomy for autologous transfusion should be determined by the blood bank physician, the interval between donations is usually one week, with the final unit not to be drawn within 72 hours of the anticipated operation or transfusion. Usually two, but up to a total of five, units of whole blood may be collected, providing the patient's hemoglobin/hematocrit remain above 33%. Iron supplementation should be prescribed (ferrous sulfate 300 mg t.i.d.).

**Directed Donations**

Directed donations accounted for 2.5% of the blood supply in 1989. Some patients, anticipating the need for trans-

fusion, have turned to family and friends as a potential means of protecting themselves against blood-borne infectious diseases. In most cases, this is futile. With the exception of spousal donations, directed donations have been found to be no safer than transfusions from random allogeneic donors.

Some of the advantages (Table 2-8) of directed donation include a reduction in the anxiety a patient or family may have about the safety and availability of blood and an increase in donor participation, which extends the general availability of blood and components to all patients.

A disadvantage of directed donations is that donors are under pressure to donate, which might motivate them to conceal information about exposure to high-risk behaviors. Another disadvantage is that directed donors often do not realize that they forgo donor confidentiality and

**Table 2-8. Advantages and Disadvantages of Directed Blood Transfusion Practice**

| Advantages |
| --- |
| Positive psychological effect |
| Increases overall blood supply |
| Possible decreased litigation |
| Decreased risk of fetal-maternal alloimmunization (with maternal donors) |

| Disadvantages |
| --- |
| Possible increased risk of infectious-disease transmission |
| Increased risk of graft-versus-host disease (GVHD) |
| Increased risk of fetal-maternal alloimmunization (with paternal donors) |
| Increased cost |
| Possible increased litigation |

Source: Adapted from Yomtavian, R. Is directed blood transfusion a good idea? *Med. Lab. Observer* 24(11): 31–34, November 1992.

**Table 2-9. Two Anticoagulant-Preservative Solutions in General Use**

|  | CPD[A] | CPDA-1[B] |
| --- | --- | --- |
| Na$_3$ citrate | 26.3 gm | 26.3 gm |
| Citric acid | 3.27 gm | 3.27 gm |
| Dextrose | 25.2 gm | 31.9 gm |
| NaH$_2$PO$_4$. H$_2$O | 2.22 gm | 2.22 gm |
| Adenine | — | 0.275 gm |
| Water | 1000 mL | 1000 mL |
| Volume per 100 mL blood | 14 mL | 14 mL |
| Storage limit | 21 days | 35 days |

Source: Perkins, H. A.: Strategies for massive transfusion, in *Clinical Practice of Blood Transfusion,* Lawrence D. Petz and Scott N. Swisher, New York: Churchill Livingstone, 1981, pp. 485–499.
[A] CPD citrate-phosphate-dextrose solution
[B] CPDA-1 citrate-phosphate-dextrose-adenine solution

may be liable if the recipient experiences an adverse reaction such as contracting an infectious disease. In addition to the cited disadvantages, the nonutilization rate of directed donations is very high.

## STORAGE AND PROCESSING OF DONOR BLOOD

### Types of Anticoagulants

The storage of blood has evolved since the initial preservation of whole blood in glass bottles. These bottles contained a sufficient concentration of acid-citrate-dextrose (ACD) to bind the ionized calcium of a unit of whole blood, with excess citrate remaining available to complex with calcium in the recipient. A variety of anticoagulants and anticoagulant-preservative media are now available, and plastic collection bags have replaced glass bottles.

Anticoagulants and/or anticoagulant preservatives for whole blood and red cell concentrate storage include:

1. ACD (acid-citrate-dextrose)
2. CPD (citrate-phosphate-dextrose)
3. Heparin
4. CPD-A1 and CPD-A2 (citrate-phosphate-dextrose-adenine)
5. Adsol (AS-1)

The composition of two anticoagulant-preservative solutions in general use today is presented in Table 2-9.

### Approved Storage Times

The approved storage time (expiration date) of a blood product is the last day on which the blood or blood component is considered useful for ordinary transfusion purposes. Because different media produce distinct effects on stored blood at 4° C, the approved length of storage differs. Whole blood or red cells collected without breaking the hermetic seal and stored in CPD or ACD have an expiration date not exceeding 21 days after phlebotomy. Whole

blood or red cells collected and stored in CPD-A1 shall have an expiration date not exceeding 35 days after phlebotomy. Whole blood or red cells collected and stored in heparin solution shall have an expiration date not exceeding 48 hours after phlebotomy.

Red blood cells that are separated and frozen at −65° C have an approved storage time of 10 years. Other components have variable storage times (see Chapter 10, Blood Components). The use of rejuvenation solutions for red blood cells is an area that has been studied. Anticoagulant-preservative additive solutions, such as Adsol (AS-1) or Nutricel (AS-3), have not been licensed for use with rejuvenation solutions.

### The Effects of Anticoagulants on Stored Blood

Although the use of plastic bags improved red cell respiration and viability compared to glass bottles, and research on the effects of anticoagulants on red cell metabolism has led to improved anticoagulant preservatives, whole blood or red blood cells exhibit changes (Table 2-10) when stored at 4° C. The critical changes include a decrease of essential components such as 2,3 diphosphoglycerate (2,3 DPG), and an increase in toxic materials (e.g. plasma potassium).

**Table 2-10. Changes in Bank Blood on Storage at 4° C**

| Decrease of Essential Components |
| --- |
| 1. RBC viability |
| 2. Platelet viability |
| 3. Granulocyte viability |
| 4. Coagulation Factors: Factor V and Factor VIII |

| Increase in Toxic Materials |
| --- |
| 1. Plasma potassium |
| 2. Free hemoglobin |
| 3. Plasma lactate |
| 4. Plasma ammonium |
| 5. Plasticizers |

| Formation of microaggregates |
| --- |

Source: Modified from Perkins, H. A.: Strategies for massive transfusion, in *Clinical Practice of Blood Transfusion,* Lawrence D. Petz and Scott N. Swisher, New York: Churchill Livingstone, 1981, pp. 485–499.

When one of the anticoagulant-preservative solutions, such as CPDA-1, is used in a normal blood donation, 63 mL of anticoagulant-preservative is mixed with 450 mL of donor whole blood. This solution dilutes the whole blood constituents to 88% of their original concentration. The solution also adds 18 mEq of sodium and 3 mEq of phosphorous to each unit, and alters the pH of freshly collected blood to between 7.0 and 7.2. When using anti-coagulants designed for long-term storage, a certain amount of hemolysis occurs whenever RBCs are stored 35 days or more. However, additives will protect RBC membranes against hypotonic shock and will reduce the degree of hemolysis during storage.

## Red Cell Viability

When blood is collected in a plastic bag with a standard anticoagulant-preservative solution and stored at 4° C, the red cells slowly undergo metabolic changes in vitro that lead to a loss of red cell function—primarily the capacity to off-load oxygen normally. In order to decrease metabolic demands, red blood cells are stored at 4° C. This temperature slows down enzyme activity, which partially protects hemoglobin or the red blood cell membrane. The proportion of viable, transfused red blood cells remaining in the circulation of the recipient 24 hours after transfusion is referred to as *posttransfusion viability*.

Factors leading to the loss of posttransfusion viability and contributing to extravascular catabolism include the following:

1. A decrease of surface area to volume ratio. This may be caused by a loss of surface area or a volume increase, which leads to entrapment because of the inability of the red blood cells to pass through the microcirculation of the reticuloendothelial system.
2. Changes in membrane deformability, either from intrinsic conditions (sickled hemoglobin) or extrinsic factors (low pH, or changes in membrane surface properties).
3. Decreases in pH to between 4.5 and 5.5 induces an immediate decrease in the deformability of intact red blood cells and cessation of ATP generation occurs.

Regulations of the FDA require that at least 70% of the red blood cells in a donor unit remain viable in the anticoagulant-preservative solution at the end of the approved storage period. For example, viability of red blood cells in CPD solution after 21 days of storage averages 80 to 85%, and red blood cells in AS-1 solution demonstrate a mean posttransfusion recovery of 83% after 42 days of storage. Increased survival of red cells in liquid storage can be achieved by rejuvenation of adenosine triphosphate (ATP) levels with adenosine, which produces an improvement in membrane-related functions.

There is considerable variability in the percentage of viable RBCs because of the characteristics of the anticoagulant preservatives, such as the initial osmolarity and pH of the solution and the ability of the solution to support ATP levels. The characteristics of the RBCs of individual donors can also affect viability. Female donors often have been found to have better RBC survival rates. It has been suggested that this may be related to higher concentrations of steroid hormones, which may act as RBC membrane-stabilizing agents during storage.

When RBCs are allowed to settle without agitation during the storage of whole blood, poorer posttransfusion survival has been observed. Storage of packed RBCs with a hematocrit greater than 75% limits the availability of substrate around each cell and leads to shortened survival, even with high concentrations of glucose or the presence of purine nucleotides.

## Storage Lesion

The ATP-independent, irreversible loss of surface area of the red cell is referred to as *storage lesion. Viability* (posttransfusion survival) is believed to relate to the structural and metabolic status of the red cell membrane, including ATP level, red cell shape, and red cell deformability. The disruption of normal membrane architecture—a membrane lesion—can lead to recognition and destruction of transfused RBCs (extravascular catabolism) by the reticuloendothelial system.

## RBC Membrane Changes and ATP Depletion

Red cells undergo changes in shape and membrane structure during metabolic depletion. These changes include:

**Early stage:** shape changes, cellular swelling
**Middle stage:** oxidation of hemoglobin
**Middle–late stage:** binding of cytoplasmic proteins to the membrane, increased intracellular $Ca^{++}$, loss of $K^+$ and $H_2O$
**Late stage:** irreversible membrane protein crosslinking, loss of lipid vesicles, echinocyte-sphero-echinocyte shape change

The basic RBC membrane structure includes the lipid bilayer, the proteins spanning it (integral membrane proteins), and a filamentous meshwork of proteins along the cytoplasmic surface (peripheral membrane proteins) that form a membrane skeleton for the RBC. Membrane changes are considered to be involved in RBC destruction. These include:

1. Loss of phospholipid asymmetry influences the adherence of RBCs to endothelial surfaces, and may stimulate recognition and phagocytosis by monocytes.
2. Modification of cell-surface antigens—including glycoproteins, glycolipids, and proteolipids—or rearrangement of their topography, can alter RBC survival. An antibody in the plasma appears to be directed against antigens that only reveal themselves in aged RBCs in vivo or during in vitro storage.

When ATP levels in the red cell fall below 10 to 15% of normal, RBCs begin to develop spicules, and the shape changes. Change in shape is reversible for up to 20 hours of ATP depletion by incubation with glucose and purine nucleotides. This treatment returns ATP levels to normal or supernormal. However, after 28 hours of ATP depletion, the formation of spheroechinocytes with reduced surface area–to–volume ratio occurs.

The mechanism by which ATP depletion produces permanent surface area loss has not been completely described, but it is known that it directly or indirectly promotes the loss of lipid-rich vesicles. This loss of lipid from the membrane begins immediately upon storage and represents the major lethal injury—irreversible deformability of the membrane—to the RBC.

## Antigen Preservation

The major focus of research in anticoagulant preservatives for the past decade has been on increasing the shelf-life of liquid blood. However, it is important that blood stored for increasing amounts of time retain reactive antigens in order to continue to be grouped and typed and to be suitable for compatibility testing. It would be useless to extend RBC viability if the blood could not be reliably tested to prevent an in vivo clinical transfusion reaction. Fortunately, no significant changes in the ABO and Rh antigens during storage have been detected with any of the currently approved anticoagulant-preservative solutions. Although a moderate decrease in antigenic strength of the Lewis and P antigens has been demonstrated, the loss of antigenic reactivity of clinically significant antigens, to the point where they would give unreliable serologic reactions and be dangerous to the recipient, has not been observed.

## STORAGE, TRANSPORTATION, AND ISSUING OF BLOOD

Immediately after collection, blood must be placed in storage at a temperature between 1° C and 6° C. However, if the blood is to be used as a source of components, up to 8 hours may elapse before storage. For harvesting platelets, blood should be placed in storage at a temperature of about 20–24° C. A detailed discussion of the storage requirements (Table 2-11) of whole blood and blood components is presented in Chapter 10, Transfusion Therapy: Blood and Blood Components.

If blood collected intraoperatively is stored, it must be handled like any unit of blood intended for autologous use only, except that testing for disease markers may be waived. If blood collected by intraoperative means is not used immediately, units collected and processed under sterile conditions, with a device for intraoperative blood collection that washes with 0.9% saline USP shall be stored

**Table 2-11. Storage Temperatures for Blood and Blood Components**

| Product | Required Temperature (°C) |
| --- | --- |
| Whole blood and liquid | 1 to 6 |
| Platelets | 20 to 24 |
| Granulocytes | 20 to 24 |
| Fresh frozen plasma | ≤ −18 |
| Cryoprecipitated AHF | ≤ −18 |
| Red blood cells | |
| Frozen in 40% glycerol | ≤ −65 |
| Frozen in 20% glycerol | ≤ −120 |

Source: Adapted from *Standards for Blood Banks and Transfusion Services*, 15th ed. American Association of Blood Banks: Bethesda, MD, 1993, 15.

under one of two conditions prior to the initiation of transfusion. These two requirements are:

1. Storage at room temperature for up to 6 hours
2. Storage at 1–6° C for up to 24 hours, provided storage begins within 6 hours of initiating the collection

Transfusion of blood collected intraoperatively by other means shall begin within 6 hours of initiating the collection.

If blood is collected by the process of isovolemic hemodilution, it may be stored prior to initiation of transfusion. However, this blood must meet one of two requirements for reinfusion: It may be stored at room temperature for up to 8 hours; or it may be stored at 1–6° C for up to 24 hours, provided that storage at 1–6° C is begun within 8 hours of initiating the collection.

Transfusion of shed blood collected under postoperative or posttraumatic conditions shall begin within 6 hours of initiating collection.

When a unit of blood is collected, the integral donor tubing must be filled with anticoagulated blood and sealed into segments to be available for testing and compatibility examination. These segments should be able to be separated from the collection bag without breaking the sterility of the container. If the sterility of the collection bag is broken during processing or pooling, the blood or components must be stored between 1° C and 6° C and have an expiration time of 24 hours. If sterility of components that are stored between 20° C and 24° C is compromised, the unit must be transfused as soon as possible, or within a maximum of 4 hours.

If the seal is broken during processing of components that are to be stored frozen, place the component in the freezer within 6 hours after the seal is broken. When the component is thawed, it must be used within 6 hours after thawing, if stored between 20° C and 24° C, or within 24 hours if stored at 1–6° C.

Whole blood, modified whole blood, and all liquid red blood cell components must be transported in a manner that will ensure maintenance of a temperature of 1–10° C. Components ordinarily stored at 20–24° C should be transported at 20–24° C. Components ordinarily stored frozen should be kept frozen while being transported.

Blood and blood components must be inspected immediately before shipment. If a unit is abnormal in appearance, it should not be shipped. In addition, autologous units of blood cannot be shipped if the unit is HIV-1 confirmed positive, HIV-2 repeatedly reactive, or HBsAg confirmed reactive, unless a written statement from the attending physician confirms the acceptability of the blood.

## Processing and Labeling of Blood

### In-House Donor Blood

***Testing.*** Donor blood on a sample from each donation collected in-house needs to be tested for ABO grouping and Rh typing (these blood group systems are discussed in Chapters 4 and 5). If the initial test with anti-D is negative, the blood must be tested for weak D (D$^u$). If both the D and weak D tests are negative, the donor is Rh negative. If either the D or weak D tests are positive, the donor is Rh positive.

For almost 50 years, the only test for infectious diseases present in donor blood performed by blood banks was the test for syphilis. In the early 1970s, the test for hepatitis B surface antigen (HbsAg), originally referred to as the Australian antigen, was added to the protocol for the screening of donor blood. Because of the lack of a specific test for hepatitis C (HCV)—previously called non-A, non-B hepatitis—surrogate tests were used to screen blood for hepatitis C. The surrogate tests are alanine aminotransferase (ALT) and antibody to hepatitis B core antigen (anti-HBc). Since the late 1980s, additional donor laboratory screening tests have been added (Table 2-12). The addition of these tests has improved the safety of the blood supply. For example, the rate of infection with HCV has decreased by more than 90%, from 0.45% per unit transfused before the introduction of surrogate hepatitis marker testing to 0.03% after the introduction of anti-HCV test-

**Table 2-12. Required Infectious Diseases Screening Tests on Donated Blood**

| Screening Test | Rate of Positivity (Percentage) |
| --- | --- |
| Syphilis | 0.20 |
| HBsAg | 0.04 |
| ALT | 0.17 |
| Anti-HBc | 2.15 |
| Anti-HCV | 0.29 |
| Anti-HIV-1 | 0.02 |
| Anti-HTLV-1 | 0.05 |
| Anti-HIV-2 | <0.01 |

*Key:* HBsAg = hepatitis B surface antigen, ALT = alanine aminotransferase, HBc = hepatitis B core antigen, HCV = hepatitis C virus, HIV-1 = human immunodeficiency virus, HTLV = human T-cell leukemia/lymphoma virus.
Source: Adapted from McCullough, J.: The nation's changing blood supply system, *JAMA 269*(17):May 5, 1993.

ing. The introduction of a second generation anti-HCV test is estimated to prevent an additional 40 cases of HCV infection per day in the United States.

The FDA recommended that all donated blood be screened for antibodies to human immunodeficiency virus type 2 (HIV-2) beginning no later than June 1, 1992. Because epidemiologic data indicate that the prevalence of HIV-2 infections in persons in the United States is extremely low compared to the West African nations plus Angola and Mozambique, where the prevalence of HIV-2 is reported to exceed 1% in the general population, the CDC does not recommend routine testing for HIV-2 in settings other than blood centers. However, the 15th edition of the *Standards* of the American Association of Blood Banks requires that HIV-2 testing be done on all donor units in accredited facilities.

Tests required by the AABB *Standards,* not performed by the on-site blood bank or transfusion service, must be performed in a laboratory accredited by the AABB, CAP, or JCAHO, and certified by the Health Care Financing Administration (HCFA).

Additional testing should include serum or plasma testing of previously transfused persons or pregnant women for clinically significant antibodies. If antibodies are detected, the blood should be processed into components containing only minimal amounts of plasma.

In addition to testing, all units must meet the general requirements for labeling (see Table 2-4). If the blood product is a blood component, additional requirements must be met (see Table 2-5).

### Donor Blood from Outside Sources

The hospital blood bank must assume that the collection agency from whom the blood was obtained has vigorously applied all appropriate standards of practice to the collection of blood. The appropriate criteria include patient history and physical examination, ABO grouping and Rh typing, unexpected antibody screening, screening tests for infectious diseases, and correct labeling and identification of the unit.

Upon receipt of the blood by the hospital blood bank, it is placed in the hospital's provisional inventory. The tests that are repeated are usually the ABO group and Rh type. It is not necessary to repeat the screening test for unexpected antibodies or tests for infectious diseases.

### Autologous Blood

The processing of blood for autologous transfusion within the collecting facility must have the ABO group and Rh type determined by the collecting facility. Other testing is optional. In the case of autologous blood, or any component thereof, that will be transfused outside of the collecting facility, tests for HBsAg, anti HIV-1, anti HIV-2, anti-HCV, anti-HBc, a serologic test for syphilis, and any other tests recommended or required by the FDA should be performed on the first unit from a given donor during a 30-day period.

In addition to the labeling requirements described for the processing of in-house donor blood, proper identification of autologous units is of critical importance. The unit must have a label or tag bearing specific information. This information should include: autologous donor label; the patient's name; the name of the transfusing facility; and the patient's hospital number, social security number, birthdate, or other identifying information. The label should state the date of expiration of the unit (Figure 2-9). This unit must also have a label stating "For Autologous Use Only" (Figure 2-10B), if the blood is not suitable for allogeneic use. Blood that has been collected intraoperatively must be labeled with the patient's first and last name, hospital identification number, date and time of collection initiation, and the statement "For Autologous Use Only," if the blood is removed from the presence of the donor-patient.

When additional testing has been performed, a biohazard label should be applied to each patient-donor unit if the HIV-1 is confirmed positive, HIV-2 is repeatedly reactive, HBsAg is confirmed reactive, the anti-HBc or anti-HCV are repeatedly reactive, or if a reactive serologic test for syphilis is confirmed to be positive or not further tested.

If the HIV-1 is confirmed positive, HIV-2 is repeatedly reactive, or HBsAg is confirmed reactive, a unit of blood or component cannot be shipped unless a written statement from the attending physician is obtained confirming the acceptability of the donor blood.

If repeatedly reactive results are obtained for anti-HBc or anti-HCV or a reactive serologic test for syphilis is con-

firmed to be positive or not further tested, the patient-donor's physician should be informed.

If the unit is made available for allogeneic transfusion, the donor classification label must not be removed or obliterated. However, labeling information that identifies the donor-patient must be removed or obliterated. Autologous units must be segregated and used solely for this purpose unless the donor-patient and the donated blood meet all of the requirements of normal donations. The exceptions to the normal requirements include: the interval between donations; the donor-patient's age, pulse, blood pressure and weight; and pregnancy status.

### Processing Blood Components

Processing of blood components must follow the protocol described above for either in-house donor collection or units imported from other sources. In addition, the blood bank records of the preparing facility must include the identification number of each unit in the pool and the identification of the facility for each unit in the pool. Other information regarding blood components can be found in Chapter 10, Transfusion Therapy: Blood and Blood Components.

## ISSUING BLOOD FOR TRANSFUSION

Blood must be inspected for abnormalities in appearance, such as hemolyis, immediately before issue from the blood bank. If any abnormality is observed, the unit should not be used unless specific authorization is granted by the medical director.

A transfusion requisition similar to the form (Fig. 2-10) must be completed for each requested unit. This form must minimally indicate the following:

1. Intended recipient's name, identification number, and ABO group and Rh type
2. Donor unit or pool identification number, and the donor ABO group and Rh type
3. Compatibility results, if performed

A label or tag with the recipient's first and last names, patient identification number, patient ABO group and Rh type, unit number assigned by transfusing or collecting facility, donor ABO group and Rh type, and interpretation of compatibility tests, if performed, must be attached securely to each unit of donor blood, component, or pooled component before release for transfusion.

In order to detect possible errors, interpretations of current tests must be compared with patient records for ABO grouping and Rh typing done during the past 12 months. In addition, difficulty in blood typing, detection of clinically significant unexpected antibodies, or severe adverse reactions to transfusions in the past 5 years should be checked.

```
Patient's Name: _____

Unit Number: _____ Physician: _____

Sex _____ Birth Date _____ S.S. No. _____

Date Collected:_____ Date of Surgery:_____

Date this unit expires _____

    Patient's Signature ▶_____

AUTOLOGOUS BLOOD TRANSFUSION

A
- - - - - - - - - - - - - - - - - - - - - - - - - - -
NOT DONOR BLOOD
FOR AUTOLOGOUS
TRANSFUSION ONLY

B
```

**Figure 2-9.** A, Autologous donor label. B, Autologous donor sticker.

**Figure 2-10.** Transfusion requisition.

Both the blood bank technologist and the nurse to whom the blood is being issued should check the patient's identifying information, the blood group and type of both the patient and donor unit, and the expiration date of the unit. Both individuals should sign appropriate forms or the blood bank ledger.

A copy of the transfusion form needs to be attached to the recipient's chart. The record system must make it possible to:

1. Trace any unit of blood or any blood component from the source (the donor or collecting facility) to the final disposition (transfused, shipped, or discarded)
2. Recheck the records applying to the specific component
3. Investigate adverse reactions manifested by the recipient

If a unit of blood is returned to the blood bank, it cannot be reissued unless certain requirements have been met (see page 46 for reissue requirements).

Transfusions must be administered under medical direction. The patient must be observed for any adverse reaction. If a patient is not available for direct medical observation after a transfusion, the patient must be given specific instructions regarding possible adverse reactions. There must be a written protocol for the administration of blood and blood components and the use of infusion devices and ancillary equipment. All products must be transfused through sterile, pyrogen-free transfusion sets with a filter designed to retain particles that are potentially harmful to the recipient.

If warming of blood is desired, such as in a massive transfusion, this must be done during the passage of the blood through the transfusion set. Blood must not be warmed above 38° C; the warming system must be equipped with a visible thermometer.

No drugs or medications of any kind can be added to blood or blood components. Solutions, such as 0.9% NaCl injection USP may be added to blood or blood components. However, other intravenous solutions may be used in an administration set or added to blood or blood components, if approved for this use by the FDA or if documentation exists that the addition of the solution to blood or blood components is safe and effective.

**Urgent Requirement for Blood**

Blood may be urgently needed. In such cases, a delay in beginning to transfuse a patient could be detrimental and blood may be issued without a crossmatch. However, the ABO group and Rh type of the patient and all units for transfusion must be verified using a segment attached to each unit. If a patient's ABO group is unknown, the patient must receive group O red blood cells. If the patient's ABO group has been determined by the blood bank without reliance on past records, the patient may receive ABO group-specific whole blood or ABO group-compatible red blood cell components before other tests for compatibility have been completed. Routine compatibility testing should be completed as soon as possible. If the patient expires due to the nature of the emergency, compatibility testing may be discontinued or abbreviated to the extent deemed necessary by the physician responsible for the transfusion service.

The tag or label on the unit of blood shall indicate in a conspicuous fashion that compatibility testing has not been completed at the time of issuance of the unit. In an urgent situation, blood bank records shall contain a statement from the requesting physician indicating that the clinical situation was sufficiently urgent to require release of blood before completion of standard compatibility testing.

Whole blood and blood components cannot be used for transfusion unless the results of the screening tests for blood-borne infectious diseases are negative. In an emergency, most states allow for blood to be transfused before testing is completed. However, an attached label must indicate incomplete testing. If a test is subsequently positive or reactive, the recipient's physician must be notified.

### Retention of Blood Samples

A stoppered or sealed sample of each donor's blood, and a similar sample of the recipient's blood, must be stored at 1–6° C for at least 7 days posttransfusion. Some facilities prefer to save samples for up to 2 weeks.

Donor and recipient specimens are retained in case retesting is needed. Retesting, such as ABO grouping or unexpected antibody screening, may be needed if a transfusion reaction is suspected.

### Reissue of Blood

If a unit of blood is returned to the blood bank, it cannot be reissued unless certain requirements have been met:

1. The container closure has not been disturbed.
2. The blood has not been allowed to warm above 10° C or cool below 1° C during storage or transportation. If the temperature of off-site storage (e.g., operating room refrigerator) cannot be documented, the blood should not be away from the blood bank for more than 30 minutes.
3. The records indicate that the blood has been reissued.
4. The blood is inspected prior to reissue.
5. A sealed segment of integral donor tubing has remained attached to the container if the blood has left the premises of the issuing facility.
6. If the blood has remained on the premises of the issuing facility, a removed sample may be reidentified by confirming that the originally attached label and identification correspond with the identification on the container.

## TRANSPORTATION OF BLOOD AND COMPONENTS

Blood and blood components must be inspected immediately before shipment. If a unit is abnormal in appearance, it should not be shipped. In addition, autologous units of blood cannot be shipped if the unit is HIV-1 confirmed positive, HIV-2 repeatedly reactive, or HBsAg confirmed reactive, unless a written statement from the attending physician confirms the acceptability of the blood.

Whole blood, modified whole blood, and all liquid red blood cell components must be transported in a manner that will ensure maintenance of a temperature of 1° C to 10° C. Components ordinarily stored at 20–24° C should be transported at 20–24° C. Components ordinarily stored frozen should be kept frozen while being transported. The FDA requires that frozen components be transported at −18° C or colder. Proper storage and shipment of specific blood components is included in Chapter 10, Transfusion Therapy: Blood and Blood Components.

Periodic temperature checks of received blood or components under all encountered conditions must be performed and documented. One method to check arriving units is to measure the temperature of two bound-together components after 60 seconds. Other suitable methods for monitoring shipments include using a time/temperature tag (3-M Company, St. Paul, MN). This system will record if the temperature has exceeded 10° C. A "high-low" thermometer is available (Taylor Instruments, Rochester, NY). This reusable thermometer measures and records the highest and lowest temperature during any time period. A bead system for monitoring temperatures exceeding 10° C is available (Chek Lab Inc., Aurora, IL).

Blood or components issued for infusion and returned must also meet transportation and storage requirements. Because blood at 1–6° C warms to 10° C or above in approximately 30 minutes at room temperature, transfusion should ordinarily be started or the unit returned to the blood bank within 30 minutes. If a longer time must elapse, individual units of blood may be placed in an insulated, pre-cooled (1–6° C) bag. Blood being held in the operating room can be placed in an insulated plastic chest with a lid, if a monitored blood bank refrigerator is not available.

Blood exposed to temperatures above 10° C is not necessarily unsuitable for transfusion. The disposition of the unit is best decided by experienced personnel.

## CHAPTER SUMMARY

### Patient Blood Specimen Collection

A properly collected blood specimen is essential to the accuracy and safety of blood transfusion. Major potential sources of error are identification errors involving either the patient or the specimen.

The collection of blood must follow a carefully prescribed protocol. Patient identification is the *critical* first step in blood collection. The other steps in properly collecting a specimen include checking the test requisitions, assembling the appropriate equipment, and washing your hands before putting on a pair of disposable gloves. After selecting an appropriate site and performing the venipuncture, all specimens should be properly labeled *immediately after* the specimen is drawn and *before* leaving the patient's bedside. The label must state the recipient's first and last names, identification number, date, and name or initials of the phlebotomist. The specimen label and request form must agree. Any contaminated disposable supplies and the used needle should be placed immediately in appropriate biohazard containers.

Occasionally, problems are encountered in obtaining a blood specimen. If two attempts are unsuccessful, notify the appropriate supervisor.

## Donor Blood Collection

Although many hospitals receive donor blood from large regional collection agencies, many hospital blood banks also maintain active donor facilities for specialized purposes such as autologous predeposit of blood, emergency donors, or hemapheresis. Standard procedures must be followed in the processing of donors prior to blood collection.

Sterility must be maintained while collecting donor blood intended for recipient transfusion. To maintain aseptic conditions, a sterile, closed system is used and a single venipuncture is performed. After selection of an appropriate vein, the intended venipuncture site must be properly prepared and the phlebotomy procedure correctly followed. Each unit collected must be labeled with a numeric or alphanumeric system in order to trace any unit of blood or component from the donor source to the final disposition.

Postphlebotomy care is essential to the blood donation process. The blood bank physician must provide written instructions for handling donor reactions.

Hemapheresis is a unique type of blood donation. In this process, whole blood from either a healthy donor or patient is separated. Desired cellular elements or plasma are retained and the remaining products are recombined and returned to the donor or patient.

Autologous donation or self-donation may take the form of predeposit or autotransfusion. Predeposit of autologous blood has many benefits including the elimination of sensitization to cellular blood components and allergic reactions; it also has the potential for eliminating blood-borne exposure to infectious diseases. The most common adverse effects of autologous blood donation are anemia and hypovolemia.

Some patients, anticipating the need for transfusion, have turned to directed donations from relatives and friends. Although having blood donated by persons known to the patient may alleviate anxiety about the safety and availability of blood, directed donations are no safer than screened blood from allogeneic donors.

## Storage and Processing of Donor Blood

Plastic bags have replaced glass bottles, and several types of anticoagulants or anticoagulant-preservative media are now used. The approved length of storage at $4°$ C depends upon the anticoagulant or anticoagulant-preservative solution. Red blood cells that are separated and frozen can be stored for a considerably longer period than blood in the liquid state.

Red blood cells exhibit changes when stored at $4°$ C. Critical changes include a decrease of red blood cell viability and 2,3 diphosphoglycerate (2,3 DPG) levels. At least 70% of the red blood cells must remain viable at the end of the permitted storage period. The ATP-independent, irreversible loss of surface area of the red cell is referred to as *storage lesion.*

Immediately after collection, blood must be refrigerated at 1 to $6°$ C. If platelets are to be harvested, the unit of blood should be stored at $20–24°$ C and the platelets must be separated from the unit within 8 hours. If the sterility of a donor unit is compromised, the unit must be transfused promptly.

Allogeneic donor blood must be tested for ABO group, Rh type, and weak D ($D^u$). In addition, tests for infectious disease markers must be performed. Additional testing should include serum or plasma testing of previously transfused persons or pregnant women for clinically significant unexpected antibodies. Modifications in the processing of blood are appropriate for autologous donors and blood received from other donor collection sources.

## Issuing Blood for Transfusion

Blood must be inspected for abnormalities in appearance immediately prior to issue from the blood bank. All relevant patient and donor information must be checked. Compatibility results, if performed, must also be checked. A label or tag with this information must be attached securely to the blood bag before release for transfusion.

An integral segment from the blood bag and a sealed sample of the recipient's blood must be stored at $1–6°$ C for at least 7 days after transfusion.

---

## REVIEW QUESTIONS

1. The characteristics of EDTA include:
   A. Chelates $Ca^{++}$, which results in plasma in a test tube
   B. Chelates $Ca^{++}$, which results in serum in a test tube
   C. Forms an insoluble calcium salt that prevents blood coagulation
   D. Both A and C

2–6. Organize the appropriate steps in blood procurement:
   2. _____
   3. _____
   4. _____
   5. _____
   6. _____

A. Label the specimen tubes
B. Palpate venipuncture site
C. Identify the patient
D. Put on disposable gloves
E. Check the test requisition and assemble the appropriate equipment

**7–10.** Match the following phlebotomy situation with its respective correct solution:

7. _____
8. _____
9. _____
10. _____

7. Movement of the vein
8. Sudden movement that causes the needle to come out of the patient's arm
9. Refusal by patient to have blood drawn
10. For prevention of a hematoma:

A. Immediately remove tourniquet and place gauze pad on venipuncture site
B. Move needle around until the vein is located
C. Politely excuse yourself and note refusal on requisition
D. Avoid piercing both sides of blood vessel and apply pressure to oozing venipuncture site
E. Always place firm pressure on arm below intended venipuncture site

**11–13.** Order the steps in the process of collecting blood from donors:

11. _____
12. _____
13. _____

A. Conduct a brief physical examination
B. Interview the prospective donor
C. Collect the unit of blood

**14.** The usual acceptable age for homologous blood donation is:
A. 15 through 65
B. 17 through 65
C. 18 through 70
D. 21 through 75

**15.** The acceptable interval between allogeneic whole-blood donation is:
A. 4 weeks
B. 6 weeks
C. 8 weeks
D. 10 weeks

**16.** If a prospective allogeneic donor has received blood or blood components known to be sources of hepatitis due to conditions (e.g., surgery), the donor should be deferred from donating for _____ after the transfusion.
A. 6 weeks
B. 3 months
C. 6 months
D. 12 months

**17.** If a prospective donor is taking a prescription or nonprescription medication, the donor should be:
A. Deferred until 10 days after stopping the medication
B. Accepted, if the drug is on the list of permitted drugs
C. Accepted on an individual basis by a physician
D. Either B or C

**18.** A reason or reasons for permanent donor deferral include:
A. A reactive test for hepatitis B surface antigen (HBsAg)
B. A person involved in a high-risk behavior associated with acquired immunodeficiency syndrome (AIDS)
C. A history of malaria
D. Both A and B

**19.** If a donor weighs 105 lb, how much blood can safely be drawn?
A. 450 mL
B. 440 mL
C. 432 mL
D. 427 mL

**20.** The acceptable pulse rate for a homologous donor is _____ beats per minute.
A. 20–40
B. 50–75
C. 50–100
D. 100–180

**21.** The lowest acceptable fingertip hematocrit from a female donor is:
A. 32
B. 34
C. 36
D. 38

**22.** In the copper sulfate hemoglobin method, the correct specific gravity of the solution is:
A. 1.051
B. 1.053
C. 1.055
D. 1.057

**23.** All of the following are acceptable solutions for one of the two methods of donor arm preparation except:
A. 70% ethyl alcohol
B. 15% aqueous soap
C. 10% acetone in 70% isopropyl alcohol
D. 3% tincture of iodine

**24.** The appropriate method of applying solutions to a donor's arm in preparation for venipuncture is:
A. Liberally apply all solutions
B. Allow all solutions to remain in contact with the skin for 20 seconds
C. Apply solutions at the intended venipuncture site and move the applicator outward in a ring

**D.** Apply solutions about 1 inch from the intended venipuncture site and move the applicator toward the site

**25–29.** Correctly sequence the following steps in the phlebotomy procedure of a blood donor.

**25.** _____
**26.** _____
**27.** _____
**28.** _____
**29.** _____

**A.** Apply a tourniquet or blood-pressure cuff to the donor's arm.
**B.** Strip the donor tubing.
**C.** Perform the venipuncture.
**D.** Have the donor drink fluids.
**E.** Inspect the anticoagulant bag for leaks and cloudiness.

**30–33.** Match the following possible donor reactions with the appropriate initial first-aid procedure:

**30.** Fainting
**31.** Nausea and vomiting
**32.** Hyperventilation
**33.** Hematoma
**A.** Divert the donor's attention with conversation.
**B.** Place the donor on back and raise feet above level of the head.
**C.** Remove the tourniquet and needle from the donor's arm.
**D.** Instruct the donor to breathe slowly and deeply.

**34–37.** Match the following terms with their respective definitions:

**34.** Predeposit autologous donation
**35.** Intraoperative autotransfusion
**36.** Hemodilution
**37.** Postoperative autotransfusion
**A.** The collection of blood from a body cavity or wound, processing, and return to donor-patient
**B.** The removal and storage of blood or blood components from a donor-patient
**C.** Collection of blood and retransfusion following open heart and traumatic hemothorax
**D.** Collection of blood with replacement using a crystalloid or colloid solution

**38.** Which of the following is *not* a benefit of autologous donation?
**A.** Completely eliminates homologous transfusion
**B.** Can decrease health care costs
**C.** No risk of alloimmunization
**D.** No transfusion-related reactions

**39.** The only generally accepted criterion for autologous donation is:
**A.** Over 18 years of age

**B.** Absence of all medications
**C.** Blood pressure not above 180/100
**D.** Hematocrit at least 33%

**40–42.** Match the anticoagulant with the respective approved maximum storage time:
**40.** CPD or ACD      **A.** 35 days
**41.** CPD-A1          **B.** 21 days
**42.** heparin          **C.** 48 hours

**43.** FDA regulations require that at least _____% of erythrocytes remain viable in an anticoagulant-preservative solution at the end of the permitted storage period:
**A.** 35
**B.** 50
**C.** 65
**D.** 70

**44.** All of the listed factors, except _____, lead to the loss of posttransfusion viability.
**A.** Increased pH
**B.** Decreased pH
**C.** Changes in membrane surface properties
**D.** A decrease of surface area to volume ratio

**45.** The proper storage temperature for whole blood is _____° C.
**A.** −20 to −10
**B.** 0 to 4
**C.** 1 to 6
**D.** 2 to 10

**46.** Allogeneic donor blood collected and processed from outside sources must have the following tests repeated by the hospital blood bank:
**1.** ABO
**2.** Rh
**3.** HBsAg
**4.** anti-HIV-1
**5.** Alloantibodies
**A.** 1 and 2
**B.** 1, 2, and 5
**C.** 3 and 4
**D.** 3, 4, and 5

**47.** Autologous blood donor units must be tested for:
**1.** ABO
**2.** Rh
**3.** HBsAg
**4.** anti-HIV-1
**5.** Alloantibodies
**A.** 1 and 2
**B.** 1, 2, and 5
**C.** 3 and 4
**D.** 3, 4, and 5

**48.** Samples of recipient's blood and donor units must be stored for _____ days after transfusion.
**A.** 1
**B.** 3
**C.** 5
**D.** 7

**49.** Which of the following is the exception? If a unit of blood is returned to the blood bank after issue, it cannot be reissued unless:

    **A.** The closure has not been opened

    **B.** The records indicate that it has been reissued

    **C.** The blood is inspected prior to reissue

    **D.** It is administered to the same patient

## Bibliography

Advance for Medical Laboratory Professionals: Autologous donation risk in seriously ill less dangerous than thought, *5*(22):14, May 3, 1993.

Bello, K.: Managing an autologous blood program, *Medical Laboratory Observer,* 63–66, February 1987.

Brecher, M.E., Borchers, B., Rosen, N.R., and Lord, M.: Directed donations: An underutilized blood donor resource, *Laboratory Medicine 19*(2):103–105, February 1988.

Bull, M.H., Bull, B.S.: The use of autologous blood, *JAMA 263*(23): 3150, June 20, 1990.

Button, L., Kruskall, M.S., Scanlan, A., and Kevy, S.: Rejuvenation of red cells drawn in adsol to extend autologous red cell storage, *Transfusion 26*(6):558, 1986.

Coleman, P.F.: Detecting and differentiating HIV-2, *American Clinical Laboratory 11*(10):10, October 1992.

Council on Scientific Affairs: Autologous blood transfusions, *JAMA 256*(17):2378–2380, November 7, 1986.

Cowell, H.R.: Prior deposit of autologous blood for transfusion, *J Bone Joint Surg. 69-A*(3):319, March 1987.

Greenwalt, T.J.: Autologous and Aged Blood Donors, *JAMA 257*(9):1220–1221, March 6, 1987.

Huestis, D.W., Bove, J.R., Case, J.: Blood Donation, in *Practical Blood Transfusion,* 4th ed., Boston: Little, Brown, 1988, 1–54.

Kruskall, M.S. et al.: Utilization and effectiveness of a hospital autologous preoperative blood donor program, *Transfusion 26*(4): 335–340, 1986.

Kumar, B.: The haemonetic cell saver, *Anaesthesia 41*(7):774–775, July 1986.

Leitman, S.F. et al.: Allergic reactions in healthy plateletpheresis donors caused by sensitization to ethylene oxide gas, *Transfusion 26*(6):580, 1986.

Marwick, C.: Will more donor questions make blood safer? *JAMA 265*(7):838–839, February 20, 1991.

Matsui, Y. et al.: Effects of frequent and sustained plateletapheresis on peripheral blood mononuclear cell populations and lymphocyte functions of normal volunteer donors, *Transfusion 26*(5): 446–452, 1986.

McCullough, J.: The nation's changing blood supply, *JAMA 269*(17):2239–2245, May 5, 1993.

Meryman, H.T., Hornblower, M.L-S., and Syring, R.L.: Prolonged storage of red cells at 4° C, *Transfusion 26*(6):500–505, 1986.

National Blood Resource Education Program, National Heart, Lung, and Blood Institute, Bethesda, MD. The use of autologous blood, *JAMA 263*(3):414–417, January 19, 1990.

Nightingale, S.L.: Test for HIV-2 antibody licensed, *JAMA 264*(2): 168, July 11, 1990.

Oberman, H.A.: Surgical blood ordering, blood shortage situations, and emergency transfusion, in *Clinical Practice of Blood Transfusion,* Lawrence D. Petz and Scott N. Swisher, New York: Churchill Livingstone, 1981, 393–404.

Popovsky, M.A.: Autologous patients with localized infections, *AABB News Briefs 11*(6):9–10, July 1988.

Schmidt, P.J.: Autologous blood transfusion, *JAMA 257*(7): 928–929, February 20, 1987.

Schoenleber, D.G.: Everybody wins with this autologous donor program, *Med. Lab. Observer,* 39–42, August 1987.

Silvergleid, A.J.: Safety and effectiveness of pre-deposit autologous transfusions in pre-teenage and adolescent children, *Transfusion 26*(6):580, 1986.

Starkey, J.M. et al.: Markers for transfusion-transmitted disease in different groups of blood donors, *JAMA 262*(24):3452–3454, December 22/29, 1989.

Toy, P.T.C.Y. et al.: Predeposited autologous blood for elective surgery, *N. Engl. J. Med. 316*(9):517–520, February 26, 1987.

U.S. Dept. of Health and Human Services, Public Health Service, Centers for Disease Control, *MMWR 42*(9):173–175, 1993.

U.S. Dept. of Health and Human Services, Public Health Service, Centers for Disease Control, *MMWR 41*(RR-12):1–9, 1992.

Walker, R.H. (ed.): Standards for blood bank and transfusion services. 15th ed. Bethesda, MD. American Association of Blood Banks, 1993.

Wasman, J. and Goodnough, L.T.: Autologous blood donation for elective surgery, *JAMA 258*(21):3135–3137, December 4, 1987.

Widmann, F.K. (Ed.): *Technical Manual of the American Association of Blood Banks,* 11th ed. Bethesda, MD: American Association of Blood Banks, 1993.

Wolfe, L.C.: The membrane and the lesions of storage in preserved red cells, *Transfusion 25*(3):185–201, May–June, 1985.

Yomtovian, R.A.: Is directed blood transfusion a good idea? *Med. Lab. Observer 24*(11):31–34, November 1992.

Yomtovian, R.A.: Autologous blood transfusion: Past performance and current concerns, *Minnesota Medicine 69*:353–356, June 1986.

Yomtovian, R.A.: Predeposit autologous blood transfusion: An analysis of donor attitudes and attributes, *Q.R.B. 13*(2):45–50, February 1987.

# Principles of Antigens and Antibodies

At the conclusion of this chapter, the reader should be able to:

- Briefly describe the process of hematopoiesis.
- Describe the organization and functions of the immune system.
- List cell types and effector mechanisms triggered by or involved in immune reactions.
- Describe the structure of the organs that house immunologic cells.
- Explain the general characteristics of the specific immune response.
- Compare and contrast humoral immunity to cell-mediated immunity.
- Discuss the formation of cell products of the specific immune response.
- Explain the role of the thymus in self-recognition.
- Describe the chemical composition of antigens and antibodies.
- Define the terms *agglutination, immunity, isotype, allotype,* and *idiotype.*
- List the classes of immunoglobulins.
- Explain the physical and chemical properties of IgM antibodies.
- Explain the physical and chemical properties of IgM and IgG antibodies.
- Compare the characteristics of IgM, IgG, IgA, IgD, and IgE.
- Contrast the characteristics of a primary and secondary (anamnestic) response.
- Describe the production of monoclonal antibodies.
- Name the four types of noncovalent bonds formed in antigen-antibody reactions.
- State the most commonly used technique to detect and measure the consequences of antigen-antibody interaction.
- Name the four major methods commonly used in routine blood banking to enhance the agglutination of erythrocytes and describe the purpose of the AHG test.
- Explain the method of grading the strength of agglutination reactions.
- State the reason for pseudoagglutination and describe the results of the prozone phenomenon.
- Explain the role of the complement system in blood banking.

## Chapter Outline

## PRINCIPLES OF ANTIGENS AND ANTIBODIES

An *antigen* can be defined as a foreign substance that is able to elicit an *antibody* response. Not all foreign substances are capable of stimulating an antibody response, however, and the production of antibodies in response to antigenic stimulation depends on two major factors:

1. A person's immunologic ability both to recognize an antigen as foreign or non-self and to respond to this foreignness.
2. The physical and chemical nature of the antigen.

## THE IMMUNE SYSTEM

The ability of the body to recognize the foreignness of a substance and produce antibodies in response depends on several body cells, including several kinds of lymphocyte-type leukocytes, plasma cells, and macrophages. Lymphocytes recognize foreign antigens and/or produce antibodies, whereas plasma cells only produce antibodies. Macrophages, which are phagocytic cells, are important in the processing of antigens.

### Hematopoiesis

Hematopoiesis is the process of blood cell production, differentiation, and development. The hematopoietic system consists of the bone marrow, liver, spleen, lymph nodes, and thymus.

#### Hematopoietic Growth Factors

The hematopoietic growth factors are glycoprotein hormones that regulate the proliferation and differentiation of hematopoietic progenitor cells and the function of mature blood cells. Hematopoietic growth factors were originally referred to as "colony-stimulating factors (CSF)" because they stimulated the formation of colonies of cells derived from individual bone marrow progenitors.

Erythropoietin, granulocyte-macrophage colony-stimulating factor (GM-CSF), granulocyte colony-stimulating factor (G-CSF), macrophage colony-stimulating factor (M-CSF), and interleukin-3 are representative factors that have been identified, cloned, and produced through recombinant DNA technology. The hematopoietic growth factors interact with blood cells at different levels in the cascade of cell differentiation from the multipotential progenitor to the circulating mature cell. Each growth factor is encoded by a single gene. The gene for erythropoietin is located on chromosome 7. The genes for GM-CSF, interleukin-3, and M-CSF are clustered on the long arm of chromosome 5. Chromosome 17 is the location of the G-CSF gene. The cellular sources and other characteristics of growth hormones are presented in Table 3-1.

Protein molecules that work in conjunction with hematopoietic growth factors to stimulate proliferation and dif-

**Table 3-1. Characteristics of Human Hematopoietic Growth Factors**

| Growth Factor | Cellular Source | Progenitor-Cell Target* | Mature Cell Target |
|---|---|---|---|
| Erythropoietin | Peritubular cells of the kidney, Kupffer cells | CFU-E, late BFU-E, CFU-Meg | None |
| Interleukin-3 | Activated T-lymphocytes | CFU-Blast, CFU-GEMM, CFU-GM, CFU-G, CFU-M, CFU-Eo, CFU-Meg CFU-Baso, BFU-E | Eosinophils, Monocytes |
| G-CSF | Monocytes, Fibroblasts, Endothelial cells | GFU-G | Granulocytes |
| M-CSF | Monocytes, Fibroblasts, Endothelial cells | CFU-M | Monocytes |
| GM-CSF | T-lymphocytes, Monocytes, Fibroblasts, Endothelial cells | CFU-Blast, CFU-GEMM, CFU-GM, CFU-G, CFU-M, CFU-Eo, CFU-Meg, BFU-E | Eosinophils, Monocytes, Granulocytes |

* CFU = colony-forming unit-blast; CFU-GEMM = colony forming unit-granulocyte, erythrocyte, monocyte, and megakaryocyte; CFU-GM = colony-forming unit-granulocyte and macrophage; CFU-Eo = colony forming unit-eosinophil; CFU-Meg = colony-forming unit-megakaryocyte; BFU-E = burst-forming unit-erythroid; CFU-G = colony-forming unit-granulocyte; CFU-M = colony-forming unit-macrophage; CFU-E = colony-forming unit-erythroid; and CFU-Baso = colony-forming unit-basophil.

ferentiation of specific cell lines are the interleukins: IL-1 to IL-7. Interleukins are cytokines that act independently or in conjunction with other ILs to encourage hematopoietic growth. The interleukins are described in Table 3-2. This interacting network of inflammatory stimuli and cytokines suggests that these growth factors may have a limited role in hematopoietic homeostasis, but a major role in host responses to infection or antigenic challenge. The major role of the hematopoietic growth factors appears to be regulating the proliferation and differentiation of hematopoietic progenitor cells as well as regulating the survival and function of mature blood cells.

### Biologic Effects of Growth Factors

The biologic effects of hematopoietic growth factors are mediated through specific binding to receptors on the surface of target cells. Hematopoietic growth factors are being used and tested in clinical trials for the treatment of a variety of hematologic disorders. Specific factors are being used as adjunct therapy in a wide variety of diseases (e.g., to stimulate production of granulocytes or lymphocytes).

## Development and Differentiation of Lymphocytes

During embryonic development, lymphocytes arise from progenitor cells. Later, in fetal development and throughout the life cycle, the bone marrow becomes the sole provider of progenitor cells, which can further develop into lymphocyte precursors. Continued cellular development of these cells and their subsequent proliferation occurs as the cells travel to specific sites, with the majority of cells differentiating into the two major categories of lymphocytes, *T lymphocytes* (T cells) or *B lymphocytes* (B cells).

### Primary Lymphoid Tissues

In humans, both the *bone marrow* and *thymus* are classified as primary or central lymphoid tissues (Fig. 3-1). Progeni-

tor cells migrate to the thymus to proliferate and differentiate. These cells acquire thymus-dependent characteristics to become *immunocompetent* (able to function in the immune response) T lymphocytes. Mature T cells leave the thymus with one of two phenotypes (CD4 + 8 − or CD4 − 8 +). It is believed that the bone marrow functions as the bursal equivalent in humans. It is from the term *bursa* that the B lymphocytes derive their name. B cells have the capacity to synthesize heavy and light immunoglobulin chains and assemble them into an immunoglobulin molecule. Most of the cells produced in the primary sites die before leaving, with only a small percentage migrating to the secondary tissues.

### Secondary Lymphoid Tissues

The secondary lymphoid tissues include the *lymph nodes, spleen,* and *Peyer's patches* in the intestine (Fig. 3-1). Proliferation of the T and B cells in the secondary or peripheral lymphoid tissues depends primarily on antigenic stimulation. The T cells (Fig. 3-2) populate the perifollicular and paracortical regions of the lymph node, the medullary cords of the lymph nodes, the periarteriolar regions of the spleen, and the thoracic duct of the circulatory system. The B cells (Fig. 3-2) multiply and populate the follicular and medullary (germinal centers) of the lymph nodes, the primary follicles and red pulp of the spleen, the follicular regions of gut-associated lymphoid tissue (GALT), and the medullary cords of the lymph nodes.

## Cellular Activities of the Immune System

### Macrophages

Macrophages exist as either "fixed" or "wandering" cells. Fixed macrophages line the endothelium of the capillaries and the sinuses of organs such as the bone marrow, spleen, and lymph nodes. These cells, along with the network of reticular cells of the spleen, thymus, and other lymphoid

**Table 3-2. Origin and Immunoregulatory Activity of Cytokines**

| Cytokines | Origin | Prominent Biological Activities |
|---|---|---|
| *Interleukins* | | |
| IL-1 | Macrophages, keratinocytes, etc. | Activates resting T cells; induces fever, acute phase response, and inflammation |
| IL-2 | T cells | Proliferation and clonal expansion of activated T cells; activates cytotoxic cells; induces other lymphokines |
| IL-3 | Activated T cells | Promotes the growth of early hematopoietic cell lines |
| IL-4 | T cells; mast cells | Growth factor for early activation of resting B cells; induces HLA-DR molecules on B cells and macrophages; governs B cell isotype switching to $IgG_1$ and IgE; growth and differentiation of T cells, mast cells, granulocytes, megakaryocytes, and erythrocytes |
| IL-5 | T cells, mast cells, ? B cells | Growth and differentiation inducing factor for activated T and B cells; eosinophil differentiation and proliferation; induces class-specific B cell differentiation (IgA production) |
| IL-6 | Macrophages, mitogen-activated T cells, fibroblasts | Growth and final differentiation factor for B cells; induces acute phase response; growth factor for T and B cells; T cell activation; cytolytic T cell activation factor |
| IL-7 | Bone marrow stroma | Early T and B cell differentiation and maturation |
| IL-8 | Monocytes, keratinocytes, fibroblasts | Chemotaxis and activation of neutrophils |
| IL-9 | T cells | Proliferation of T cells; thymocytes; mast cells |
| IL-10 | T cells, mast cells, ? B cells | Inhibition of cytokine synthesis in various cells; proliferation of mast cells |
| IL-11 | Bone marrow stroma | Regulator of hematopoiesis; stimulates the production of megakaryocyte and myeloid progenitors; Increases the number of Ig-secreting B lymphocytes |
| IL-12 | B cells | Enhances the activity of cytotoxic effector T cells; acts as a growth factor for activated NK/lymphokine activated killer cells and for activated T cells of both the CD4+ and CD8+ subsets |
| INF alpha | Leukocytes | Augments natural killer cell activity; induces class I antigen expression; anti-proliferation activity |
| INF beta | Fibroblasts, epithelial cells | Identical to IL-6 |
| INF gamma | Activated T cells | Major macrophage activator; induces MHC class II molecules on many cells and can synergize with tumor necrosis factor; augments NK cell activity; antagonist to IL-4 |
| *Tumor Necrosis Factors* | | |
| TNF alpha | Activated macrophages | Directly cytotoxic for some tumor cells; mediates acute phase response, inflammation, and septic shock |
| TNF beta | Activated lymphocytes | Lymphotoxin; properties similar to TNF alpha |
| *Colony Stimulating Factors* | | |
| Multi CSF | Identical to IL-3 | |
| GM CSF | Activates neutrophils; promotes granulocyte and macrophage colonies | |
| G CSF | Promotes granulocyte colonies | |
| M CSF | Promotes macrophage colonies | |
| *Transforming Growth Factors* | | |
| TGF beta | Chemotactic for monocytes; induces secretion of inflammatory mediators; suppresses IL-1 induced T cell proliferation | |

Adapted from D. H. Beezhold, Immune Regulation, *Guthrie J., 59*(1):5, winter 1990, and H. N. Claman, The Biology of the Immune Response, *JAMA, 268*(20): 2791, November 25, 1992.

tissues, comprise the *mononuclear phagocytic system* (Fig. 3-3). Macrophages and their known precursors, the monocytes, migrate freely into the tissues from the blood to replenish and reinforce the macrophage population.

The immunologic functions of the macrophage cells are to phagocytize, process, and present antigens to T cells. Hence, the name antigen-presenting cells has been applied to cells such as the macrophages and dendritic cells. Enzymes released by the macrophages degrade engulfed antigens, antigen processing, and the antigenic determinants seem to be preserved. These processed antigens are located on the surface of antigen-presenting cells. T cells receive RNA or other messages from macrophages and extracts from macrophages containing an RNA-antigen determinant-linked complex that can be used to stimulate IgG synthesis by lymphocytes. Antigen modification may not be required of all antigens. Low molecular weight antigens may activate T and B cells directly.

## Lymphocytes

Several major categories of lymphocytes are recognized as functionally active. These categories are the *T cells, B cells,* and the *natural killer (NK)* and *K-type* lymphocytes.

*T-Cells.* T cells are responsible for foreign antigen recognition or cellular immune responses, which include chronic rejection in organ transplantation, the regulation of antibody reactions by either helping or suppressing the activation of B lymphocytes, and the secretion of soluble mediators.

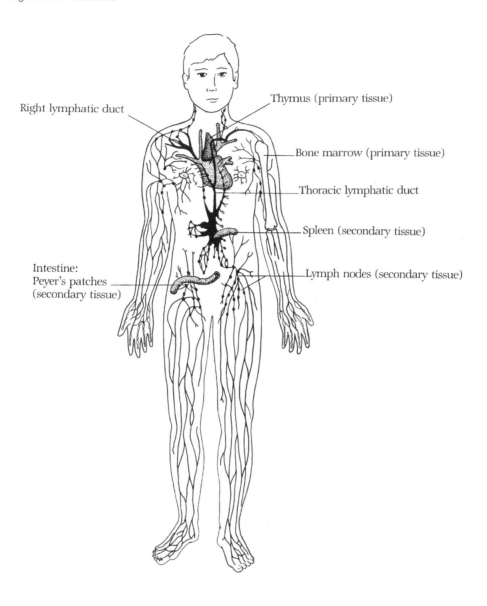

**Figure 3-1.** The primary and secondary lymphoid tissues. The primary lymphoid tissues are the bone marrow and the thymus. The secondary tissues consist of the spleen, lymph nodes, and Peyer's patches of the small intestine. (Illustration from Turgeon, M.L.: *Clinical Hematology: Theory and Procedures.* Boston; Little, Brown and Company, 2nd ed., 1993, p. 155).

Within the figure, the following labels appear:
- Right lymphatic duct
- Thymus (primary tissue)
- Bone marrow (primary tissue)
- Thoracic lymphatic duct
- Spleen (secondary tissue)
- Lymph nodes (secondary tissue)
- Intestine: Peyer's patches (secondary tissue)

T cells are divided into two subsets, the *helper/inducer* subset and the *suppressor/cytotoxic* subset. Functionally, the helper/inducer subset signals B cells to generate antibodies, to control production and switching of types of antibodies that are formed, and to activate suppressor cells. The suppressor-cytotoxic lymphocytes control and inhibit antibody production by either suppressing helper cells or turning off B-cell differentiation.

T cells are also associated with the production of soluble mediators, *lymphokines,* which provide the language for cell-to-cell communication.

***B Cells.*** B cells serve as the primary source of cells responsible for humoral (antibody) responses. Participa- tion of B cells in the humoral immune response is accomplished by their maturation into plasma cells, which subsequently synthesize and secrete immune antibodies (immunoglobulins). Circulating unstimulated resting B lymphocytes have immunoglobulin molecules, usually monomeric IgD and IgM, on their surface. This feature makes them easy to identify in mixed cell populations or tissue. B cells also have surface receptors for complement and express HLA-DR antigens. Stimulation of B cells to produce antibodies is a complex process, usually requiring interactions between *macrophages, T cells,* and *B cells.* The condition of hyperacute rejection of transplanted organs is mediated by the B cell.

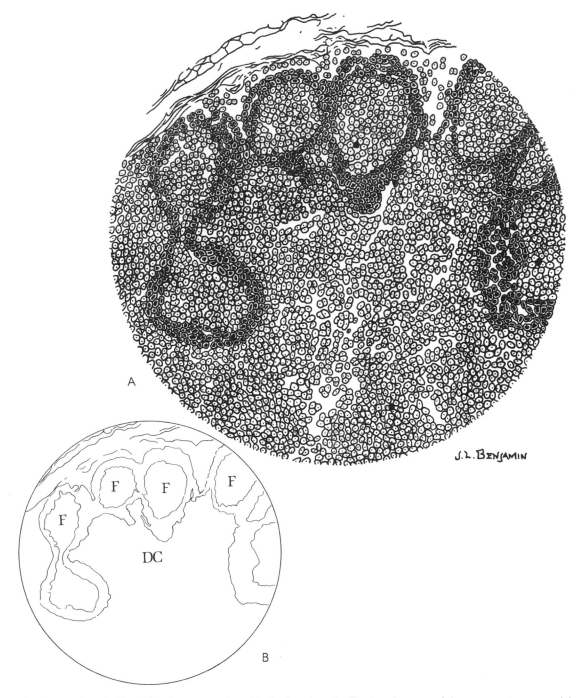

A

B

F  F  F  F
F
DC

**Figure 3-2. A, B.** Lymph node. T and B cell areas are found in the lymph node. The lymphocytes of the outer cortex are mainly arranged in lymphoid follicles (F), which are the major sites of B lymphocyte localization and proliferation. The deep cortical zone (DC), or paracortex, is composed mainly of T lymphocytes that are never arranged in follicles. The number of cortical follicles and the depth of the deep cortical zone vary, both according to the immunologic state of each lymph node and in each individual. (Illustration from Turgeon, M.L.: *Clinical Hematology: Theory and Procedures.* Boston; Little, Brown and Company, 2nd ed., 1993, p. 156.)

***Natural Killer and K-type Lymphocytes.*** These cells, which lack the recognizable surface markers of mature T or B lymphocytes, include the *natural killer (NK)* and *K-type.* The NK and K cells destroy target cells through an extracellular nonphagocytic mechanism referred to as a cytotoxic reaction.

NK-cells have the ability to nonspecifically attack certain types of tumor cells and cells infected with a number of different viruses. NK-cells are classified as a population of effector lymphocytes that produce such mediators as *interferon* and *interleukin 2.* These cells have long been classified as *null* cells, but monoclonal antibodies have re-

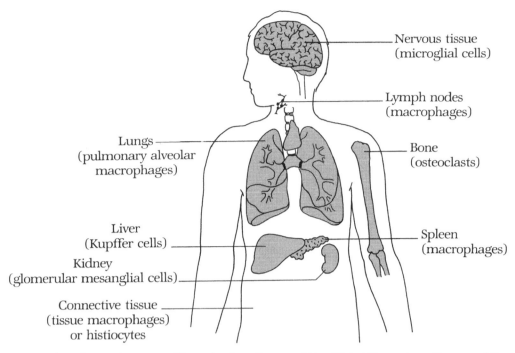

**Figure 3-3.** The mononuclear phagocytic system. (Illustration from Turgeon, M.L.: *Clinical Hematology: Theory and Procedures.* Boston; Little, Brown and Company, 2nd edition, 1993, p. 156.)

vealed several membrane markers that affirm their T-cell nature. They cannot be absolutely classified as T cells, however, because they have an unmistakably primitive lineage.

K-type cells exhibit a different kind of cytotoxic mechanism from NK cells. The target cell must be coated with low concentrations of IgG antibody (to be discussed later in this chapter). This is referred to as an *antibody-dependent, cell-mediated, cytotoxicity (ADCC)* reaction. An ADCC reaction may be exhibited by both K cells and phagocytic and nonphagocytic myelogenous-type leukocytes. K cells are capable of lysing tumor cells. The precise lineage of the K cell is uncertain.

*Plasma Cells.* The pathway from the B lymphocyte to the antibody-synthesizing plasma cell (Fig. 3-4) occurs when the B cell is antigenically stimulated and undergoes *blast transformation.* The immune antibody response begins when B lymphocytes encounter antigens that bind to their specific immunoglobulin surface receptors. After receiving an appropriate "second signal" provided by interaction with helper T cells, these antigen-bound B lymphocyte cells undergo blast cell transformation and proliferation to generate a clone of mature plasma cells, which secrete a specific type of antibody.

## Cellular Membrane Marker Development

The development of T and B lymphocytes is traditionally separated into sequential phases of *antigen-independent* and *antigen-dependent* maturational phases. Lymphocyte

development in the thymus and bursal-equivalent are antigen-independent. Antigen-dependent maturation involves exposure of the T or B cell to a specific antigen that results in the expression of surface receptor molecules that can

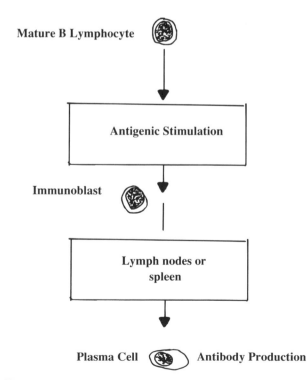

**Figure 3-4.** Plasma cell development from B lymphocytes. (Illustration from Turgeon, M.L.: *Clinical Hematology: Theory and Procedures.* Boston; Little, Brown and Company, 2nd ed., 1993, p. 163).

recognize the foreign antigen upon re-presentation. Lymphocytes in the peripheral lymphoid organs—including the lymph nodes, spleen, and other lymphoid tissues—remain in a resting state until they are stimulated to undergo antigen-dependent development.

### T Cell Maturation

Maturation of T cells is recognized by the presence of surface markers CD9 and CD10. Early cells share an enzyme, terminal deoxynucleotidyl transferase (TdT), that is lost during maturation. This marker is used to identify the lineage of immature cells in acute leukemias.

Committed pre-T cells mature into early thymocytes which express the CD11 antigen. Further maturation and differentiation result in expression of the CD4, CD6, and CD8 antigens. CD6 will be lost as the cell matures, but CD4 and CD8 persist. In addition, the immunocompetent T cell acquires two new markers, CD1 and CD3, in the common immunocyte phase of development. Further differentiation in the medulla and mitotic division produces a subset of cells expressing either CD4 or CD8. Both populations express a new marker CD12.

### B Cell Maturation

Certain immunologic characteristics are associated with B cell development. The early pre-B cell is TdT positive and expresses HLA-DR, CD19, CD20, and usually CALLA (CD10) antigen. The first unique feature that identifies pre-B cells is the appearance of immunoglobulin chains in the cytoplasm. Immunoglobulins consist of light and heavy molecular-weight chains. The heavy chain (u) of IgM is synthesized first and characterizes the pre-B cell. During the next stage of maturation, the early or immature B cell has cytoplasmic (cIg) and surface immunoglobulin (sIg) in the form of complete heavy and light chain molecules of IgM. The surface-bound IgM is structurally different from the IgM molecules that normally circulate in the plasma. Receptors for complement proteins and the Fc portion of an immunoglobulin (IgG) also appear. All of this occurs while the cells reside in the bone marrow, prior to antigen stimulation.

Circulating, unstimulated, resting, mature B cells have two types of immunoglobulin—usually monomeric IgM and IgD on their surface. This feature makes them easy to identify in mixed-cell populations or tissue. In addition, mature B cells express CD19 and CD20 cell surface markers, HLA-DR antigens, and surface receptors for complement. When activated, B cells undergo clonal expansion, producing daughter cells that retain the same antibody idiotype (antigen-binding region). Some daughter cells become memory cells and regain the small mature B-cell morphology and phenotype; others continue development into a short-lived antibody-secreting cell, the plasma cell.

## ANTIGEN CHARACTERISTICS

Foreign substances, such as erythrocytes, can be *immunogenic* or *antigenic* (capable of provoking an immune response) if their membrane contains a number of areas recognized as foreign. These areas are called *antigenic determinants* or *epitopes*. A single antigen may possess many different epitopes. Each epitope (5–6 amino acids) is capable of eliciting an antibody response and each can be the target of these antibodies. Not all surface areas act as antigenic determinants. Only prominent determinants on the surface of a protein are normally recognized by the immune system, and some of these are much more immunogenic than others. An immune response is directed against specific determinants and resultant antibodies bind to them, with much of the remainder of the molecule being nonimmunogenic. Functionally, immunogenic determinants are said to be *immunodominant*.

### Cell Surface Antigens

The cellular membrane of all mammalian cells consists of proteins, phospholipids, cholesterol, and traces of polysaccharide. The most popular hypothesis to explain the arrangement of these molecular components is the *fluid mosaic model*. According to this model, the cell membrane is a dynamic fluid structure with globular proteins floating in lipids. The lipids, as phospholipids, are arranged in two layers. The polar (charged) phosphate ends of the phospholipids are oriented toward the inner and outer surfaces, whereas the nonpolar (fatty acid) ends point toward each other in the interior of the membrane. Protein molecules may be either intrinsic (incorporated into the lipid bilayer) or extrinsic (associated with either the outer or the inner surface of the membrane). Polysaccharides (carbohydrates) in the form of either glycoproteins or glycolipids can be found attached to the lipid and protein molecules of the membrane. Most of these proteins are immunogenic when injected into an individual of another species or even into a different individual of the same species.

Cellular antigens of importance to immunohematologists are blood group antigens, histocompatibility (HLA) antigens, and autoantigens.

### Blood Group Antigens

Blood group substances are widely distributed throughout the tissues, blood cells, and body fluids. The literature does not agree on the presence of the major blood group antigen systems on certain cells, particularly leukocytes. Recent studies (Table 3-3) have documented the fact that many erythrocyte antigens are not as widely distributed as previously thought. Some blood group antigens are restricted to specific types of cells. For example, Kell blood

**Table 3-3. Erythrocyte Antigen Incidence on Leukocytes**

| Investigator(s) | Date | Occurrence of Major RBC Antigens on Leukocytes |
|---|---|---|
| Gaidulis et al. | 1985 | Not detectable on human granulocytes: A, B, D, U, Gerbich, Jk$^a$, Jk$^b$ (Jk3), and Cartwright (Yt$^a$) |
| Kelton and Bebenek | 1985 | Granulocytes do not have surface A or B antigens |
| Dunstan | 1986 | Lymphocytes expressed A, B, Le$^a$ and Le$^b$ depending on the secretor status |
| | | ABH and Lewis antigens are not detectable on monocytes and segmented neutrophils (PMNs) regardless of secretor (Se) status |
| | | Lymphocytes, monocytes, and PMNs do not express D, E, e, C, c, Fy$^a$, Fy$^b$, Fy$^5$, Jk$^a$, Jk$^b$, K, k, M, m, S, s, U, Vel, Co$^a$, Lan, Jk3, Yt$^a$, Di$^b$, Ge, Sc:1 or Lu$^b$ antigens |
| | | Lymphocytes, monocytes, and PMNs all express I, i, P and P$_1$ antigens |

group antigens, with one exception, are found only on erythrocytes.

Certain antigens, especially those of the Rh system, are integral structural components of the erythrocyte membrane. If these antigens are missing, the erythrocyte membrane is defective and causes hemolytic anemia. When antigens do not form part of the essential membrane structure such as A, B and H (ABH), the absence of antigen has no effect on membrane integrity. The Lewis antigens are passively adsorbed by selective uptake onto erythrocytes from the plasma.

## Histocompatibility Antigens (HLA)

***General Characteristics.*** The histocompatibility complex that encodes cell surface antigens was first discovered in graft rejection experiments with mice. When the antigens were matched between donor and recipient, the ability of a graft to survive was remarkably improved. These antigens are second in importance only to the A and B antigens in influencing the survival or graft rejection of transplanted organs. The term *histocompatibility antigens* was coined for these antigens.

A comparable genetic system of alloantigens was later identified in humans. The presence of histocompatibility antigens was first recognized when multiply transfused patients experienced transfusion reactions despite proper crossmatching. It was discovered that these reactions resulted from leukocyte antibodies rather than antibodies directed against erythrocyte antigens. These same antibodies were subsequently discovered in the sera of multiparous women.

In humans, the major histocompatibility complex is referred to as human leukocyte antigen (HLA). It is the

most complex immunogenetic system presently known in humans and is controlled by a major histocompatibility complex, or supergene, which includes several loci closely linked on the short arm of chromosome 6. Each of these loci involves numerous alleles, having at least 10 to 40 alleles per locus that control the production of their corresponding antigens. The antigens are found on body cells such as leukocytes, platelets, and other tissue cells as well as on some non-nucleated cells, and in body fluids. Some groups of these antigens exhibit cross-reacting characteristics that further increase the complexity of the system.

Although HLA was originally identified by its role in transplant rejection, it is now recognized that proteins encoded in this region are involved in many aspects of immunologic recognition, including interaction between different lymphoid cells and between lymphocytes and antigen-presenting cells.

The products of HLA genes play a crucial role in our immune system. The HLA genes encode for three classes of molecules: class I, class II, and class III. The class I major transplantation antigens are serologically defined. HLA-A, B, and C genes are responsible for the corresponding Class I HLA antigens. In addition to the classical genes, HLA-A, HLA-B, and HLA-C, other gene loci exist, including HLA-E, HLA-F, HLA-G, and HLA-A. The class II immune response gene region antigens are encoded in the HLA-D region and can be subdivided into three families, called HLA-DR, -DC (DQ), and -SB (DP). Class I and class II molecules are surface membrane proteins. Class I molecules are transmembrane glycoproteins, but the class II dimer molecule differs from class I in that both dimers span the cell membrane. Class I and class II gene products are biochemically distinct, although they appear to be distantly related through evolution. Both class I and class II antigens function as targets of T lymphocytes that regulate the immune response. The presence of self-class I antigens is a requisite for cytotoxic T lymphocytes to recognize and lyse virus-infected cells. Another function of class II molecules is to restrict the activity of regulatory T cells (T helper, suppressor, and amplifier subsets). Class II molecules are normally expressed by only a few types of cells such as B lymphocytes and macrophages; they may also appear under certain circumstances on activated T lymphocytes and epithelial cells. Many of the genes in both class I and class II gene families have no known functions. Class II genes code for the production of the complement proteins as well as cytokine (tumor necrosis factor). Class III molecules bear no clear relation to class I and II molecules aside from their genetic linkage. Located between the Class I and Class II genes is a group of genes coding for the HLA Class III molecules.

Class I antigens are determined by several techniques; the most popular and reproducible is the lymphocyte microcytotoxicity method. With this technique, a living lymphocyte suspension from peripheral blood or lymphatic tissue is mixed with antisera and complement. In the presence of the corresponding antigen, complement is fixed and the cells are killed. Cell death is determined by staining. A stain such as trypan blue penetrates dead cells but not living ones. Unaffected cells remain brilliantly refractile when observed microscopically. Other methods of analysis include leukocyte agglutination and complement fixation on platelets in suspension.

*HLA Applications.* HLA matching is of value in organ transplantation as well as in the transplantation of bone marrow. HLA-matched platelets are useful to patients who are refractile to random donor platelets. In paternity testing, HLA typing, along with the determination of ABO, Rh, MNSs, Kell, Duffy, and Kidd erythrocyte antigen, is used. In the past, most laboratories involved in testing individuals in disputed parentage cases used only the ABO, Rh, and MNSs systems. The chance of identifying a falsely accused man with these tests was 58%. Additional testing for Kell, Duffy, and Kidd erythrocyte antigens, and HLA typing offers an exclusion rate estimated at 92%. HLA typing is also useful in forensic medicine, anthropology, and basic research in immunology.

HLA testing is being used increasingly as a diagnostic and genetic counseling tool. An intriguing peculiarity of certain HLA alleles is that they appear to be genetically linked to the predisposition to various diseases, mainly of an autoimmune nature.

### Autoantigens

In some situations (not always abnormal), antibodies may be produced in response to normal self-antigens. This failure to recognize self-antigens can result in autoantibodies directed at hormones, such as thyroglobulin, and cell-membrane antigens, such as the Ii blood group system. Antibodies of this type are discussed in detail in Chapter Five.

### The Chemical Nature of Antigens

Antigens or *immunogens* are usually large organic molecules that are either proteins or large polysaccharides, and rarely (if ever) lipids. Antigens, especially cell surface or membrane-bound antigens, can be composed of combinations of the biochemical classes, for example, glycoproteins or glycolipids. For example, HLA antigens are glycoprotein in nature and are found on the surface membranes of nucleated body cells comprising both solid tissue and most circulating blood cells. The Lewis antigens are glycolipids, ceramide pentasaccharides (Le$^a$), or hexasaccharides (Le$^b$), which are absorbed from the plasma where they circulate on lipoproteins.

Proteins are excellent antigens because of their high molecular weight and structural complexity; lipids are considered inferior antigens because of their relative simplicity and lack of structural stability. When lipids are linked to proteins or polysaccharides, they may function as antigens. Nucleic acids are poor antigens because of their relative simplicity, molecular flexibility, and rapid degradation. Antinucleic acid antibodies can be produced by artificially stabilizing these acids and linking them to an immunogenic carrier. Carbohydrates (polysaccharides) by themselves are considered too small to function as antigens. However, in the case of erythrocyte blood group antigens, protein or lipid carriers may contribute to the necessary size and the polysaccharides present in the form of side chains, confer the immunologic specificity (immunodominant carbohydrate) and are considered the *antigenic determinant* groups or combining sites with which antibodies react.

### The Physical Nature of Antigens

For antigens to function effectively, the following factors are important: foreignness, degradability, molecular weight, structural stability, and complexity.

### Foreignness

The more foreign the antigenic determinant or the greater the degree to which it is recognized as non-self by an individual's immune system, the more antigenic it is. The immunogenicity of a molecule depends greatly on its degree of foreignness. Normally, an individual's immune system does not respond to self-antigens.

### Degradability

For an antigen to be recognized as foreign by an individual's immune system, a sufficient amount of antigen must be present to stimulate an immune response. Foreign molecules, which are rapidly destroyed, will not be present for enough time to provide the necessity antigenic exposure.

### Molecular Weight

The higher the molecular weight, the better the molecule functions as an antigen. The number of antigenic determinants on a molecule is directly related to its size. Although large foreign molecules (molecular weight greater than 10,000) are better antigens; *haptens,* which are very small molecules, can bind to a larger carrier molecule and behave as antigens. If a hapten is chemically linked to a large molecule, a new surface structure is formed on the large molecule, which may function as an antigenic determinant.

### Structural Stability

If a molecule is to function as an effective antigen, structural stability is an essential characteristic. Molecules such as gelatin are poor antigens because of their structural instability. Totally inert molecules are also poor antigens.

## Complexity

The more complex an antigen is, the more effective it will be. Complex proteins are better antigens than large repeating polymers such as lipids, carbohydrates, and nucleic acids, which are relatively poor antigens.

## ANTIBODY CHARACTERISTICS

Antibodies, chemically classified as globulins, can be found in blood plasma and many body fluids such as tears, saliva, and breast milk. These specific glycoproteins are referred to as *immunoglobulins,* abbreviated Ig. Five distinct classes of immunoglobulin molecules are recognized in most higher mammals: IgM, IgG, IgA, IgD, and IgE.

The immunoglobulin classes differ from each other in characteristics such as molecular weight, sedimentation coefficient, and carbohydrate content (Table 3-4). In addition to the differences between classes, the immunoglobulins also vary within each class.

### Antibody Response to Antigen

Production of antibodies is induced when the host's immune system comes into contact with a foreign antigenic substance and reacts to this antigenic stimulation. When an antigen is initially encountered, the cells of the immune system recognize the antigen as non-self and either elicit an immune response or become tolerant to it, depending on the circumstances. An immune reaction can take the form of cell-mediated immunity (immunity dependent on T cells and macrophages) or involve the production of antibodies directed against the antigen. Whether a cell-mediated response or an antibody response takes place depends on the way in which the antigen is presented to the lymphocytes; many immune reactions display both kinds of responses. The antigenicity of a foreign substance is also related to the route of entry. Intravenous and intraperitoneal routes are stronger stimuli than subcutaneous and intramuscular routes. Subsequent exposure to the same antigen produces a memory response, also known as a secondary or *anamnestic response,* and reflects the out-

come of the initial challenge. In the case of antibody production, both the quantity and class of immunoglobulins produced varies.

### The Primary Antibody Response

Following a foreign antigen challenge, the primary IgM antibody-producing response proceeds in four phases (Fig. 3-5) but the actual time period and levels of antibody (titer) depend on the characteristics of the antigen and the individual. The four phases are the following:

1. A *lag* phase, when no antibody is detectable
2. A *log* phase, in which the antibody titer rises logarithmically
3. A *plateau* phase, during which the antibody titer stabilizes
4. A *decline* phase, in which the antibody is catabolized

### The Secondary Antibody (Anamnestic) Response

Subsequent exposure to the same antigenic stimulus produces an antibody response that exhibits the same pattern as a primary response. Repeated exposure to an antigen can take place many years after the initial exposure, but clones of the T memory cells will be stimulated to proliferate, with subsequent production of antibody by the individual. Thus an anamnestic response, differs from a primary response in several important aspects (Fig. 3-6). The major differences between a primary and secondary response include the following:

*Time.* A secondary response has a shorter lag phase, a longer plateau, and a more gradual decline.
*Type of Antibody.* IgM-type antibodies are the principal class formed in the primary response. Although some IgM antibodies are formed in a secondary response, IgG antibodies are the predominant type of antibody formed.
*Antibody Titer.* In a secondary response, antibody levels attain a higher titer. The plateau levels in a secondary response are typically ten-fold more, or greater, than the plateau levels in the primary response.

### Antibody Structure

Antibodies exhibit diversity among the different classes, which suggests that they perform different functions in

## Table 3-4. Comparison of Characteristics of the Five Immunoglobulin Classes

| Characteristic | IgM | IgG | IgA | IgE | IgD |
|---|---|---|---|---|---|
| Molecular weight | 900,000 | 160,000 | 360,000 | 200,000 | 160,000 |
| Sedimentation coefficient | 19S | 7S | 11S | 8S | 7S |
| Percent carbohydrate | 12 | 3 | 7 | 12 | 12 |
| Subclasses | None | IgG1–4 | alpha 1, 2 | None | None |
| Serum concentration, mg/100 mL | 50 to 200 | 800 to 1600 | 150 to 400 | 0.002 to 0.05 | 1.5 to 40 |
| Half-life days | 5 | 21 | 6 | 2 | 3 |

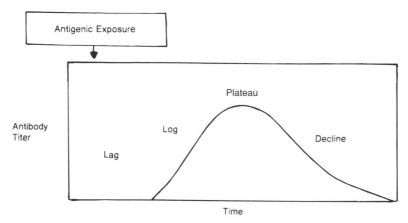

**Figure 3-5.** The four phases of an antibody response. Following an antigenic challenge, the antibody response in an immunocompetent proceeds in four phases: lag, log, plateau and decline.

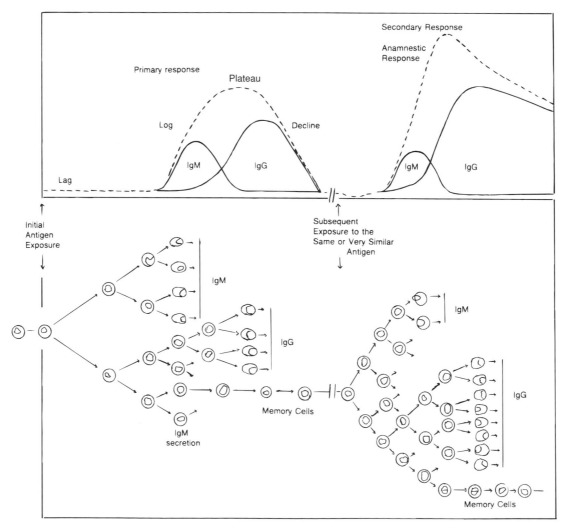

**Figure 3-6.** The primary and secondary (anamnestic) response. The differences between a primary and secondary response include the length of the lag phase, the type of antibody produced, and the antibody titer.

addition to their primary function of antigen binding. Essentially, each immunoglobulin molecule is bifunctional. One region of the molecule is concerned with binding to an antigen, whereas a different region mediates binding of the immunoglobulin to host tissues, including cells of the immune system and the first component (C1q) of the classical complement system.

The primary structure of a protein is based on the sequence of amino acid residues linked together by peptide bonds. All antibodies have a common, basic polypeptide structure that has a three-dimensional configuration. The polypeptide chains are linked together by covalent and noncovalent bonds, which produce a unit composed of a four-chain structure based on pairs of identical heavy and light chains. The immunoglobulins IgG, IgD, and IgE occur only as monomers of the four-chain unit. IgA occurs in both monomeric and polymeric forms; IgM occurs as a pentamer with five four-chain subunits linked together.

## A Typical Immunoglobulin Molecule

A classic model of antibody structure is displayed by the IgG molecule. Using electron microscopy, it can be seen to be Y-shaped (Figure 3-7). If the molecule is treated with a compound, such as 2-mercaptoethanol, which breaks interchain disulfide bonds, the molecule separates into four separate polypeptide chains. The basic molecule consists of two identical light polypeptide chains and two identical heavy polypeptide chains linked together by disulfide bonds. The light chains are found in the N-terminal half of the molecule. Light chains are small chains (MW 25,000) and are common to all classes of immunoglobulins. The light chains are of two subtypes termed kappa ($\kappa$) and lambda ($\lambda$), which have very different

**Figure 3-7.** Basic immunoglobulin molecule configuration. The basic structure of an immunoglobulin molecule consists of two identical light polypeptide chains and two identical heavy polypeptide chains linked together by disulfide bond (heavy dark bars). At one end of the molecule, the amino (N) terminal ends are located; the opposite end has carboxy (C) terminals.

amino acid sequences and are antigenically different. In humans, about 65% of immunoglobulin molecules have kappa chains, while 35% have lambda. The larger, heavy chains (MW, 50,000–77,000) extend the full length of the molecule.

A general feature of the immunoglobulin chains is their amino acid sequence. The first 110 to 120 amino acids of both the light and heavy chains have a variable sequence and form the variable (V) region; the remainder of the light chains represent a constant (C) region with an amino acid sequence that is similar for each type and subtype. The remaining portion of the heavy chain is also constant for each type and has a hinge region. The class and subclass of an immunoglobulin molecule are determined by its heavy chain type (Fig. 3-8).

## The Fab, Fc, and Hinge Molecular Components

A typical monomeric IgG molecule consists of three globular regions (two Fab regions and an Fc portion) linked by a flexible hinge region. If the molecule is digested with a proteolytic enzyme (Fig. 3-9) such as papain, it splits into three approximately equal-sized fragments. Two of these fragments retain the ability to bind antigen and are referred to as *antigen-binding (Fab) fragments.* The third fragment, which is sometimes crystallizable, is referred to as the *Fc portion.* If IgG is treated with another proteolytic enzyme, pepsin, the molecule separates in a somewhat different manner. The Fc portion is split into very small peptides and completely destroyed. The two Fab fragments remain joined together to produce a structure called F(ab)′2. This structure has two antigen-binding sites. If F(ab)′2 is treated to reduce its disulfide bonds, it breaks into two Fab fragments with only one antigen binding site each. Further disruption of the interchain disulfide bonds in the two Fab fragments demonstrates that each contains a light chain and half of a heavy chain, the *Fd portion.*

## Immunoglobulin Classes and Subclasses

Five major immunoglobulin classes exist. Each is unique and possesses its own characteristic antigenic determinants.

### IgG

The most prominent immunoglobulin in normal serum is IgG. It is a 7S molecule with a molecular weight of approximately 150,000. IgG accounts for 70 to 75% of the total immunoglobulin pool. One of the subclasses, IgG₃, is slightly larger (MW 170,000) than the other subclasses.

***Subclasses of IgG.*** Within the major immunoglobulin classes are variants known as subclasses and subtypes. These subclasses differ in their heavy chain composition

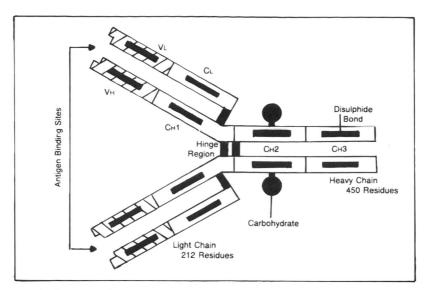

**Figure 3-8.** The basic structure of IgG. In the IgG molecule, the amino terminal end is characterized by sequence variability (V) in both the light (L) and heavy (H) chains. These are referred to as the $V_L$ and $V_H$ regions. The sites where antibody binds to antigen are located in these variable regions. The remainder of the molecule has a relatively constant (C) structure. The constant region of the light chain is the $C_L$ region; the constant region of the heavy chain is $C_H$. The $C_H$ regions are divided into three distinct regions: $C_H1$, $C_H2$, and $C_H3$. These sections are stabilized by intrachain disulfide bonds. The hinge region is a segment of heavy chain between the $C_H1$ and $C_H2$ domains. The flexibility of the hinge region permits variation in the distance between the two antigen-binding sites; therefore, they can react independently.

**Figure 3-9.** Enzymatic cleavage of human IgG1.

**Figure 3-10.** The molecular structures of the polypeptide chains of the four human IgG subclasses. The subclasses have different numbers and arrangements of the interchain disulfide bonds. In IgG1, the disulfide bond linking the light and heavy chains goes to the hinge region. In IgG2, IgG3, and IgG4, the bond goes to the junction between the variable and constant regions.

(Fig. 3-10) and in some of their characteristics such as biologic activities (see Table 3-5). Four IgG subclasses (IgG$_1$, IgG$_2$, IgG$_3$, IgG$_4$) exist. The subclasses occur in the approximate proportions of 66, 23, 7, and 4%, respectively, in humans.

## IgM

IgM accounts for about 10% of the immunoglobulin pool. It is largely confined to the intravascular pool, and is the predominant antibody produced in a primary immune response. In humans, it is found in smaller concentrations than IgG or IgA. The pentamer configuration of the molecule has individual heavy chains with an MW of 65,000; the whole molecule has an MW of 970,000 and a sedimentation coefficient of 19S.

The IgM molecule is structurally composed of five basic subunits. Each basic subunit consists of two kappa or two lambda light chains and two mu heavy chains. The individual monomers of IgM are linked together by disulfide bonds in a circular fashion (Fig. 3-11). A small cysteinrich polypeptide called the J chain must be considered an integral part of the molecule. IgM has carbohydrate residues attached to the C$_{H3}$ and C$_{H4}$ domains. The site for complement activation by IgM is located on this C$_{H4}$ region. IgM is more efficient than IgG in activities, such as the activation of complement cascade and agglutination.

## IgA

IgA represents 15 to 20% of the total circulatory immunoglobulin pool. It is the predominant immunoglobulin in

secretions, such as tears, saliva, colostrum, breast milk, and intestinal secretions. IgA is synthesized largely by plasma cells located on body surfaces. If the IgA is produced by cells in the intestinal wall, it may pass directly into the intestinal lumen or diffuse into the blood circulation. As IgA is transported through intestinal epithelial cells or hepatocytes, it binds to a glycoprotein called the secretory piece. This secretory piece protects IgA from digestion by gastrointestinal proteolytic enzymes and forms a complex molecule named secretory IgA (SIgA). Secretory IgA is of critical importance in protecting body surfaces against invading microorganisms.

In humans, more than 80% of IgA occurs as a typical four-chain structure consisting of paired kappa or lambda chains and two heavy chains. The basic four-chain monomer has an MW of 160,000. However, in most mammals plasma IgA occurs mostly as a dimer. In dimeric IgA, the molecules are joined by a J-chain linked to the Fc regions. Secretory IgA exists mainly in the 11S, dimeric form and has an MW of 385,000. In humans, variations in the heavy chains account for the subclasses IgA$_1$ and IgA$_2$.

## IgD

IgD, found in very low concentrations in plasma, accounts for less than 1% of the total immunoglobulin pool and is susceptible to proteolysis. This is primarily a cell membrane immunoglobulin found on the surface of B lymphocytes in association with IgM. The molecule has an MW of 184,000 and consists of two kappa or lambda light chains and two delta heavy chains. It has no interchain disulfide bonds between its heavy chains and it has a very exposed hinge region.

## IgE

IgE is a trace plasma protein in the blood plasma of nonparasitized individuals. It has an MW of 188,000. IgE is of major importance because it mediates some types of

**Table 3-5. Variations in Subclasses of IgG**

| Characteristic | IgG$_1$ | IgG$_2$ | IgG$_3$ | IgG$_4$ |
|---|---|---|---|---|
| % of total IgG in serum | 65 | 24 | 7 | 4 |
| Complement fixation | 4+ | 2+ | 4+ | (+) |
| Half-life in days | 23 | 23 | 8 | 23 |
| Placental passage | + | ? | + | + |

**Figure 3-11.** Pentameric polypeptide chain structure of human IgM.

allergic reactions, allergies, and anaphylaxis, and is generally responsible for an individual's immunity to invading parasites.

The IgE molecule is composed of paired kappa or lambda light chains and two epsilon heavy chains. It is unique in that its Fc region binds strongly to a receptor on mast cells and basophils and, together with antigen, mediates the release of histamines and heparin from these cells.

**Other Immunoglobulin Variants**

An antigenic determinant is the specific chemical determinant group or molecular configuration against which the immune response is directed. Immunoglobulins can function as effective antigens when used to immunize mammals of a different species because they are proteins. When the resulting anti-immunoglobulins or antiglobulin antibodies are analyzed, three principal categories of antigenic

determinants (Table 3-6) can be recognized: isotype, allotype, and idiotype determinants (Fig. 3-12).

**Isotypic Determinants**

This class of antigenic determinants is the dominant type found on the immunoglobulins of all animals of a species. The heavy-chain, constant-region structures associated with the different classes and subclasses are termed *isotypic variants*. Genes for isotypic variants are present in all healthy members of a species. Determinants included in this category include those that are specific for each immunoglobulin class, such as gamma for IgG, mu for IgM, and alpha for IgA, as well as the subclass-specific determinants, kappa and lambda.

**Allotypic Determinants**

The second principal group of determinants is found on the immunoglobulins of some, but not all, animals of a

**Table 3-6. Principal Categories of Antigenic Determinants**

| Variant | Distribution | Variant | Location | Examples |
|---------|-------------|---------|----------|----------|
| Isotypic | All variants in normal persons | Classes, subclasses, types | $C_H$, $C_H$, $C_L$ | IgM, IgE, IgA$_1$, IgA$_2$, kappa, lambda |
| Allotypic | Genetically controlled alternate forms—not present in all persons | Allotypes | Mainly $C_H/C_L$, sometimes $V_H/V_L$ | Gm groups in humans |
| Idiotypic | Individually specific to each immunoglobulin molecule | Idiotypes | Variable regions | Probably one or more hypervariable regions forming the antigen-combining site |

C = constant regions  V = variable regions
Modified from Roitt, Ivan M.: *Essential Immunology*, Fifth edition. Oxford, England, Blackwell Scientific Publications, 1984, p. 42.

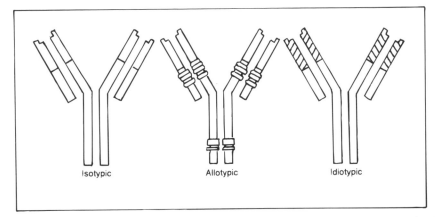

**Figure 3-12.** Variants of antibodies. Isotypic variation refers to the different heavy and light chain classes and subclasses. These variants are present in all healthy members of a species. Allotypic variations are not all present in all healthy members of a species. This type of variation occurs mostly in the constant region of the molecule. Idiotypic variations are specific to each antibody molecule. These variations occur only in the variable region of the molecule.

species. Antibodies to these allotypes (*alloantibodies*) may be produced by injecting the immunoglobulins of one animal into another member of the same species. The allotypic determinants are genetically determined variations representing the presence of allelic genes at a single locus within a species. Typical allotypes in humans are the Gm specificities on IgG (Gm = marker on IgG). In humans, the following five sets of allotypic markers have been found: Gm, Km, Mm, Am, and Hv.

### Idiotypic Determinants

Idiotypes exist as a result of the unique structures on light and heavy chains. These individual determinants characteristic of each antibody are termed the *idiotypes.* The idiotypic determinants are located in the variable part of the antibody associated with the hypervariable regions that form the antigen-combining site.

### The Functions of Antibodies

The principal function of an antibody is to bind antigen. Antibodies, however, may exhibit secondary effector functions, as well as behaving as antigens. The significant secondary effector functions of antibodies (Table 3-7) are complement fixation and placental transfer. The activation of complement (discussed in detail later in this chapter) is one of the most important effector mechanisms of IgG$_1$ and IgG$_3$ molecules. IgG$_2$ seems to be less effective in activating complement; IgG$_4$, IgA, IgD, and IgE are ineffective in terms of complement activation. In man, most of the IgG subclass molecules are capable of crossing the

placental barrier. It is not universally agreed whether or not IgG$_2$ crosses the placenta. Passage of antibodies across the placental barrier is an important mechanism in hemolytic disease of the newborn (HDN, discussed in Chapter 10) and in conferring passive immunity to the newborn during the first few months of life.

### Antibody Avidity

Each four-polypeptide-chain antibody unit has two antigen binding sites that allow the unit to be potentially multivalent in its reaction with an antigen. The strength with which a multivalent antibody binds a multivalent antigen is termed *avidity;* this term contrasts with *affinity,* which is the bond between a single antigenic determinant and an individual combining site. When a multivalent antigen combines with more than one of an antibody's combining sites, the strength of the bonding is significantly increased. For the antigen and antibody to dissociate, all of the antigen-antibody bonds must be broken simultaneously.

Decreased avidity can result from the fact that an antigen has only one antigenic determinant (monovalent). Additionally, a hapten is monovalent and therefore can react only with one antigen combining site.

### Antibody Specificity and Cross-Reactivity

Antigen-antibody reactions can show a high level of *specificity.* Specificity refers to the fact that the binding sites of antibodies directed against determinants of one antigen are not complementary to determinants of another dissimilar antigen. When some of the determinants of an antigen

**Table 3-7. Properties of Immunoglobulins**

|  | IgG$_1$ | IgG$_2$ | IgG$_3$ | IgG$_4$ | IgM | IgA | IgD | IgE |
|---|---|---|---|---|---|---|---|---|
| Complement fixation | 2+ | 1+ | 3+ | 0 | 3+ | 0 | 0 | 0 |
| Placental transfer | 1+ | ± | + | 1+ | 0 | 0 | 0 | 0 |

are shared by similar antigenic determinants on the surface of apparently unrelated molecules, a proportion of the antibodies directed against one kind of antigen will also react with the other kind of antigen. This is called *cross-reactivity*. Antibodies directed against a protein in one species may also react in a detectable manner with the homologous protein in another species, which is also an example of cross-reactivity.

Examples of cross-reactivity also occur between bacteria that possess cell-wall polysaccharides in common with mammalian erythrocytes. Intestinal bacteria and other substances found in the environment possess A- or B-like antigens similar to the A and B erythrocyte antigens. If A or B antigens are foreign to an individual, production of anti-A or anti-B occurs even though the person has never been exposed to these erythrocyte antigens. Cross-reacting antibodies of this type are *heterophile antibodies*.

## Monoclonal Antibodies

Monoclonal antibodies are purified antibodies that are cloned from a single cell and engineered to bind to a single specific antigen. Monoclonal antibodies to cell surface antigens now provide a method for classifying and identifying specific cellular membrane characteristics, such as in the typing of erythrocyte and leukocyte antigens, and as a reagent in the detection of coating of erythrocyte antigens in the antihuman globulin (AHG) test.

### Discovery of the Technique

In 1975, George Kohler, a postdoctoral student at Cambridge University, was examining cell hybrids developed from different lines of cultured myeloma cells (plasma cells derived from malignant tumor strains) by using Sendai

virus to induce the cells to fuse together. (Sendai virus is an influenza virus that characteristically causes cell fusion.)

Initially, he immunized donors with sheep erythrocytes to provide a marker for the normal cells. After making the hybrids, he tested them to see if they still produced antibodies against the sheep erythrocytes and discovered that some of the hybrids were manufacturing large quantities of specific antisheep erythrocyte antibodies.

This technique is referred to as *somatic cell hybridization*. The resulting hybrid cells secrete the antibody characteristic of the parent cell, antisheep erythrocyte antibodies. The multiplying hybrid cell culture is called a *hybridoma*. Hybridoma cells can be cloned (the process in which single cells are selected and grown). The immunoglobulins derived from a single clone of cells are named *monoclonal antibodies*.

### Monoclonal Antibody Production

Modern methods for producing monoclonal antibodies (Fig. 3-13) are refinements of the original technique developed by Kohler. Basically, hybridoma technique enables scientists to inoculate crude antigen mixtures into mice and then select clones producing specific antibodies, each directed against a single cell surface antigen. The process of producing monoclonal antibodies takes from 3 to 6 months to complete.

To initiate the production of monoclonal antibodies, mice are immunized with a specific antigen. Several doses of the antigen are given to ensure a vigorous immune response. From 2 to 4 days later, spleen cells are then mixed with cultured mouse myeloma cells. Myeloma parent cells, which lack the enzyme hypoxanthine phosphoribosyl transferase, are selected because these cells cannot

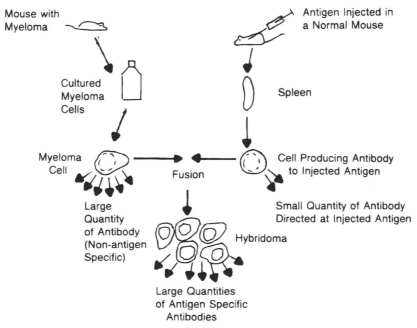

**Figure 3-13.** Monoclonal antibody production. Monoclonal antibodies are produced from hybridoma cells. The cells result from the fusion of neoplastic myeloma cells and specific antibody-producing cells.

use hypoxanthine derived from the culture medium to manufacture purines and pyrimidines, and if unfused, will not survive in the culture medium. Additionally, the mouse myeloma cell lines usually do not secrete immunoglobulins, which simplifies the purification process.

Polyethylene glycol rather than Sendai virus is added to the cell mixture to promote cell-membrane fusion. Only 1 in every 200,000 spleen cells actually forms a viable hybrid with a myeloma cell. Normal spleen cells do not survive in culture. The fused-cell mixture is placed in a medium containing hypoxanthine, aminopterin, and thymidine (HAT medium). Aminopterin is a drug that prevents myeloma cells from making their own purines and pyrimidines, and because they cannot use hypoxanthine from the medium, the cells die.

Hybrids resulting from the fusion of spleen cells and myeloma cells contain transferase provided by the normal spleen cells. Consequently, the hybridoma cells are able to use the hypoxanthine and thymidine in the culture medium and survive. They divide rapidly in HAT medium, doubling their numbers every 24 to 48 hours. About 300 to 500 different hybrids can be generated from the cells of a single mouse spleen, although not all make the desired antibodies. After the hybridomas have been growing for 2 to 4 weeks, the supernatant is tested for specific antibody, using methods such as the enzyme-linked immunoabsorbent assay (ELISA) or radioimmunoassay (RIA). Clones that produce the desired antibody are grown in mass culture and recloned to eliminate nonantibody-producing cells.

Antibody-producing clones lose their ability after being cultured for several months. It is usual to freeze and store hybridoma cells in small aliquots. They may then be grown in mass culture or injected intraperitoneally into mice. Because hybridomas are tumor cells, they grow rapidly and induce the effusion of large quantities of fluid into the peritoneal cavity. This ascites fluid is rich in monoclonal antibody and can be easily harvested.

In the case of the production of Anti-Human Globulin Murine Monoclonal BioClone (by Ortho Diagnostic Systems, Inc.), the reagent is prepared from a pool of mouse monoclonal anti-C3b and anti-C3d. The mouse anti-C3b and anti-C3d portions are obtained by intraperitoneally injecting a group of mice with an anti-C3b-secreting hybridoma and another group of mice with an anti-C3d-secreting hybridoma. After a suitable time, the mouse ascitic fluid is harvested from each of the groups, pooled, and manufactured into the specific anti-C3b, -C3d anti-human globulin (AHG) reagent.

### Applications of Monoclonal Antibodies in Blood Banking

The greatest impact of monoclonal antibodies in blood banking has been on the analysis of cell-membrane antigens. Because monoclonal antibodies have a single speci-

ficity compared to the range of antibody molecules present in the serum, they are useful in erythrocyte typing, leukocyte typing (lymphocyte subsets), and tissue typing.

The use of monoclonal antibodies can potentially reduce the overall cost of erythrocyte antigen determinations. Monoclonal antibodies produced by individual murine hybridomas to human blood group A cells can be used to detect A antigens as well as weak subgroups of A. Although not all anti-D monoclonal antibodies may be sensitive enough to detect weak D ($D^u$) reactions, the use of monoclonal anti-D can eliminate the need for supplemental weak D ($D^u$) testing.

Occasional instances of incorrect ABO typing have been observed because of inappropriate monoclonal antibody sensitivity. In these reported cases, inaccurate reactivity with some group B specimens has been noted with anti-A reagent.

## THE MOLECULAR BASIS OF ANTIGEN-ANTIBODY REACTIONS

The basic Y-shaped immunoglobulin molecule is a bifunctional structure. The V domains are primarily concerned with antigen binding. When an antigenic determinant and its specific antibody combine, they interact through the chemical groups found on the surface of the antigenic determinant and on the surface of the *hypervariable* regions of the immunoglobulin molecule. Although the C domains do not form the antigen binding sites, the arrangement of the C domains and hinge region give the molecule segmental flexibility, which allows it to combine with separated antigenic determinants.

### Types of Bonding

The bonding of an antigen to an antibody takes place because of the formation of multiple reversible intermolecular attractions between an antigen and amino acids of the binding site. These forces require close proximity of the interacting groups. The optimum distance separating the interacting groups varies for different types of bonds. Bonds form across short distances and weaken very rapidly as the distance increases (Fig. 3-14).

The bonding of antigens to antibodies is exclusively *noncovalent*. The attractive force of noncovalent bonds is weak when compared to covalent bonds; however, the formation of multiple noncovalent bonds produces considerable total binding energy. The strength of a single antigen-antibody bond is termed the *antibody affinity* and is produced by the summation of the attractive and repulsive forces. The types of noncovalent bonds involved in antigen-antibody reactions are the following:

1. Hydrophobic bonds
2. Hydrogen bonding
3. Van der Waals forces
4. Electrostatic forces

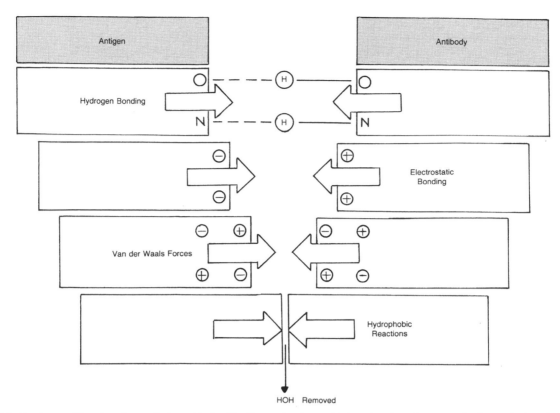

**Figure 3-14.** The types of bonds or forces that can bind antibodies and antigens. Various bonds or forces can be formed when the interacting groups of antigens and antibodies closely approach each other. The distance between interacting groups of molecules that produces optimum binding varies for different bond types.

### Hydrophobic Bonds

The major bonds formed between antigens and antibodies are hydrophobic. Many of the nonpolar side chains of proteins are hydrophobic. When antigen and antibody molecules come together, these side chains interact and exclude water molecules from the area of the interaction. The exclusion of water eliminates some of the constraints imposed by the proteins, which results in a gain in energy and forms an energetically stable complex.

### Hydrogen Bonding

Hydrogen bonding results from the formation of hydrogen bridges between appropriate atoms. Common hydrogen bonds in antigen-antibody interactions are O-H-O, N-H-N, and O-H-N.

### Van der Waals Forces

Van der Waals forces are nonspecific attractive forces that are generated by the interaction between electron clouds and hydrophobic bonds. These bonds occur as a result of a minor asymmetry in the charge of an atom because of the position of its electrons. Van der Waals forces rely on the association of nonpolar, hydrophobic groups so that contact with water molecules is minimized. Although

these forces are very weak, they may become collectively important in an antigen-antibody reaction.

### Electrostatic Forces

Electrostatic forces develop because of the attraction of oppositely charged amino acids located on two protein side chains. The relative importance of electrostatic bonds is unclear.

### Goodness of Fit

The strongest bonding develops when antigens and antibodies are in close proximity to each other and when the shapes of both the antigenic determinants and the antigen-binding site conform to each other. The complementary matching of determinants and binding sites is referred to as "goodness of fit."

A good fit creates ample opportunities for the simultaneous formation of several noncovalent bonds and few opportunities for disruption of the bond. If a poor fit exists, repulsive forces can dominate any small forces of attraction. Variations from the ideal complementary shape produce a decrease in the total binding energy because of increased repulsive forces and decreased attractive forces. Therefore, "goodness of fit" is important in determining the binding of an antibody molecule to a particular antigen.

## IN VITRO DETECTION OF ANTIGEN-ANTIBODY REACTIONS

### Laboratory Tests

In vitro tests detect the combination of antigens and antibodies. Tests such as the RIA and ELISA measure immune complexes formed in an in vitro system. Tests such as agglutination tests are the most widely used to detect and measure the consequences of antigen-antibody interaction. Other test types include precipitation reactions, hemolysis testing, and inhibition of agglutination. Because of the widespread use of agglutination testing in blood banking procedures, such as blood grouping and compatibility testing, agglutination reactions are presented in detail in the following section. The reader should consult an immunology text for detailed descriptions of the other types of serologic procedures that have applications to transfusion therapy, such as hepatitis testing.

### The Mechanism of Agglutination

Agglutination is the clumping of particles with antigens on their surface, such as erythrocytes, by antibody molecules that form bridges between the antigenic determinants. This is the endpoint for most tests involving erythrocyte antigens and blood group antibodies. Agglutination, which is influenced by a number of factors, is believed to occur in two stages: *sensitization* and *lattice formation.*

### Sensitization—The First Phase

The first phase of agglutination, *sensitization,* represents the physical attachment of antibody molecules to antigens on the erythrocytic membrane. In this initial reversible interaction, antibodies combine rapidly with antigenic particles. The amount of antibody that will react is affected by the equilibrium constant, or affinity constant, of the antibody. In most cases, the higher the equilibrium constant, the higher the rate of association and the slower the rate of dissociation of antibody molecules. The degree of association of antigen with antibody is affected by a variety of factors and can be altered in some cases in vitro by altering some of these factors. The factors influencing antigen-antibody association include the following:

1. The antigen-antibody ratio or the number of antibody molecules in relation to the number of antigen sites per cell.
2. Physical conditions such as pH, temperature, and length of time of incubation, ionic strength, and steric hindrance.

*Antigen-antibody Ratio.* Under conditions of antibody excess, a surplus of molecular antigen-combining sites which are not bound to antigenic determinants exists.

The outcome of excessive antibody concentration is known as the *prozone phenomenon,* which can produce false-negative reactions. This phenomenon can be overcome by serially diluting the antibody-containing serum until optimum amounts of antigen and antibody are present in the test system.

*pH.* Although the optimum pH for all reactions has not been determined, a pH of 7.0 is used for routine laboratory testing. It is known that some antibodies such as anti-M and anti-D react best at a lower pH. For example, anti-D reacts best at a pH between 6.5 and 7.0.

*Temperature and Length of Incubation.* The optimum temperature for reaching equilibrium in an antibody-antigen reaction differs for different antibodies. IgM (19S) type antibodies are cold-reacting (thermal range 4 to 22° C) and IgG (7S) antibodies are warm reacting with an optimum temperature of reaction of 37° C. The length of time of incubation required to achieve maximum results depends upon the rate of association and dissociation of each specific antibody. In laboratory testing, incubation times range from 15 to 60 minutes. The optimum time of incubation varies according to the class of immunoglobulin and how tightly an antibody attaches to its specific antigen.

*Ionic Strength.* The concentration of salt in the reaction medium has an effect on antibody uptake by the membrane-bound erythrocyte antigens. Sodium ($Na^+$) and chloride ($Cl^-$) ions in a solution have a shielding effect. These ions cluster around and partially neutralize the opposite charges on antigen and antibody molecules, which hinders the association of antibody with antigen. Reducing or lowering the ionic strength of a reaction medium with agents such as low ionic strength saline (LISS) or polybrene enhances antibody uptake.

*Steric Hindrance.* Steric hindrance is an important physiochemical effect that influences antibody uptake by cell surface antigens. If dissimilar antibodies with approximately the same binding constant are directed against antigenic determinants located in close proximity to each other, they will compete for space in reaching their specific receptor sites. The effect of this competition can be mutual blocking or *steric hindrance,* and neither antibody type will be bound to its respective antigenic determinant. Steric hindrance can occur whenever a conformational change in the relationship of an antigenic receptor site to the outside surface occurs. In addition to antibody competition, competition with bound complement, other protein molecules, or the action of agents that interfere with the structural integrity of the cell surface can produce steric hindrance.

Knowledge of the physical conditions on the uptake of antibody is important to the blood bank technologist. Because the combination of antigen and antibody is a reversible chemical reaction, altering the physical conditions can cause the release of antibody from the antigen-binding site. When physical conditions are purposely manipulated

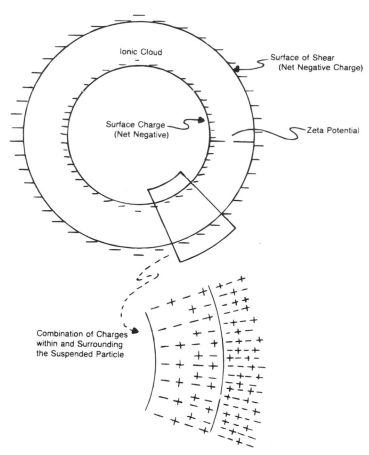

**Figure 3-15.** Zeta potential. Particles, such as erythrocytes, in suspension have a net negative surface charge. The zeta potential is the difference in electrostatic potential between the net charge at the cell membrane and the charge at the surface of shear.

to break the antigen-antibody complex with subsequent release of the antibody into the surrounding medium, the procedure is referred to as an *elution procedure* (see Chapter 14). The product of this procedure, antibody suspended in a medium, is called an *eluate*. This procedure is of practical application in the investigation of positive direct anti-human globulin (DAT) tests and in alloantibody investigation.

### Lattice Formation—The Second Phase

Lattice formation, or the establishment of crosslinks between sensitized particles such as erythrocytes and antibodies resulting in aggregation (clumping), is a much slower process than the sensitization phase. The formation of chemical bonds and resultant lattice formation depend on the ability of a cell with attached antibody on its surface to come close enough to another cell to permit the antibody molecules to bridge the gap and combine with the antigen receptor site on the second cell. Crosslinking is influenced by factors such as the *zeta potential*.

*Zeta Potential.* In the blood circulation, erythrocytes have a net negative surface charge (Fig. 3-15). Because like charges repel one another, erythrocytes in suspension remain separated from each other. The actual distance of

separation is governed by the effective net surface charge density. When erythrocytes are suspended in electrolyte solutions such as sodium chloride, the ions in a suspending solution arrange themselves about the surface of the cell and become more diffuse as the distance from the cell surface increases. As an erythrocyte floats in an electrolyte solution, some ions remain with it. The diffuse double layer surrounding the cell is called the *ionic cloud* and the outer edge of this layer is referred to as the *surface of shear*.

A difference in electrostatic potential exists between the net charge at the cell membrane and the charge at the surface of shear. This electrostatic potential is referred to as the *zeta potential*. Zeta potential is believed to depend on the actual net surface charge density at the surface of the cell membrane and the *dielectric constant* of the surrounding medium (dielectric constant is a measure of the electrical conductivity of a suspending medium). The zeta potential as well as the distance between adjacent cells can be manipulated by altering the net surface charge density of the cells or the dielectric constant of the medium.

*The Influence of Antibody Types on Agglutination.* Immunoglobulins are relatively positively charged, and following sensitization or coating by particles, they reduce the zeta potential. Antibodies can bridge charged particles by extending beyond the effective range of the zeta potential, which results in the erythrocytes closely approaching each other, binding together, and agglutinating.

Antibodies differ in their ability to agglutinate. IgM antibodies, sometimes referred to as *complete antibodies,* are considerably more efficient than IgG or IgA antibodies in exhibiting in vitro agglutination when the antigen-bearing erythrocytes are suspended in physiologic (0.85%) sodium chloride (saline). Antibodies that do not exhibit visible agglutination of saline-suspended erythrocytes even when bound to the cell's surface membrane are considered nonagglutinating antibodies and may be called *incomplete antibodies.* Incomplete antibodies may fail to exhibit agglutination because the antigenic determinants are located deep within the surface membrane or may demonstrate restricted movement in their hinge region, causing them to be functionally *monovalent.*

***The Effect of Antigen Dosage.*** The term "double dose" is sometimes used to depict the homozygous genotypic expression of an antigen (such as "cc"), in comparison to the heterozygous genotypic expression of an antigen (such as "Cc"), which is referred to as a single dose. In some blood group systems, the presence of a homozygous genotype expresses itself with more antigen than the heterozygous genotype. The consequence of possessing a double dose of some blood group antigens (such as "c"), is that a greater proportion of erythrocytes is agglutinated. This variation in strength of agglutination is referred to as the *dosage effect.*

***Methods of Enhancing Agglutination.*** Several methods are commonly used in routine blood banking to enhance agglutination. These techniques include centrifugation, treatment with proteolytic enzymes, use of colloids, and addition of anti-human globulin (AHG) reagent.

CENTRIFUGATION. Centrifugation at high speed is a common technique incorporated into the protocol of many blood banking methods. Centrifugation attempts to overcome the problem of distance by subjecting sensitized cells to a high gravitational force, which counteracts the repulsive effect and physically forces the cells together.

ENZYME TREATMENT. Alteration of the zeta potential to enhance the chances of demonstrable agglutination is commonly used in the blood bank. Treatment with a weak proteolytic enzyme can strip off some of the negative charges on the cell membrane by removing surface sialic acid (cleaving sialoglycoproteins from the cell surface) residues; thereby reducing the surface charge on the cells, lowering the zeta potential, and permitting the cells to come closer together for chemical linking by specific antibody molecules. The risk of enzyme treatment is that it destroys some blood group antigens such as M, N, and Duffy ($Fy^a$ and $Fy^b$).

COLLOIDAL MEDIA. In 1945, Cameron and Diamond established that certain anti-D (anti-$Rh_o$) sera would agglutinate Rh positive erythrocytes suspended in a colloid, bovine albumin. In 1964, Pollack first investigated the mechanism of action of bovine albumin. He concluded that agglutination of sensitized erythrocytes depended on factors such as the characteristics of the reaction medium. Therefore, some IgG antibodies, especially those with Rh-hr specificity, agglutinate if the zeta potential is carefully adjusted by the addition of colloids and salts. Although colloids can enhance agglutination, the effectiveness of the medium depends on the chemical properties and composition of the specific type of colloidal medium. The most frequently used colloidal reagent is bovine albumin solution. This product is manufactured from raw bovine serum. Processing results in a solution with a 22% protein concentration and a pH of 7.2, specifically designed for laboratory use. The solution additionally contains 0.1% sodium azide as a preservative.

OTHER ENHANCEMENT MEDIA. Additional enhancement media can be used to detect low-titered antibodies in routine alloantibody screening or compatibility testing. These media include low ionic strength saline (LISS), polybrene, and polyethylene glycol (PEG).

The principle of LISS is that the rate of antibody association increases as the ionic strength of the medium decreases. The use of LISS not only increases the sensitivity of antibody detection compared to bovine albumin, but also allows a shortened period of incubation. The most frequent disadvantage of a LISS technique is the increased number of nonspecific or false positive reactions observed. A more serious problem is the difficulty in detecting some examples of anti-Kell using low ionic strength solutions.

Enhancement of erythrocyte agglutination can also be achieved by using a low ionic strength medium with added positively charged macromolecules, such as polybrene or protamine. Although this technique was originally used in automated antibody detection systems, it has been adapted to manual procedures. With this technique, serum and erythrocytes are incubated in a low ionic strength medium, followed by aggregation of the cells with polybrene. The principle of this technique is that the addition of the macromolecule brings the red cells closer together to facilitate strong crosslinking by cell-bound antibodies. The use of enhancement media, such as polybrene, displays ABO incompatibility as effectively as a room temperature cross match and offers the added benefit of detecting most other clinically significant blood group alloantibodies reported to have been missed by saline-albumin screening techniques.

The addition of polyethylene glycol to serum-cell test mixtures has been reported to be more effective in detecting weak antibodies than LISS and manual polybrene. In general, polyethylene glycol does not produce nonspecific reactions.

CHEMICALLY MODIFIED ANTISERA. Chemical modification of antisera involves the conversion of some "incomplete" IgG antibodies, which are not capable of causing direct agglutination of saline-suspended erythrocytes, into saline agglutinins. This modification is achieved by reducing the disulfide bond near the hinge region of the IgG molecule with dithiothreitol, followed by an alkylation step to make the change permanent. Reduction of the disulfide bond enables the two IgG Fab structures to span a greater distance. The modified molecules can bridge the space separating erythrocyte suspended in saline and agglutinate them. Chemically modified antisera are available for detection of D and Kell antigens. Chemically modified anti-D sera are also suitable for the weak D (D$^u$) test.

## The Antiglobulin Test

In some cases, antigens may be so deeply imbedded in the membrane surface that the previously described techniques will not bring the antigens and antibodies close enough to crosslink. The antiglobulin test is frequently incorporated into the protocol of many laboratory techniques to facilitate agglutination. Two forms of antiglobulin testing are used in blood banking: the direct antiglobulin test (DAT) and the indirect antiglobulin test (IAT). The DAT can be used to demonstrate in vivo coating of red blood cells with antibody and/or antibody complement. The IAT can be used to demonstrate in vitro reactions between red blood cells and coating antibodies.

### Reagent Preparation

Because immunoglobulins are proteins, they function as effective antigens when injected into mammals of a different species. For example, human immunoglobulins promote a strong antibody response when injected into a rabbit. In the traditional preparation of antiglobulin reagent, one colony of rabbits is injected with purified human gamma globulin and a second colony of rabbits is injected with purified components of human beta globulin. After a suitable time, plasma is harvested from the whole blood of the rabbits as the raw material. It is pooled and manufactured into a specific reagent for use in detecting human gamma globulin or components of complement. The product is buffered with bovine albumin and 0.1% sodium azide is added as a preservative. If color is added, such as in Ortho Anti-Human Globulin (green), FD&C Blue No. 1 and FD&C Yellow No. 5 dye are added.

Reagents, such as AHG, can be produced through genetic engineering. The synthesis of antibodies through biotechnology is discussed in detail in the section on monoclonal antibodies.

Using either the classic method or biotechnology, the resulting anti-immunoglobulin is useful in demonstrating that erythrocytes have been sensitized but fail to produce visible agglutination. The sensitizing globulins may be gamma globulin (antibody) and/or beta globulin (components of complement).

### Principles of the Procedure

The principle of the antiglobulin (AHG) technique was rediscovered by Coombs in 1945; therefore the procedure was called the *Coombs' test* for many years. The AHG

**Table 3-8. A Comparison of the Direct and Indirect Antiglobulin Procedures**

| Type of Test | Patient's Erythrocytes | Patient's Serum |
|---|---|---|
| Direct antiglobulin test (DAT) | Tested for in vivo coating of erythrocytes | — |
| Indirect antiglobulin test (IAT) | — | Tested for the presence of unexpected antibodies |

method is routinely applied in direct and indirect testing (Table 3-8). The DAT is used to detect in vivo sensitization or coating. If it is necessary to test for the presence of incomplete antibodies or complement on the surface of erythrocytes as in cases of suspected hemolytic anemia the DAT is used. A patient's washed erythrocytes are mixed with AHG, and if incomplete antibodies are present, agglutination occurs. To test for the presence of incomplete antibodies in a serum, an IAT is used. In the indirect technique, the serum containing antibodies is initially incubated with erythrocytes containing antigens that adsorb the incomplete antibodies. After washing with saline to remove unbound antibodies, the coated erythrocytes are mixed with AHG. On reacting with bound antibody, the AHG crosslinks and produces agglutination.

### Types of Antiglobulin Reagent

Two types of antiglobulin reagent can be used in laboratory testing procedures (Tables 3-9 and 3-10): broad-spectrum (*polyspecific*) sera and *monospecific* sera.

Polyspecific serum is the basic type of reagent used in routine blood banking procedures, such as compatibility testing or antibody screening. A polyspecific serum is defined as one that must contain anti-IgG and anti-C3d (anticomplement component). The reagent may contain antibodies of other specificities, such as anti-IgM, anti-IgA, anti-C3b, or anti-C4. If the test is positive with polyspecific sera, a monospecific sera may be used for follow-up testing.

Monospecific sera such as anti-IgG and anticomplement containing C3b + C3d (previously called anti-non-gamma) are the most commonly used types of monospecific sera. Anti-IgG can detect most clinically significant antibodies. This type of reagent is useful in differentiating agglutination produced by IgG antibodies rather than agglutination due to complement fixation produced by cold agglutinins. Although various components of complement can sensitize erythrocytes, the C3d component is associated with immune hemolysis; therefore, it is important that this component be included in anticomplement reagents to facilitate the investigation of immune hemolytic anemias. Monospecific sera containing anti-IgM or anti-IgA are not routinely used in clinical laboratories because the need for them is rare, but they are used by reference and research immunohematology laboratories.

**Table 3-9. Indications for Use and Limitations of AHG Reagents with Direct Antiglobulin Test (DAT)**

| Disorder | Polyspecific | Anti-IgG (Rabbit) | Indications for Use Anti-C3b, C3d (Murine Monoclonal BioClone) | Anti-C3d (Murine Monoclonal BioClone) |
|---|---|---|---|---|
| Hemolytic disease of the newborn (HDN) | Yes | Yes | | |
| Transfusion reactions | Yes | Yes* | Yes* | Yes* |
| Drug-induced RBC sensitization | Yes | Yes* | Yes* | Yes* |
| Autoimmune hemolytic anemia | Yes | Yes* | Yes* | Yes* |
| Differentiation of immunoglobulin from complement coating of RBCs | | Yes | Yes† | |
| Specific identification of coating substance | | Yes | | Yes |

* This reagent should not be used as the sole antiglobulin reagent. To avoid false negative results, both IgG and C3d need to be included in the testing protocol.
† Except for C4.
Modified from Anti-Human Globulin (Rabbit and Murine Monoclonal BioClone® Product Brochure, June, 1986. Ortho Diagnostic Systems, Inc., Raritan, New Jersey.

## Sources of Error

False-negative and false-positive results can be obtained with antiglobulin testing. These errors in either the DAT or IAT procedures are discussed in Chapter 13, Basic Procedures.

## Grading Agglutination Reactions

In the blood bank, it is important to observe the strength of agglutination when it occurs. The combining of antigens (also referred to as *agglutinogens*) on the surface of erythrocytes and their corresponding antibodies (also referred to as *agglutinins*) should result in agglutination (synonymously referred to as hemagglutination if the cells are erythrocytes).

Observation of agglutination is initially made by gently shaking the test tube containing the serum and cells and viewing the lower portion, *the button,* as it is dispersed with a magnifying glass. Because agglutination is a reversible reaction, the test tube must be treated delicately and hard shaking must be avoided; however, all the cells in the button must be resuspended before an accurate observation can be determined. Observations are made both *macroscopically* (using a magnifying lens) and *microscopically* (using a microscope). Attention should also be given to observing whether or not discoloration of the fluid above the cells, *the supernatant,* is present. If the erythrocytes have been *hemolyzed,* this is as important a finding as agglutination.

The strength of agglutination, called *grading,* uses a scale of 0 or negative (meaning no agglutination) to 4+ (meaning all the erythrocytes are clumped). A standardized system has been developed by the American Association of Blood Banks for the grading of macroscopic agglutination reaction (Table 3-11).

Pseudoagglutination, or false appearance of clumping, may occur because of the presence of *rouleaux formation.* Rouleaux formation can be encountered in patients with high or abnormal types of globulins in their blood, such as in multiple myeloma or after receiving dextran as a plasma expander. If this condition is present, the erythrocytes microscopically resemble rolls of stacked coins. To disperse pseudoagglutination, a few drops of physiologic sodium chloride can be added to the reaction tube, remixed, and re-examined. This procedure, *saline replacement,* should be performed carefully if pseudoagglutination is suspected. It should never be done before the initial testing protocol is followed because the dilutional effect of the saline may produce a false negative result.

**Table 3-10. Indications for Use and Limitations of AHG Reagents with Indirect Antiglobulin Tests (IAT)**

| Disorder | Polyspecific | Anti-IgG (Rabbit) | Anti-C3b, C3d (Murine Monoclonal BioClone) |
|---|---|---|---|
| Pretransfusion compatibility testing (X-match) | Yes | Yes* | |
| Unexpected antibody screening | Yes | Yes* | |
| Antigen detection | Yes | Yes | |
| Serum antibody identification | Yes | Yes | Yes |
| Identification of antibody in an elution | Yes | Yes | |

* The results of some studies indicate that anti-IgG may occasionally fail to detect antibodies, which are demonstrable only with polyspecific AHG reagent. Therefore, anti-IgG should not be used exclusively for the detection of clinically significant antibodies in antibody screening or pretransfusion compatibility testing. Anti-IgG should be used in conjunction with a polyspecific type of AHG.
Modified from Anti-Human Globulin (Rabbit and Murine Monoclonal BioClone® Product Brochure, June, 1986. Ortho Diagnostic Systems, Inc., Raritan, New Jersey.

**Table 3-11. Grading Agglutination Reactions**

| Grade | Description |
|---|---|
| Negative | No aggregates. |
| Mixed field (MF) | Few isolated aggregates, mostly free floating cells, supernatant, appears red |
| Weak (+) | Tiny aggregates that are barely visible macroscopically, many free erythrocytes, turbid and reddish supernatant |
| 1+ | A few small aggregates just visible macroscopically, many free erythrocytes, turbid and reddish supernatant |
| 2+ | Medium-sized aggregates, some free erythrocytes, clear supernatant |
| 3+ | Several large aggregates, some free erythrocytes, clear supernatant |
| 4+ | All the erythrocytes are combined into one solid aggregate, clear supernatant |

## THE COMPLEMENT SYSTEM

Complement is a complex series of at least 25 different glycoproteins. Most of these molecules circulate in an inactive precursor form and develop proteolytic activity upon activation. Collectively, these proteins are a major fraction of the beta 1 and beta 2 globulins. In the laboratory, it is often desirable to inactivate complement for certain tests. To inactivate serum, it must be heated for 30 minutes at 56° C. The sequential activation of the complement enzymes and products formed during the reaction chain, referred to as the complement cascade, has a variety of physiologic and cellular consequences. The physiologic consequences include blood vessel dilation and increased vascular permeability. The cellular effects of complement activation include the following:

1. Cell activation, e.g., chemotaxis
2. Cytolysis or hemolysis, if the cells are erythrocytes. The most important biologic role of complement in blood group serology is the production of cell membrane lysis of antibody-coated targets.
3. Opsonization, which renders cells vulnerable to phagocytosis.

The complement system is composed of two interrelated enzyme cascades, the *classical* and *alternative pathways* (Fig. 3-16). The classical pathway is initiated by the complexing of antigen to its specific antibody, either IgG or IgM, and is the primary amplifier of the biologic effects of humoral immunity. The alternative pathway is activated by contact with a foreign surface, such as the polysaccharide coating of a microorganism, and amplifies nonimmune defense against microbial infection and other biologic alterations. It is probable that under normal physiologic conditions, activation of one pathway also leads to activation of the other. Either of the two routes

leads to a common final pathway. Both pathways convert C3 to C3b, the central event of the common final pathway, which in turn leads to the activation of the lytic complement sequence, C5-C9, and cell destruction. A third set of plasma proteins, which function as the membrane attack complexes, become assembled into the structures responsible for lytic lesions in the lipid bilayer of the cell membrane and disrupt membrane integrity.

Once complement is initially activated, each enzyme precursor is activated by the previous complement component or complex, which is a highly specialized proteinase. This converts the enzyme precursor to its catalytically active form by limited proteolysis. During this activation process, a small peptide fragment is cleaved, a membrane-binding site is exposed, and the major fragment binds. As a consequence, the next active enzyme of the sequence is formed. It is important to note that because each enzyme can activate many enzyme precursors, each step up to C3 is amplified; therefore, the system forms an *amplifying cascade*.

### The Classical Pathway

The principal components of the pathway are numbered C1 through C9. The sequence of component activation does not follow the expected numeric order. The sequence is C1, C4, C2, C3, C5, C6, C7, C8, and C9.

C3 is present in the plasma in the largest quantities and fixation of C3 is the major quantitative reaction of the complement cascade. Although the principal source of synthesis of complement in vivo is debatable, the majority of the plasma complement components are synthesized in hepatic parenchymal cells, except for C1, which is primarily manufactured in the epithelium of the gastrointestinal and urogenital tracts.

The classical pathway is composed of the following 3 stages:

1. Recognition
2. Enzymatic activation
3. Membrane attack leading to cellular destruction

#### Fixation of the C1 Complex

The recognition unit of the complement system is the C1 complex: C1q, C1r, and C1s, an interlocking enzyme system. The C1 complex is a unique feature of the classical pathway leading to C3 conversion. C1 fixation occurs when the C1q subcomponent binds directly to an Fc position of the immunoglobulin molecules that have the appropriate binding site in the $C_H2$ domain of the heavy chain. The other two subcomponents, C1r and C1s, do not bind to the immunoglobulin but are involved in subsequent activation of the classical pathway. Whether or not C1 fixation occurs depends on a number of factors. These conditions include the following:

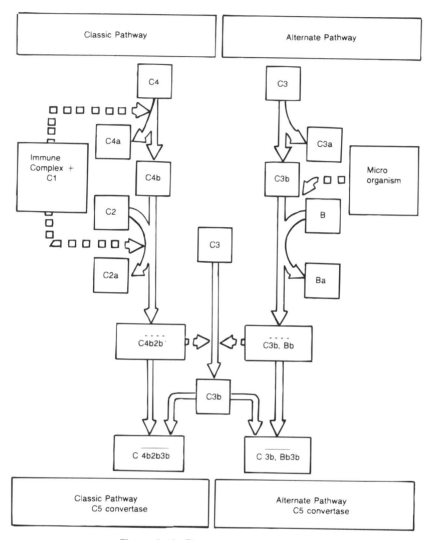

**Figure 3-16.** The complement cascade.

1. Subclass of immunoglobulin. Only certain subclasses of immunoglobulin, such as IgM, and most of the IgG subclasses, can fix C1 even under optimal conditions.
2. Spatial or configurational constraints.

A single IgM molecule is potentially able to fix C1, but at least a pair of IgG molecules is required for this purpose. The amount of C1 fixed is directly proportional to the concentration of IgM antibodies; however, this is not true for IgG molecules.

The C1q molecule is potentially multivalent for attachment to the complement fixation sites of immunoglobulin. The structures of C1q peptide chains are formed into 3 subunits of 6 chains each. Each subunit consists of a Y-shaped pair of triple helices joined at the stem and ending in a globular head. The globular ends are assumed to be the sites for multivalent attachment to the complement-fixing sites in immune-complexed immunoglobulin. The sites on the IgG molecule are on the $C_{H2}$ domains and probably the $C_{H4}$ domain of IgM. The complement-fixing site may become exposed following complexing of the im-

munoglobulin, or the sites may always be available but need multiple attachments by C1q with critical geometry to achieve the necessary avidity.

C1r and C1s are chemically similar, but C1r forms dimers whereas C1s binds monovalently to C1r. C1r and C1s form a tetrad complex that binds to C1q in the presence of Ca ion. The binding mechanism of C1r by C1q is unknown because C1q is not known to have enzymatic activity. However, it is known that C1r and C1s activate in sequence while attached to C1q, and that both proteins become typical serine-histidine esterases on activation. C1s is the only substrate for C1r. C1s activates C4 and C2, the next components in the classical complement sequence, but C1r does not.

### Fixation and Activation of C4 by the C1qrs Complex

C1s splits a peptide C4a from the N-terminal part of the alpha chain of the C4 component, leaving a large fragment, C4b. This reaction occurs in the fluid phase of the plasma around the C1s catalytic site and a reactive internal thioester bond is revealed on C4b. The stable binding of C4b molecules to membranes is less than 10% efficient. Binding occurs in close proximity to the site of activation, to either the C1qrs complex or the adjacent erythrocyte membrane. C4b molecules, which fail to bind, become inactive and decay.

C1s is weakly proteolytic for free intact C2 but highly active against C2, which has complexed with C4b molecules in the presence of Mg$^{++}$ ions. This reaction will occur only if the C4b, C2 complex forms close to the C1s. The resultant C2b fragment joins with C4b to form the new C4b2b enzyme, the classical pathway C3 convertase. The catalytic site of the C4b2b complex is probably in the C2b peptide. A smaller, C2a fragment from the C2 component is lost to the surrounding environment. The C4b2b enzyme is unstable and decays with a half-life of 5 minutes at 37° C because of the release and decay of C2b.

There are two chief constraints on the activities of C1s on C4 and C2, and on the stable formation of the C4b2b complex:

1. The action of the proteinase inhibitor, C1 esterase
2. The effect of C3b inactivator

C1 esterase inhibitor binds to C1s and C1r. This activity may not be important in restraining the action of C1s at a local membrane site, but is extremely important in preventing the excessive action of free C1 on C4 and C2 in the fluid phase.

C3b-inactivator has the ability to disintegrate membrane-bound C4b. This action destroys the acceptor site for C2, which prevents the formation of C4b2b convertase.

### The Action of C4b2b Complex on C3

The complement cascade reaches its full amplitude at the C3 stage, which represents the heart of the system. The C4b2b complex, referred to as the classical pathway C3 convertase, activates C3 molecules by splitting a peptide, the C3 anaphylatoxin, from the N-terminal end of the peptide of C3. This exposes a reactive binding site on the larger fragment, C3b. Consequently, clusters of C3b molecules are activated and bound near the C4b2b complex. Each catalytic site can bind several hundred C3b molecules, although the reaction is very inefficient. Only one C3b molecule combines with C4b2b to form the final proteolytic complex of the complement cascade.

### Action of C3b on C5

C3b splits C5a from the alpha chain of C5 to initiate C5b fixation and the beginning of the membrane attack complex. No further proteinases are generated in the classical complement sequence. Other bound C3b molecules not involved in the C4b2b3b complex form an opsonic macromolecular coat on the erythrocyte or other target cell, which renders it susceptible to immune adherence by C3b receptors on phagocytic cells.

### The C5-9 Membrane Complex

The fixation of C5b to biologic membranes is followed by the sequential addition of C6, C7, C8, and C9. When fully assembled in the correct proportions, they form the membrane attack complex. The C5b-C6 complex is hydrophilic, but with the addition of C7 to the C567 complex, the complex has additional detergent and phospholipid binding properties as well. This occurrence of both hydrophobic and hydrophilic groups within the same complex may account for its tendency to polymerize and form small protein micelles (a packet of chain molecules in a parallel arrangement). In free solution, uncombined C567 has a half-life of about 0.1 seconds. It can attach to any lipid bilayer within its effective diffusion radius, which produces the phenomenon of "*reactive lysis*" on innocent bystander cells. Once membrane-bound, C567 is relatively stable and can interact with C8 and C9.

C5-8 polymerizes C9 to form a tubule, known as the membrane attack complex, which bridges the membrane. This is a hollow cylinder (15 nm in length and 10 nm in diameter), which is inserted at one end into the lipid bilayer with the other end projecting from the membrane. Although the micellar arrangement of the membrane insertion region has not been positively established, a structure of this form can be assumed to disturb the lipid bilayer sufficiently to allow the free exchange of ions as well as water molecules across the membrane. The consequence in a living cell is that the influx of Na$^+$ and H$_2$O leads to disruption of osmotic balance, which produces cell lysis.

### The Alternate (Properdin) Pathway

The alternate pathway shows points of similarity with the classical sequence and both pathways generate a C3 convertase, which activates C3 to provide the pivotal event in the final common pathway of both systems. However, in contrast to the classic pathway which is initiated by the formation of antigen-antibody reactions, the alternate complement pathway is predominantly a nonantibody-initiated pathway.

A key feature of the alternate pathway is that the first three proteins of the classic activation pathway, C1, C4, and C2, do *not* participate in the cascade sequence. The C3a component is considered the counterpart of C2a in the classic pathway, and C2 of the classic pathway structurally resembles factor B of the alternate pathway. The omission of C1, C4, and C2 is possible because activators of the alternate pathway catalyze the conversion of another series of normal serum proteins, which lead to the activation of C3. It was previously believed that *properdin,* a normal protein of human serum, was the first protein to function in the alternate pathway; thus, the pathway was originally named after this protein.

Activators of the alternative pathway are now known usually to be polysaccharides or carbohydrate-containing molecules such as lipopolysaccharides or glycoproteins. Known activators of the alternative pathway include zymosan, a polysaccharide complex from the surface of yeast cells, bacterial endotoxin, and aggregated IgA or IgE. In paroxysmal noctural hemoglobinuria (PNH), the patient's erythrocytes act as an activator, and the result is excessive lysis of the patient's erythrocytes.

The uptake of factor B onto C3b occurs when C3b is bound to an activator surface. However, C3b in the fluid phase or attached to a nonactivator surface preferentially binds to factor H and so prevents C3b,B formation. C3b and factor B combine to form C3b,B, which is converted into an active C3 convertase, C3b,Bb. This occurs because of the loss of a small fragment, Ba (a glycine-rich alpha$_2$ globulin which is believed to be physiologically inert) through the action of the enzyme, factor D. The C3b,Bb complex is able to convert more C3 to C3b, which binds more factor B and so the feedback cycle continues.

The major controlling event of this pathway is factor H, which prevents the association between C3b and factor B. Factor H blocks the formation of C3b,Bb, the catalytically active C3 convertase of the feedback loop. Factor H (previously Beta$_1$H) competes with factor B for its combining site on C3b, eventually leading to C3 inactivation. Factors B and H apparently occupy a common site on C3b. The factor that is preferentially bound to C3b depends on the nature of the surface to which C3b is attached. Polysaccharides are called activator surfaces and favor the uptake of factor B on the chain of C3b with the corresponding displacement of factor H. In this situation, binding of factor H is inhibited and consequently factor B replaces H at the common binding site. When factor H is excluded, C3b is thought to be formed continuously in small amounts. Another controlling point in the amplification loop depends on the stability of the C3b, Bb convertase. Ordinarily, C3b,Bb decays because of the loss of Bb with a half-life of approximately 5 minutes. However, if properdin (P) binds to C3b,Bb, forming C3b,BbP, the half-life is extended to 30 minutes.

The association on the surface of an aggregate of protein or the surface of a microorganism of numerous C3b units, factor Bb, and properdin has potent activity as a C5 convertase. With the cleavage of C5, the remainder of complement cascade continues as in the classical pathway.

## CHAPTER SUMMARY

### The Immune System

An antigen can be defined as a foreign substance that can elicit an antibody response. Production of antibodies in response to antigenic stimulation depends on a person's immunologic ability to recognize an antigen as foreign and on the physical and chemical nature of the antigen.

Recognition of foreign antigens and production of antibodies depend on several T and B lymphocytes, plasma cells, and macrophages.

Hematopoiesis is the process of blood cell production, differentiation, and development. Hematopoietic growth factors are glycoprotein hormones that regulate the proliferation and differentiation of progenitor cells and the function of mature blood cells.

### Antigen Characteristics

Foreign substances such as erythrocytes can be immunogenic if the membrane contains a number of antigenic determinants or epitopes. An immune response is directed against these determinants, and resultant antibodies bind to them. Most cellular membrane proteins are immunogenic. Cellular antigens of importance to immunohematologists are the blood group antigens, histocompatibility (HLA) antigens, and auto-antigens. Some of these antigens are much more potent than others in provoking an immune response and are called the major histocompatibility (HLA) antigens.

Antigens are usually large organic molecules that are either proteins or large polysaccharides and rarely, if ever, lipids. Proteins are excellent antigens because of their high molecular weight and structural complexity. Polysaccharides by themselves are considered too small to function as antigens. In the case of erythrocyte antigens, protein or lipid carriers may contribute to the necessary size and the polysaccharides present in the form of side chains, confer the immunologic specificity and function as the combining sites with which antibodies react. For antigens to function effectively, several factors are important: foreignness, degradability, molecular weight, structural stability, and complexity.

### Antibody Characteristics

Antibodies can be found in blood plasma and many body fluids such as tears, saliva, and breast milk. These specific glycoproteins are referred to as immunoglobulins, abbreviated Ig. Five distinct classes of immunoglobulin molecules are recognized in most higher mammals: IgM, IgG, IgA, IgD and IgE. These immunoglobulin classes differ from each other in characteristics such as molecular weight, sedimentation coefficient, and carbohydrate content.

After a foreign antigen challenge, an IgM antibody response proceeds in four phases, but the actual time period and titer depend on the characteristics of the antigen and the individual. The four phases of an antibody response are the lag, log, plateau, and decline phases. Subsequent exposure to the same antigenic stimulus produces an anamnestic antibody response that exhibits the same four phases as the primary responses. An anamnestic response differs from a primary response in the length of time of the response and the type and titer of antibody produced.

Each of the five major immunoglobulin classes is unique and possesses its own characteristic antigenic determinants. IgG accounts for 70 to 75% of the total immuno-globulin pool. The subclasses of IgG differ in their heavy chain composition and in some of their characteristics and biologic activities. IgM accounts for about 10% of the immunoglobulin pool. It is the largest molecule and the predominant antibody found in a primary immune re-sponse. IgA represents 15 to 20% of the total circulatory immunoglobulin pool. It is the predominant immuno-globulin in secretions, such as tears, saliva, colostrum, breast milk, and intestinal secretions. Secretory IgA is of critical importance in protecting body surfaces against in-vading microorganisms. IgD is found in very low concen-trations in plasma and accounts for less than 1% of the total immunoglobulin pool. This immunoglobulin is pri-marily a cell membrane immunoglobulin found on the surface of B lymphocytes in association with IgM. IgE is a trace plasma protein in the blood plasma of unparasitized individuals. It is of major importance because it mediates some types of allergic reactions, allergies, and anaphylaxis, and is generally responsible for an individual's immunity to invading parasites.

The principal function of an antibody is to bind anti-gen, but antibodies may exhibit secondary effector func-tions as well as behaving as antigens. The significant sec-ondary effector functions of antibodies are complement fixation and placental transfer.

## The Molecular Basis of an Antigen-Antibody Reaction

The basic Y-shaped immunoglobulin molecule is a bifunc-tional structure. The V domains are primarily concerned with antigen binding. Although the C domains do not form antigen-binding sites, the arrangement of the C do-mains and hinge region give the molecule segmental flexi-bility that allows it to combine with separated antigenic determinants.

Bonding of an antigen to an antibody takes place be-cause of the formation of multiple reversible intermolecu-lar attractions between an antigen and amino acids of the binding site. Various types of noncovalent bonds are formed in antigen-antibody reactions. These bond types include hydrophobic bonds, hydrogen bonding, Van der Waals forces, and electrostatic forces. Hydrophobic bonds are the most common.

## In Vitro Detection of Antigen-Antibody Reactions

Agglutination tests are the most commonly used technique to detect and measure the consequences of antigen-anti-body interaction. Agglutination is the clumping of parti-cles that have antigens on their surface, such as erythro-cytes, by antibody molecules that form bridges between the antigenic determinants. Agglutination is believed to occur in two stages: sensitization and lattice formation. Sensitization represents the physical attachment of anti-body molecules to antigens on the erythrocytic membrane.

Lattice formation or the establishment of crosslinks be-tween sensitized particles such as erythrocytes, and anti-bodies results in clumping.

Antibodies differ in their ability to agglutinate. IgM-type antibodies or complete antibodies are considerably more efficient than IgG or IgA antibodies in exhibiting in vitro agglutination when the antigen-bearing erythro-cytes are suspended in physiologic saline. Antibodies that do not exhibit visible agglutination of saline suspended erythrocytes even when bound to the cell's surface mem-brane are considered nonagglutinating or incomplete anti-bodies.

Several methods are commonly used in routine blood banking to enhance the agglutination of erythrocytes. These procedures include centrifugation, treatment with proteolytic enzymes, the use of colloids and other enhance-ment agents, such as low ionic strength saline solution, and the antiglobulin (AHG) test.

## The Complement System

Complement is a complex series of proteins, many of which are enzymes. Complement enzymes and products formed during the reaction chain, referred to as the com-plement cascade, have various physiologic and cellular consequences. The most important biologic role of com-plement in blood bank testing is the production of cell membrane lysis of antibody-coated cells.

## REVIEW QUESTIONS

1. Production of antibodies depends on:
   A. An individual's immunologic ability to recog-nize an antigen as non-self
   B. An individual's immunologic ability to respond to a foreign antigen
   C. The physical nature of an antigen
   D. All of the above
2. The hematologic cells of importance in an immu-nologic response are:
   A. Lymphocytes, plasma cells, and macrophages
   B. Plasma cells, neutrophils, and macrophages
   C. Macrophages, neutrophils, and monocytes
   D. Neutrophils, lymphocytes, and monocytes
3. Erythrocytes can be antigenic if their membrane contains:
   A. Foreign antigenic determinants
   B. Epitopes
   C. Lipid-rich surface areas
   D. Both A and B
4. In blood banking, cellular antigens of importance include:
   A. Blood group antigens
   B. Histocompatibility (HLA) antigens
   C. Interferon
   D. Both A and B

5. The Lewis blood group antigens are unique among blood group antigens because they:
   A. Are generally restricted to erythrocytes
   B. Are absorbed on the red cells from the plasma
   C. Are an integral part of the red cell membrane
   D. Result in hemolytic anemia if they are missing from the red cell membrane
6. The histocompatibility (HLA) antigens are important in:
   A. Production of IgM antibodies
   B. Production of IgG antibodies
   C. Survival of transplanted organs
   D. Activation of complement
7. One of the characteristics of proteins that makes them excellent antigens is their:
   A. High molecular weight
   B. Structural simplicity
   C. Structural stability
   D. Molecular flexibility
8. In the primary antibody response to a foreign antigen, the type of antibody initially formed is:
   A. IgM
   B. IgG
   C. IgD
   D. IgA
9. In a secondary (anamnestic) response, the predominant type of antibody formed is:
   A. IgM
   B. IgG
   C. IgD
   D. IgA
10–13. Match the following phases of an antibody response with the appropriate description:
   10. Plateau
   11. Lag
   12. Decline
   13. Log
   A. No detectable antibody is present
   B. Antibody titer stabilizes
   C. Antibody titer rises
   D. Antibody is catabolized
14–15. Match the following antibody characteristics (use an answer only once).
   14. IgM
   15. IgG
   A. Molecular weight of 900,000
   B. Half-life of 3 days
   C. 11S (sedimentation coefficient)
   D. Four subclasses
   E. Serum concentration (1.5-40 mg/100mL)
16–20. Match the following antibody characteristics (use an answer only once):
   16. IgM
   17. IgG
   18. IgA
   19. IgD

20. IgE
   A. Predominant immunoglobulin in secretions
   B. Primarily a cell membrane immunoglobulin found on the surface of B lymphocytes
   C. Mediates some types of allergic reactions
   D. A pentamer configuration
   E. Important in immune responses
21–23. Match the following antigenic determinants with their respective descriptors:
   21. Isotype
   22. Allotype
   23. Idiotype
   A. Determinants found on the immunoglobulins of some, but not all, animals of a species
   B. Result from unique structures on light and heavy chains
   C. The heavy chain constant region structures associated with the different classes and subclasses
25. The principal function of an antibody is to:
   A. Bind antigen
   B. Fix complement
   C. Pass through the placenta to provide passive immunity to the newborn infant
   D. Stimulate the inflammatory response
25. The term "avidity" refers to:
   A. The bond between a single antigenic determinant and an individual combining site
   B. The strength of an AHG reaction
   C. The pattern of agglutination displayed by HTLA antibodies
   D. The strength with which a multivalent antibody binds to a multivalent antigen
26. The major bond(s) formed between antigens and antibodies is/are:
   A. Hydrophobic
   B. Hydrogen bonding
   C. Van der Waals forces
   D. Electrostatic forces
27. Which of the following is *not* a factor that influences antigen-antibody association?
   A. The number of antibody molecules in relation to the number of antigen sites per cell
   B. The subclass of IgG molecules
   C. pH
   D. Temperature and length of time of incubation
28. The *prozone phenomenon* can:
   1. Result from excessive antibody concentration
   2. Result in a false positive reaction
   3. Result in a false negative reaction
   4. Be overcome by serially diluting the antibody-containing serum
   5. Be influenced by the length of incubation
   A. 1 only
   B. 1 and 2
   C. 2 and 3
   D. 1, 3 and 4

**29.** Lattice formation is the establishment of cross-links between _____ and antibodies.
- **A.** Antigens
- **B.** Erythrocytes
- **C.** Leukocytes
- **D.** Sensitized erythrocytes

**30.** Zeta potential is:
- **A.** The same as the ionic cloud around a particle (e.g., RBC)
- **B.** The outer edge of the ionic cloud surrounding an RBC in solution
- **C.** The difference between net charge at the cell membrane and the charge at the surface of shear
- **D.** Net surface charge density at the surface of the cell membrane

**31.** The term "complete antibody" is sometimes used to refer to:
- **A.** IgM
- **B.** IgG
- **C.** IgD
- **D.** IgA

**32.** Which of the following genotypic expressions could produce a "dosage effect?"
- **A.** Mm
- **B.** Le$^a$Lb$^b$
- **C.** Cc
- **D.** cc

**33.** Which of the following methods would *not* potentially enhance agglutination?
- **A.** Increasing the speed of centrifugation
- **B.** Decreasing the speed of centrifugation
- **C.** Treatment with proteolytic enzymes
- **D.** Extended incubation time
- **E.** The use of AHG sera

**34–37.** Match each of the following grading of agglutination reactions with the appropriate description:
- **34.** Mixed field
- **35.** Weak (+/−)
- **36.** 1+
- **37.** 3+
- **A.** Medium-sized aggregates, some free erythrocytes, clear supernatant
- **B.** Few isolated aggregates, mostly free floating cells, supernatant appears red
- **C.** Several large aggregates, some free erythrocytes, clear supernatant
- **D.** Tiny aggregates that are barely visible macroscopically, many free erythrocytes, turbid and reddish supernatant.
- **E.** A few small aggregates just visible macroscopically, many free erythrocytes, turbid and reddish supernatant.

**38.** The direct antiglobulin test (DAT) detects:
- **A.** In vivo sensitization of erythrocytes
- **B.** In vivo sensitization of leukocytes
- **C.** In vitro sensitization of erythrocytes
- **D.** A or C

**39.** A polyspecific antiglobulin sera contains:
- **A.** Anti-IgG
- **B.** Anti-C3d
- **C.** Anti-IgE
- **D.** Both A and B

**40.** To disperse pseudoagglutination, which of the following can be done?
- **A.** Add a few drops of albumin
- **B.** Add a few drops of saline
- **C.** Add a few drops of proteolytic enzyme
- **D.** Shake the reaction tube vigorously

**41.** To inactivate complement in serum, the serum should be:
- **A.** Frozen at −18° C
- **B.** Incubated at 37° C for 15 minutes
- **C.** Incubated at 37° C for 30 minutes
- **D.** Incubated at 56° C for 30 minutes

**42.** The physiologic or cellular components of complement activation produce all of the following except:
- **A.** Blood vessel dilation
- **B.** Increased vascular permeability
- **C.** Cell membrane lysis
- **D.** Initiation of antibody production

**43.** The classical pathway of the complement system is initiated by:
- **A.** The complexing of antigen and its specific antibody
- **B.** The presence of IgM in the circulation
- **C.** The presence of IgG in the circulation
- **D.** Contact with a foreign surface, e.g., the polysaccharide coating of a microorganism

**44.** The classic complement pathway is characterized by:
- **A.** Recognition
- **B.** Enzymatic activation
- **C.** Membrane attack
- **D.** All of the above

**45.** Which classes of immunoglobulin can fix complement?
- **A.** IgM
- **B.** IgG
- **C.** IgD
- **D.** Both A and B

**46.** The membrane attack unit is composed of:
- **A.** C5b, C6, C7, C8, and C9
- **B.** C5, C6, C7, C8, and C9
- **C.** C5, C6, and C7
- **D.** C1r, C1s, C1q, C4, and C2

**47.** Which complement components *do not* participate in the alternate (Properdin) pathway?
- **A.** C1r, C1s, and C1q
- **B.** C1, C4, and C2
- **C.** C4, C2, and C3
- **D.** C3, C5, and C6

## Bibliography

Auffray, C., and Strominger, J.L.: Molecular genetics of the human major histocompatibility complex, Adv. Hum. Genet., *15:* 197–247, 1986.

Barrett, J.T.: Textbook of Immunology (4th ed). St. Louis, Mosby, 1983, pp. 29–40.

Beck, M.L., Hardman, J.T., and Henry, R.: Reactivity of a licensed murine monoclonal anti-A reagent with group B cells. Transfusion, *26*(6):572, 1986.

Callicoat, P.A., Hall, C., and Brenner, N.: Evaluation of monoclonal anti-A and anti-B for routine ABO grouping in microplates, Transfusion, *26*(6):549, 1986.

Carpenter, P.L.: Immunology and Serology. Philadelphia, W.B. Saunders, 1975, 8, 20–22, 38, 239–245.

Dannenberg, A.M., Jr. Macrophages and Monocytes. In Fundamentals of Clinical Hematology. Edited by Jerry L. Spivak. Hagerstown, Md., Harper and Row, 1980, pp. 137–153.

Dunstan, R.A.: Status of major red cell blood group antigens on neutrophils, lymphocytes and monocytes. Br. J. Haematol., *62:* 301–309, 1986.

Duran, L.W., and Pease, L.R.: Relating the structure of major transplantation antigens to immune function, Transplantation, *41*(3):279–285, 1986.

Epley, K.M., Line, L.M., and Severns, M.L.: Evaluation of a monoclonal anti-D for D$^u$ testing. Transfusion, *26*(6):549, 1986.

Ersley, A.J., and Gabuzda, T.G.: Phagocytes. In Pathophysiology of Blood. Philadelphia, W.B. Saunders, 1975, pp. 100–118.

Gaidulis, L., Branch, D.R., Lazar, G.S., et al.: The red cell antigens A, B, D, U, Ge, Jk3 and Yt$^a$, are not detected on human granulocytes, Br. J. Haematol., *60:*659–668, 1985.

Hall, S., Olekna, D., and Davies, D.: Production of unique monoclonal ABO blood grouping antisera, Transfusion, *25*(5):448, 1986.

Hubbard, M.: Paternity testing. In Complements, edited by William G. Cannady Rogers, Arkansas, Pel-Freeze Biologicals, *2*(1): 1–2, June, 1982.

Keller, R.H., et al.: Monoclonal antibodies: Clinical utility and the misunderstood epitope, Lab. Med. *15*(12):795–802, 1984.

Kelton, J.G., and Bebenek, G.: Granulocytes do not have surface ABO antigens, Transfusion, *25*(6):567–569, 1985.

McElligott, M.C., Menitove, J.E., and Aster, R.H.: Recruitment of unrelated persons as bone marrow donors, Transfusion, *26*(4): 309–314, 1986.

Meyers, M.A., Walker, R.H., and Phillips, L.M.: The usefulness of histocompatibility antigens (HLA-A,B) in parentage testing, Transfusion, *25*(5):481, 1985.

Moheng, M.C.: Blood banking: State of the art. In Approaches to Serological Problems in the Hospital Transfusion Service. Edited by Pierce, S.R., and Wilson, J.K., Arlington, Va., American Association of Blood Banks, 1985, pp. 1–27.

Monoclonal Antibodies, St. Louis, Sigma Diagnostics, 1985.

Nehlsen-Cannarella, S.: The wonderment of HLA. In Complements, edited by Nehlsen-Cannarella, S. Brown Deer, Wisconsin, Pel-Freeze Biologicals, *4*(1):2–4, April, 1984.

Ortho Product Brochure: Anti Human Globulin (Rabbit and Murine Monoclonal BioClone®) (Clear or Green) Anti-OgG, − C3d, Polyspecific, Ortho Diagnostic Systems Inc., Raritan, NJ, revised June 1986.

Ortho Product Brochure: Ortho Bovine Albumin Solution 22% Protein Concentration pH 7.2, Ortho Diagnostic Systems Inc., Raritan, NJ, revised November 1985.

Pliska, C.: Low ionic strength solution, Lab. Med. *11*(3):159–164, 1980.

Rivera, R., and Scornik, J.C.: HLA Antigens on Red Cells, Transfusion, *26*(4):375–381, 1986.

Roitt, I.: Essential Immunology (Fifth Edition). Oxford, England, Blackwell Scientific Publications, 1984, pp. 76–85.

Sebring, E.S., Polesky, H.F., and Schanfield, M.S.: GM and KM allotypes in disputed parentage, A. J. C. P., *71*(3):281–285, 1979.

Snyder, E.L., and Falast, G.A.: Significance of the direct antiglobulin test, Lab. Med., *16*(2):89–96, 1985.

Spitalnik, P.F., and Spitalnik, S.L.: Selective uptake by erythrocytes of Lewis antigens based on ceramide composition. Abstract of papers presented at AABB 39th Annual Meeting, Nov., 1986.

*Standards for Blood Banks and Transfusion Services,* 12th ed., Arlington, Va., American Association of Blood Banks, 1987, pp. 21, 87, 103, 181.

Steane, E.A., et al.: A proposal for compatibility testing incorporating the manual hexadimethrine promide (Polybrene) test, Transfusion *25*(6):540–544, 1986.

Tizard, I.R.: Immunology: An Introduction. Philadelphia, W.B. Saunders, 1984, pp. 14, 22, 93, 97, 105, 127, 197.

Turgeon, M.L.: Clinical Hematology: Theory and Procedures. Boston, Little, Brown and Co., 1988, pp. 97–105.

Vengelen-Tyler, V., and Choy, C.: A comparative study of antibody enhancement techniques, Transfusion, *26*(6):570, 1986.

Wenk, R.E., and Brooks, M.: Paternity probabilities of biologic fathers and unexcluded falsely-accused men, Transfusion, *26*(6): 548, 1986.

Zmijewski, C.M.: Immunohematology. 2nd ed., New York, Appleton Century Crofts, 1972, pp. 20, 38–40.

Part **II**

# Erythrocyte Blood Group Systems

# The ABO Blood Group System

At the conclusion of this chapter, the reader will be able to:

- Describe the history of the discovery of the ABO system.
- Contrast the antigens and antibodies found in the blood in the ABO system.
- Discuss the patterns of inheritance of *A* and *B* genes.
- State the phenotypic frequencies of groups A, B, and O.
- Name the specific transferase for the *A, B,* and *H* genes.
- Identify the immunodominant monosaccharide residual for *A, B,* and *H* genes.
- Describe the synthesis of H, A, and B antigens.
- State the percentage of persons in the United States who are secretors of water-soluble ABH substances.
- Identify the product or products found in the saliva of persons of various ABO groups.
- State the characteristic genotype of a nonsecretor.
- Describe the subgroups of group A.
- Explain the importance of A subgroups in the clinical situation.
- Describe the purpose of absorbed anti-$A_1$.
- Name the ethnic population with the highest frequency of the superactive *B* gene.
- State the genotype of individuals with the Bombay phenotype.
- Explain the causes of acquired A antigen and acquired B antigen.
- Describe the characteristics of anti-A and anti-B.
- Analyze some of the types of problems that can be encountered in ABO grouping.

## Chapter Outline

## INTRODUCTION

The ABO, H, P, I, and Lewis blood group antigens are constructed on structurally related carbohydrate molecules. It is possible for these carbohydrate molecules to express determinants for more than one of these blood groups. Therefore, the activities of the genes of one of these groups may impact the expression of the antigens of another.

## HISTORICAL ASPECTS OF THE ABO SYSTEM

In the early 1900s, Landsteiner recognized the presence of two separate erythrocyte antigens, the A and B antigens. Based on his observations of the agglutination reaction of erythrocytes and the presence of serum antibodies in the serum of individuals directed against these antigens, he established the existence of the first known blood group system, the ABO system. He proposed three separate groups: A, B, and O. Shortly hereafter, von Decastello and Sturli identified a fourth group, AB. The serologic

**Table 4-1. Classification of the ABO Blood Types**

| Blood Group | Erythrocyte Antigens | Serum Antibodies |
|---|---|---|
| A | A | Anti-B |
| B | B | Anti-A |
| AB | A and B | None |
| O | None | Anti-A, anti-B, anti-A, B |

reactions of the ABO blood groups are presented in Table 4-1.

## GENETIC INHERITANCE

As early as 1908, Epstein and Ottenberg suggested that the ABO blood groups were inherited. It was not until 1924 that Bernstein postulated the existence of three allelic genes, *A, B,* and *O.* He proposed that an individual inherited two genes, one from each parent, and that these genes determined which ABO antigens would be present on a person's erythrocytes. The O gene was defined as *amorphic* because no detectable antigen is produced in response to the inheritance of this gene. In 1930, Thompson proposed a four-allele theory of inheritance based on the discovery of von Dungern and Hirszfeld in 1911, which demonstrated that the A antigen could be divided into A$_1$ and A$_2$ subgroups. Thompson's four-allele theory encompassed the four allelic genes, $A_1$, $A_2$, *B* and *O.*

Expression of A and B genes in erythrocytes or body fluids results from the independently inherited *Hh, Sese,* and *A* and *B* genes. The ABO locus resides on chromosome 9 in humans; the remaining two loci, Hh and Sese (secretion), have been demonstrated in family studies to be closely linked on chromosome 19. Under normal circumstances, if either the *A* or *B* genes are present on either chromosome, the gene can be phenotypically demonstrated on erythrocytes. Examples of exceptional cases of expression of *A* or *B* genes on erythrocytes and other alterations of genetic expression are discussed later in this chapter. The H allele produces an enzyme that acts at the cellular level to construct the H antigen, the precursor substance on which A and B antigens are built. The Se gene is directly responsible for the expression of H on the glycoproteins in epithelial secretions such as saliva.

The four allelic genes of the ABO system ($A_1$, $A_2$, *B* and *O*) and resulting phenotypes are presented in Table 4-2. Inheritance of the ABO genes follows Mendelian

**Table 4-2. The Major ABO Genotypes and Phenotypes**

| Phenotype | Possible Genotypes |
|---|---|
| $A_1$ | $A_1/A_1$, $A_1/A_2$, $A_1/O$ |
| $A_2$ | $A_2/A_2$, $A_2/O$ |
| $A_1B$ | $A_1/B$ |
| $A_2B$ | $A_2/B$ |
| B | $B/B$ or $B/O$ |
| O | $O/O$ |

principles, with the *A* and *B* genes being codominant. Two examples of genetic crosses involving the ABO system, with the resultant genotypes and phenotypes of the off-spring, are presented in the Appendices.

## DEVELOPMENT AND DISTRIBUTION OF THE ABO GROUPS

### Development of the A and B Antigens

The A and B antigens are not fully developed in newborn infants, but some antigenic development can be detected on embryonic erythrocytes as early as 5 weeks of gestational age. Although the strength of A and B antigens does *not* increase during fetal life, these antigens do gain strength shortly after birth. Weaker agglutination reactions are observed with fetal and newborn infants' erythrocytes compared to the mature erythrocytes of adults.

It has been proposed that the differences in cellular A, B, and H activity between infants and adults may be related to the number of branched structures carried on the cellular membranes of each group. The number (Table 4-3) and strength of antigen sites are lower in infants than adults.

The A, B, and H antigens are thought to be constructed of predominantly linear oligosaccharides with only one terminal point for the addition of H and then A or B. In contrast, the red blood cells of adults contain a high proportion of branched oligosaccharides with additional points that can be converted to H precursor and then A and B antigens.

Group A infants may type as $A_2$ at birth, but subsequently demonstrate type $A_1$ reactions by the time they are 6 to 18 months old. It should also be noted that A and B antigens as well as H, $P_1$, and D antigens produce significantly weaker or negative reactions in reticulocyte-rich blood preparations.

**Table 4-3. Examples of the Number of A and B Antigen Sites on Erythrocytes**

| | Antigen | Number of Sites |
|---|---|---|
| Adult blood | $A_1$ | 810,000 to 1,170,000 A antigen sites |
| | $A_2$ | 240,000 to 290,000 A antigen sites |
| | $A_3$ | 35,000 A antigen sites |
| | $A_X$ | 4,800 A antigen sites |
| | $A_m$ | 700 A antigen sites |
| | $A_1B$ | 460,000 to 850,000 A antigen sites |
| | | 310,000 to 560,000 B antigen sites |
| | $A_2B$ | 120,000 A antigen sites |
| | B | 610,000 to 830,000 B antigen sites |
| Newborn cord blood | $A_1$ | 250,000 to 370,000 A antigen sites |
| | $A_2$ | 140,000 A antigen sites |
| | $A_1B$ | 220,000 A antigen sites |
| | B | 200,000 B antigen sites |

Economidous J., Hughes-Jones, N.C., and Gardner, B.: Quantitative measurements concerning A and B antigen sites. Vox Sang. *12*:321, 1967.

**Table 4-4. Representative ABO Frequencies**

| Phenotype | Genotype | White (%) | Black (%) | Oriental (%) |
|---|---|---|---|---|
| $A_1$ | $A_1A_1$, $A_1A_2$, $A_1O$ | 32 | 19 | 27 |
| $A_2$ | $A_2$, $A_2$, $A_2O$ | 9 | 8 | (Rare) |
| B | BB, BO | 9 | 19 | 25 |
| $A_1B$ | $A_1B$ | 3 | 3 | 5 |
| $A_2B$ | $A_2B$ | 1 | 1 | (Rare) |
| O | OO | 45 | 49 | 40 |

### Distribution of ABO Groups

In 1919, Hirszfeld and Hirszfeld discovered that the distribution of ABO blood groups differed for various populations. Mourant conducted a comprehensive survey of the world blood type distribution (Table 4-4). Although this information is mostly of academic interest, an awareness of these differences is a helpful guide to blood bank inventory management.

## BIOCHEMICAL ACTIVITIES RELATED TO THE DEVELOPMENT OF A, B, AND H ANTIGENS

Inheritance of *A* and *B* genes usually results in the expression of *A* and *B* gene products (antigens) on erythrocytes, but H, A, and B antigens are *not* the direct products of the *H, A,* and *B* genes, respectively. Each gene codes for the production of a specific *transferase* enzyme (Table 4-5), which catalyzes the transfer of a monosaccharide molecule from a donor substrate to the precursor substance.

### Expression of H, A, and B Antigens

The H gene codes for the production of α-L-fucosyl transferase that catalyzes the addition of L-fucose, the immunodominant structure of H antigen, to two slightly different structures known as the type 1 and 2 precursor chains. Once the H gene-specified transferase has acted and L-fucose has been added to the chains, the A and B gene-specified products can then act to add a monosaccharide to these preformed H-bearing chains (Fig. 4-1). If a person does not inherit at least one H gene, L-fucose is *not* transferred to the precursor substance and the A and B immunodominant sugars *cannot* be added subsequently. This is the basis of explanation for the Bombay or $O_h$ phenotype (see page 95 for a discussion of the Bombay phenotype).

**Table 4-5. ABH Genes and Their Enzymatic Products**

| Gene | Enzyme |
|---|---|
| H | α-L-fucosyltransferase |
| A | α-3-N-acetyl-D-galactosaminyl transferase |
| B | α-3-D-galactosyl transferase |
| O | None |

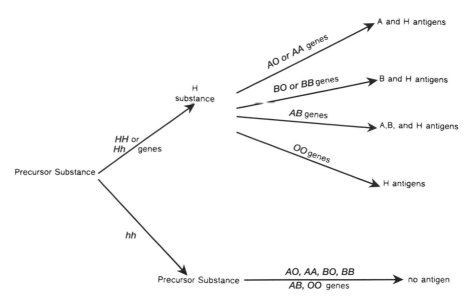

**Figure 4-1.** Genetic pathway of expression of ABH substances on erythrocytes.

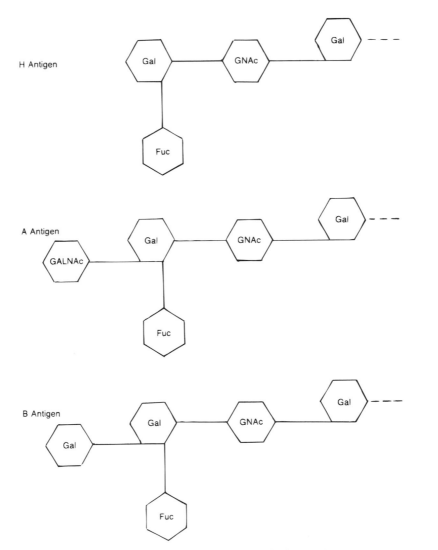

**Figure 4-2.** Biochemical configurations conferring antigenic specificity. The carbohydrate residual attached to the third carbon of galactose determines antigenic activity. N-acetyl-galactosamine confers A specificity and galactose confers B specificity. If the fucose residual that confers H specificity is not attached to the 2nd carbon, the galactose residual cannot react with either galactose or N-acetyl-galactosamine at the third carbon. Gal = Galactose, GNAc = N-acetyl-glucosamine; Fuc = Fucose; GALNAc = N-acetylgalactosamine.

Specific transferase enzymes are the products of *A* or *B* genes. The A and B antigens result from the actions of these transferases, which attach specific monosaccharides to the H substrate. The immunodominant monosaccharides of the A and B antigens are shown in Figure 4-2. The *A* gene produces an α-3-N-acetyl-D-galactosaminyl transferase that attaches N-acetyl-D-galactosamine to the acceptor molecule; the *B* gene produces an α-3-D-galactosyl transferase, which attaches D-galactose to the acceptor molecule. Because the A and B transferases convert the same acceptor molecule, they compete with one another for the substrate. Both A₁ and B cells have many immunodominant sugars added, resulting in a low level of detectable H antigen on $A_1$ and B erythrocytes.

## Variations in Transferase Enzymes

The level of $A_1$-specified transferase enzyme is higher in serum from cord blood than in the sera of $A_1$ (nonpregnant) adults. In pregnancy, the level of $A_1$ specified transferase enzyme in the serum drops to less than half the amount present in the sera of nonpregnant $A_1$ adults.

Although they are specific for the same monosaccharide and use the same acceptor molecule, the transferases produced by the $A_1$ and $A_2$ genes are both quantitatively and qualitatively different. It has been demonstrated that the levels of transferase are 5 to 10 times higher in $A_1$ persons than in $A_2$ individuals and the transferases differ in their chemical requirements, such as optimum pH.

Studies of transferase indicate that in two individuals with an $A_2B$ erythrocyte phenotype but an $A_1B$ genotype, each has a strong B transferase capable of incorporating more [14]C-labelled galactose onto structures with H activity and attaching more galactose onto group O cells at a rate more rapid than normal. Previous investigations provided evidence for the existence of an atypical "superactive" *B* gene. It has also been suggested that in $A_1B$ persons, a hybrid AB gene-specified transferase may also be made.

Detection and measurement of H, A, and B gene-specified transferases in sera are often important in the investigation of complex problems involving the ABO system.

## The Molecular Configuration of A, B, and H

Glycosphingolipids carrying A or B oligosaccharides are integral parts of the membranes of red blood cells, and epithelial and endothelial cells. These oligosaccharides are also present in soluble forms in plasma. Glycoproteins that carry identical oligosaccharides are responsible for the A and B activity of secreted body fluids such as saliva. A and B oligosaccharides that lack carrier protein or lipid molecules are found in milk and urine.

### Type I and Type 2 Chains

H antigens are synthesized on precursor (core) oligosaccharide chains ending in Type 1 and Type 2 linkages

**Table 4-6. Comparison of Type 1 and Type 2 Chains**

|  | Type 1 | Type 2 |
|---|---|---|
| Linkage | Beta 1, 3 | Beta 1, 4 |
| Origin | Plasma | Synthesized on erythrocytic precursors |
| Controlling genes | H, A, B, Se, and Lewis | H, A and B genes |

(Table 4-6). The chains differ only in the linkage of B-galactose to a terminal β-N-acetylglucosamine residual. The carbon 1 of galactose can be attached to either carbon 3 or carbon 4 of β-N-acetylglucosamine (Fig. 4-3). The beta-1,3 linkage represents a type 1 chain; the beta-1,4 linkage represents a type 2 chain. The H, A, and B immunodominant sugars can be added to either of these chains.

Type 1 chains are the main carriers of A, B, and H in body fluids and secretions. Type 1 A, B, and H antigens

Precursor Substance

Type 1 Chain beta (1-3) Linkage

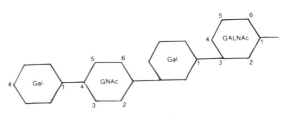

Type 2 Chain beta (1-4) Linkage

**Figure 4-3.** Chain types. Gal = Galactose; GNAc = N-acetylglucosamine; GALNAc = N-acetylgalactosamine.

are carried on free oligosaccharides in milk and urine and on glycolipids in plasma. In saliva, A, B, and H antigens are carried on glycoproteins with type 1 and type 2 chains. Type 2 chains almost exclusively form the glycolipid A, B, and H antigens produced by red blood cells. Recent studies suggest that more complex core molecules, called type 3 and type 4 chains, may also be involved.

### Antigen Acquisition

Most of the H, A, and B antigens of erythrocytes are synthesized by the erythrocytic precursors; some are acquired from the plasma. The antigens acquired from the plasma are of the type 1 variety and are glycosphingolipids. This attachment of A, B, and H antigens to erythrocytes from the plasma occurs because glycolipids can be inserted into the membrane of the cells. The H, A, and B structures synthesized on erythrocytic precursors are exclusively of the type 2 variety, which are attached to both glycoproteins and glycosphingolipids. The H, A, and B, as well as Lewis determinants on type 1 chains that reach the erythrocytes by way of the plasma, are dependent on the H, A, B, Lewis, and secretor genes. The site of synthesis of plasma H, A, B, and Lewis antigens is not known. The type 2 chains are controlled (in terms of both presence and quantity) simply by the *H, A,* and *B* genes.

Glycosphingolipids carrying A or B oligosaccharides are integral parts of the red blood cell membrane, and epithelial and endothelial cells. These substances are also present in soluble form in plasma. Glycoproteins that carry identical oligosaccharides are responsible for the detectable A and B activity of secreted body fluid, such as saliva. A and B oligosaccharides that lack carrier protein or lipid molecules are found in fluids, such as milk and urine.

Lymphocytes and platelets acquire H, A, and B antigens from the plasma by insertion of preformed glycosphingolipids into the membrane. It is currently believed that little, if any, H, A, or B is synthesized during lymphocyte development. Therefore, all the lymphocyte membrane-borne H, A, and B antigens are acquired from the plasma. There is disagreement as to whether all the platelet-borne H, A, and B antigens are acquired from plasma or some acquired and some synthesized during platelet development.

Until recently, it was believed that addition of A and B sugars to core molecules terminated chain growth. Glycosyltransferase was not believed to use A or B antigens as acceptor substrates. The discovery of glycolipids, in which two A structures appeared linked in tandem (type 3A antigen structures), altered this view.

## SECRETORS AND NONSECRETORS

### The Secretor State

The terms *secretor* and *nonsecretor* only refer to the presence of water-soluble ABH antigen substances in body fluid.

**Table 4-7. The Relationship of ABH Substances and ABO Group**

| ABO Group Secretors | ABH Substances in Saliva | | |
|---|---|---|---|
| | A | B | H |
| A | much | none | some |
| B | none | much | some |
| O | none | none | much |
| AB | much | much | some |

This condition is influenced by the independently inherited, regulator Se gene. Approximately 78% of the population possess at least one Se gene and secrete A, B, or H water-soluble antigens. The presence of the Se gene allows the H gene to function in secretory cells.

These secretions have the property of reacting with their corresponding antibodies, and neutralize or inhibit the ability of the antibody to agglutinate erythrocytes possessing the corresponding antigen. This reaction is termed *hemagglutination inhibition* and provides a means of assaying the relative activity or potency of these water-soluble blood group substances (see Chapter 14, Procedures).

The production of A, B, and H antigens in saliva or other body fluids (Table 4-7) is controlled by the secretor gene, which is inherited independently of the *ABO* and *H* genes. Both the locus of the secretor gene *(Se)* and its allele *(se),* which is amorphic, and the exact mechanism of inheritance are unknown. At least one *Se* gene (genotype *SeSe* or *Sese*) is essential for the expression of the ABH antigens in secretions. Individuals who are homozygous for se (sese) do *not* secrete H, A, or B antigens regardless of the presence of *H, A,* or *B* genes. The secretions of sese persons contain type 1 and type 2 chains, but no H, A, or B activity. At least one *H* gene is necessary for H, A, or B antigens to be manufactured.

The enzyme produced by the H gene acts primarily on type 2 chains and in the red blood cell membranes. The enzyme produced by Se prefers type 1 chains and acts primarily in the secretory glands. The suggested role for the Se-specified transferase (L-fucosyltransferase) is transfer of L-fucose to the terminal galactose of type 1 chains, which forms H substance into the secreted material. It is the presence of L-fucosyltransferase that subsequently determines whether ABH soluble substances will be secreted, because H substance must be synthesized before the formation of A or B substances. The Se gene does *not* bring about the formation of A, B, or H antigens on erythrocytes, nor does it control the presence of A, B, or H transferases in hematopoietic tissue. In contrast, the A or B transferase enzymes, unlike A or B antigens, are found in the secretions of $A_1$ or B persons regardless of secretor status.

Secretor status can be determined by the inhibition (neutralization) test described in Chapter 14. Testing for ABH secretion is helpful in establishing the true ABO group of an individual. The detection of small amounts of A or B antigens in the saliva of a secretor can be a useful confirmatory test when establishing a phenotype that involves a subgroup of A or B.

## TYPE A

### The A₁ and A₂ Subgroups

Group A antigens can be differentiated into two principal subgroups, $A_1$ and $A_2$. Approximately 80% of group A individuals are $A_1$, most of the others belong to the $A_2$ subgroup. Inheritance patterns of $A_1$ and $A_2$ phenotypes, as well as $A_1B$ and $A_2B$ phenotypes, suggest that the $A_1$ and $A_2$ genes code for different transferases. Some biochemical studies appear to have produced evidence that there are different patterns of N-acetyl-D-galactosamine attachment on $A_1$ and $A_2$ erythrocytes, which suggests that the acceptor sites for the $A_1$ and $A_2$ gene-specified transferases might be different.

Four different types of A-active and H-active glycolipids have been isolated from erythrocytes. The H-bearing chains are classified as $H_1$, $H_2$, $H_3$, and $H_4$; the A-bearing chains are referred to as $A_a$, $A_b$, $A_c$, and $A_d$. These chains vary considerably in length and complexity of branching (Table 4-8).

The A-immunodominant carbohydrate and the $H_1$ and $H_2$ glycolipids are converted to $A_a$ and $A_b$ glycolipids by the transferase produced by the $A_1$ or $A_2$ genes. The $H_3$ and $H_4$ glycolipids are converted to $A_c$ and $A_d$ when the $A_1$ gene-specified transferase is made. Some $A_2$ cells may lack $A_d$ altogether and carry only small amounts of $A_c$. This means that $H_3$ and $H_4$ are much more readily available when $A_2$ erythrocytes are tested with anti-H. Thus, the high level of A and low level of H on $A_1$ cells and the lower level of A and higher level of H on $A_2$ cells are demonstrable.

Immunodominant sugars are attached to erythrocyte membrane-borne glycoproteins and glycolipids. On the erythrocytes of adults, some of the glycoproteins and glycolipids are straight chains; others are complex branched chains with several different sites at which the H, A, and B, specific carbohydrates can be added. On erythrocytes from cord blood samples, the complex branched chains are not well developed, so that the number of sites to which immunodominant carbohydrates can be added are fewer than on the erythrocytes of adults. The decreased number of A and B antigens on fetal erythrocytes acts as a defense against hemolytic disease of the newborn (HDN) even when large amounts of maternal antibody enter the fetal circulation.

The serologic distinction between $A_1$ and $A_2$ antigens

is based on the reactions of erythrocytes with various antisera. Reagent anti-A sera from human sources rarely differentiates $A_1$ from $A_2$ subtypes but anti-A,B sera of human origin can detect common subgroups of A and B and IgM antibodies produced by individual murine hybridomas (monoclonal antibodies) can detect weak subgroups of A.

If anti-A from a group B person is adsorbed with $A_2$ cells, a typing serum (adsorbed anti-$A_1$) can be prepared that will agglutinate $A_1$ but not $A_2$ erythrocytes. Probably the most practical way to differentiate between $A_1$ and $A_2$ subgroups is by use of lectin anti-$A_1$, which is made from *Dolichos biflorus* seeds. Lectin anti-$A_1$ agglutinates $A_1$ but not $A_2$ erythrocytes. Dolichos lectin is not totally specific for $A_1$ because it also agglutinates some group O or group B erythrocytes that carry Cad and other antigens that are polyagglutinable. Such reactions, are rare enough that they do not significantly reduce the usefulness of Dolichos lectin as an anti-$A_1$ reagent.

For routine transfusion, it is not necessary to distinguish between patients or donors as $A_1$ or $A_2$ except when working with an $A_2$ or $A_2B$ individual whose serum contains anti-$A_1$. Estimates of the frequency of anti-$A_1$ in sera vary between 1 and 8% of $A_2$ persons and 22 and 35% of $A_2B$ persons. Although anti-$A_1$ is considered clinically insignificant unless it reacts at 37° C, it can cause ABO discrepancies between cell and serum tests and may also cause crossmatch incompatibilities.

### Infrequent Subgroups of A

Genetically controlled subgroups of A result from the inheritance of rare alleles at the ABO locus. The distribution and characteristics of the uncommon subgroups of the A antigen, from the strongest $A_3$ to the weakest $A_{end}$, comprise a continuum.

Classification of these subgroups of A is based on the reactivity of patient erythrocytes with anti-A, anti-A,B, anti-$A_1$ (*Dolichos biflorus*), and anti-H; the presence or absence of anti-$A_1$ in the serum; and the presence of H and/or A substance in the saliva of secretors (Table 4-9).

**Table 4-8. A and H Chain Complexity**

| Straighter Chains | More Branched Chains |
|---|---|
| $H_1$ and $H_2$ | $H_3$–$H_4$ |
| $A_a$ and $A_b$ | $A_c$ and $A_d$. |

**Table 4-9. Serologic Reactions of A₁, A₂, A₁B and A₂B Phenotypes**

| | | Phenotypes | | | |
|---|---|---|---|---|---|
| | | $A_1$ | $A_2$ | $A_1B$ | $A_2B$ |
| | Anti-A | + | + | + | + |
| Erythrocyte | Anti-$A_1$ | + | 0 | + | 0 |
| Reactions | Anti-B | 0 | 0 | + | + |
| | Anti-A,B | + | + | + | + |

| | | $A_1$ | $A_2$ | $A_2$ with anti-$A_1$ | $A_1B$ | $A_2B$ | $A_2B$ with anti-$A_1$ |
|---|---|---|---|---|---|---|---|
| | $A_1$ cells | 0 | 0 | + | 0 | 0 | + |
| Serum | $A_2$ cells | 0 | 0 | 0 | 0 | 0 | 0 |
| Reactions | B cells | + | + | + | 0 | 0 | 0 |
| | O cells | 0 | 0 | 0 | 0 | 0 | 0 |

**Table 4-10. A Comparison of the Serologic Reactions of A$_1$, A$_{int}$, and A$_2$ Phenotypes**

| Phenotype | Erythrocyte Reactions* | | | | | Serum Reactions† | | | | Saliva of Secretors |
|---|---|---|---|---|---|---|---|---|---|---|
|  | A | B | A,B | H | A$_1$ | A$_1$ | A$_2$ | B | O |  |
| A$_1$ | 4+ | 0 | 4+ | 0 | 4+ | 0 | 0 | 4+ | 0 | A & H |
| A$_{int}$ | 4+ | 0 | 4+ | 3+ | 2+ | 0 | 0 | 4+ | 0 | A & H |
| A$_2$ | 4+ | 0 | 4+ | 2+ | 0 | ‡ | 0 | 4+ | 0 | A & H |

Reactions of patient's erythrocytes with reagent antiserum
† Reactions of patient's serum with reagent erythrocytes
‡ The occurrence of anti-A$_1$ is variable in these phenotypes

Failure to detect a weak A antigen usually results in the blood being mistakenly typed as group O. If a unit of erythrocytes of a weak subgroup of A is transfused to a group O recipient, a transfusion reaction is possible, although significant in vivo erythrocyte destruction may not occur.

### The Subgroup A$_{int}$

Originally, this subgroup of A was described as being intermediate between A$_1$ and A$_2$ in terms of its reactions with anti-A and anti-A$_1$. In 1970, it was agreed that blood would be classified as A$_{int}$ based on the reaction with anti-A$_1$ (Table 4-10) but A$_{int}$ erythrocytes react more strongly with anti-H than either A$_1$ or A$_2$ cells. This is indicative of the genetic control of H antigen production that is independent of the effects of the ABO genes.

### Additional Subgroups of A

A variety of subgroups of A have been identified but are rare in occurrence. Serologic reactions of these groups are presented in Table 4-11. It is important to rule out condi-

tions such as *chimeras* or weakening of the A antigen before considering these subgroups during laboratory testing.

Many subgroups are believed to result from the inheritance of a specific allele; others are considered to result from genetic interaction (Table 4-12).

### TYPE B

Subgroups or variants of type B blood, such as the B$_3$ phenotype, are much rarer than subgroups of A, but the incidence of B antigen subgroups is more frequent in some racial groups. For example, 24% of the Chinese population of Taiwan have type B blood and the frequencies of B$_3$ and A$_1$B$_3$ blood are about 1:900 and 1:1800, respectively.

The classification of B subgroups by Race and Sanger is divided into three categories (Table 4-13) based on serologic characteristics. Subgroups of B are usually recognized by variations in the strength of the reaction using human anti-B and anti-A,B reagent antisera. It has been suggested that qualitative as well as quantitative differences exist in the B antigen. These differences have been noted because of the significantly lower avidity of subgroup B and subgroup A$_1$B with both polyclonal and monoclonal antisera, compared to normal group B cells.

B(A) is the designation used to describe the small number (0.1 to 1.0%) of type B individuals whose red blood cells react with anti-A blood grouping reagent partially formulated with murine monoclonal antibody. In addition, their serum contains excessively high concentrations of B gene-specific galactosyltransferase.

**Table 4-11. Serologic Reactions of Uncommon A Phenotypes**

| Phenotype | A$_{int}$ | A$_3$ | A$_x$ | A$_m$ |
|---|---|---|---|---|
| Anti-A | 4+ | 2+* | Weak/0 | +/weak |
| Anti-A,B | 4+ | 2+* | 2+ | +/weak |
| Anti-A$_1$† | 2+ | 0 | 0 | 0 |
| Anti-H | 3+ | 4+ | 4+ | 4+ |
| Saliva (secretor) | A,H | A,H | H | A,H |

**Reactions of Serum Against Known Reagent Erythrocytes**

| Phenotype | A$_{int}$ | A$_3$ | A$_x$ | A$_m$ |
|---|---|---|---|---|
| A$_1$ cells | 0 | *† | 2+ | 0 |
| A$_2$ cells | 0 | 0 | 0/+ | 0 |
| B cells | 4+ | 4+ | 4+ | 4+ |
| O cells | 0 | 0 | 0 | 0 |

**Reactions of Erythrocytes Against Known Antisera**

| Phenotype | A$_{end}$ | A$_{el}$ | A$_{bantu}$ | A$_{iae}$ | A$_{finn}$ |
|---|---|---|---|---|---|
| Anti-A | Weak | 0 | 1–2+* | 0 | Weak |
| Anti-A,B | Weak | 0 | 1–2+* | 0 | Weak |
| Anti-A$_1$† | 0 | 0 | 0 | 3+ | 0 |
| Anti-H | 4+ | 4+ | 4+ | 4+ | 4+ |
| Saliva (secretor) | H | H | H | H | H |

* Mixed field
† Dolichos biflorus

### ABNORMALITIES ENCOUNTERED IN THE EXPRESSION OF ABH ANTIGENS ON ERYTHROCYTES

The expression of ABH antigens on erythrocytes may be altered by a variety of factors, which include

1. Modifying genes
2. Acquired antigens
3. Altered antigens
4. High levels of soluble ABH substances
5. Depression of A, B, and H antigens in disease
6. Mixtures of blood

**Table 4-12. Characteristics of Uncommon A Subgroups**

| Phenotype | Date Identified | Characteristics |
|---|---|---|
| $A_x$ | 1935 | Some are possibly inherited as an allele, $A_x$, at the ABO locus. Others appear to result from modifying genes |
| $A_3$ | 1936 | Believed to be an allele, $A_3$, at the ABO locus |
| $A_m$ | 1942 | Originally called $A_x$. Some result from inheritance of a gene $A_m$, an allele at the ABO locus. Others demonstrate that the phenotype can result from a double dose (homozygous state) of a rare, recessive, modifying gene, y. Serologically, RBCs of the $A_y$ phenotypes are indistinguishable from the $A_m$ phenotype |
| $A_{end}$ | 1959 | Results from the inheritance of an allele at the ABO locus |
| $A_{el}$ | 1964 | Thought to result from inheritance of an allele at the ABO locus |
| $A_{bantu}$ | 1966 | Controlled by a variant gene that resides at the ABO locus. |
| $A_{finn}$ | 1973 | This subgroup is very likely $A_{end}$ |

## Modifying Genes

### A Superactive *B* Gene

In some AB people with relatively few A antigen sites on their erythrocytes, the deficit of A antigen is believed to be caused by the presence of a superactive B transferase, coded for by a superactive *B* gene, that competes with normal $A_1$ or $A_2$ transferase. Predominantly Black populations have the highest frequency of this atypical B gene.

### $O_h$: The Bombay Phenotype

In 1952, a new phenotype within the ABO system was recognized. It was initially believed that in normal persons an additional gene was necessary for the *A* or *B* gene to be expressed as A or B antigen. This gene, originally called X by Levine, was viewed as possibly acting as a suppressor. In Bombay, it was hypothesized that the X (H) gene was not present, but its allele x (h) (in a homozygous state) prevented the production of A or B antigenic expression.

Defining the biochemical composition of the H, A, and B antigens was essential to interpreting the identity of the *X* and *H* genes. When the roles of H gene-specified transferase in adding L-fucose to precursor substance and A and B gene-specified transferase in adding the immunodominant monosaccharides of A and B antigens were understood, it was concluded that the X and H genes were the same.

The gene was designated Bombay. Afflicted persons of the Bombay type have an *hh* genotype and an $O_h$ phenotype. The alleles Hh and ABO have been demonstrated to segregate independently. The $O_h$ phenotype can carry *A* or *B* genes, but these genes do not express themselves

**Table 4-13. Race and Sanger Classification of Erythrocyte Reactions of B Subgroups**

| | Category I | Category II | Category III |
|---|---|---|---|
| Anti-B | Weak | Weak | Weak |
| Anti-A,B | Weak | Weak | Weak |
| Serum | Anti-B | Absent | Absent |
| Saliva (of secretors) | B,H | B,H | H |
| | | | B* |

* B may be present in decreased amounts but is usually negative.

as A or B antigens on the erythrocytes of the $O_h$ persons because of the lack of *H* gene and consequent lack of H-bearing structures on the erythrocytic membrane. Therefore, the lack of demonstrable A or B antigens on $O_h$ erythrocytes is a function of the lack of a suitable acceptor site. If, however, an *A* or *B* gene is transmitted to offspring with an *H* gene being received from the other parent, the offspring can have normal A or B antigenic expression (see Fig. 4-1).

The $O_h$ phenotype erythrocytes have normal in vivo survival. There is also no reason to assume that $O_h$ erythrocytes lack anything but the terminal carbohydrates normally attached to the erythrocytic membrane-borne glycolipids and glycoproteins.

In the laboratory, the erythrocytes of the $O_h$ phenotype are not agglutinated by anti-A, anti-B, anti-A,B, or anti-H reagent antisera. The H gene-specified fucosyl transferase is not present in the sera of $O_h$ persons. If anti-H is produced by $O_h$ persons, it is usually more potent at 37° C, in comparison to anti-H produced by $A_1$ or B persons, which is typically a cold-reacting antibody of no clinical significance. Group O erythrocytes must *never* be transfused to an $O_h$ person because of the potential of sensitization and subsequent anti-H production in $O_h$ persons from the H antigen of group O donors.

### $A_h$ and Similar Phenotypes

A or B antigens may, on rare occasions, develop in the absence of H. Different groups of investigators claim to have found hidden H (and/or A and B) antigens on $O_h$ erythrocytes with traces of A and B antigens that are detectable in direct tests.

In 1961, Levine et al. described a person in whom the erythrocytes failed to react with anti-H, but did react weakly with anti-A. The serum contained anti-B and an anti-H antibody that was active at 37° C, but the saliva did not contain ABH substances. Other family members were secretors. The name $A_h$ was applied to this phenotype as parallel to $O_h$.

Levine hypothesized that the $A_h$ phenotype was caused by a partial suppressor at the Hh locus that prevented normal quantities of H substance from being produced.

He concluded that whatever H substance was produced was converted to A substance by action of the *A* gene. This theory provided an explanation for the absence or decreased amount of detectable H substance. Most transferase assays have supported this line of reasoning, but a deficiency of erythrocytic membrane-borne H antigen can occasionally occur even though a person has a normal level of H gene-specified transferase enzyme in the serum. It is possible that variants in the H gene also exist.

Some investigators theorize that an alternative pathway exists for the formation of A (and perhaps B) antigens on the erythrocyte membrane. It is believed that in the absence of H substance, the A and perhaps B gene-specified transferases can add small quantities of A- and perhaps B-immunodominant monosaccharides.

## $A_m$ Phenotype

Families have been identified that are believed to be genetically $A_1$ or $A_2$ but do not express the $A_1$ or $A_2$ phenotype. Individuals from these families have been classified as $A_m$ phenotype, which results from a homozygous state of a rare, recessive, modifying gene, y. This modifying gene is inherited independently of the *ABO* genes. The common gene, Y, is necessary for normal expression of the A antigen, and the absence of a *Y* gene (*yy*) results in decreased expression of A antigen on erythrocytes. The absence of a *Y* gene does not usually affect the secretion of A substance, nor is the expression of B antigen on erythrocytes usually altered.

## A Dominant Suppressor Gene

In 1973, the presence of a dominant suppressor of A and B was noted. In the presence of this dominant suppressor, erythrocytes were typed as group O, but the serum lacked anti-A. Saliva of secretors contained both A and H substances. It is believed that afflicted persons are genetically $A_1 O$.

## The *AB* cis Gene

Individuals carrying an *AB*-cis gene were first observed because of an anomaly of inheritance of the ABO groups. In these cases, the *A* and *B* genes seem to have been inherited on a single chromosome (Fig. 4-4). The term *AB*-cis gene is used to describe this rare situation, which is be-

lieved to result from unequal crossing over at the *ABO* locus. Both an *A* gene on one chromosome and a *B* gene on the other are involved. The resultant new *AB* cis gene is composed of part of the genetic information normally carried by the *A* gene and part of the *B* gene. *AB* cis gene products include the transferases normally expected as products of *A* and *B* genes.

The A and B antigens on erythrocytes of persons genetically AB/O are not as strong as those on the erythrocytes of persons genetically A/B. Many of the phenotypes resulting from the AB cis gene have been characterized as $A_2B$, with the B antigen reacting more weakly than usual.

Other instances of similar phenotypes caused by AB cis can include an $A_{weak}B$ phenotype, in which a B gene-specified transferase enzyme was so productive that it added galactose to most of the H-bearing receptors before the slower-acting $A_2$ gene-specified transferase could add galactosamine.

## Acquired Antigens

### Acquired A Antigen

Acquired A antigen has been reported in persons of type O or type B in association with severe aseptic infections caused by *Proteus mirabilis*. In these conditions, reactions with anti-A reagent are visible microscopically as mixed-field agglutination.

Tn-activated erythrocytes can demonstrate the presence of an acquired A antigen. The reason that group O or group B Tn-activated erythrocytes react with some anti-A reagents is that, like the A antigen, the immunodominant monosaccharide of Tn is N-acetyl-galactosamine. This phenomenon is rare and represents a type of polyagglutinability. Tn activation of erythrocytes is permanent and not associated with bacterial or viral infections.

### Acquired B Antigen

Acquired B-like antigen was first recognized in 1959 in association with conditions such as carcinoma of the colon or rectum, intestinal obstruction, massive infection of the lower gastrointestinal tract, and septicemia caused by *Proteus vulgaris*. After recovery from the condition or infection, the acquired B-like antigen is lost and the patient reverts to normal blood status. This phenomenon is infrequently observed in healthy individuals.

The acquisition of B antigen usually occurs in persons of the $A_1$ phenotype. It is infrequent in those of the $A_2$ phenotype, and is not known to occur in type O persons. One theory of acquisition of the acquired B antigen is that deacetylation of the $A_1$ antigen by bacterial enzymes takes place and causes a change in the antigen. The number of A receptor sites diminishes as the number of B receptor sites increases. Acetylation of the acquired B antigen results

**Figure 4-4.** Cis-AB phenotype. The cis-AB phenotype results from the inheritance of both A and B genes from one parent and a normal O gene from the other parent.

in the loss of B activity and the reappearance of the $A_1$ antigen that has been deacetylated. Because the difference between the A and B antigens involves the substitution of only the terminal immunodominant monosaccharide, the change from $A_1$ antigen to B antigen by deacetylation can be explained. The greater number of antigen sites on $A_1$ compared to $A_2$ erythrocytes explains why acquired B antigens are almost always found in group $A_1$ individuals.

A second mechanism of antigen formation may exist. An acquired B antigen can result from increased permeability of the intestinal wall and subsequent adsorption of the bacterial polysaccharide (*Escherichia coli* $O_{86}$) on the erythrocyte. Some types of bacteria produce lipopolysaccharides that include B-like structures. The passive adsorption of these materials by erythrocytes can result in the cells acquiring a B-like antigen with no reduction of A antigen in the case of $A_1$ and $A_2$ erythrocytes. It should be noted that this mechanism has never been established as a route for the in vivo acquisition of B antigen.

The presence of acquired B-like antigen is occasionally associated with polyagglutination of erythrocytes. A state of polyagglutination involving acquired B-like antigen may be restricted to cases in which the acquired antigen represents deacetylation of A. B-like antigen can be suspected when observing a very slowly-reacting and weak appearing agglutination pattern with anti-B typing sera compared to true group B erythrocytes. In these cases, the patient's serum contains a form of anti-B that fails to react with autologous cells or with those from others with an acquired B-like antigen, but reacts with all normal group B erythrocytes. Eluates made from erythrocytes that have acquired B-like antigen do not usually contain anti-B. An anti-B lectin, *Bandeirae simplicifolia* (modified BS-1 lectin), has the ability to differentiate true B antigens from acquired B-like antigens on erythrocytes. Modified BS-1 lectin does not agglutinate acquired B antigens but does agglutinate true B antigens. This lectin is not widely available. If anti-B typing sera is acidified to pH 6.0, it agglutinates only true B antigens.

## Altered Antigens

All normal adult sera contain varying levels of naturally occurring antibodies such an anti-T, anti-Tn, and anti-Cad. These antibodies rarely react with erythrocytes that may have inherited or acquired surface abnormalities that produce polyagglutination. Polyagglutination is defined as the agglutination of erythrocytes by most normal human sera. Three types of polyagglutination include the following:

1. T-activation
2. Tn-activation
3. Cad polyagglutinability

Polyagglutinable cells react with these antibodies either because they have acquired antigenic reactivity or because the donor has inherited an unusual antigen such as Cad.

## T Activation

All normal erythrocytes possess antigens that are not usually detectable by routine blood banking methods. T activation or the unmasking of these "hidden antigens" is usually a temporary condition caused by the removal of sialic acid and exposure of the T antigen because of the action of microbial neuraminidase. Organisms that produce neuraminidase include bacteria, particularly *Bacteroides* and *Clostridium*, as well as protozoa, yeast, and viruses (predominantly influenza). When the causative infection subsides, the erythrocytes are usually no longer T-activated or polyagglutinable.

All normal adult sera contain anti-T; therefore T-activated erythrocytes are polyagglutinable. The reaction of T-activated erythrocytes and serum demonstrates a pattern of mixed-field agglutination. T-activated erythrocytes are not agglutinated by cord serum because the latter lacks anti-T; nor are they agglutinated by the person's own serum, because the serum antibody is not an autoantibody. Additionally, T-activated erythrocytes fail to be aggregated by polybrene. It is possible to obtain a correct ABO typing by preparing T-activated cells and allowing them to absorb the anti-T from the typing sera.

## Tn Activation

The Tn antigen is not demonstrated on normal erythrocytes, and all normal sera contain the corresponding antibody. The activation of the Tn antigen is rather uncommon and possibly results from insufficient addition of sialic acid during erythrocyte maturation. Conditions associated with Tn activation include hematologic abnormalities such as hemolytic anemia, leukocytopenia, and thrombocytopenia.

Tn activation of erythrocytes is a permanent alteration and cannot be simulated in vitro. Although these altered cells are agglutinated by *Dolichos biflorus* extract, Tn activation can be identified by using extracts for *Salvia sclarea* or *Salvia haematodes* seeds.

Tn-activated cells and T-activated cells share the following characteristics

1. Reduced erythrocytic membrane sialic acid content
2. A mixed-field agglutination pattern with all normal adult sera
3. No agglutination with cord serum
4. No agglutination with polybrene
5. Reduced M and N surface antigen

The correct ABO status of a person can be determined by treating the Tn-activated cells with 1% ficin or papain to destroy the Tn receptor sites.

## Cad Polyagglutinability

Cad cells are polyagglutinable because they carry an extraordinary quantity of the $Sd^a$ antigen; most cells have a much smaller amount of this antigen. Most sera contain trace amounts of anti-Sd$^a$; therefore, Cad cells are readily agglutinated because of the large quantity of Sd$^a$ surface antigen present. Cad cells are more strongly agglutinated by *Dolichos biflorus* extract than group A$_1$ erythrocytes. Unlike Tn-activated cells, the Cad receptor is not destroyed by enzyme treatment, but may actually be enhanced. The diagnosis of Cad polyagglutination is made by exclusion, aided by the reaction of the seed extract of *Salvia horminum*. This extract agglutinates both Tn and Cad polyagglutinable erythrocytes.

### High Levels of Soluble ABH Substances

Rarely, in conditions such as ovarian cysts, carcinoma of the stomach or pancreas, or intestinal obstruction, excess amounts of blood group-specific substances can be observed. The level of ABH substance in a person's serum may be so high that it inhibits the anti-A or anti-B reagent serum. This interference with ABO grouping is caused by neutralization of the reagent anti-A or anti-B by the specific soluble substances, which leaves no unbound antibody to react with the person's erythrocytes. This situation can produce false-negative or weak reactions in the antigen typing of erythrocytes. Washing the patient's red cells can prevent neutralization.

### Depression of A, B, and H Antigens

#### Antigenic Weakening Caused by Disease

Weakening of the A antigen has been noted in patients with leukemia or lymphoma. The subscript g as in A$_g$ has been used to indicate an antigen weakened by the leukemic process. The B and H antigens can also be depressed, but, in some cases, as the level of A or B antigen has decreased, the level of H antigen detectable on erythrocytes has been seen to increase. In addition to antigenic alteration associated with leukemia, similar findings have been observed in Hodgkin's and non-Hodgkin's lymphoma and in refractory anemias associated with abnormal erythrocytic enzymes.

#### Antigenic Weakening in Group AB

Errors of interpretation can occur in cases of subgroups of A antigen in association with the B antigen in the AB phenotype. The phenotype A$_2$B is sometimes mistakenly designated as A$_3$B because of the weakening of the A antigen in the presence of B.

The weakened form of A in A$_2$B blood is caused by transferase activity. It has been found that in the genotype A$_1$B, the A$_1$ and B gene-specified transferases are about equal in terms of efficiency in adding immunodominant sugars to H-bearing chains. In the genotype A$_2$B or other weak forms of A and B, (A$_x$B) the *B* gene-specified trans-

ferase is more efficient than A. Consequently, more H-bearing chains receive galactose (the B immunodominant monosaccharide) than receive galactosamine (the A immunodominant monosaccharide). In the absence of B gene-specified transferase such as the genotype A$_2$O, no competition exists and more galactosamine is added to H chains. Therefore, A$_2$ erythrocytes carry more A antigen sites than the A$_2$B phenotype.

The most reliable way of correctly determining affected AB persons is to carry out family studies. In some of these cases, the products of the A gene may be found in a family member who lacks the B gene.

#### Mixtures of Blood

In 1975 it was found that some individuals who were not genetic blood group *chimeras* had two populations of erythrocytes, group O and group A. Alleles at the ABO locus were found to be responsible. The ABO-mos phenotype, as these cases are designated, is transmitted to different generations within the families.

## ANTIBODIES OF THE ABO BLOOD GROUP SYSTEM

Landsteiner reasoned from his observations that most individuals possess antibodies directed against the antigens that are absent from their own cells (see Table 4-1). These antibodies were called "naturally occurring," but this term is really a misnomer. Scientific evidence supports the fact that anti-A and anti-B are stimulated by agents such as bacteria, pollen, or other substances present in the internal or external environment that have molecular configurations similar to the A and B antigen. The wide distribution of these agents ensures constant exposure to A, B, and H-like antigens. Consequently, the immune response to noncellular antigenic stimulation results in the production of the complementary IgM antibodies (anti-A and/or anti-B) in immunologically competent individuals. The predictable relationship between antigens and antibodies in the ABO system permits the use of both serum and cell tests in ABO grouping.

### Development of Anti-A and Anti-B

Antibody production is initiated at birth by exposure to foreign substances such as bacteria, pollen, and dust. Initially, antibody titers are usually too low for serologic detection and do not increase until the age of 3 to 6 months. If antibodies are detected in a newborn or young infant, they are probably of maternal origin. Serum from newborn infants may contain IgG antibodies passively acquired by placental transfer from the mother if she has IgG anti-A or anti-B. Anti-A and anti-B production increases for the first 5 or 6 years and then remains fairly constant until late in adult life. In elderly people, the titer of anti-A and anti-B is often much lower than in young adults.

The strength (titer) of antibodies varies considerably from sera to sera. In general, the strength of anti-A in group B and group O sera tends to be greater than anti-B in group A and group O sera. With the exception of group AB serum, complete absence of anti-A, anti-B, or both is rare.

## Antibody Characteristics

The antibodies of the ABO blood group system have similar characteristics, including the following:

1. Agglutination of saline suspended erythrocytes.
2. Reactivity at room temperature.
3. Production of hemolysis in vivo and in vitro. Both IgM and IgG anti-A and anti-B are capable of binding complement. All examples of IgG anti-A and about 90% of IgM anti-A have been demonstrated to be hemolytic.
4. Inactivation of IgM anti-A and anti-B with 2-mercaptoethanol (2-ME).

Antibodies to the A and B antigens are generally divided into two classes: IgM, if environmentally stimulated, and IgG, if stimulated by foreign erythrocytes. IgG stimulation can result from the transfusion of ABO-incompatible erythrocytes, receipt of plasma containing blood group substances, or maternal-fetal ABO incompatibility.

Anti-A produced by group B individuals and anti-B produced by group A individuals are predominantly composed of IgM molecules, with small quantities of IgG molecules also being presented in the sera of these two groups. IgG is the predominant form of anti-A and anti-B in the sera of group O persons.

If complement is present, erythrocytes may be hemolyzed because of the presence of A or B antigens and their corresponding antibodies. ABO antibodies that produce hemolysis bind to short-chain structures on the erythrocytic membrane and act as hemolysins both in vivo and in vitro. Anti-A and anti-B efficiently activate complement because complement is activated close to the cell membrane, which facilitates the binding of many of the activated complement components to the membrane before they decay.

In vitro hemolysis can produce either a pink discoloration of the supernatant fluid or total destruction of the erythrocytes after centrifugation. Because hemolysis requires complement, it will not occur if an anticoagulant such as calcium-chelating EDTA is present (see Chapter 3 for a discussion of complement).

Anti-A and anti-B can coat erythrocytes without producing agglutination. Coating antibodies are usually IgG. When a patient's serum contains both coating and agglutinating antibodies of the same specificity, agglutination is the only detectable end point unless the agglutinating antibodies are neutralized or inactivated in some way.

## Anti-A,B (Group O)

Serum from type O persons contains the antibody anti-A,B. When type A erythrocytes are used for absorbing anti-A from type O serum, the eluate contains anti-A and anti-A,B, which reacts with both A and B erythrocytes. Similar reactions are observed when B cells are used for absorption. Saliva from group A or group B secretors inhibits the reaction of this antibody with either A or B erythrocytes.

Anti-A,B from group O serum reacts more strongly than anti-A or anti-B with erythrocytes of some A and B subgroups. Although AABB standards do not require the use of anti-A,B or any other procedure to detect weak A or B phenotypes, some laboratories use reagent anti-A,B to check ABO groupings. This procedure is performed to avoid labelling blood as group O when it is a subgroup of A or B. Anti-A,B can be used alone as the required procedure to reconfirm the ABO status of group O erythrocytes before transfusion.

## Anti-A$_1$

The anti-A in group O and group B sera has been observed to contain separable anti-A and anti-A$_1$. By absorbing anti-A serum with A$_2$ erythrocytes, reactivity against A$_1$, but no A$_2$ cells remains. The apparent anti-A$_1$ remaining in serum after absorption with A$_2$ erythrocytes is believed to be a weakened form of anti-A. It is believed that individuals with A$_2$ cells that carry A$_a$ and A$_b$, but no or only low levels of A$_c$ and A$_d$, might form anti-A$_1$. Anti-A$_1$ might possibly have an anti-A$_{cd}$ specificity, and A$_c$ and A$_d$ might be missing or present in small amounts more often in A$_2$B erythrocytes than in A$_2$ cells. This theory might explain the higher incidence of anti-A$_1$ in persons who are A$_2$B than in persons who are A$_2$.

## Anti-H

There are two kinds of human anti-H. One type is a cold-reacting type antibody in the serum of persons with small amounts of H on their erythrocytes, usually group A$_1$ or AB. The other type is produced by individuals with the rare O$_h$ (Bombay) phenotype whose erythrocytes have no H antigen.

Cold-reactive anti-H is uncommon. Although all blood groups have some H substance on the erythrocytes, it is believed to be blocked by the added sugars of the A and B antigens. Group O and A$_2$ phenotypes are not associated with the production of anti-H. Occasionally, group A$_1$, A$_1$B or, less commonly, group B erythrocytes have such a small amount of unconverted H substance that individuals with this phenotype can produce weakly reacting anti-H. The concept that H is covered on A$_1$ and B cells is supported by the finding that erythrocytes of the subgroups of A lower than A$_2$ have levels of H roughly similar to those on O cells, which have none of the H chains covered by other carbohydrates.

Quantities of H Antigen in Diminishing Order

$$O > A_2 > A_2B > B > A_1 > A_1B$$

As expected, group O erythrocytes react more strongly with anti-H reagent sera than do group $A_2$ cells. In the case of $O_h$ persons, who completely lack the H antigen, anti-H is a frequent alloantibody. This form of anti-H reacts between 4 and 37° C and agglutinates all erythrocytes other than $O_h$. This type of anti-H binds complement and causes hemolysis. $O_h$ persons *must* be transfused with $O_h$ blood because their anti-H rapidly destroys normal group O erythrocytes.

## EXAMPLES OF DISCREPANCIES IN ABO FORWARD AND REVERSE GROUPING

Technical errors and various clinical conditions or diseases can contribute to a discrepancy between erythrocyte and serum results in ABO grouping. When the expected *forward grouping,* using known sources of reagent antisera (antibodies) to detect antigens on erythrocytes, or *reverse grouping,* using known reagent erythrocytes to test patient serum, do not produce the complementary matching of ABO antigens and antibodies, the possibility of technical error must first be excluded. Technical and clerical problems leading to falsely positive results include:

1. Contaminated reagents or dirty glassware
2. Overcentrifugation
3. Incorrect interpretation or recording of tests results

False negative results can be attributable to technical or clerical problems, such as:

1. Lack of specimen or reagents in the test system
2. An incorrect serum : cell ratio
3. Undercentrifugation or incorrect incubation temperature
4. Old or otherwise inactive reagents
5. Incorrect interpretation, such as failure to recognize hemolysis as a positive reaction, or an error in the recording of test results

If carefully controlled repeat testing yields the same agglutination patterns, the variation can be assigned to one of four categories:

1. Weak or missing antigen reactions
2. Unexpected antigen reactions
3. Weak or missing antibody reactions
4. Unexpected antibody reactions

In this section, conditions that can produce discrepancies and examples of the laboratory findings in these discrepancies are presented. This section reviews previously presented material; however, technical information and laboratory findings that have not been previously discussed are also presented. The protocol for conducting further

**Table 4-14. Example of a Weak or Missing Antigen Reaction**

| Forward Grouping | | | Reverse Grouping | | | |
|---|---|---|---|---|---|---|
| Patient's erythrocytes + Reagent antisera | | | Patient's serum + Reagent erythrocytes | | | |
| Anti-A | Anti-B | Anti-A,B | $A_1$ | B | O | Autocontrol |
| 0 | 0 | 1+ | 0 | 3+ | 0 | 0 |

In contrast to the strong reactions normally observed on forward typing, this patient demonstrated a weak reaction. Based on the reverse grouping, the patient would be expected to demonstrate A antigen activity. The weak agglutination of erythrocytes with anti-A,B, and the absence of agglutination with anti-A suggest a weak subgroup of A.

Additional Laboratory Testing

Absorption and elution tests produced anti-A from the erythrocytes. The patient's saliva contains A and H substances, although the ratio of A to H is significantly reduced.
The conclusion derived from these results is that this patient is a subgroup of A ($A_2$ phenotype).

investigations of each of these problems is presented in Chapters 14 and 15.

### Missing or Weak Antigen Reactions

Examples of conditions contributing to missing or weak antigen (Table 4-14) expression on erythrocytes include the following:

1. Subgroups of A or B antigens
2. Disease states such as leukemias
3. Excess blood group-specific soluble substances

Weak antigen reactions may be caused by the inheritance of a subgroup of A or B. Weakened A antigen expression may also result from acquired characteristics such as the changes observed in acute leukemias. The weakening of antigenic strength can occur with B and H antigens as well as antigens of other blood group systems.

### Unexpected Antigen Reactions

Examples of conditions (Table 4-15) producing unexpected reactions on forward grouping can be caused by the following:

1. Acquired A or B antigen
2. Altered antigens (T-activation, Tn-activation; Cad polyagglutinability)
3. Erythrocytes coated with antibody
4. Additives to antisera (acriflavin)
5. Mixtures of blood
6. Low incidence antigen and antibody reaction

Acquired A Antigen

Group O or group B persons with Tn-activated erythrocytes can manifest an acquired A antigen.

**Table 4-15. Example of a Typical Unexpected Antigen Reaction**

| Forward Grouping | | | Reverse Grouping | | | |
|---|---|---|---|---|---|---|
| Patient's erythrocytes + Reagent antisera | | | Patient's serum + Reagent erythrocytes | | | |
| Anti-A | Anti-B | Anti-A,B | A₁ | B | O | Autocontrol |
| 4+ | 2+ | 4+ | 0 | 4+ | 0 | 0 |

Observation of the 4+ forward and reverse grouping reactions is typical in a group A person. However, the 2+ reaction of erythrocytes with anti-B cannot be ignored. Note that the autocontrol (patient's serum + patient's cells) is negative.

Additional Laboratory Testing

A substance but not B substance was present in the saliva of the patient. Additionally, this patient had been admitted to the hospital for a severe gastrointestinal infection.

The conclusion was that the patient was group A with an acquired B-like antigen.

## Acquired B-like Antigen

The characteristics of an acquired B-like antigen are that the erythrocytes react as a group AB, while the serum contains only anti-B. The strength of the forward grouping reaction is much greater for A than B antigen, an autocontrol (patient's serum + patient's cells) is negative, and A substance is present in the saliva of secretors but B substance is not.

## Altered Antigens

In testing with *Dolichos biflorus* extract, it should be noted that lectin agglutinates Cad Sd(a⁺⁺) and Tn-activated Sd(a⁺) erythrocytes irrespective of ABO group.

## Erythrocytes Coated with Antibody

Erythrocytes that are heavily coated with antibody exhibit a positive direct antiglobulin reaction. This may produce mixed-field or weak agglutination in the forward grouping. Conditions causing this situation include autoimmune hemolytic anemia, drugs such as alpha-methyldopa, transfusion reactions, and hemolytic disease of the newborn.

This type of spontaneous agglutination reacts more weakly at room temperature during ABO testing. It is possible to remove the antibody by elution techniques, after which anti-A and anti-B can reliably be used for ABO grouping.

## Additives to Antisera

Acriflavin, the yellow dye used in some commercial anti-B reagents, can produce agglutination in some persons. This false agglutination results from antibodies against acriflavin in the serum combining with the dye and attaching to the erythrocytes of the individual.

## Mixtures of Blood

Mixture of cell types in recently transfused patients or recipients of bone marrow transplants can produce unexpected reactions in forward typing.

## Low-Incidence Antigens-Antibody Reaction

Antibodies to low-incidence antigens may be present in reagent antisera such as anti-A or anti-B. A low-incidence antibody in antisera rarely reacts with the corresponding low-incidence antigen present on a patient's or donor's erythrocytes; however, this situation should be considered when an unexpected reaction mimics the presence of a weak antigen.

## Weak and Missing Antibody Reactions

Missing or weak isoagglutinins result from depressed or absent antibody production. Missing antibody reactions (Table 4-16) on reverse grouping can be caused by the following:

1. Age
2. Hypogammaglobulinema
3. Agammaglobulinemia
4. Chimerism

### Age

Newborn and young infants and the elderly may exhibit weak or missing isoantibodies. Reverse grouping is not routinely performed on serum from newborn infants because it is unlikely that they have started to produce antibodies. Detectable antibodies in newborn or young infants are acquired in utero from the mother.

### Hypogammaglobulinemia

Decreases in the gamma globulin fraction of plasma protein, (hypogammaglobulinemia) can lead to weak or miss-

**Table 4-16. Example of a Typical Missing Antibody Reaction**

| Forward Grouping | | | Reverse Grouping | | | |
|---|---|---|---|---|---|---|
| Patient's erythrocytes + Reagent antisera | | | Patient's serum + Reagent erythrocytes | | | |
| Anti-A | Anti-B | Anti-A,B | A₁ | B | O | Autocontrol |
| 0 | 0 | 0 | 1+ | 0 | 0 | 0 |

The absence of agglutination in forward grouping suggests a group O; however, the reverse grouping suggests a group B.

Additional Laboratory Testing

Incubation of the forward and reverse typing for 30 minutes at room temperature and at 4° C demonstrated additional agglutination in the A₁ reverse grouping cells. The autocontrol remained negative.

The conclusion of this testing was that the patient was a group O with a low titer anti-A isoagglutinin.

ing antibodies. Conditions in which hypogammaglobuli-nemia may be demonstrated include the use of immunosuppressive drugs, lymphomas, leukemias, immunodeficiency disorders, and following bone marrow transplantation.

### Agammaglobulinemia

Agammaglobulinemia (absence of plasma gamma globulins) can be either congenital or acquired. Disorders such as Burton's agammaglobulinemia, immune deficiency disorders, and the effects of physical agents such as radiation exposure and cytotoxic drugs can all contribute to a state of agammaglobulinemia.

### Chimerism

Chimerism is an infrequent cause of a weak or missing ABO isoagglutinin. True chimerism is rarely found and occurs mostly in twins in whom two cell populations exist in one individual throughout his lifetime. The two cell populations are both recognized as self; consequently, these individuals do not make anti-A or anti-B and no detectable isoagglutinins are present in the serum. Chimerism in a person who has no twin may be caused by dispermy (two sperm fertilizing one egg) and indicates *mosaicism.*

Artificial or transient chimeras can be detected when group O erythrocytes are transfused to a group A or B patient after bone marrow transplant, exchange transfusion, or fetal-maternal bleeding.

### Unexpected Antibody Reactions

Conditions producing unexpected reactions on reverse grouping (Tables 4-17 through 4-19) can be caused by

1. Rouleaux formation
2. Cold autoantibodies

**Table 4-17. Example 1 of a Typical Unexpected Antibody Reaction**

| Forward Grouping | | | Reverse Grouping | | | |
|---|---|---|---|---|---|---|
| Patient's erythrocytes + Reagent antisera | | | Patient's serum + Reagent erythrocytes | | | |
| Anti-A | Anti-B | Anti-A,B | A₁ | B | O | Autocontrol |
| 4+ | 0 | 4+ | 1+ | 4+ | 0 | 0 |

The strong (4+) forward agglutination with anti-A and anti-A,B and reverse agglutination with B cells represents a typical group A reaction. The reaction with A₁ cells suggests the presence of an additional weakly reacting antibody.

Additional Laboratory Testing

The serum was tested against three examples each of A₁, A₂, and O red cells. Agglutination was observed in all of the A₁ erythrocytes but none of the A₂ or O cells. Additionally, the patient's erythrocytes were tested with anti-A lectin. The anti-A₁ lectin was negative.

The conclusion was that this patient was a group A₂ phenotype with an anti-A₁ antibody.

**Table 4-18. Example 2 of a Typical Unexpected Antibody Reaction**

| Forward Grouping | | | Reverse Grouping | | | |
|---|---|---|---|---|---|---|
| Patient's erythrocytes + Reagent antisera | | | Patient's serum + Reagent erythrocytes | | | |
| Anti-A | Anti-B | Anti-A,B | A₁ | B | O | Autocontrol |
| 4+ | 0 | 4+ | 0 | 4+ | 3+ | 0 |

Based on the 4+ agglutination pattern, a group A₁ blood is suspected; however, a slightly weaker reaction with Group O cells suggests the presence of an additional antibody.

Additional Laboratory Testing

Testing of the patient's erythrocytes with anti-A₁ lectin yielded a positive reaction. The patient's serum was tested with additional group O, A₂, A₁ cells and group O cord cells. All of the group O cells and the A₂ cells demonstrated agglutination. The additional A₁ cells were negative.

The conclusion was that the patient was a group A₁ phenotype with anti-H.

3. Unexpected ABH isoagglutinins
4. Unexpected antibodies

### Rouleaux Formation

If erythrocytes are suspended in their own serum, rouleaux formation or aggregation of erythrocytes may simulate agglutination. A variety of conditions can produce rouleaux, including abnormal concentrations of serum proteins, elevated globulin levels in diseases such as multiple myeloma, Waldenstrom's macroglobulinemia, increased fibrinogen levels, the presence of plasma expanders such as dextran, and Hodgkin's lymphoma. In cord blood samples from newborn infants, the presence of Wharton's jelly can also cause rouleaux formation.

Washing a patient's red blood cells four times in saline is usually sufficient to remove proteins that cause rouleaux. A drop of saline added to an agglutinated cell suspension may also disperse rouleaux formation.

**Table 4-19. Example 3 of a Typical Unexpected Antibody Reaction**

| Forward Grouping | | | Reverse Grouping | | | |
|---|---|---|---|---|---|---|
| Patient's erythrocytes + Reagent antisera | | | Patient's serum + Reagent erythrocytes | | | |
| Anti-A | Anti-B | Anti-A,B | A₁ | B | O | Autocontrol |
| 4+ | 4+ | 4+ | 2+ | 2+ | 2+ | 2+ |

The presence of a positive autocontrol (patient's serum + patient's erythrocytes) invalidates the initial testing results.

Additional Laboratory Testing

A cold autoabsorption method was performed and the absorbed serum was tested against A₁, B, and group O cells. No agglutination was observed with the absorbed serum and these reagent cells. The conclusion was that the patient was a group AB phenotype with an auto anti-I.

### Cold Autoantibodies

There may be unexpected autoantibodies in the serum that reacts with antigens other than the $A_1$ or B cells used for reverse grouping. Anti-I is the most commonly encountered autoantibody in reverse grouping. Anti-I usually agglutinates all erythrocytes from adult donors, including the patient's own and those used in reverse grouping. Except in fulminant cold hemagglutinin disease, the agglutination caused by anti-I is usually weaker than that caused by anti-A and anti-B. Cord cells that have less I antigen development are generally not agglutinated.

### Unexpected Isoagglutinins

Unexpected isoagglutinins in the serum can react at room temperature with the corresponding antigen present on the reagent erythrocytes. Examples of this include $A_2$ and $A_2B$ individuals who can produce "naturally occurring" anti-$A_1$, or $A_1$, and $A_1B$ individuals who may produce "naturally occurring" anti-H. Anti-$A_1$ in serum from $A_2$ or $A_2B$ persons may strongly agglutinate $A_1$ erythrocytes. Anti-H in serum from $A_1$ or $A_1B$ persons rarely causes a problem in reverse grouping because $A_1$ and B cells used for serum grouping have relatively little H.

The serum of most cis-AB persons contains a weak anti-B, which leads to an ABO discrepancy in the reverse grouping. The anti-B formed reacts with all ordinary B erythrocytes, but not with cis-AB erythrocytes.

### Unexpected Antibodies

Unexpected antibodies other than ABO isoagglutinins in a person's serum may cause a discrepancy in the reverse grouping. Reverse grouping erythrocytes possess antigens in addition to the A, B, and I antigens previously discussed. It is possible that other unexpected antibodies present in the serum will react with reagent cells. In these cases, if the screening test for antibodies with group O erythrocytes (see Chapter 7) is negative, the reverse grouping with several other examples of $A_1$ and B cells should be repeated. If the antibody reacts with an antigen so uncommon that the group O cells do not possess it, randomly selected $A_1$ and B cells can also be expected to lack the antigen.

## CHAPTER SUMMARY

### Historical Aspects of the ABO System

Landsteiner identified two erythrocyte antigens, the A and B antigens, and established the first blood group system, proposing three groups, A, B, and O. Von Decastello and Sturli identified a fourth group, AB.

### Genetic Inheritance

In 1924 Bernstein postulated the existence of three allelic genes, *A, B,* and *O.* In 1930 Thompson proposed a four-allele theory of inheritance, encompassing the four allelic genes *A1, A2, B,* and *O.*

Expression of *A* and *B* genes in erythrocytes or body fluids results from the independently inherited *Hh, Sese,* and *A* and *B* genes. Under normal circumstances, if either the *A* or *B* gene is present on either chromosome, the gene can be phenotypically demonstrated on erythrocytes. Inheritance of the *ABO* genes follows Mendelian principles with the *A* and *B* genes codominant.

### Development and Distribution of the ABO Groups

The A and B antigens are not fully developed in newborn infants but gain in strength shortly after birth. Although group O is the most common blood type, the distribution of groups A and B varies according to racial groups.

### Biochemical Activities Related to the Development of A, B, and H Antigens

Inheritance of the *A* and *B* genes usually results in their expression on erythrocytes, but the H, A, and B antigens are not direct products of the *H, A,* and *B* genes respectively. Each gene codes for the production of a specific transferase enzyme that catalyzes the transfer of a monosaccharide molecule from a donor substrate to the precursor substance.

### Secretors and Nonsecretors

Approximately 78% of persons in the United States secrete water-soluble H, H and A, or H and B antigens. Lewis system antigens can also be found in saliva. The manifestation of A, B, and H antigens in saliva or other body fluids is controlled by a secretor gene that is inherited independently of the *A, B,* and *H* genes. At least one Se gene is essential for the expression of ABH antigens in secretions.

The Se gene does not affect the formation of A, B, or H antigens on erythrocytes, nor does it control the presence of A, B, or H transferases in hematopoietic tissue. In contrast, the A or B transferase enzymes, unlike A or B antigens, are found in the secretions of $A_1$ or B persons regardless of secretor status.

The detection of small amounts of A or B antigens in the saliva of a secretor can be a useful confirmatory test in establishing a phenotype that involves a subgroup of A or B.

### Group A

Group A antigens can be differentiated into two principal subgroups, $A_1$ and $A_2$. Approximately 78% of type A individuals are $A_1$, with most of the others belonging to the $A_2$ subgroup.

The serologic distinction between $A_1$ and $A_2$ is based on the reactions of erythrocytes with various antisera. Reagent anti-A serum from human sources rarely differentiates $A_1$ and $A_2$ subtypes, but anti-A,B serum of human origin can detect common subgroups of A and B.

The distribution and characteristics of the uncommon

subgroups of the A antigen, from the strongest $A_3$ to the weakest $A_{end}$, comprise a continual curve.

### Group B

Subgroups or variants of group B are less common than subgroups of A. The incidence of B antigen subgroups is more frequent in certain racial groups.

### Abnormalities Encountered in the Expression of ABH Antigens on Erythrocytes

The expression of ABH antigens on erythrocytes may be altered by various factors. In some AB individuals, the deficit of A antigen is believed to be caused by the presence of a superactive B transferase that competes with normal $A_1$ or $A_2$ transferase. In the rare Bombay $O_h$ phenotype, individuals can carry A or B genes, but these genes do not express themselves as A or B antigens on the erythrocytes because of the lack of H gene and consequent lack of H-bearing structures on the erythrocytic membrane.

Examples of acquired A antigen have been reported in persons of group O or B in association with severe infections caused by *Proteus mirabilis*. Tn-activated erythrocytes can also demonstrate the presence of the acquired A antigen. Acquired B-like antigen has been observed in association with conditions such as carcinoma of the colon or rectum, intestinal obstruction, massive infection of the lower gastrointestinal tract, and septicemia caused by *Proteus vulgaris*. Erythrocytes may have inherited or acquired surface abnormalities that produce polyagglutination. The three types of polyagglutination are T activation, Tn activation, and Cad polyagglutinability.

Weakening of the A antigen has been noted in leukemia. The B and H antigens can also be depressed but, in some cases, as the level of A or B antigen has decreased, the level of H antigen detectable on erythrocytes has been seen to increase.

### Antibodies of the ABO Blood Group System

Landsteiner observed that most individuals possess antibodies directed against the ABH antigens that are absent from their own cells. Although these antibodies were named "naturally occurring," scientific evidence supports the fact that anti-A and anti-B are stimulated by agents such as bacteria, pollen, or other substances present in the internal or external environment that have molecular configurations similar to the A and B antigens. The immune response to noncellular antigenic stimulation results in the production of the complementary IgM antibodies (anti-A and/or anti-B) in immunologically competent individuals, and a predictable relationship between antigens and antibodies in the ABO system permits the use of both serum and cell tests in ABO grouping.

The antibodies of the ABO blood group system are characterized by agglutination of saline-suspended erythrocytes, reactivity at room temperature, and production of hemolysis in vivo and in vitro.

There are two kinds of human anti-H. One is a cold-reacting type antibody in the serum of persons with relatively little H on their erythrocytes, usually group $A_1$ or AB. The other type is produced by individuals with the rare $O_h$ (Bombay) phenotype whose erythrocytes have no H antigen.

Technical errors and various clinical conditions or diseases can contribute to a discrepancy between erythrocyte and serum results in ABO grouping. When the expected forward and reverse results do not produce the complementary matching of ABO antigens and antibodies, the possibility of technical error must first be excluded. If technical error is excluded, the discrepancy may be due to weak or missing antigen reactions, unexpected antigen reactions, weak or missing antibody reactions, or unexpected antibody reactions.

### Examples of Discrepancies in ABO Forward and Reverse Grouping

Examples of conditions contributing to missing or weak antigen expression on erythrocytes include subgroups of A or B antigens, disease states, and excess blood group-specific soluble substances. Unexpected antigen reactions can be due to acquired A or B antigen, altered antigens, erythrocytes coated with antibody, additives to antisera, mixtures of blood, and low-incidence antigen and antibody reactions.

Weak or missing antibody reactions can be caused by depressed or absent antibody production. Conditions producing missing antibody reactions include age, hypogammaglobulinemia, agammaglobulinemia, and chimerism.

Unexpected antibody reactions can be caused by rouleaux formation, cold autoantibodies, unexpected ABH isoagglutinins, and unexpected antibodies.

### REVIEW QUESTIONS

1. The discoverer of the ABO system was:
   A. Weiner
   B. Landsteiner
   C. von Decastello
   D. Sturli

2–5. Match the following blood types with the respective erythrocytic antigens:

| Blood Type | Antigen(s) |
|---|---|
| 2. A | A. Both A and B antigens |
| 3. B | B. A antigen |
| 4. AB | C. Neither A nor B antigens |
| 5. O | D. B antigen |

6–9. Match the following blood types with their complementary antibodies:

| Blood Type | Antibody/Antibodies |
|---|---|
| 6. A | A. anti-A |
| 7. B | B. anti-B |
| 8. AB | C. Both anti-A and anti-B |
| 9. O | D. Neither anti-A nor anti-B |

**10–12.** Match the given phenotypes with their respective genotypes:

| Phenotype | Genotype |
|-----------|----------|
| **10.** $A_1$ | **A.** $A_2/A_2$ |
| **11.** $A_2$ | **B.** $A_1/A_2$ |
| **12.** O | **C.** O/O |

**13.** From the following ABO mating, what are the probabilities of the ABO phenotypes of potential offspring? Mother: Group O; Father: Group B (heterozygous)
   **A.** 50% BO, 50% OO
   **B.** 100% BO
   **C.** 50% B, 50% O
   **D.** 50% BO, 50% AO

**14.** The greatest number of antigen sites on erythrocytic membranes is found in _____ phenotype.
   **A.** Cord blood $A_1$        **C.** Adult $A_1$
   **B.** Cord blood B        **D.** Adult $A_2$

**15.** The most frequent phenotype in all races is type:
   **A.** A        **C.** O
   **B.** B        **D.** $A_1B$

**16.** The frequency of phenotype B is more than 15% in:
   **A.** Whites
   **B.** Blacks
   **C.** Orientals
   **D.** Both B and C

**17–20.** Match the genes with their specific transferase.

| Genes | Enzymes |
|-------|---------|
| **17.** H | **A.** [α]-L-fucosyltransferase |
| **18.** A | **B.** α–3–N–acetylgalactosaminyltransferase |
| **19.** B | **C.** α–3–D–Galactosyltransferase |
| **20.** O | **D.** None |

**21–23.** Referring to the figure below, match the immunodominant monosaccharide residual with the appropriate antigen.

| Antigen | Immunodominant monosaccharide |
|---------|-------------------------------|
| **21.** H | **A.** N-acetyl-D-galactosamine |
| **22.** A | **B.** D-galactose |
| **23.** B | **C.** L-fucose |

**Figure for Questions 21–23:**

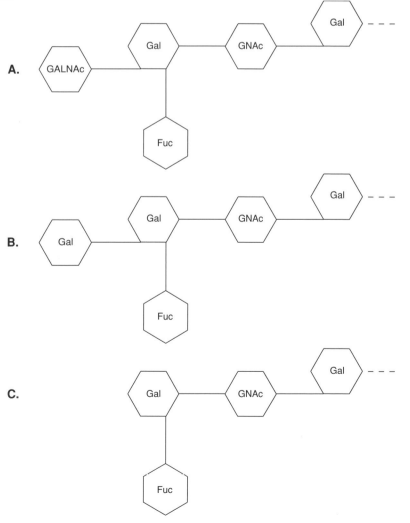

**24.** Most of the H, A, and B antigens that are synthe-
sized on the erythrocytic membrane are attached
to:
   **A.** Glycospingolipids
   **B.** Glycoconjugates
   **C.** Glycoproteins
   **D.** Either A or C

**25.** Referring to the figure below, identify the type 1
chain present in blood group active substances.

**26.** A, B, and H antigens are acquired by:
   **A.** Synthesis by erythrocytic precursors
   **B.** Synthesis during lymphocytic development
   **C.** Insertion into the erythrocytic membrane
        from the plasma
   **D.** Both A and C

**27.** Approximately _____% of persons in the
United States are secretors of water soluble ABH
substances.
   **A.** 10%
   **B.** 20%
   **C.** 50%
   **D.** 80%

**28.** Which of the following genotypes is characteris-
tic of a nonsecretor?
   **A.** SeSe
   **B.** Sese
   **C.** sese
   **D.** Both A and B

**29–32.** Identify the product(s) found in the saliva of the
following:
   **A.** B, H
   **B.** A, B, H
   **C.** H only
   **D.** No A, B, or H

**Figure for Question 25:**

beta (1–3) Linkage

beta (1–4) Linkage

ABO
| Group | Secretor Status | Secretion |
|---|---|---|
| O | SeSE or Sese | No. 29 |
| $A_1$ | sese | No. 30 |
| AB | SeSe or Sese | No. 31 |
| $O_h$ | SeSe | No. 32 |

**33.** The $A_1$ phenotype comprises approxi-
mately _____% of all A phenotypes.
   **A.** 15%
   **B.** 35%
   **C.** 56%
   **D.** 78%

**34.** Adsorbed anti-$A_1$ will agglutinate _____ eryth-
rocytes.
   **A.** $A_1$
   **B.** $A_2$
   **C.** Weak subgroups of A
   **D.** Both A and B

**35.** The frequency of anti-$A_1$ is highest in type:
   **A.** $A_1$
   **B.** $A_2$
   **C.** B
   **D.** $A_2B$

**36.** With a few exceptions, secretors of the infre-
quent subgroups of A have _____ in their sa-
liva.
   **A.** Only H
   **B.** A and H
   **C.** A, B and H
   **D.** A, B, H, and Se

**37.** A mixed-field agglutination pattern with anti-B
and anti-A,B typing sera is characteristic of type:
   **A.** B
   **B.** $B_3$
   **C.** $B_m$
   **D.** $B_x$

**38.** The highest frequency of the superactive *B* gene
occurs in the _____ population.
   **A.** Oriental
   **B.** Oriental in Taiwan
   **C.** Black
   **D.** Caucasian

**39.** Individuals with the Bombay phenotype have the
following genotype:
   **A.** HH
   **B.** Hh
   **C.** hh
   **D.** Either HH or Hh

**40.** The $A_m$ phenotype is believed to result from:
   **A.** Absence of an H gene
   **B.** Absence of a Y gene
   **C.** Inheritance of the yy genotype
   **D.** Both B and C

**41.** The AB cis genotype is:
   **A.** AB
   **B.** $A_xB$

**C.** A$_3$B
**D.** ABO

**42–46.** Match the following conditions with answer **A** or answer **B.**
  **A.** Acquired A antigen
  **B.** Acquired B antigen
  **42.** Demonstrated by Tn-activated erythrocytes
  **43.** Can be associated with *Proteus vulgaris*
  **44.** Can be associated with *Proteus mirabilis*
  **45.** Usually associated with the A$_1$ phenotype
  **46.** Represents deacetylation of A antigen

**47–50.** Match the following characteristics with the respective altered antigen condition. An answer may be used more than once.
  **A.** T activation
  **B.** Tn activation
  **C.** Both T and Tn activation
  **47.** Is a permanent alteration
  **48.** Fails to react with cord serum
  **49.** Demonstrates a mixed-field agglutination with all normal sera
  **50.** Produced by bacteria or viruses

**51.** The Cad receptor is:
  **A.** Not destroyed by enzyme treatment
  **B.** Possibly enhanced by enzyme treatment
  **C.** Not agglutinated by *Dolichos biflorus*
  **D.** Both A and B

**52.** Weakening of the A antigen may be observed in:
  **A.** Leukemia
  **B.** Tn-activated erythrocytes
  **C.** Cad polyagglutinability
  **D.** Bacterial infections

**53–56.** Match the following characteristics:
  **53.** "Naturally occurring" antibodies   **A.** Low antibody titer
  **54.** Infants up to 6 months of age   **B.** Anti-A titer higher than anti-B titer
  **55.** IgG   **C.** Dust, pollen, bacteria
  **56.** Group O persons   **D.** Stimulated by foreign erythrocytes

**57–61.** Select either answer **A** (true) or **B** (false) for whether the following are characteristics of Anti-A *and* anti-B.
  **57.** Agglutinate in saline-suspended erythrocytes
  **58.** Require 37° C to agglutinate
  **59.** Do not produce in vivo or in vitro hemolysis
  **60.** Are capable of binding complement
  **61.** Can be inactivated by treatment with 2-mercaptoethanol (2-ME)

**62.** The phenotype with the greatest amount of H antigen on the erythrocytic membrane is:
  **A.** O
  **B.** A$_2$

**C.** A$_2$B
**D.** B

**63–66.** Match the following conditions with the reaction they can produce or simulate:
  **63.** Additives to antisera   **A.** Missing or weak antigen
  **64.** Hypogammaglobulinema   **B.** Unexpected antigen
  **65.** Rouleaux formation   **C.** Missing or weak antibody
  **66.** Subgroups of A   **D.** Unexpected antibody

**67–70.** Match the following conditions with the appropriate reactions.
  **67.** Tn activation   **A.** Missing or weak antigen
  **68.** Related to age   **B.** Unexpected antigen
  **69.** Excess blood group specific soluble substances   **C.** Missing or weak antibody
  **70.** Cold autoantibodies   **D.** Unexpected antibody

**Bibliography**

Dracker, R.A., Lavenstein, K.J., and Davey, F.R.: Immunohematology, in Clinical Diagnosis and Management by Laboratory Methods, 18th ed. John B. Henry (Ed.), Philadelphia, Saunders, 1991, 976–1011.
Drozda, E.A., Jr., and Dean, J.D.: Another example of the rare A$_y$ phenotype. Transfusion, 25(3):280–281, 1985.
Economidous, J., Hughes-Jones, N.C., and Gardner, B.: Quantitative measurements concerning A and B antigen sites. Vox Sang., 12:321, 1967.
Eversole, M.B., Nonemaker, K., Zurek, S., and Simon, T.: Uneventful administration of plasma products in a recipient with T-activated red cells. Transfusion, 26(2):182–185, 1986.
Frederick, J., Hunter, J., Greenwell, P., et al.: the A$^1$B genotypes expressed A$^2$B on the red cells of individuals with strong B gene-specific transferases. Transfusion, 25(1):30–33, 1985.
Gergal, A., Maslet, C., and Salmon, C.: Immunological aspects of the acquired B antigen. Vox Sanguin. 28:398–403, 1975.
Hall, S., Olekna, D., and Davies, D.: Production of unique monoclonal ABO blood grouping antisera. Transfusion, 25(5):448, 1985.
Lin-Chu, M., Broadberry, R.E., and Chiou, P.W.: The B$_3$ phenotype in Chinese. Transfusion, 26(5):428–430, 1986.
Mallory, D.M.: Problems in the hemagglutination reactions. Part 1: False positive reactions due to drugs, dyes, and interfering substances. *In* A Seminar on Polymorphisms in Human Blood. Washington, D.C., American Association of Blood Banks, 1975. pp. 129–141.
Mollison, P.L.: Blood Transfusion in Clinical Medicine. 7th Ed. Oxford, Blackwell Scientific Publications, 1983.
Vengelen-Tyler, V., and Gonzalez, B.: Reticulocyte rich RBCs will give weak reactions with many blood typing antisera. Transfusion, 25(5):476, 1985.
Wittels, E.G., and Lichtman, H.C.: Blood group incidence and *Escherichia coli* bacterial sepsis. Transfusion, 26(6):533–535, 1986.

# The Rh Blood Group System

## THE Rh SYSTEM

Many of the blood group systems in humans are highly complex. The purpose of this chapter is to present and discuss these systems at the level of general use.

The Rh system was identified in 1940 by Landsteiner and Wiener. This discovery followed the detection of an antibody by Levine and Stetson in 1939 in the mother of a stillborn infant who had been transfused with her husband's blood during pregnancy. Originally, Landsteiner and Wiener found that human erythrocytes were agglutinated by this antibody to an antigen apparently common to all rhesus monkeys and 85% of humans. This factor was named the Rh factor. Later the antigens detected by the rhesus antibody and by the human antibody were established as dissimilar, but the system had already been named. This contribution to medical science was the most significant event in blood group systems research since the discovery of the ABO system 40 years before.

The Rh-hr blood group system is probably the most complex of all erythrocyte blood group systems, with more than 40 different Rh antigens. The descriptive terms Rh positive and Rh negative refer *only* to the presence or absence of the red cell antigen D. The early name given to the D antigen, $Rh_o$, is less frequently used.

Four additional genes (*C, E, c,* and *e*) are recognized as belonging to the Rh system. The major allelic pairs are *C/c* and *E/e.* Many variations or combinations of the five principal genes and their products (antigens) have been recognized. These antigens and their corresponding antibodies characterize the Rh blood group system and account for the majority of Rh antibodies encountered in blood banking.

### Genetic Basis of the Rh System

Five major antigens have been observed in the Rh system: D, C, c, E, and e. C and c, as well as E and e, are antithetical but the antithetical antigen for D has never been demonstrated. The term *antithetical* refers to two antigens controlled by a pair of allelic genes. For convenience, the allelic gene to D is expressed as d.

The Rh genes reside on chromosome 1 with the *D* gene acting as an autosomal dominant. These genes that

ERYTHROCYTE BLOOD GROUP SYSTEMS

**Figure 5-1.** Theories of Rh inheritance.

determine the Rh antigens are transmitted as discrete units (Wiener) or as haplotypes (Fisher and Race). An Rh haplotype may be thought of as a single "gene" composed of nucleotide sequences within the gene that encodes multiple individual epitopes. The Fisher-Race theory states that there are three closely-linked loci, inherited as a unit, that rarely exhibit crossing over. Each of these loci contains a primary set of codominant allelic genes: *D* and the theoretic *d*, *C* and *c*, or *E* and *e* (Fig. 5-1). The gene complex of an individual is referred to as the genotype that produces an antigen complex with multiple specificities.

An alternate proposal of Rh gene inheritance by Wiener remains controversial. He proposed that multiple alleles were positioned at a single complex locus.

### Nomenclature of the Rh System

The unmodified descriptive terms Rh+ and Rh− refer to the presence or absence of the ud cell antigen D. An earlier name for D, $Rh_o$, has fallen into disuse but is of historical interest.

The CDE and Rh-hr systems of nomenclature in the Rh system are equivalent (Table 5-1). The CDE nomenclature of Fisher and Race is used almost exclusively, but it is sometimes necessary to use a combination of CDE and Rh-Hr (Weiner's Theory) terminology. In the CDE terminology of Fisher and Race, the same letter is used for both gene and gene product, but the symbols for genes are printed in italics. Traditionally, the Rh genes (and phenotypes) are expressed in the sequence *CDE*. Although the subloci sequencing is almost certainly *DCE*, both expressions of the *CDE* arrangements are acceptable. The

combination of the major Rh genes used in both the Fisher-Race and Wiener systems, their shorthand notations, and their respective frequencies, are presented in Table 5-2.

### Rh Phenotypes

In the clinical laboratory, only five reagent antisera are commonly available. Routine testing involves only the use of anti-D, although other antisera are used to resolve antibody problems or conduct family studies. The agglutination reactions of an individual's erythrocytes with specific Rh antisera produce a variety of patterns. These reactions represent the Rh phenotype (Table 5-3).

No reliable serologic method exists to distinguish between red cells with D antigen resulting from one gene and those with D antigen as the product of two genes. A person whose erythrocytes are D positive can be assigned a genotype only by inference from the frequencies with which the individual Rh gene complexes occur in the population. The racial origin of the person in question should influence deductions regarding the genotype because the frequencies of the Rh genes differ based on ethnic origin. The patient's agglutination reactions allow estimations of the probabilities of an individual Rh genotype (Table 5-4).

### Biochemical Composition of Rh Antigens

Multiple research studies agree that the Rh antigens are present on a protein structure and are probably all on the

**Table 5-1. Examples of Equivalent Nomenclature**

| Fisher-Race | Wiener | Rosenfield |
|---|---|---|
| CDE | Rh-Hr | |
| D | $Rh_o$ | Rh1 |
| C | rh′ | Rh2 |
| E | rh″ | Rh3 |
| c | hr′ | Rh4 |
| e | hr″ | Rh5 |
| f (ce) | hr | Rh6 |

**Table 5-2. Rh Nomenclature**

| Fisher-Race Terms | Shorthand Symbols | Antigens Expressed | Freq. (U.S.) | |
|---|---|---|---|---|
| | | | White | Black |
| *CDe* | $R^1$ | C, D and e | 0.42 | 0.17 |
| *cDE* | $R^2$ | c, D and E | 0.14 | 0.11 |
| *cDe* | $R^o$ | c, D and e | 0.04 | 0.44 |
| *CDE* | $R^z$ | C, D and E | rare | rare |
| *cde* | *r* | c and e | 0.37 | 0.26 |
| *Cde* | *r′* | C and e | 0.02 | 0.02 |
| *cdE* | *r″* | c and E | <0.01 | rare |
| *CdE* | *r^y* | C and E | rare | rare |

**Table 5-3. Rh Phenotypes Based on Reactions of Antisera with Erythrocytes**

| Antisera | | | | | Phenotypes | |
|---|---|---|---|---|---|---|
| Anti-D | Anti-C | Anti-E | anti-c | anti-e | Wiener | Fisher-Race |
| + | + | 0 | + | + | Rh₁rh | CcDe |
| + | + | 0 | 0 | + | Rh₁ | CDe |
| + | + | + | + | + | Rh₁Rh₂ | CcDEe |
| + | 0 | 0 | + | + | Rhₒ | cDe |
| + | 0 | + | + | + | Rh₂rh | cDEe |
| + | 0 | + | + | 0 | Rh₂ | cDE |
| + | + | + | 0 | + | Rh₂Rh₁ | CDEe |
| + | + | + | + | 0 | Rh₂Rh₂ | CcDE |
| + | + | + | 0 | 0 | Rh_z | CDE |
| 0 | 0 | 0 | + | + | rh | ce |
| 0 | + | 0 | + | + | rh'rh | Cce |
| 0 | 0 | + | + | + | rh"rh | cDe |
| 0 | + | + | + | + | rh'rh" | CcEe |

same polypeptide chain. It appears probable that membrane lipids are restricted to a supporting role at the phenotypic level. Simple antigens such as D, C, and E presumably represent certain amino acid sequences; however, antigens like G represent some of the amino acids of D and some others. Antigens such as rh are thought to represent repressed amino acids of C and e that are located adjacent in the $R^1$ and r' specified folded polypeptide, but apart when $R^2$ and r make separate polypeptides for the same cell membrane. The Rh antigens exhibit numerous serologic complexities that undoubtedly represent an extremely complicated polypeptide.

## Expression of CDE Antigens

The production or nonproduction of D, as well as the production of either C or c and E or e antigens, is genetically determined. Rh antigen sites are believed to be randomly distributed on the red cell membrane. Based on computer analysis, the distance between sites appears to be orderly, but the number of Rh antigen sites varies with

genotype (Table 5-5). The number of antigen sites can potentially influence the strength of antigenic expression. The number of D antigen sites varies from 10,000 to 33,500 per erythrocyte.

### Alteration of Genetic Expression

The expression of an inherited gene can be affected by the interaction between genes. When an Rh gene on one chromosome affects the action of another Rh gene on the same chromosome (in terms of increased or decreased antigen production), it is referred to as a *cis* effect. When an Rh gene on one of the chromosomes of a homologous pair affects the action of an Rh gene on the other homolog, it is called a *trans* effect.

The cis effect produces a weaker expression of the E antigen in the genotype cDE/cde than in cdE/cde. The most dramatic Rh trans position effect known occurs when C is trans to D (CDe/Cde), which weakens the D antigen.

***Weak Expression of D.*** Weak reactivity with anti-D antisera was previously designated by the collective term Dᵘ. Red blood cells that carry weak forms of D antigen are now called weak D. The phenotype can be written D + w. The weak D (Dᵘ) phenotype can arise in 3 different ways:

1. Suppression of D antigen expression because of genetic interaction.
2. Inheritance of a gene that codes for less D antigen
3. Absence of a genetically determined epitope that comprises the D antigen, partial D.

***Gene Suppression.*** One form of the weak D (Dᵘ) phenotype results from an alteration in genetic expression, gene suppression. It occurs when a person has a C gene on one chromosome that affects the expression of the D gene on the other. The effect of this trans position, whereby a gene on one chromosome affects the expression

**Table 5-4. Estimation of Probabilities in Rh Genotyping**

| Antisera | | | | | Possibilities | |
|---|---|---|---|---|---|---|
| Anti-D | Anti-C | Anti-E | Anti-c | Anti-e | 1st Choice | 2nd Choice |
| + | + | 0 | + | + | Cde/cde (R¹r) | CDe/cDe (R¹R⁰) |
| + | + | 0 | 0 | + | CDe/CDe (R¹R¹) | CDe/Cde (R¹r') |
| + | + | + | + | + | CDe/cDE (R¹R²) | CDe/cdE (R¹r")
CDE/cde (R²r)
cDE/cDe (R²R⁰) |
| + | 0 | 0 | + | + | cDe/cde (R⁰r) | cDe/cDe (R⁰R⁰) |
| + | 0 | + | + | + | cDE/cde (R²r) | cDE/cDe (R²R⁰) |
| + | 0 | + | + | 0 | cDE/cDE (R²R²) | cDE/cdE (R²r') |
| + | + | + | 0 | + | | |
| + | + | + | + | 0 | | |
| + | + | + | 0 | 0 | | |
| 0 | 0 | 0 | + | + | cde/cde (rr) | — |
| 0 | + | 0 | + | + | | |
| 0 | 0 | + | + | + | | |
| 0 | + | + | + | + | | |

**Table 5-5. Representative Examples of the Number of Antigen Sites on Erythrocytes***

| Phenotype | D | C | E | c | e |
|---|---|---|---|---|---|
| CDe/CDe | 14,500 to 19,500 | 46,000 to 56,500 | 0 | 0 | 18,000 to 24,500 |
| CDe/cde | 10,000 to 15,000 | 21,500 to 40,000 | 0 | 37,000 to 53,000 | 18,000 to 24,500 |
| cDE/cDE | 16,000 to 33,500 | 0 | 25,500 | 70,000 to 85,000 | 0 |
| cde/cde | 0 | 0 | 0 | 70,000 to 85,000 | 18,000 to 24,500 |

* Modified from Issitt, P.D.: Applied Blood Group. Serology, 3rd ed. Miami, FL, Montgomery Scientific, 1985.

of a gene on the paired autosome, was discussed in the preceding section.

***Genetic Inheritance.*** Some Rh genes appear to code for a weakly reactive D antigen. This form of weak D ($D^u$) is the least frequent type and simply codes for the production of less D antigen. Weak D antigen expression exhibits a pattern of Mendelian dominance. It is fairly common in Blacks. Transmission of a weak form of D is considerably less common in Whites. When it does occur, however, it is more often the product of a deviant $R^1$ (*CDe*) or $R^2$ (cDE) gene. A genetically determined weak D antigen exhibits negative or very weak reactions in direct agglutination tests with most anti-D sera but is readily detectable with anti-human globulin (AHG).

***Partial D.*** The concept of a number of genetically determined epitopes was developed and advanced to explain the fact that some people with D positive erythrocytes produced anti-D that was nonreactive with their own cells. Wiener originally proposed that the D antigen on normal D positive erythrocytes included all of the epitopes. If one or more components are missing from D positive cells, some demonstrate a positive reaction with anti-D sera and others may react weakly with anti-D. In the past, red blood cells lacking parts of the D antigen complex were referred to as "D mosaic" or "D variant." Present terminology would indicate that such red blood cells are deficient in epitopes of D; therefore, the term "partial D" is used. The important distinction between red blood cells lacking part of the D antigen, partial D or D- epitope-deficient phenotype, compared to inheritance of the weak D gene is that antigens of the epitope-deficient type are qualitatively different from normal, but weak D is quantitatively different from normal D.

Another antigen, $Go^a$, is part of the Rh system of antigens and is found on erythrocytes that lack part of the D epitope. This antigen was originally discovered in 1955 and named $D^{cor}$. When anti-$Go^a$ was described in 1967, it was not immediately recognized that the $D^{cor}$ and $Go^a$ antigens were the same and the $Go^a$ terminology persisted. The $Go^a$ antigen, which probably represents a single point mutation, is found in 1.9 to 2.8% of American Blacks. In instances of anti-$Go^a$ formation, the antibody may cause severe hemolytic disease of the newborn.

Rh positive blood very rarely lacks any of the epitope components. However, the concept that the D antigen is a structure composed of a number of genetically determined epitopes was developed to explain why some individuals

with D positive red blood cells produced anti-D that was nonreactive with their own red blood cells. Correct terminology would indicate that such red blood cells are deficient in epitopes of D, therefore, the term "partial D" is used.

### Rh Deletion Phenotypes

There are some rare *Rh* genes that behave as if portions of the genetic material have been deleted or rendered nonfunctional. The first recognized case was the D-deletion gene (D--). Since the first example, many others have been reported. Presumably the multitude of Rh genes arose from mutation. In some cases, it is assumed that some mutations arose as new mutations of previous mutants. It is also commonly believed that even the most bizarre-acting Rh genes have a close relative, or a series of predecessors, among the more common Rh genes.

***The D Deletion Gene (D--).*** D-- genes do not code for the production of some common Rh antigens such as the Cc or Ee series, but they do code for the production of D and G antigens. Homozygous individuals immunized to antigen-positive erythrocytes by means of transfusion or pregnancy can and do form antibodies of similar but not identical specificity to the missing antigens. Most often, the -D- phenotype is identified as the result of alloantibody investigations. Evans, a low-frequency antigen, is also present on the erythrocytes of individuals who inherit genes somewhat similar to D--.

***Other Gene Deletions.*** Rare genes exist that code for Rh polypeptides lacking activity at the E/e site, or at the sites of both C/c and E/e. In some cases, only D (or D and C/c) are detectable. In addition to -D-, examples of this situation are seen in the haplotypes $C^wD^-$, $cD^-$, and .D. These haplotypes are extremely uncommon. Recognition of erythrocytes that lack Rh antigens may be detected during routine testing because the D antigen may show exceptionally strong D reactivity.

***Rh Null Syndrome and Rh Mod.*** When no Rh antigens are expressed on the erythrocyte membrane, the term Rh null is used. If a less complete type of suppressed Rh gene expression is observed, the term Rh mod is used. In both of these situations, erythrocytes lacking Rh antigens have membrane abnormalities that shorten the in vivo red cell survival time. The severity of the hemolytic anemia resulting from the production of red cells with a defective protein portion in the lipoprotein molecule in the membrane varies, but Rh null persons exhibit stomatocytosis (cup-shaped red cells), and have different reaction patterns with other blood group antigens, such as S, s, and U.

rh NULL SYNDROME. This condition has been observed in at least 43 persons in 14 different families. It is produced by two different genetic mechanisms. In the more common regulator-type of Rh null, the absence of a very common regular gene $X^1$ prevents expression of normal Rh genes. Rh null persons are thought to be homozygous for $X^Q r$, a rare allele of $X^1 r$ that segregates independently of genes of the Rh system. In these cases, individuals appear to transmit normal Rh genes to their offspring, but in some cases, parents or children of individuals with the regulator-type of Rh null show overall depression of their Rh antigens.

The other, extremely rare form of Rh null occurs in persons homozygous for an amorphic gene ($\bar{r}$) at the Rh locus. The gene appears to have no detectable gene product with Rh antisera. In these cases, parents and children are heterozygous for the amorph. Their phenotypes invariably reflect the presence of a single Rh haplotype, the one inherited from the parent with normal Rh antigens. Therefore, the erythrocytes of obligate $\bar{r}$ heterozygotes will never be both C positive and c positive, nor E positive and e positive.

rh MOD. The Rh mod phenotype shares a similar genetic basis with the regulator Rh null. The term $X^Q$ has been given to the unlinked recessive modifier gene thought to be responsible for the condition. Unlike Rh null cells, those classified as Rh mod do not completely lack Rh and LW antigens (to be discussed later in this chapter); expression, however, is reduced and sometimes variable in expression.

## The e Epitope

The e antigen of some Blacks may lack one or more of the epitopes. The appearance of e-like antibodies made by e positive individuals is analogous to the anti-D made by individuals lacking a D epitope.

The e antigen is of high incidence and, in most cases, the relationship of e and anti-e is straightforward. If antibody is formed by E + e − (usually $R^2 R^2$) persons, it typically reacts with all e positive erythrocytes. In Blacks, however, the situation is different; some have red cells that type as e + but made antibodies that closely resemble anti-e (or anti-f or anti-rh₁) but do not react with the person's own red cells. The e, $hr^S$, $Hr^B$, and $hr^S$-like (Santiago antibody defined) portions of the epitope have been studied and characterized, but do not fully explain the complexity of the e epitope.

## Other Rh Antigens

Of the more than 40 identified Rh antigens (Table 5-6) only a few additional and variant antigens will be discussed in this section.

**Table 5-6. Summary of Selected Rh Antigens and Variants**

| CDE Term | Year Antigen Reported | Frequency in Population % White | Black |
|---|---|---|---|
| D | 1939 | 85 | 92 |
| C | 1941 | 70 | 33 |
| $C^w$ | 1946 | 1–2 | <1 |
| E | 1943 | 30 | 21 |
| c | 1941 | 80 | 97 |
| e | 1945 | 98 | 99 |
| V | 1955 | 2 | 30 |

## The G Antigen

In 1958, the G antigen, which does not fit neatly into the concept of three subloci of the Rh system, was defined. Almost all genes that made C or D antigens make G antigen as well. Conversely, the genes that do not make C or D usually do not make G. Some examples of erythrocytes that express at least a part of the D antigen but lack G antigen have been demonstrated. Rare cells have been discovered that possess G antigen, but lack D antigen and exhibit diminished or altered expression of C antigen.

Before 1958, questions arose about the production and serologic reactions of antibodies with apparent anti-C plus anti-D (anti-CD) specificity in rr individuals exposed to cDE or Cde erythrocytes via pregnancy or transfusion. Superficially, these antibodies appeared to be anti-C positive, D but were actually anti-G, which cannot be separated into anti-C and anti-D (Table 5-7). The fact that G appears to exist as an entity common to D and C explains why D − persons immunized by C −, D + erythrocytes sometimes appear to make anti-C + D. It may also explain why D − persons who are exposed to C + D − erythrocytes may develop antibodies appearing to contain an anti-D component.

The G antigen appears to be no more immunogenic than the C antigen. For potent anti-G to be produced, rr individuals who have already made anti-C and anti-D must be exposed to additional G positive erythrocytes before anti-G is synthesized in significantly detectable amounts.

**Table 5-7. Adsorption-Elution Technique to Recognize Anti-G**

| Process | Serum No. 1 | Serum No. 2 |
|---|---|---|
| Antibodies Present: | Anti-D, -C | Anti-D, -C, -G |
| Phenotype of RBCs for first adsorption | cDeG | cDeG |
| Antibodies in eluate | Anti-D | Anti-D, -G |
| Phenotype of RBCs for second adsorption | CdeG | CdeG |
| Antibodies in eluate | None | Anti-G |

## Compound Antigens

The term compound antigen is used to communicate the idea that certain combinations of Rh antigens demonstrate a combined effect, such as the ce or f antigen. Other examples of compound antigens include Ce, cE, and CE. These combined gene products are cis gene products and are expressed when two Rh genes are carried on the same chromosome. The CDe gene creates the C and e antigen and also produces Ce when located in the cis position. The product of the gene CDe possesses antigenic activity defined as D, C, and e. It also includes Ce, a compound product that always accompanies C and e when they are determined by the same gene. Cells having C and e determined by separate genes, for example CDE/cde, do not have the Ce antigen.

Antibodies against these compound antigens are not rare but are encountered less frequently than antibodies with single specificities. Antibodies directed against compound antigens may be concealed in serums containing antibodies of the more obvious specificities. Only absorption with erythrocytes of selected phenotypes will demonstrate their presence.

## Variant Antigens

In 1955, the V antigen was discovered. This antigen is always the product of $R^o$, $R^{ou}$ or r genes. V antigen is present on the erythrocytes of almost 30% of random American Blacks and up to 40% of individuals in other Black populations. Very few Whites have the V antigen.

Although erythrocytes from most individuals with common alloantibodies give straightforward reactions, some produce atypical reactions and others stimulate the production of alloantibodies that do not react with erythrocytes of common Rh phenotypes. Unexpected reactions in this category usually represent subtle differences in composition among various Rh gene products.

By considering C and c or E and e as expressing antithetical products, the concept can be expanded to include alternate antigenic activities. If the genes are together at the same site but are determined by genes coding for products distinct from the common Rh determinants, variant activity can be observed. In Blacks, atypical activity at the e antigen site is common. Several patterns have been identified ($hr^{s-}$ and $hr^{B-}$).

The antigen $C^w$ is an example of a variant antigen that usually functions as an allele in the antithetical relationship of C/c. This antigen is expressed in approximately 1 to 2% of some White populations. $C^w$ was first described in 1962. Characteristics of $C^w$ antibody include demonstration of a ''dosage effect'' (see p 115 for a discussion of dosage effect). This antibody has the capability of causing hemolytic transfusion reactions and hemolytic disease of the newborn.

## The LW Antigen

The LW ($LW^a$) antigen, which was demonstrated with the original animal anti-rhesus sera, was named in honor of Landsteiner and Wiener. It is now recognized as distinct from the D antigen. This antigen is present on rhesus monkey erythrocytes and on the majority of human erythrocytes. In human adults, D− individuals display comparatively weaker LW activity, but umbilical cord bloods from both D+ and D− babies are strongly reactive. In general, the amount of LW antigen demonstrated on a person's erythrocytes is related to the presence or absence of D antigen. The classifications $LW_1$ and $LW_2$ describe the strong LW reactivity of D+ erythrocytes and the weaker LW reactivity of adult D− erythrocytes. The category $LW_3$ represents the phenotype of individuals who produce anti-LW but have nonreactive erythrocytes with the LW antibody. The classification $LW_4$ (LW a− b−) has been applied to the extremely rare case of having $LW^-$ erythrocytes with serum containing a potent form of anti-LW that agglutinated $LW_3$ erythrocytes as well as $LW_1$ and $LW_2$ erythrocytes.

There is a strong phenotypic association between the Rh and LW blood group systems; but the CDE and LW genes control different blood group antigens and segregate independently. LW is a very high incidence antigen. All erythrocytes of the Rh null phenotype, however, are LW−. Rare cases have been documented in which normal Rh antigens, with or without D antigen, are present but LW antigen is absent. The LW ($LW^a$) gene appears to require for its expression some product of Rh gene activity.

As the LW subclassifications demonstrate, LW− individuals can form alloanti-LW. The antibody displays the same degree of reactivity with D+ and D− erythrocytes as the animal antisera. Anti-LW has sometimes been identified in the sera of LW positive persons whose erythrocytes at the time of antibody formation were either transiently LW− or exhibited very weak reactivity with anti-LW sera. In these transient cases, the normal LW+ status of the erythrocytes has been documented to return to a positive status as the antibody disappears.

In 1981, a new blood group antigen, $Ne^a$, was reported with a frequency of approximately 5% in the Finnish population. Anti-$Ne^a$ displayed a variation in the strength of reactivity similar to anti-LW that suggested a relationship between $Ne^a$ and LW. It is now known that $Ne^a$ and LW are products of allelic genes. Therefore, the antigen formerly called LW has become $LW^a$ and $Ne^a$ becomes $LW^b$.

## Rh Antibodies

The Rh antibodies are predominantly of the immunoglobulin class IgG. The production of these antibodies is consistent with the classical immune response that initially elicits IgM antibody followed by IgG. Some examples of

**Table 5-8. Characteristics of Selected Rh Antibodies**

| Antibody | Mode of Reactivity | | | Usual Immunoglubulin Subclass | | | Usual Form of Stimulation | |
|---|---|---|---|---|---|---|---|---|
| | Sal. | AHG | Enz. | IgM | IgG | IgA | RBCs | Other |
| Anti-D | | X | X | Some | Most | Few | X | Rare |
| Anti-C | | X | X | | Most | | X | Rare |
| Anti-E | X | X | X | Some | Most | | X | Some |
| Anti-c | | X | X | | Most | | X | |
| Anti-e | | X | X | | Most | | X | |
| Anti-C^w | X | X | X | Some | Most | | X | Some |

IgA have been identified. When IgG antibodies are synthesized, most of them are IgG1 or IgG3. The IgG1 subclass of anti-D is more common if immunization results from pregnancy. Although Rh antibodies are associated with both hemolytic transfusion reactions and hemolytic disease of the newborn, in vitro binding of complement is rare. The lack of in vitro complement fixation is believed to be hampered by the small number of Rh antigen sites, the distance of the antigen from the erythrocyte membrane, and the lack of exposure of the combining site of the complement C1q component on the immunoglobulin molecule.

## Antibody Characteristics and Frequencies

Except for some examples that occur without a known red cell stimulus, most Rh antibodies result from erythrocyte immunization subsequent to pregnancy or transfusion. Therefore, the majority of these antibodies are IgG. The characteristics of selected Rh antibodies are presented in Tables 5-8 and 5-9. The D antigen is the most potent Rh immunogen. Of D− patients who receive a single unit of D+ blood, 50 to 75% can be expected to develop anti-D; but 25 to 30% of D− individuals are nonresponders, which makes them unable to produce anti-D. Additionally, some weak D (D^u) recipients can form anti-D if transfused with D+ blood.

In studies of deliberate immunization to induce alloantibody production, the C, c, E, and e antigens were demonstrated to be much less immunogenic than D. Anti-E is the most common antibody associated with these four antigens, followed by anti-c. Anti-E can be found in the absence of erythrocyte antigen exposure. Some examples of anti-E react only with protease-modified erythrocytes, while others are reactive at temperatures below 37° C. Anti-C as a single antibody is rare in both Rh positive and negative persons. Anti-e is rarely found because only about 2 individuals in 100 are able to synthesize anti-e.

Some Rh antibodies commonly occur together. For example, an $R_1R_1$ person who has made immune anti-E has probably been exposed to the c antigen as well as E. In these cases, anti-c is usually present in addition to anti-E, although the titer of anti-c may be low and not detectable when the anti-E is demonstrated. Anti-c can produce a hemolytic transfusion reaction following the administration of compatible E negative, c positive blood. When selecting blood for transfusion to $R_1R_1$ recipients with detectable anti-E who might also produce anti-c, transfusing with $R_1R_1$ blood should be considered. A patient with detectable anti-c may not have a concurrent anti-E because exposure to c antigen is more probable than exposure to E antigen.

## Dosage Effects

Anti-D seldom exhibits any difference in reactivity between erythrocytes with homozygous or heterozygous expression of the D antigen. Variably strong reactions, however, may be observed with red cells representing certain genotypes. The (cDE/cDE) dosage effect can be observed with antibodies having specificities for the E, c, or e antigens. Dosage may occasionally be observed with anti-C.

**Table 5-9. Serologic Characteristics of Blood Group Antibodies**

| System | Antibody | Reactive Phases | | | | Comments |
|---|---|---|---|---|---|---|
| | | R.T. | 37° C | A.H.G. | Enzyme | |
| Rh-hr | Anti-D | Some | Most | Most | Most | |
| | Anti-C | Few | Most | Most | Most | Often found with anti-D, anti-Ce, or anti-C^w |
| | Anti-E | Some | Most | Most | Most | Often found with anti-c |
| | Anti-c | Rare | Most | Most | Most | Often found with anti-E |
| | Anti-e | Rare | Most | Most | Most | Often found with anti-C |
| | Anti-C^w | Some | Most | Most | Most | |
| | Anti-V | Rare | Most | Most | Most | |

## CHAPTER SUMMARY

The Rh system was identified in 1940 by Landsteiner and Wiener, who originally found that human erythrocytes were agglutinated by an antibody apparently common to all rhesus monkeys and 85% of humans. This factor was named the Rh factor. The Rh-hr blood group system is probably the most complex of all red cell blood group systems, with more than 40 different Rh antigens. The descriptive terms, Rh positive and Rh negative, refer *only* to the presence or absence of the red cell antigen, D. Four additional genes (C, E, c, and e) are recognized as belonging to the Rh system.

The CDE and Rh-hr systems of nomenclature in the Rh system are equivalent. In the clinical laboratory only five reagent antisera are commonly available for the D, C, c, E, and e antigens. Routine testing involves only the use of anti-D, but other antisera are used to resolve antibody problems or to conduct family studies.

Multiple research studies agree that the Rh antigens are present on a protein structure and are probably all on the same polypeptide chain. It appears that membrane lipids are restricted to a supporting role at the phenotypic level. Simple antigens (e.g., D, C, E, etc.) presumably represent certain amino acid sequences. However, antigens like G represent some of the amino acids of D and some others. Antigens such as rh are thought to represent repressed amino acids of C and e that are located adjacent in the $R^1$ and r′ specified folded polypeptide, but apart when $R^z$ and r make separate polypeptides for the same cell membrane. The Rh antigens exhibit numerous serological complexities that undoubtedly represent an extremely complicated polypeptide.

The production or nonproduction of D, as well as the production of either C or c and E or e antigens is genetically determined. Rh antigen sites are believed to be randomly distributed on the red cell membrane. The expression of an inherited gene can be affected by the interaction between genes. When an Rh gene on one chromosome affects the action of another Rh gene on the same chromosome, by either increased or decreased antigen production, it is referred to as a *cis* effect. When an Rh gene on one of the chromosomes of a homologous pair affects the actions of an Rh gene on the other homolog, it is called a *trans* effect. The most dramatic *Rh trans* position effect known occurs when C is in trans to D (CDe/Cde), which weakens the D antigen. This is one reason for the weak D (Dᵘ) phenotype, but it is now recognized that the weak D phenotype can also arise in two other ways: the inheritance of a gene that codes for less D antigen, and the absence of a portion or portions of the total material that comprise the D epitope.

Rh positive blood very rarely lacks any of the epitope components. However, a system of classifying D positive persons who produce anti-D was devised in 1962. The six categories of antibody formers are referred to as: I, II, III, IV, V, and VI based on the reactions of erythrocytes with anti-D from these individuals, as well as the specificity of the anti-D produced.

The e antigen of some Blacks is an epitope structure. The appearance of e-like antibodies made by e positive individuals is analogous to the anti-D made by individuals with D variations. More than 40 other Rh antigens have been identified, including the G and V antigens. The term *compound antigen* is used to communicate the idea that certain combinations of Rh antigens demonstrate a combined effect. An example of a compound antigen is the ce or f antigen. Variant antigens also exist. The antigen, $C^w$, is an example of a variant antigen. There are some rare Rh genes that behave as if portions of the genetic material have been deleted or rendered nonfunctional. The first recognized case was the D-deletion gene (D⁻⁻). When no Rh antigens are expressed on the red cell membrane, the term Rh null is used to describe this phenotype; if a less complete type of suppressed Rh gene expression is observed, the term *Rh mod* is used. The LW antigen, which was demonstrated with the original animal anti-rhesus sera, was named in honor of Landsteiner and Wiener. It is now recognized as being distinct from the D antigen. This antigen is present on rhesus monkey erythrocytes and on the majority of human erythrocytes.

The Rh antibodies are predominantly of the immunoglobulin class IgG. Most Rh antibodies result from erythrocyte immunization due to pregnancy or transfusion. Some Rh antibodies commonly occur together.

## REVIEW QUESTIONS

1. The term *Rh positive* refers to the presence of:
   A. Anti-D
   B. D antigen
   C. C antigen
   D. E antigen
2. The symbol *R* is used for haplotypes that include:
   A. c
   B. E
   C. r
   D. D
3–7. Match the following examples of equivalent nomenclature:

| Fisher-Race | Wiener |
|---|---|
| 3. D | A. hr′ |
| 4. c | B. rh′ |
| 5. E | C. Rh₀ |
| 6. e | D. rh″ |
| 7. C | E. hr″ |

**8–13.** Match the following Fisher-Race terms with their respective shorthand symbols:

    **8.** CDe         **A.** $R^2$
    **9.** cDE         **B.** $R^o$
   **10.** cDE         **C.** r
   **11.** CDE         **D.** $R^Z$
   **12.** cde         **E.** $R^1$
   **13.** CdE         **F.** $r^y$

**14.** The most common Rh genotype in Whites is:

    **A.** $R^1R^1$
    **B.** $R^1R^2$
    **C.** $R'r$
    **D.** $rr$

**15.** The most common Rh genotype in Blacks is:

    **A.** $R^or$
    **B.** $R^oR^o$
    **C.** $R'R^o$
    **D.** $R'r$

**16.** Based on the following reactions, what is this person's most probable genotype?

*Antisera*

| Anti-D | Anti-C | Anti-E | Anti-c | Anti-e |
|--------|--------|--------|--------|--------|
| + | 0 | + | + | 0 |

    **A.** $R^1r$
    **B.** $R^2R^2$
    **C.** $R^zR^z$
    **D.** $R^or$

**17.** The highest number of D antigen sites is found on erythrocytes of which genotype?

    **A.** *cDE/cDE*
    **B.** *CDe/CDe*
    **C.** *CDe/cde*
    **D.** *cde/cde*

**18.** When an Rh gene on one chromosome affects the action of another Rh gene on the same chromosome, in terms of increased or decreased antigen production, it is referred to as:

    **A.** Cis effect
    **B.** Trans effect
    **C.** Either cis or trans effect

**19.** A weak D ($D^u$) phenotype resulting from gene suppression is characterized by:

    **A.** The action of a C gene
    **B.** A trans position effect
    **C.** Low grade $D^u$ activity
    **D.** Both A and B

**20.** Phenotypically erythrocytes of the partial D type react similarly to:

    **A.** Low grade weak D ($D^u$)
    **B.** High grade weak D ($D^u$)
    **C.** D positive RBCs
    **D.** Weak D ($D^u$) negative RBCs

**21.** The D_____ phenotype does not code for the production of _____ antigen(s).

    **A.** D
    **B.** C
    **C.** E
    **D.** Both B & C

**22.** When no Rh antigens are expressed on the RBC membrane, the term _____ is used to express the phenotype

    **A.** Rh mod
    **B.** Rh null
    **C.** $-D-$
    **D.** CD$-$
    **E.** None of the above

**23–26.** Match the following:

   **23.** G antigen      **A.** Compound antigen
   **24.** V antigen      **B.** Antibodies resemble anti-C + anti-D
   **25.** f antigen      
   **26.** $C^W$            **C.** Example of a variation antigen
                     **D.** Product of $R^o$, $R^{OU}$, or r genes

**27.** The LW antigen:

    **A.** strength is related to the presence or absence of D antigen.
    **B.** is negative in cases of Rh null phenotype.
    **C.** is a high-incidence antigen of human RBCs.
    **D.** All of the above.

**28.** Rh antibodies are predominantly:

    **A.** IgM
    **B.** IgG
    **C.** IgD
    **D.** IgA

**29–34.** A = true, B = false.

   **29.** Most Rh antibodies are stimulated by RBC antigens.
   **30.** In vitro binding of complement is common in the Rh system.
   **31.** The c antigen is the most potent immunogen of all of the Rh antigens.
   **32.** Anti-e is a frequently encountered antibody.
   **33.** Anti-E + anti-c are commonly found together.
   **34.** Dosage effects may be observed with E, c, or e.

**35.** A person of the genotype rr could potentially produce antibodies of the following Rh specificity, if appropriately stimulated:

    **A.** Anti-D
    **B.** Anti-C
    **C.** Anti-E
    **D.** All of the above.

## Bibliography

Ceppellini, R., Dunn, L.C., and Turri, M.: An interaction between alleles at the Rh locus in man which weakens the reactivity of the $Rh_o$ factor ($D^u$). Proc. Nat. Acad. Science USA, *41:* 283–288, 1955.

Dracker, R.A., Lauenstein, K.J., and Davey, F.R.: Immunohematology. *In* Clinical Diagnosis and Management by Laboratory

Methods. Edited by J.B. Henry. Philadelphia: Saunders, 1992, 988–992.

Giblett, E.: Blood group antibodies causing hemolytic disease of the newborn. Clin. Obstet. Gynecol., *7*:1044–1055.

Levine, P.: On Hr factor and Rh genetic theory. Science, *102*:1–4, 1945.

Marsh, W.L. et al.: Mapping human autosomes: Evidence supporting assignment of rhesus to the short arm of chromosome No. 1. Science, *183*:966–968, 1974.

Mournat, A.E.: A new rhesus antibody. Nature, *155*:542, 1945.

Pollack, W. et al.: Studies on Rh prophylaxis after transfusion with Rh-positive blood. Transfusion, *11*:340–344, 1971.

Race, R.R., and Taylor, G.L.: A serum that discloses the genotype of some Rh-positive people. Nature, *152*:300, 1943.

Race, R.R., Taylor, G.L., Cappell, D.F., and McFarlane, M.M.: Recognition of a further common Rh genotype in man. Nature, *153*:52–53, 1944.

Ruddle, F. et al.: Somatic cell genetic assignment of peptidase C and the Rh linkage group to chromosome A-1 in man. Science, *176*:1429–1431, 1972.

Vos, G.H., et al.: A sample of blood with no detectable Rh antigens. Lancet, *i*:14, 1961.

Walker, R.H. (Ed.): Technical Manual, 11th ed. Bethesda, MD: American Association of Blood Banks, 1993, 229–258.

# Lewis and Other Blood Group Systems

At the conclusion of this chapter, the reader should be able to:

- Describe the mode of inheritance of Lewis and secretor genes.
- Compare the phenotypes and genotypes in the Lewis blood group system.
- Describe the relationship of *H, A,* and *B* genes and their expression in secretions and on erythrocytes.
- Diagram the mode of inheritance of the Lewis phenotypes and explain the clinical significance of the Lewis system.
- State the most common Lutheran phenotype or phenotypes.
- Describe the mode of inheritance within the M, N, S, and P blood group systems.
- List the incidence of the most frequent genes within the M, N, S, and P systems and describe the significance of these systems.
- Explain the physical and chemical properties of the M, N, S, and P blood group systems.

- Explain the inheritance and development of the Ii blood group system.
- Describe the techniques used in working with "nonspecific antibodies."
- Cite the major antigens and their incidence, describe the characteristics, and discuss the clinical significance of the Kell blood system.
- List the incidence of Kell antigens.
- Explain the mode of reaction of the Duffy and Kidd systems.
- Describe the clinical significance of Duffy and Kidd antigens and antibodies.
- Cite the incidence of Duffy and Kidd antigens.
- Briefly explain the characteristics of other blood group system antigens and antibodies.
- Name the HLA antigen that is not uncommonly detected on erythrocytes.
- List at least four antigens that are associated with antibodies to high-incidence antigens.

## Chapter Outline

## THE LEWIS BLOOD GROUP SYSTEM

The two common antigens of the Lewis system are Lewis$^a$ (Le$^a$) and Lewis$^b$ (Le$^b$). The first antibody of this system, anti-Le$^a$, was identified in 1946. The antibody to the corresponding allele, anti-Le$^b$, was recognized in 1948. The Lewis blood group system is unlike other blood group systems in that genetic control of the two antigens, Le$^a$ and Le$^b$, appear to reside in a single gene, called Le. This system, which represents a complex interaction between the independent Lewis, ABO, and secretor genes, is best understood by thinking of it as a system of genetically determined water-soluble antigens that are present in body fluids and secretions, such as saliva. Lewis antigens are adsorbed onto the surface of cells such as erythrocytes.

The Lewis system differs from other blood group systems in three significant ways. The differences include the following:

1. Erythrocytes acquire the Lewis phenotype by adsorbing Lewis substances from the plasma, rather than being membrane-bound antigens.
2. Although the Lewis and secretor genes are inherited independently, the Lewis phenotype is influenced by the secretor status. Inheritance of the nonsecretor (sese) genes and Lewis genes results in the phenotype Le(a + b −); while inheritance of at least one secretor gene, Sese or SeSe, and the Lewis gene results in the phenotype Le(a − b +).
3. The Lewis phenotype may be modified by the ABO phenotype (such as $A_1$), which may interfere with the expression of the Le$^a$ antigen in Le(b +) individuals.

### The Secretor Status

The terms secretor and nonsecretor refer only to the presence of water-soluble ABH antigen substances in body fluid. This condition is influenced by the independently inherited regulator Se gene. Approximately 78% of humans possess at least one Se gene and secrete A, B, or H water-soluble antigens (Table 6-1). The presence of the Se gene allows the H gene to function in secretory cells.

These secretions have the property of reacting with their corresponding antibodies to neutralize or inhibit the ability of these antibodies to agglutinate erythrocytes possessing the corresponding antigen. This reaction is termed hemagglutination inhibition and provides a means of as-

**Table 6-1. The Relationship of ABH Substances and ABO Group**

| ABO Blood Group Secretors | ABH Substances in Saliva | | |
|---|---|---|---|
| | A | B | H |
| A | Much | None | Some |
| B | None | Much | Some |
| O | None | None | Much |
| AB | Much | Much | Some |

**Table 6-2. Blood Group Substances**

| Genes[1] | In Secretions | On Erythrocytes |
|---|---|---|
| H, Se, A, Le | H,A, Le$^a$, Le$^b$ | H, A, Le$^b$ |
| H, Se, OO, Le | H, Le$^a$, Le$^b$ | H, Le$^{a2}$, Le$^b$ |
| H, Se, A, lele | H, A | H,A |
| H, sese, A, Le | Le$^a$ | H, A, Le$^a$ |
| hh[3], Se, A, Le | Le$^a$ | Le$^a$ |

[1] The H, Se, A(or B), and Le genes produce their effect when present in either the homozygous or heterozygous state. When the amorphic genes h, O, le and se are present in a homozygous state, no detectable effect is produced.
[2] In some group O (and A₂) individuals who have the genes H, Se, and Le. Le$^a$ as well as Le$^b$ can be detected on the erythrocytes.
[1] The H gene is necessary for the formation of H, A, and Le$^b$ substances.

saying the relative activity or potency of these water-soluble blood group substances (see Chapter 14).

The water-soluble form of the Le$^a$ and Le$^b$ antigens can be present in saliva. Individuals who possess the Se gene are Le(a−), but these subjects can secrete ABH substance in a water-soluble form. Their erythrocytes type as Le(a−). All Le(a−b−) individuals are nonsecretors of ABH substance (Table 6-2). However, Le$^c$ and Le$^d$ antigens exist in individuals with Lewis (a−b−) phenotypes. Le$^c$ is present in nonsecretors (se se) and Le$^d$ in secretors (Se se or Se Se).

## Mode of Inheritance

The inheritance of an *Le* gene produces Le$^a$ antigen. The inheritance of the amorph gene, *le,* in a homozygous state (*lele*) prevents the production of any Lewis antigen and results in the null phenotype. The Le$^b$ antigen is the product of the interaction of the dominant Lewis gene and the *H* gene in the presence of the *Se* gene (Fig. 6-1). This explains why an *Le$^b$* gene is not required for the formation of the Le$^b$ antigen.

The Lewis gene does not directly code for the production of Lewis antigens. Without the *Le* gene, no Lewis substances can be formed, and the erythrocytes are Le(a−b−), regardless of the secretor status. If the *Le* gene is inherited, antigens are produced by the action of a specific glycosyl transferase, L-fucosyl transferase, which adds L-fucose to the basic precursor substance. It should be noted that Lewis genes compete with A and B genes in the addition of L-fucose to the N-acetylglucosamine sugar of the common precursor structure manufactured by tissue cells.

The result of the Lewis gene activity is the production of an $\alpha$-4-L-fucosyltransferase that catalyzes the transfer of fucose to the carbon-4 position of N-acetylglucosamine produces the Le$^a$ active structure. The Le$^a$ soluble antigen is then secreted and adsorbed onto the erythrocyte membrane. In the absence of the secretor gene, Le$^a$ is not converted to Le$^b$; therefore, body fluids contain abundant Le$^a$ and no Le$^b$ and the erythrocytes are Le(a+b−).

If both the H and Le gene products are present, the addition of fucose to the carbon 4 position of N-acetylglucosamine results in an Le$^b$ active structure (Fig. 6-2), because the H gene has transferred fucose to the carbon-2 position of galactose. This Le$^b$ substance will be present on erythrocytes as well as in body fluids. The small amount of the initial Le$^a$ that was not converted can be detected in body fluids but is insufficient to attach to erythrocytes. In this case, the phenotype is Le(a−b+).

To further understand the Lewis system, it is important to realize that there are two types of carbohydrate chains ending in the glycoprotein of the precursor substance. The same sugars are present in each type of chain, although they have different linkages. In Type I chains, the terminal galactose has a $\beta$-1,3 linkage with N-acetylglucosamine and in Type II chains, the sugar has a $\beta$-1,4 linkage. The

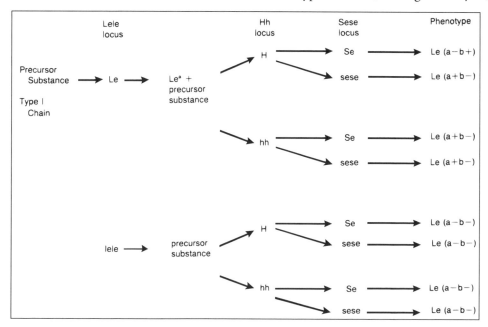

**Figure 6-1.** Mechanism of expression of Lewis phenotypes.

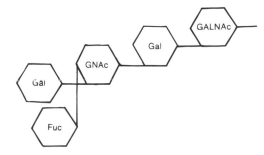

A molecule with Le$^a$ specificity

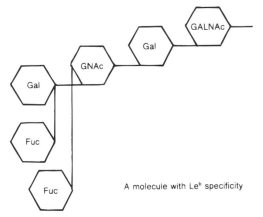

A molecule with Le$^b$ specificity

**Figure 6-2.** Molecules with Lewis specificity. Key:
Gal = D-Galactose
GNAc = N-acetylglucosamine
Fuc = Fucose
GALNAc = N-acetylgalactosamine

fucosyltransferase produced by the Le gene is unable to act on a type II chain because the number 4 carbon atom is already occupied by the galactosyl structure. Two antigens, Le$^c$ and Le$^d$, are postulated to be derived from the precursor substance of the type II chains. These antigens exist in the Lewis (a−b−) phenotype.

The Le$^x$ antigen probably represents the action of a fucosyltransferase adding a fucose to a shorter carbohydrate chain. This antigen is present in all individuals who type as Le(a+b−) and Le(a−b+). Le$^x$ is also found on cord red blood cells from approximately 90% of Whites who originally phenotyped as Le(a−b−).

## The Biochemical Nature of Lewis Antigens

The water-soluble Lewis antigens found in secretions are glycoproteins, as are the ABH substances from secretors.

These glycoproteins are composed of approximately 80% carbohydrates and 15% amino acids. Lewis specificity that is similar to ABH antigens resides in the carbohydrate portion of the molecule. In the blood plasma, the Lewis antigens as well as the ABH substances are glycosphingolipids.

Le$^a$ and Le$^b$ antigens are absent or extremely weak at birth. Cord blood specimens are essentially Le(a−b−). The Le$^a$ antigen develops more rapidly than Le$^b$. By 3 months of age, more than 80% of children produce an Le(a+) reaction, but this reactivity, decreases with age, and by about 2 years of age, the adult level of 20% reactivity is established. The expression of the adult frequency of approximately 70% reactivity of Le$^b$ antigen on erythrocytes is reached at about 6 years. Antigenic strength is also known to vary during pregnancy for unknown reasons. In cases of diminished activity, normal reactivity returns after pregnancy.

Lewis antigens readily adsorb to and elute from the red blood cell membrane. Transfused red blood cells shed their Lewis antigens and assume the Lewis phenotype of the recipient within a few days of entering the circulation.

## Lewis Phenotypes

The expression of Lewis antigens results from the continuous exchange of glycosphingolipids between the plasma and the erythrocyte membrane. Because erythrocytes adsorb Lewis antigens in vivo, the Lewis phenotype depends entirely on the uptake of antigens from the plasma.

Three major Lewis phenotypes exist in adults (Table 6-3):

1. Le(a+b−)
2. Le(a−b+)
3. Le(a−b−)

### The Le(a+b−) Phenotype

Characteristics of this phenotype, Le(a+b−), include the presence of Le$^a$ antigen in plasma and saliva and agglutination of erythrocytes with anti-Le$^a$ reagent sera. Le(a+b−) erythrocytes do not react with anti-Le$^b$ because of the absence of Le$^b$ antigen. Although these individuals produce large amounts of Le$^a$ substance, they do not secrete ABH substances in their saliva. Only saliva from Le(a+b−) individuals forms a precipitate with an anti-Le$^a$ serum produced in rabbits.

### Table 6-3. Lewis Phenotypes in Adults

| Red Cell Phenotype | Genotype | Lewis Substance (Saliva) | H Substance (Saliva) | Frequency (Approximate) White (%) | Frequency (Approximate) Black (%) |
|---|---|---|---|---|---|
| Le(a+b−) | H, sese, Le very rare hh, Se or sese, Le | Le$^a$ | Absent | 22 | 23 |
| Le(a−b+) | H, Se, Le | Le$^b$ + Le$^a$ | Present | 72 | 55 |
| Le(a−b−) | H, Se, lele | Absent | Present | 6 | 22 |
| | H, sese, lele very rare hh, Se or sese, lele | Absent | Absent | <1 | ? |

## The Le(a−b+) Phenotype

This is the most common phenotype in adults. Individuals of the phenotype Le(a−b+) have the genes H, Se, and Le and their secretions contain H, Le$^a$ and Le$^b$. If Le(a−b+) individuals have an A (or B gene), they will also have A or B substances, respectively, in their secretions. The plasma of Le(a−b+) individuals contains predominantly Le$^b$ substances, but trace amounts of Le$^a$ may also be detected. The phenotype Le(a+b+) can be observed with erythrocytes of rare O and A$_2$ persons. These anti-Le$^a$ reactions are weak and detectable only with antihuman globulin (AHG) testing. The phenotype Le(a+b+) has not been found in A$_1$ adults, probably because they make less Le$^a$ substance as a result of competition between the A$^1$ and Le gene products for the basic precursor substance.

## The Le(a−b−) Phenotype

This uncommon phenotype, Le(a−b−), has the genotype lele, which results in erythrocytes with the phenotype Le(a−b−). These erythrocytes react with either anti-Le$^c$ or anti-type I H (previously anti-Le$^d$). Persons with the genotype lele have traces of Le$^a$ in their serum.

### Lewis (Anti-Le$^a$ and Anti-Le$^b$) Antibodies

The Lewis antibodies (anti-Le$^a$ and anti-Le$^b$) are frequently found in individuals who have never been transfused or received any other known erythrocyte antigen stimulus. As many as 20% of Le(a−b−) individuals have a Lewis antibody. Anti-Le$^a$ and anti-Le$^b$ are especially common in pregnant women. The Lewis antibody incidence in Le(a−b−) persons is 4 times more common in Blacks than Whites. Lewis antibodies in a recipient's serum are readily neutralized by Lewis blood group substance in donor plasma. Lewis antibodies have been cited as the cause of posttransfusion hemolysis. This reflects the rare situation in which Lewis antibodies cause hemolysis of transfused Le(a+) or Le(b+) red blood cells. Antibodies that cause hemolysis in vitro or produce a strong AHG reaction in crossmatching have been associated with posttransfusion hemolysis. Lewis antibodies have been cited as the cause of posttransfusion reactions.

Anti-Le$^a$ is more common as an individual antibody than anti-Le$^b$ and is found only in individuals who are genetically Lewis-negative, lele, and have the phenotype Le(a−b−). Anti-Le$^b$ is usually a weakly reactive antibody in serum which contains a relatively potent anti-Le$^a$. The incidence of anti-Le$^b$ as a single antibody is infrequent. Producers of anti-Le$^b$ (without anti-Le$^a$) are nonsecretors of ABH and always of the phenotype Le(a−b−). It is very rare for Le(a+b−) individuals to form anti-Le$^b$; but there is no theoretic reason why they should not be able to do so, because they are completely lacking in Le$^b$ antigen. Almost all Lewis antibodies are of the IgM variety. Rare examples of anti-Le$^a$ are solely IgG. The in vitro stability of these antibodies in serum is unpredictable, even when they are frozen.

Sera containing anti-Le$^a$ usually agglutinate Le(a+) cells suspended in saline and react more strongly at room temperature or colder temperatures. Erythrocytes agglutinated by anti-Le$^a$ characteristically have a "stringy" appearance. This agglutination may not be obvious with saline-suspended erythrocytes. Hemolysis of erythrocytes, particularly cells treated with a proteolytic enzyme, may be observed at 37° C because the antibody almost always binds complement. Some examples of Le$^a$, and less frequently anti-Le$^b$, are detectable only with antihuman globulin (AHG) testing, if complement is present in the test mixture and a polyspecific antiserum is used.

Some examples of anti-Le$^b$ fail to react with A$_1$ cells but react strongly with group O or A$_2$ erythrocytes. Two kinds of anti-Le$^b$ exist. Those that are neutralized by the saliva of all ABH secretors, including those of Le(a−b−) individuals. These anti-Le$^b$ antibodies are referred to as anti-Le$^{bH}$. The other form, referred to as anti-Le$^{bL}$ (true anti-Le$^b$), is neutralized by the saliva of Le(a−b+) persons. This form of anti-Le$^b$ reacts with A$_1$, erythrocytes almost as well as with erythrocytes of other blood groups.

### Other Lewis Antibodies

Two additional antibodies have been named in the Lewis blood group system. These antibodies are anti-Le$^c$ and anti-Le$^d$. Anti-Le$^c$ reacts with the erythrocytes of Le(a−b−) nonsecretors, from individuals of genotype *lele, sese,* and also with those of genotype *lele, hh.* This antibody is inhibited by the saliva of individuals of the same genotypes. Anti-Le$^d$ reacts with erythrocytes of Le(a−b−) secretors.

A summary of the typical serologic behavior of Le$^a$ and Le$^b$ is found in Table 6-4.

## ADDITIONAL MAJOR BLOOD GROUP SYSTEMS

Other major blood group systems exist in addition to the ABO, Rh, and Lewis blood group systems. A summary of the antigen frequencies and serologic behavior of the antibodies of the blood group systems is presented in Tables 6-5 and 6-6.

For convenience these systems can be divided into the two following categories:

1. The typically IgM antibodies that are best detected at cold temperatures [MNSsU, P, and I, and most Lutheran$^a$ (Lu$^a$) antibodies].
2. The typically IgG antibodies that are detectable by antiglobulin (AHG) testing [Kell, Duffy, Kidd, and Lutheran$^b$ (Lu$^b$) antibodies].

**Table 6-4. In Vitro Serologic Behavior of Le$^a$ and Le$^b$**

| | In Vitro Reactions | | | | | |
|---|---|---|---|---|---|---|
| | Saline | | Albumin | AGH* | Enzymes | Hemolysis |
| Antibody | 4° C | 22° C | 37° C | — | 37° C | — |
| Anti-Le$^a$ | Most | Most | Few | Many | Most | Some |
| Anti-Le$^b$ | Most | Most | Few | Some | Some | Occasional |

* AGH signifies antihuman globulin (AHG) phase of testing using a broad-spectrum (polyspecific) antisera.

**Table 6-5. Summary of Antigen Frequencies**

| Blood Group | Antigen | Frequency in Population | |
|---|---|---|---|
| | | White | Black |
| Kell | K | 9 | 2 |
| | k | 99.9 | >99.9 |
| | Kp$^a$ | 2 | Rare |
| | Kp$^b$ | >99.9 | 100 |
| | Js$^a$ | Rare | 20 |
| | Js$^b$ | >99.9 | 99 |
| Duffy | Fy$^a$ | 66 | 10 |
| | Fy$^b$ | 83 | 23 |
| Kidd | Jk$^a$ | 77 | 91 |
| | Jk$^b$ | 72 | 41 |
| Lutheran | Lu$^a$ | 8 | — |
| | Lu$^b$ | 99.9 | — |
| MNSs | M | 78 | 70 |
| | N | 72 | 74 |
| | S | 55 | 31 |
| | s | 89 | 97 |
| | U | 100 | >99 |
| Lewis | Le$^a$ | 22 | 23 |
| | Le$^b$ | 72 | 55 |
| P | P$^1$ | 79 | 94 |
| | P | 100 | 100 |
| | Tj$^a$ | 100 | 100 |
| Xg$^a$ | Xg$^a$ | 66F | 66F |
| | | 89M | 89M |
| Colton | Co$^a$ | >99 | >99 |
| | Co$^b$ | 10 | 10 |
| Dombrock | Do$^a$ | 67 | — |
| | Do$^b$ | 83 | — |
| Diego | Di$^a$ | Rare | — |
| | Di$^b$ | 100 | — |
| Wright | Wr$^a$ | <1 | — |
| Vel | Vel | 100 | — |
| Sid | Sd$^a$ | 91 | — |
| HLA | Bg$^a$ | 17 | 17 |
| | Bg$^b$ | 9 | 28 |
| | Bg$^c$ | 8 | 17 |
| Cartwright | Yt$^a$ | >99 | >99 |
| | Yt$^b$ | 8 | 8 |
| High | Ch$^A$ | Ch(a+) | Rg(a+)a |
| Incidence | Rg$^a$ | 95 | 95 |
| Antigens | Kn$^a$ | Kn(a+) | McC(a+) |
| | McC$^a$ | 97 | 95 |
| | Cs$^a$ | Cs(a+) | Yka(+) |
| | Yk$^a$ | 82 | 96 |
| | JMH | 99.9 | 99.9 |
| I | I$^a$ | See text | See text |
| | i$^a$ | | |

References:
Issitt, P. D.: Applied Blood Group Serology, 3rd Ed. Miami, FL, Montgomery Scientific, 1985.
Widmann, Frances K. (Ed.): AABB Technical Manual, 9th ed. Arlington, VA, American Association of Blood Banks, 1985.

## Typical IgM Antibody Blood Group Systems

### The Lutheran System

The first antigen of the Lutheran system was recognized in 1945. This antigen, Lu$^a$, is low in frequency. The antithetical high frequency antigen, Lu$^b$, was reported in 1956. More than 19 antigens are known to exist in this system; most are high frequency antigens. Au$^a$ (LU18), a high-incidence antigen, and its antithetical allele, Au$^b$ (LU19), have recently been shown to be part of the Lutheran system. In addition, two low-incidence antigens Mull (LU9) and LU14 have been added to the Lutheran system.

***Mode of Inheritance.*** Initially, the Lewis and Lutheran genes were erroneously believed to be linked; it was later discovered that the Lutheran genes were actually linked to the gene that controls secretor status. The Lutheran and secretor locus had the distinction of providing the first example of autosomal linkage and the first example of autosomal crossing-over in humans.

The *Lu$^a$* and *Lu$^b$* genes are codominant; however, as in other blood group systems, the expression of these genes is not straightforward (Fig. 6-3).

The rare Lu(a−b−) null phenotype is categorized as either recessive or dominant in type. The recessive null phenotype results from the homozygous inheritance of an amorphic gene. Consequently, the person lacks all Lutheran antigens. Another form of recessive inheritance is the null phenotype due to the X-borne suppressor, which is recessive in effect. The dominant type of Lu(a−b−) null phenotype results from the inheritance of a single dominant gene that prevents normal Lutheran antigen synthesis. This independently segregating inhibitor gene has been named InLu (Lutheran inhibitor). If a single InLu gene is inherited even in the presence of normal *Lu$^a$* and *Lu$^b$* genes, the resulting phenotype is Lu(a−b−). This rare gene also inhibits the production of other antigens such as P$_1$, i and Au$^a$.

***The Biochemical Nature of Lutheran Antigens.*** Lutheran antigens are probably carried on two glycoproteins, carrying both N-linked and O-linked oligosaccharides. Although the Lu$^a$ antigen is poorly developed at birth, the strength of the antigen is known to increase until about the age of 15 years. The Lu$^b$ antigen of an Lu(a−b+) cord blood is also weaker than in adults. Lutheran antigens may occasionally demonstrate dosage, but it is not as evi-

**Table 6-6. Serologic Characteristics of Blood Group Antibodies**

| System/or Antigen | Antibody | R.T. | 37° C | A.H.G. | Enzyme | Comments |
|---|---|---|---|---|---|---|
| Lewis | Anti-Le^a | Most | Few | Some | Most | Often found with anti-Le^a |
| | Anti-Le^b | Most | Rare | Some | Some | |
| Lutheran | Anti-Lu^a | Most | Few | Few | Few | Produces mixed field type of agglutination |
| | Anti-Lu^b | Few | Few | Most | Few | |
| MNSs | Anti-M | Most | Few | Some | 0 | May exhibit dosage |
| | Anti-N | Most | Rare | Rare | 0 | |
| | Anti-S | Some | Some | Most | Variable | |
| | Anti-s | Few | Few | Most | Most | |
| | Anti-U | Rare | Some | Most | Most | |
| P | Anti-P_1 | Most | Rare | Rare | Most | |
| | Anti-P | Most | Some | Some | Most | |
| | Anti-PP_1P^k (Tj^a) | Most | Some | Some | Most | |
| I | Anti-I | Most | Few | Some | Most | |
| | Anti-i | Most | Few | Some | Most | |
| Kell | Anti-K | Few | Few | Most | Most | |
| | Anti-k | Rare | Rare | Most | Most | |
| | Anti-Kp^a | Rare | Rare | Most | Most | |
| | Anti-Kp^b | Rare | Rare | Most | Most | |
| | Anti-Js^a | Rare | Rare | Most | Most | |
| | Anti-Js^b | 0 | 0 | Most | Most | |
| Duffy | Anti-Fy^a | Rare | Rare | Most | 0 | Some exhibit dosage; some may bind complement |
| | Anti-Fy^b | Rare | Rare | Most | 0 | Some exhibit dosage; some may bind complement |
| Kidd | Anti-Jk^a | Rare | Rare | Most | Most | May exhibit dosage; titers can rapidly decline; may require anti-C3 for detection |
| | Anti-Jk^b | Rare | Rare | Most | Most | May exhibit dosage; titers can rapidly decline; may require anti-C3 |
| Xg | Anti-Xg^a | Few | Few | Most | 0 | |
| Sid | Anti-Sd^a | Some | Some | Some | Most | Agglutinates have a refractile, mixed-field appearance |
| Cartwright | Anti-Yt^a | 0 | 0 | Most | Some | Usually found in combination with other antibodies |
| | Anti-Yt^b | 0 | 0 | Most | | |
| Colton | Anti-Co^a | 0 | 0 | Some | Most | |
| | Anti-Co^b | 0 | 0 | Some | Most | |
| Diego | Anti-Dj^a | Some | Some | Most | Some | |
| | Anti-Dj^b | 0 | 0 | Most | Some | |
| Dombrock | Anti-Do^a | 0 | 0 | Most | Most | |
| | Anti-Do^b | 0 | 0 | Most | Most | |
| Scianna | Anti-Sc1 | 0 | 0 | Most | 0 | Have not been implicated in transfusion reactions or HDN |
| | Anti-Sc2 | | | | | |
| HLA Related | Anti-Bg^a | 0 | 0 | Most | Some | Usually weakly reactive |
| | Anti-Bg^b | | | | | |
| | Anti-Bg^c | | | | | |
| Vel | Anti-Vel | Some | Some | Some | Some | |
| Wright | Anti-Wr^a | Most | Few | Some | Some | |
| High Incidence Antigens | Anti-Ch^a | 0 | 0 | Most | Few | All are usually weakly reactive |
| | Anti-Cs^a | | | | Most | |
| | Anti-Gy^a | | | | Most | |
| | Anti-Hy | | | | Most | |
| | Anti-JMH | | | | Few | |
| | Anti-Kn^a/Mc^a | | | | Most | |
| | Anti-Rg^a | | | | Few | |
| | Anti-Yk^a | | | | Most | |

dent as in other blood group antigens such as c and M. Enzymes do not usually affect the Lutheran antigens.

***Lutheran Phenotypes.*** The Lu(a−b+) phenotype is the most common and Lu(a−b−) is the rarest (Table 6-7). Racial differences are not apparent.

***Lutheran Antibodies.*** The Lutheran antibodies, par-

ticularly Anti-Lu^a, are infrequently observed; this is partially due to the fact that a small proportion of individuals possess the Lu^a antigen. Lutheran antibodies, however, particularly anti-Lu^a, are known to occur with no known erythrocyte stimulus in the majority of cases. Most examples of anti-Lu^b are associated with a known exposure to

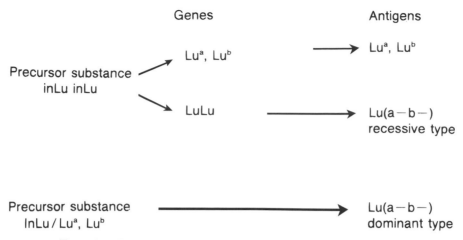

**Figure 6-3.** Theoretical mechanism of expression of Lutheran antigens.

Lu^b antigen by way of transfusion or pregnancy. Some Lutheran antibodies bind complement, but in vitro reactions are not associated with hemolysis.

The immunologic and in vitro characteristics of anti-Lu^a and anti-Lu^b are presented in Table 6-8.

Anti-Lu^a reactivity is characterized by mixed-field agglutination. Most examples of anti-Lu^a are IgM, more reactive at lower temperatures, and agglutinate saline suspended erythrocytes. Some dosage effect is exhibited. Anti-Lu^b occurs as both an IgG and IgA antihuman globulin (AHG) antibody; it is rarely an IgM antibody.

Anti-Lu3 (anti-Lu^aLu^b) is an antibody produced by individuals of the rare Lu(a−b−) phenotype. A person of this phenotype is capable of forming anti-Lu3 as well as any other Lutheran system antibody. It seems as though anti-Lu3 is made by persons of the recessive type and not by those of the dominant type of Lu(a−b−). This antibody is usually IgG or IgA and is capable of destroying incompatible erythrocytes; it reacts best with antihuman globulin (AHG) testing. Anti-Lu3 can react with all Lutheran-positive cells and is only nonreactive with other Lu(a−b−) cells.

Many other antibodies (such as anti-Lu₄) have been described. All fail to react with Lu(a−b−) erythrocytes, although they do react with the erythrocytes of other rare Lutheran phenotypes. Antibodies that fail to react with Lu(a−b−) erythrocytes of the dominant type may not belong to the Lutheran blood group system.

## The MNSs System

The M and N antigens are classically associated with paternity testing. This system was discovered in 1927 by Landsteiner and Levine when anti-M and anti-N were formed by injecting human erythrocytes into rabbits. The S and s antigens produced by a pair of allelic genes found at a locus closely linked to the MN locus were later added to this blood group system. The MNSs system includes a group of mostly low-frequency "satellite" antigens that are rarely of clinical significance. Several of these low-frequency antigens are considered interrelated and form the Miltenberger subsystem.

***Mode of Inheritance.*** The MNSs system is governed by two closely linked sets of allelic genes, MN and Ss. Because of linkage, one of four possible genetic combinations is inherited from each parent: MS, Ms, NS, or Ns. This results in 10 possible genotypes. Linkage produces disequilibrium and the gene complex Ns is 5 times more common than NS. A small proportion of Blacks are S−s− and most are also negative for the high frequency antigen, U.

The U antigen is found in all Whites and about 98.5% of Blacks. The rare phenotype S−s− is often written S^u and is the product of another allele at the Ss genetic locus.

***The Biochemical Nature of MNSs Antigens.*** M and N are glycoproteins with approximately 60% carbohydrate. The antigens of the MNS system are related to the erythrocyte membrane sialoglycoproteins referred to as glycophorin A and glycophorin B.

### Table 6-7. Frequency of Lutheran Phenotypes

| Phenotype | White (%) | Black (%) |
|---|---|---|
| Lu(a+b−) | 0.1 | 0.1 |
| Lu(a+b+) | 7.0 | 5.2 |
| Lu(a−b+) | 92.9 | 94.7 |
| Lu(a−b−) | Very rare | Very rare |

### Table 6-8. Characteristics of Lutheran Antibodies

|  | IgG | IgM | IgA | Saline Reactivity | AHG Reactivity |
|---|---|---|---|---|---|
| Anti-Lu^a | Rare | Common | Some | Common | Some |
| Anti-Lu^b | Some | Rare | Some | Few | Common |

**Table 6-9. Genotypes and Frequencies in MNSs System**

| Phenotype | Phenotypic Frequency | Possible Genotype | | Approx. Genotype Frequency (%) | Percentage Positive Anti-S | Anti-s |
|---|---|---|---|---|---|---|
| M | 30 | MS | MS | 6 | 66 | 80 |
| | | MS | Ms | 14 | | |
| | | Ms | Ms | 10 | | |
| MN | 49 | MS | NS | 4 | 53 | 92 |
| | | MS | Ns | 22 | | |
| | | Ms | NS | | | |
| | | Ms | Ns | 23 | | |
| N | 21 | NS | NS | 0.3 | 25 | 99 |
| | | NS | Ns | 5 | | |
| | | Ns | Ns | 16 | | |

M and N antigen activity resides on the glycophorin A molecule. There are approximately 500,000 copies of this molecule present on each erythrocyte. This molecule is embedded in the erythrocyte, membrane with the antigenic molecular sequence located on the external portion of the molecule. When glycophorin A carries M antigenic activity, glycophorin $A^M$, the first amino acid residual is serine and the fifth is glycine. When it carries N activity, glycophorin $A^N$, leucine, and glutamic acid replace serine and glycine at positions one and five, respectively.

Glycophorin B is a smaller molecule than glycophorin A but possesses a segment, consisting of 26 amino acids, that duplicates the sequence of glycophorin $A^N$. This characteristic accounts for the presence of an N-like antigen on almost all erythrocytes, regardless of the MN type. Approximately 100,000 copies of this molecule are present on an erythrocyte. Glycophorin B is thought to carry U, S, and s antigen activity.

*MNSs Phenotypes.* Three phenotypes, MM, NN, and MN, along with 10 genotypes, exist in the MNSs blood group system. These phenotypes, genotypes, and the frequencies of each are presented in Table 6-9.

*MNSs Antibodies.* Antibodies of the MNSs blood group system are usually considered of minor clinical significance. Anti-M can be observed in multiparous women but rarely develops during pregnancy. Anti-N is an infrequently encountered antibody. Examples of anti-N have been observed in dialysis patients. The stimulus to antibody formation in these patients is attributed to a formaldehyde-induced alteration of the N antigens resulting from the reuse of formaldehyde-sterilized dialyzer membranes.

Most examples of anti-M and anti-N are cold-reacting IgM antibodies produced by nonerythrocytic stimuli, but some rare examples are IgG-type antibodies. Because of their IgM nature, anti-M and anti-N react in saline and exhibit stronger reactivity at cold temperatures. Enzyme treatment of erythrocytes destroys reactivity due to the removal of sialic acid from glycophorin A. Anti-M reacts better at an acid pH level. Some examples of anti-M react

in anti-human globulin (AHG) testing; these antibodies should be considered potentially dangerous. When testing sera for the presence of anti-M or anti-N, the dosage effect is frequently observed. A dosage effect pattern of reactivity of suspected anti-M or anti-N displays stronger agglutination reactions with erythrocytes that are homozygous for MM or NN, respectively.

Anti-S and anti-s are usually erythrocyte-stimulated IgG antibodies. Antibodies of this type can produce hemolytic disease of the newborn (HDN) or transfusion reactions. Anti-U is rare but can be formed in S − s − individuals. These antibodies can also cause HDN and transfusion reactions. Although anti-S may react in saline or AHG tests, it does not react with enzyme enhancement. Anti-s and anti-U react in AHG tests. Anti-U is enhanced with enzyme treatment. Anti-s is not destroyed by enzymes.

### The P Blood Group System

The $P_1$ antigen, originally referred to as P, was discovered in 1927 by Landsteiner and Levine. The original P antigen was reassigned to an antigen present on almost all human erythrocytes. Recently the P blood group system was renamed P 1. A reclassification of P antigens has been conducted by the International Society for Blood Transfusion. The definitive antigen in the system is $P_1$. About 80% of Whites and more than 90% of Blacks are of the $P_1$ phenotype. Erythrocytes lacking the $P_1$ antigen but possessing the P antigen are referred to as $P_2$. Four antigens are recognized in the P system: $P_1$, P, $P^k$, and $pp_1p^k$. Another antigen, p, has not yet been assigned to the system.

*Mode of Inheritance.* The inheritance of antigens in the P blood group system is apparently complex. The $P_1$ gene is considered to be inherited as a Mendelian dominant, but the $P^k$ locus is separate from the $P_1$ locus. It is not yet known whether there is actually a p gene that codes for a sialyl transferase.

The P blood group system is related to the ABO, Ii, and Lewis blood group systems. All of the antigens of these systems share a common precursor substance, lactosyl ceramide. Antigens of these systems are synthesized by the

**Figure 6-4.** Mechanism of expression of selected P blood group system antigens.

sequential addition of carbohydrate residues to the common precursor (Fig. 6-4). In one pathway, synthesis leads to globoside, with the P antigen present on almost all erythrocytes. The other pathway produces paragloboside, which results in the $P_1$ antigen. Only the P1 antigen is derived from the same precursor substance as the A, B, H antigens. It should be noted that sialosylparagloboside, the substance recognized as p antigen, differs from paragloboside only by the addition of sialic acid residue.

Because the P blood group antigens are carbohydrates, they cannot be direct gene products. The gene products are glycosyl-transferases that transfer a specific carbohydrate to an oligosaccharide chain. Although antigens of the ABO, Ii, and Lewis systems can be glycolipid or glycoprotein, the P antigens in man have been found to be only glycolipids.

***The Biochemical Nature of P Antigens.*** Each of the antigens of the P blood group system has distinctive characteristics. In addition, the Luke (LKE) antigen has been assigned to the globoside collection of antigens.

$P_1$. $P_1$ is a glycosphingolipid on the erythrocyte membrane. This antigen results from the conversion of paragloboside. $P_1$ is poorly developed on the erythrocytes of newborn infants and may take years to reach adult levels. Antigen strength can be variable. Expression of the antigen can be drastically reduced by the inhibitor gene InLu (a gene of the Lutheran system). The $P_1$ antigen is known to deteriorate rapidly on stored erythrocytes. $P_1$ antigen is also found on leukocytes and tissue cells as well as in some secretions, such as hydatid cyst fluid.

P. This antigen is a globoside. Only the $p^k$ and p phenotypes are known to lack P antigen. In addition to the presence of P antigen on almost all erythrocytes, it is also found in plasma, on leukocytes, and on tissue cells.

$P^k$. This antigen is rare but universal. It is produced by the addition of ($\alpha$) galactose to lactosyl ceramide. The presence of $P^k$ is undetectable on erythrocytes because of the almost complete conversion of $P^k$ to P antigen. This antigen occurs on some leukocytes and tissue cells, and in plasma. The fibroblasts of all but pp individuals possess $P^k$ antigen.

p. The p gene has been considered an amorphic gene when inherited in a homozygous state. In recent years this hypothesis has been questioned. It has been suggested that a genetic abnormality exists and that an absence of $\alpha$-galactosyl transferase(s) coding for $P^k$ and $P_1$ results. Sialosylparagloboside has been designated the p antigen. It should be noted that p ($Tj^{a-}$) erythrocytes exhibit an excess of sialosylparagloboside as well as paragloboside.

***Disorders Associated with the P System.*** In cases of paroxysmal cold hemoglobinuria (PCH), the associated antibody is usually auto-anti-P. A rare example of PCH has been auto-anti-IH-induced.

***P Blood Group System Phenotypes.*** Four antigens are recognized in the P system: $P_1$, P, $P^k$, and Luke. The $P_1$ antigen is the most common. These antigens combine to form one of five phenotypes, $P_1$, $P_2$, p, $P_1^k$ $P_2^k$ The phenotypes, detectable antigens, and phenotypic frequencies are presented in Table 6-10.

***P Blood Group System Antibodies.*** Anti-$P_1$ is a common antibody. It is often found in $P_2$ persons and it is usually a cold-reacting IgM antibody. This antibody is a strong nonagglutinating, complement-binding antibody. Samples containing anti-$P_1$ that react at 4° C are considered clinically insignificant, but rare examples of IgG anti-$P_1$ as well as anti-$P_1$ with a wide thermal range can be hemolytic.

Anti-P is an extremely rare antibody in pure form. It can be produced only by individuals of the $P^k$ phenotype. Anti-P is usually a potent IgM antibody with a wide thermal range, but it may occur as an IgG antibody. Occasional cases of habitual abortion have been attributed to anti-P.

**Table 6-10. P Blood Group System Phenotypes**

| Phenotype | Detectable Antigens | Phenotypic Frequency (%) White | Black |
|---|---|---|---|
| $P_1$ | $P_1$, P, PP $P_1^k$ | 79% | 94% |
| $P_2$ | P, PP $P_1^k$ | 21% | 6% |
| $P_1^k$ | $P_1$, $P^k$, PP $P_1^k$ | very rare | |
| $P_2^k$ | $P^k$, PP $P_1^k$ | very rare | |
| p | p only | very rare | |

Anti-P^k has not been reported as a pure antibody. It has been found only as a component of anti-Tj^a using selective absorption with P_1 + cells.

Only a few examples of anti-p have been reported. Anti-p antibodies react at either 4° C or in AHG. Anti-p is neutralized by sialosylparagloboside, but enzymes, such as papain, appear to enhance agglutination reactions.

Anti-Tj^a, a very rare antibody, is also known as anti-PP_1P^k. It can be produced by persons lacking P, P_1, and P^k antigens and has been isolated in the serum of p individuals, often without prior erythrocyte exposure. This antibody can be either IgM or IgG or a combination of both. Anti-Tj^a binds complement, is a potent hemolysin, and has a wide thermal range of activity. This antibody has been associated with hemolytic disease of the newborn and severe hemolytic transfusion reactions. It has also been implicated in chronic abortions and rejection of organs subsequent to transplantation.

Examples of other antibodies encountered in the P blood group system, rarely encountered, include compound, cold-reacting antibodies such as anti-IP_1, iP_1, and anti-I^TP_1.

### The Ii System

The Ii system appears to include only two antigens, I and i. This blood group system sometimes interacts with the ABO, Lewis, and P systems, to form compound antibodies, such as anti-IP_1, anti-ILe^{bH}, and anti-IH.

Several I and i phenotypes are recognized based on genetically determined differences in the amount of I and i on erythrocytes. These phenotypes tend to be quantitative rather than qualitative; therefore, the terms I + and I − are relative terms.

*Mode of Inheritance.* It seems likely that no single I or i gene actually exists but that the presence or absence of many glycosyl transferases that attach carbohydrates result in different carbohydrate sequences. These sequences are subsequently recognized as I or i antigens by the heterogeneous antibodies designated as anti-I and anti-i. The antibody diversity of anti-I and anti-i may represent antibody recognition of a single carbohydrate, a combination of carbohydrates, or perhaps an entire chain.

With the exception of the rare i_adult phenotype (approximately 1:10,000 persons), the expression of the I + antigen status develops along a continuum. The change from the i cord blood and newborn state to the I adult status gradually changes over a period of about 18 months. This transition in Ii status reflects antigen density on the erythrocyte membrane (Table 6-11). Individuals of the O_h phenotype possess the greatest concentration of I antigen in adults.

*The Biochemical Nature of Ii Antigens.* I and i antigens reside in the subterminal portions of the oligosaccharides that eventually are converted to H and A or B anti-

**Table 6-11. Comparative Amounts of Ii Antigen Expressed on Human Erythrocytes**

| Phenotype | Antigen | |
|---|---|---|
| | i | I |
| i_cord | Elevated | Diminished |
| i_adult | Elevated | Trace |
| I_adult | Diminished | Elevated |

gens. I and i structures are found on membrane-associated glycoproteins and glycosphingolipids.

The type 2 oligosaccharide chains carrying the terminal carbohydrates that determine ABH specificity include multiple β-N-acetylglucosamine (1,3) and β-galactose (1,4) units. The i antigenic activity is formed by two disaccharides linked in a straight chain oligosaccharide. In comparison, the erythrocytes of adults demonstrate that branched chains predominate. I specificity is associated with the branched chains. The transition of Ii antigenicity in the erythrocytes of a newborn infant to those of an adult is considered a reflection of the change from predominance of straight chains to predominance of branched chains.

The Ii antigens present on erythrocytes are also demonstrated on other blood cells such as leukocytes and platelets, and probably exist on many tissue cells, as do the ABH antigens. Both I and i as soluble glycoproteins are found in plasma, serum, and secretions, such as saliva, of newborn infants and adults. Human milk (colostrum) is known to be rich in I substance.

*Disorders Associated with Ii Antigens.* It is not uncommon to detect anti-I, as an autoantibody, if the serum of normal healthy adults is tested at room temperature or cooler. However, Anti-I is usually associated with cold agglutinin syndrome (CAS) and atypical pneumonia caused by a pleuropneumonia-like organism (*Mycoplasma pneumoniae*). Potent examples of auto-anti-I are rare but may be observed in patients with some forms of autoimmune disorders, such as cold autoimmune hemolytic anemia.

Anti-i antibody is classically associated with certain viral disorders. These disorders include infectious mononucleosis caused by the Epstein-Barr virus and cytomegalovirus. It may also be seen in reticulosis, alcoholic cirrhosis, and myelogenous leukemia.

Rare examples of auto-anti-IH have been observed in cases of paroxysmal cold hemoglobinuria (PCH).

*Ii Phenotypes.* Except for unusual examples, the Ii phenotypes are straightforward. Cord blood cells demonstrate the lack of I antigen and are therefore referred to as i_cord and the erythrocytes of adults are I positive. Intermediate reactions can be observed in young children as the transition from i to I takes place. Rare examples of i and weak forms of I have been noted in adults.

*Ii Antibodies.* Most examples of anti-I are of the IgM type. This antibody is usually clinically insignificant; but

**Table 6-12. Sample Test Results with Typical Cold Antibodies**

|  | I | i | H* | IH |
|---|---|---|---|---|
| A₁ (Adult) | 4+ | 0–1+ | 0–1+ | 0–2+ |
| A₂ (Adult) | 4+ | 0–1+ | 2–3+ | 4+ |
| B (Adult) | 4+ | 0 1 I | 2 3 I | 4+ |
| O (Adult) | 4+ | 0–1+ | 4+ | 4+ |
| O (cord) | 0–2+ | 4+ | 3–4+ | 0–2+ |
| Auto | 0–4+ | 0–1+ | 0–2+ | 0–2+ |

* Anti-H is typical of the anitbody that may be formed by A₁ and A₁B persons.

it can be dangerous if it masks other significant alloantibodies. To determine if other antibodies such as anti-M or anti-Leᵃ are also present, it is useful to adsorb the patient's serum (see Chapter 14) with the patient's enzyme-treated erythrocytes and then retest the adsorbed serum.

Anti-I reacts best at 4° C. It exhibits activity in saline, albumin, and with enzyme treatment. If an antibody agglutinates all adult cells, including an autocontrol, but fails to agglutinate cord blood cells, anti-I should be suspected.

The anti-I in patients with autoimmune disorders differs from the previously described autoantibody. Individuals who are i_adult will often produce an allo-anti-I that reacts at a wider thermal range and is a more potent antibody than auto-anti-I. This antibody could reduce survival of transfused erythrocytes and may warrant the use of I− blood, if transfusion is necessary.

Anti-i shares many of the characteristics of anti-I but reacts strongly with cord blood (Table 6-12).

## Typical IgG Antibody Systems Detectable by AHG Testing

### The Kell Blood Group System

This system was first defined in 1946, when the serum of the mother of a baby with hemolytic disease of the newborn (HDN) was found to contain anti-Kell. In 1949, the Kell antigen was subsequently matched with the hypothetical allele Cellano (k) and a new blood system was established. Two other pairs of antithetical antigens were subse-

quently identified: Kpᵃ (Penney, 1957) and Kpᵇ (Rautenberg, 1958); and Jsᵃ (Sutter, 1958) and Jsᵇ (Matthews, 1963). More than 20 antigens have been identified and incorporated into this blood group system, e.g., Kpᶜ, KEL11, and KEL17.

*Mode of Inheritance.* The genes Kpᵃ, Kpᵇ, and Kpᶜ; Jsᵃ and Jsᵇ; KEL11 and KEL17; and possibly KEL14 and KEL24 are believed to be inherited as a complex or cluster together with K/k. It is further believed that Kell antigens are controlled by an inherited gene complex or by one gene that codes for several antigenic determinants. These antigens are inherited as if they are produced by alleles at closely linked loci. The extremely rare K_o phenotype represents the null phenotype of the Kell system, a condition in which none of the six antigens is expressed. It is important to remember that K_o is not an antigen; it designates a phenotype.

The mode of inheritance of Kell system antigens appears to be complex. It is assumed that a precursor substance, K_x, is coded for by a gene X¹k on the X chromosome. This K_x precursor is then converted, perhaps by enzymatic (transferase) action, to the appropriate gene products of the inherited Kell genes (see Fig. 6-5). A K_o person is negative for all the previously described; but K_o cells are rich in K_x antigens.

*The Biochemical Nature of Kell Antigens.* Kell system antigens are carried on a 93-kD glycoprotein on the red blood cell membrane. Biochemical susceptibility suggests that disulfide bonds are essential for the maintenance of antigen activity.

The Kell antigens are well-developed at birth. With the exception of K_x, the antigens seem to be restricted to the erythrocyte membrane. K_x is also found on the membranes of macrophages and neutrophilic leukocytes. The Kell system antigens are represented at the red blood cell membrane in low density (K = 3, 500, k = 2,000 to 5,000 sites).

*Disorders Associated with Kell Antigens.* Normal erythrocytes carry trace amounts of the K_x antigen. When a person lacks K_x on the red blood cell membrane, the McLeod phenotype results. In the absence of K_x, normal

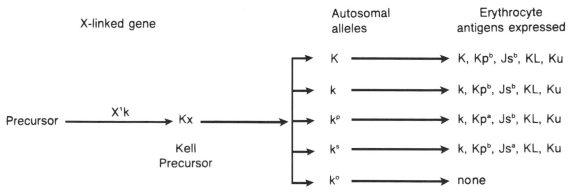

**Figure 6-5.** Theoretical mechanism of expression of selected Kell antigens.

expression of inherited Kell genes is blocked. If some synthesis does occur, the resulting antigens react weakly, if at all.

The lack of $K_x$ antigen is associated with abnormal erythrocytes (acanthocytes) that are prematurely destroyed, causing chronic hemolytic anemia. This collection of red cell abnormalities is called the McLeod phenotype. A lack of leukocytic $K_x$ is associated with chronic granulomatous disease (CGD). This appears to result from a deletion of part of the X chromosome, which includes the XK locus as well as X-CGD. Two types of CGD exist: Type I and Type II. In the Type I disorder, the usual Kell antigens, including $K_x$, are of normal strength. In Type II, many of the Kell antigens are weak and $K_x$ is undetectable. Although both types of CGD lack leukocytic $K_x$, in Type II, the erythrocytes are of the McLeod phenotype.

***Kell Phenotypes.*** The frequency of Kell blood group system antigens varies and racial differences exist. Certain combinations of antigens are common, whereas others are rare (Table 6-13).

***Kell Antibodies.*** Kell (K) antigen has an immunogenicity second only to the D antigen. Because of the potency of the K antigen, anti-K is one of the most common immune erythrocyte antibodies and accounts for almost two-thirds of non-Rh immune alloantibodies. If a K− individual receives a unit of K+ blood, the chances are 1 in 10 that an alloantibody will be produced. Cases of nonerythrocyte-stimulated anti-K are infrequent. Kell blood group system antibodies have been implicated in both hemolytic transfusion reactions and hemolytic disease of the newborn (see Chapter 10 for a further discussion of HDN).

Anti-K is usually an IgG antibody detectable with antihuman globulin (AHG). Uncommon examples of IgM anti-K can be encountered, but they must be very potent to agglutinate red cells without AHG. Additionally, some examples bind complement and therefore sensitize erythrocytes. In these cases, agglutination can be detected with anti-complement as well as by anti-IgG AHG. Anti-K and anti-Js$^b$ can also react with enzyme-treated cells.

Examples of anti-k are rare because only 2 persons in 1000 are k−. Other Kell blood group system antibodies, anti-Kp$^a$, anti-Kp$^b$, anti-Js$^a$, and anti-Js$^b$, are rare. Anti-Ku

**Table 6-13. Phenotypic Frequencies of the Major Kell Antigens**

|  | White (%) | Black (%) |
|---|---|---|
| kk | 91 | 98 |
| Kk | 8.8 | 2.0 |
| KK | 0.2 | <0.1 |
| Js (a−b+) | >99.9 | 80.5 |
| Js (a+b−) | 0.1 | 1.1 |
| Js (a+b+) | 0.1 | 18.4 |
| Kp (a−b+) | 98 | 100 |
| Kp (a+b+) | 2 | rare |
| Kp (a+b−) | 0.1 | 0 |

is found only in $K_o$ persons and reacts with all erythrocytes except those of the phenotype $K_o$. Anti-KL has been found in several patients with CGD or symptoms suggestive of it and reacts with the cells of all subjects except those of the McLeod phenotype.

### The Duffy Blood Group System

The first member of the Duffy blood group system, Fy$^a$, was identified in 1950 in a multiply transfused hemophiliac named Duffy. The corresponding allele, Fy$^b$, was described in 1951. Fy, a third allele at this locus, has a high incidence among Blacks. It produces no Fy$^a$ or Fy$^b$ antigens. In 1965 it was discovered that the erythrocytes of some Whites, previously assumed to be Fy− (heterozygous Fy$^a$− Fy$^b$−), were actually Fy$^x$. The Fy$^x$, the fourth allele in the system, makes a very small amount of Fy$^b$. In 1968, the Duffy locus was the first locus to be linked to an inherited visible abnormality, congenital cataract, on chromosome 1. The Duffy locus has the distinction of being the first locus in humans to be assigned to a particular autosome.

***Mode of Inheritance.*** The development of Duffy antigens is speculative. A proposed model suggests that a basic precursor substance is converted into an Fy precursor by the action of the hypothetical F gene. The locus of this gene is unknown, but it is believed to be independent of the Fy locus.

***The Biochemical Nature of Duffy Antigens.*** The Duffy antigens are well developed on fetal cells. The number of Fy$^a$ antigen sites on Fy$^a$Fy$^a$ erythrocytes is estimated at 12,000. These antigens are probably protein in nature and are destroyed by in vitro treatment with proteolytic enzymes, such as ficin and papain. Dosage effects are common, but not all antibodies detect the dosage effect.

***Disorders Associated with Duffy Antigens.*** It is believed that, for certain malarial parasites (*Plasmodium vivax*) to enter erythrocytes, Fy$^a$ or Fy$^b$ antigens must be present. In Africa, where malaria is endemic, natives have been found to be resistant to *Plasmodium vivax*. This resistance is undoubtedly related to the fact that in some parts of Africa all of the native population are Fy(a−b−). This phenomenon may reflect a natural defense mechanism that has persisted through natural selection. American Blacks have partially lost this characteristic because of interracial genetic mixing and the lack of need for such a defense mechanism. The gene frequency for Fy in some parts of Africa is 1.0, compared to the 0.7 incidence in Blacks in the United States.

***Duffy Phenotypes.*** The frequency of Duffy blood group system antigens (Fy$^a$ and Fy$^b$) exhibits more racial differences between Whites and Blacks than any of the other major blood group systems, but these differences are less pronounced among Blacks in the United States than in Africa. In some parts of Africa all native people are Fy(a−b−). The most predominant antigen in Whites is

**Table 6-14. Phenotypic Distribution of Duffy Antigens in the American Population**

| Phenotype | Frequency | |
|-----------|-----------|-----------|
|           | White (%) | Black (%) |
| Fy (a+b−) | 18 | 14 |
| Fy (a+b+) | 49 | 2 |
| Fy (a−b−) | 33 | 19 |
| Fy (a−b−) | 0 | 65 |

Fy$^a$. Many Blacks lack both Fy$^a$ and Fy$^b$ antigens. The phenotypic distribution in the United States is presented in Table 6-14.

*Duffy Antibodies.* Compared to the D and Kell antigens, Fy$^a$ and Fy$^b$ do not appear to be strongly antigenic; therefore the Duffy antibodies are seen about three times less frequently than anti-K. Duffy antibodies tend to occur more frequently in Whites than in Blacks. When Duffy antibodies are observed, anti-Fy$^a$ is more frequent. Anti-Fy$^b$ usually occurs in sera with multiple antibodies rather than as a single antibody. Duffy antibodies are almost always stimulated by erythrocyte antigen exposure through transfusion or pregnancy. Anti-Fy$^a$ occasionally causes hemolytic disease of the newborn, but has frequently been implicated as a cause of hemolytic transfusion reactions. Fy$^b$ can be a cause of fatal transfusion reactions.

Anti-Fy$^a$ and anti-Fy$^b$ are found mostly as IgG immunoglobulins. The most sensitive method of detecting these antibodies is AHG testing. If enzyme testing is employed, anti-Fy$^a$ may bind complement. It is important to note that the Fy$^a$ antigen is destroyed by most enzymes.

Anti-Fy3 acts like a combination of anti-Fy$^a$ + Fy$^b$ and reacts with all human erythrocytes except those of the phenotype Fy(a−b−). Fy3 is considered to be an enzyme-resistant antigen present on all Fy(a+) and Fy(b+) red blood cells but absent from Fy(a−b−) red blood cells.

Anti-Fy3 is not deteriorated by enzyme treatment and reacts with all Fy$^a$+ and Fy$^b$+ cells. It does not react with Fy(a−b−) cells. This antibody has been consistently observed in the serum of non-Black Fya−b− individuals.

Anti-Fy4 was first identified in the serum of a multiply transfused Fy(a+b+) child. It reacts with all Fy(a−b−) erythrocytes and some Fy$^a$ or Fy$^b$+ erythrocytes but not with Fy(a+b+) erythrocytes. If enzyme-treated erythrocytes are used in antibody detection, the antigen resists degradation by proteolytic enzymes. Fy4 is considered to be the product of an allele called Fy that, in the homogenous state, is responsible for the Fy(a−b−) phenotype on Blacks.

Anti-Fy5 has been identified. The antibody reacts with AHG and enzyme-treated erythrocytes. Reactivity of the antibody is similar to anti-Fy3, except that it also reacts with Fy(a−b−) erythrocytes, does not react with Rh null erythrocytes of the usual Duffy phenotypes, and reacts weakly with -D-/-D- erythrocytes. It has been postulated that Fy5 is formed by the interaction of Rh and Duffy gene products.

### The Kidd Blood Group System

The first example of the Kidd blood group system, Jk$^a$, was identified in 1951. The antithetical gene, Jk$^b$, was found in 1953. In 1959, Jk3, which is apparently a universal antigen, was discovered. Examples of the rare phenotype Jk(a−b−) Kidd null have also been recognized. It has been suggested that Jk$^a$Jk$^b$ is a distinct specific antigen in this system and probably a fundamental one in the Kidd system.

*Mode of Inheritance.* The Jk$^a$ and Jk$^b$ genes are known to be codominant alleles, but the mechanism of antigen expression in the Kidd system has not been well defined. In the case of the rare Kidd null phenotype, it is believed that it may arise from one of two mechanisms. Homozygous inheritance of an amorphic Jk gene is one explanation, and the inheritance of a suppressor gene that prevents Jk$^a$/Jk$^b$ expression on erythrocytes is the other.

*The Biochemical Nature of Kidd Antigens.* Only a limited amount of information is known about the nature and structure of the Kidd antigens, which are known to be well developed at birth. They are also low in immunogenicity. In laboratory testing, the antigens are not destroyed by enzyme treatment; in fact, ficin and trypsin have been observed to enhance reactions. Questions remain as to whether Jk$^a$ and Jk$^b$ exist on cells other than erythrocytes.

*Kidd Phenotypes.* The phenotypes and frequencies of the two antigens of the Kidd system are given in Table 6-15. The phenotype lacking both antigens is rare.

*Kidd Antibodies.* Kidd antibodies are infrequently encountered. Anti-Jk$^b$ is rarer than anti-Jk$^a$ and is usually found in sera with other immune alloantibodies. Although Kidd antibodies have been known to cause mild hemolysis, they are extremely dangerous because they disappear from the circulation rapidly and may produce violent delayed hemolytic transfusion reactions. Anti-Jk$^a$ has the reputation of causing in vivo destruction, which is much greater than might be expected from the reactions produced in vitro.

Kidd antibodies are usually of the IgG type, but may also be either IgM or a combination of both types. These

**Table 6-15. Phenotypes of Kidd System**

| Phenotype | Genotype | Frequency | |
|-----------|----------|-----------|-----------|
|           |          | White (%) | Black (%) |
| Jk (a+b−) | Jk$^a$Jk$^a$ | 25 | 75 |
| Jk (a+b+) | Jk$^a$Jk$^b$ | 50 | 34 |
| Jk (a−b+) | Jk$^b$Jk$^b$ | 25 | 9 |
| Jk (a−b−) | JkJk | 0 | 0 |

* Rare individuals of this type have been found among South American Indians and Chinese.

antibodies are often complement-dependent, very labile on storage, and most easily detected in fresh serum. All the examples of Kidd antibodies have been shown to react in AHG and not in saline, and all react with enzyme treatment. AHG reactions with anticomplement are distinctly stronger, and in some cases positive reactions are observed only with anticomplement antisera. Dosage effects may be observed. Anti-JK$^a$ frequently exhibits dosage effects and may be positive only with Jk$^a$Jk$^a$ erythrocytes.

## OTHER BLOOD GROUP SYSTEMS

### Xg

One of the most unique blood groups is the sex-linked Xg system. The Xg$^a$ antigen is the only presently recognized antigen in this system. An antithetic allele (Xg) has not been identified. Individuals are of either the Xg(a+) or Xg(a−) phenotype. Because the Xg$^a$ antigen is X-linked, it is more likely to occur in women than in men.

The frequency of the phenotype Xg(a+) is approximately 88% in women and 64% in men. The genotype of women may be Xg$^a$Xg$^a$, Xg$^a$Xg, or XgXg, but men can be only Xg$^a$ or Xg. Men who are Xg(a+) pass on Xg$^a$ to all their daughters but transmit no Xg genes to their sons. The mating of an Xg(a+) man with an Xg(a−) woman must produce all Xg(a+) daughters and Xg(a−) sons.

Anti-Xg$^a$ is an uncommon antibody. Rare examples of auto anti-Xg$^a$ in Xg(a+) individuals have been reported. Some examples of the antibody react at room temperature or 37° C, but most of these antibodies react in the AHG phase of testing. Anti-Xg$^a$ has not been associated with either hemolytic transfusion reactions or hemolytic disease of the newborn.

### Sid

Sd$^a$, the only defined antigen in this system, is inherited as an autosomal dominant character and appears to be genetically independent of most other blood group systems. Rare cases have demonstrated an enhanced erythrocyte antigen, called Sd(a++) or "Super Sid," and another form of Sd$^a$, named Cad, was originally thought to be a form of inherited polyagglutinability. The incidence of Sd$^a$ antigen is >90%. This antigen is often difficult to work with because of a wide variation in antigenic expression; it is known to be weaker during pregnancy. A possible relationship exists between Sd$^a$ and Cad antigens and the ABO system.

Sd$^a$ substance is present in most body secretions. Four times as much Sd$^a$ is found in the saliva of newborn infants as in the saliva of adults. Because the greatest concentration of Sd$^a$ occurs in the urine, it is sometimes easier to categorize apparent weak Sd(a+) persons by testing their urine.

Anti-Sd$^a$ is characteristically weakly reactive. Some Sd$^a$ antibodies react at room temperature, 37° C, and AHG. Most examples of anti-Sd$^a$ are demonstrable with enzyme-treated red cells and cells enhanced with LISS. Observable agglutinates have a characteristic refractile, mixed-field appearance.

Although a hemolytic transfusion reaction caused by anti-Sd$^a$ was reported in 1970, the antibody is not generally associated with hemolytic transfusion reactions, even if incompatible blood is transfused, or with HDN.

An autoantibody, Sd$^x$, has been described which seems to define an erythrocyte receptor related to Sd$^a$. The antibody, which is inhibited by Sd(a+) urine but not by Sd(a−) urine, has been responsible for rare cases of cold antibody autoimmune hemolytic anemia.

### Cartwright

Yt$^a$ is a common antigen, found on the erythrocytes of >99% of both the White and Black population. The Yt$^b$ antigen has a frequency of about 8% in both Whites and Blacks. The Yt$^a$ antigen was defined in 1956 and the allele, Yt$^b$, in 1964.

Anti-Yt$^a$ is not uncommon in Yt(a−) persons with a history of pregnancy or transfusion. In contrast, anti-Yt$^b$ is a rare antibody usually found in combination with other antibodies. Both anti-Yt$^a$ and anti-Yt$^b$ are usually reactive in AHG and with LISS enhancement. Some examples are reactive in enzyme-enhanced red cell suspensions.

Anti-Yt$^a$ has been implicated in both hemolytic transfusion reactions and HDN. Anti-Yt$^b$ has also been associated with HDN.

### Colton

Two antigens, Co$^a$ and Co$^b$, have been identified in this system. About 99.8% of the White population are Co(a+) and about 10% are Co(b+). American Blacks may have a lower incidence of Co(a−) than the White population.

Anti-Co$^a$ and anti-Co$^b$ were identified in 1974. These antibodies are IgG in nature and have been associated with pregnancy with an incompatible fetus. Both Co$^a$ and Co$^b$ can be detected in the AHG phase of testing. Enzyme enhancement of erythrocytes allows most examples of both antibodies to be demonstrated. Anti-Co$^a$ can cause both hemolytic transfusion reactions and hemolytic disease of the newborn. Anti-Co$^b$ has been implicated in hemolytic transfusion reactions.

### Dombrock

The antigens Do$^a$ and Do$^b$ are the two demonstrable antigens of this system. Approximately 67% of Whites are Do(a+) and about 83% are Do(b+). The incidence of Do$^a$ is lower in Blacks, American Indians, and Orientals.

Both anti-Do$^a$ and anti-Do$^b$ are infrequently encountered. Most examples of both antibodies are reactive in AHG and in enzyme and LISS enhancement. Anti-Do$^a$ has been associated with hemolytic transfusion reactions.

## Diego

Di$^a$ was identified in 1955. All Whites are Di(a−), and approximately 36% of certain South American Indians are Di(a+). Five to 15% of Japanese and Chinese are Di(a+). The Di$^b$ antigen was identified in 1967, when the first two examples of anti-Di$^b$ were described. The frequency of Di$^b$ is 100% in Whites and undetermined in other racial groups.

Some examples of anti-Di$^a$ react at room temperature, 37° C, and with enzyme enhancement. Most Di$^a$ antibodies react in the AHG phase. Anti-Di$^b$ generally reacts in AHG, but some examples are reactive with enzyme-enhanced erythrocytes. Both antibodies have been implicated in hemolytic transfusion reactions and HDN.

## Scianna

The Scianna (SC) blood group is inherited in a dominant Mendelian manner and occupies a locus on chromosome 1. SC1, a very high-frequency antigen, was originally called Sm$^1$. SC2, a very low-frequency antigen, was initially referred to as Bu$^a$ before it was realized that $Sc^1$ and Sc$^2$ were, in all probability, alleles. Sc1 and Sc2 are now considered antithetic antigens. The most frequent phenotype is Sc1,−2, but the incidence of Sc2 antigen is higher in the Mennonite population than in other Whites. Both anti-Sc1 and Sc2 are uncommon antibodies and have not been implicated in transfusion reactions or HDN.

In 1980, the existence of a third antigen in the Scianna blood group system was suggested after an alloantibody directed against a high-frequency red cell antigen was identified in a Sc−1,−2 patient. The Sc−1,−2 phenotype is rare. The findings in three cases of patients who developed IgG alloantibodies directed against red blood cell antigens that were not present on Sc null cells suggest that red cells of this phenotype may lack additional Sc antigens or have no expression of other unrelated high-frequency antigens. It is possible, however, that Sc−1,−2 red cells represent an Sc null phenotype similar to the Rh$_{null}$ phenotype of the Rh blood group system or the K$_o$ of the Kell blood group system.

## HUMAN LEUKOCYTE ANTIGENS (HLA) DETECTABLE ON ERYTHROCYTES

In the late 1950s and early 1960s, researchers identified antibodies that were contaminants in many typing sera. These antibodies were frequently found in multiparous women, often with isoleukoagglutinins. They are enhanced by the enzymes trypsin and papain but destroyed by the enzyme, bromelin, and best detected with fresh erythrocytes collected into ACD anticoagulant.

The corresponding antigens to these antibodies vary within families as well as in individuals over a period of time, and are not fully expressed at birth. These antigens were initially classified as Bg$^a$ and Bg$^b$ with the "Bennett-Goodspeed" group. Later, a third antigen, Bg$^c$, was defined.

In 1969, the erythrocyte antigen Bg$^a$ was correlated with the leukocyte antigen HLA-B7. This was the first leukocyte antigen to be demonstrated on erythrocytes. The antigen frequency on erythrocytes is about 17% in both White and Black populations. In 1971, the identification of Bg$^b$ as HLA-B17 and Bg$^c$ as HLA-A28 was reported. The frequency of Bg$^b$ is approximately 9% in Whites and 28% in Blacks. Bg$^c$ has a frequency of about 8% in Whites and approximately 17% in Blacks. Most, if not all, HLA antigens may be present on erythrocytes, but the Bg antigens, particularly Bg$^a$ and Bg$^c$, are remarkable because they give much stronger reactions than other HLA antigens. These antigens, however, cannot be detected on the erythrocytes of all individuals possessing the same antigens on their leukocytes. Enzyme treatment of red cells may depress some Bg reactivity and enhance others. Bg$^a$ is more likely than Bg$^b$ to be weakened by proteolytic enzymes.

The Bg, or hemagglutinating HLA antibodies, may be detected in multiparous or multitransfused patients. The incidence of anti-Bg$^a$ is approximately 1.5%. It is exceedingly difficult to test a high-frequency antibody for accompanying HLA antibodies, and the possibility of such contamination must be considered when discrepant or weaker than expected results are obtained. The identification of low-frequency erythrocyte antibodies is also menaced by the possible presence of HLA antibodies.

A fourth antibody has been shown to react with the red blood cells of persons with the leukocyte antigen HLA-A10.

## ANTIGENS SHARED WITH OTHER HUMAN CELLULAR ELEMENTS

### Lymphocytes and Other Tissues

The HLA antigens (see Chapter 16) exist on most tissue cells. Some HLA antigens can be demonstrated on granulocytes.

### Mature Granulocytes

Specific determinants present only on mature granulocytes have been located in the sera of persons with immune neutropenia. These include NA1 and NA2, NB1 and NB2, NC1, ND1, and NE1, and a series of related antigens called human granulocyte antigens (HGA-3a-3e).

Antibodies to the HGA-3 series of antigens are sometimes associated with febrile transfusion reactions. In addition, antibodies directed against 5a and 5b antigens occasionally occur in women after pregnancy, and may be associated with febrile transfusion reactions.

## Platelet Antigens

Platelet antigens are predominantly found on platelets. Human platelet antigens have been grouped into five divisions: HPA-1 to HPA-5. Platelet-specific antigens associated with surface glycoproteins are HPA-1 and HPA-4, which are located at the glycoprotein IIIa location: HPA-5 is located at the glycoprotein Ia location; HPA-2 is located at glycoprotein location GPIb; and HPA-3 is located at the GPIIb location.

Testing for platelet antibodies can be useful as an adjunct to HLA matching in selecting compatible platelets for recipients with alloantibodies directed at platelet antigens. Platelets express varying amounts of HLA-A and HLA-B but demonstrate no significant amounts of HLA-C and HLA-D or DR antigens.

## HIGH-INCIDENCE ANTIGENS UNRELATED TO THE PRINCIPAL BLOOD GROUP SYSTEMS

Antigens of high frequency are defined as occurring in 99.9% of the population. Examples of high-frequency antigens that are apparently unrelated to principal blood group systems include Augustine (At[a]), Cromer (Cr[a]), En[a], Gerbich (Ge), Gregory (Gy[a]) and Holley (Hy), Jacobs (Jr[a]), Joseph (Jo[a]), Langereis (Lan), Ok[a], and Vel (Ve). It should be noted, however, that the At(a−), Cr(a−), and Jo(a−) phenotypes are found predominantly in Blacks.

Antibodies to the high incidence antigens are rarely observed. Some of these, such as anti-Vel, are IgM antibodies and bind complement. Others, such as anti-Ge, are more commonly AHG-reactive. Anti-Vel and probably anti-Ge are considered clinically significant antibodies.

## OTHER RED BLOOD CELL ANTIGENS

Other red blood cells of comparatively high incidence can form antibodies formerly referred to as the high-titer, low-avidity (HTLA) antibodies. These antibodies were collectively considered because they demonstrated a similar pattern of serologic reactions. The name HTLA referred to the fact that these antibodies exhibit reactivity at high dilutions of serum, but the strength of agglutination is weak at any dilution. This characteristic differentiated the former HTLA antibodies from other blood group antibodies that demonstrate progressively weaker reactivity with increased dilution of the antibody-containing serum.

Antibodies most frequently encountered are those directed at the high-frequency antigens York (Yk[a]) and Cost-Stirling (Cs[a]), Knops-Helgeson (Kn[a]) and McCoy

(McC[a]), Chido (Ch[a]) and Rodgers (Rg[a]), John Milton Hagen (JMH), Holley and Gregory (Gy[a]). The Chido and HLA loci are linked. Rodgers, like Chido, is also linked to the HLA-B locus. It has recently been shown that Chido (Ch 1-6) and Rodgers (Rd 1,2) antigens are part of the $C_4$ molecule of human complement.

Antibodies to these antigens characteristically exhibit varying degrees of reactivity with different samples of antigen-positive erythrocytes. This variability is particularly marked with Ch[a] and Rg[a]. Most of these antibodies are reactive in the AHG phase of testing.

Chido antibody is not an uncommon cause of difficulty in crossmatching in previously transfused patients. This antibody is adsorbed by the leukocytes of Ch(a+) individuals and neutralized by the plasma and serum but not saliva of Ch(a+) individuals. Anti-Ch[a] does not reduce the survival of Ch(a+) erythrocytes in vivo. Both anti-Ch[a] and anti-Rg[a] react more weakly with enzyme-treated cells than with untreated cells. In addition, Chido and Rodgers are the only antibodies in this grouping that are neutralizable. A characteristic of Rg(a+) erythrocytes is that cells stored as a clot react more strongly than fresh cells.

The clinical significance of these antibodies is questionable, but for the most part there is little evidence that they cause hemolytic transfusion reactions. Anti-McC[a] has been associated with hemolytic transfusion reactions and probably with hemolytic disease of the newborn. It is important, however, to distinguish these antibodies from low-titered antibodies to high-incidence antigens, such as Kp[b], Lan, and Vel.

## LOW-INCIDENCE ANTIGENS UNRELATED TO THE PRINCIPAL BLOOD GROUP SYSTEMS

Low-incidence antigens unrelated to the principal blood group systems are defined as antigens with an incidence of less than 1%. Examples of this type of antigen include the Wright blood group system, which is independent of all other blood group systems, as well as the Swann (Sw[a]), By, Mt[a], and Tr[a] antigens. In general, these antigens are unimportant in blood transfusion because it is easy to find compatible blood for patients who develop corresponding antibodies to these antigens.

### Wright Blood Group System

The antigen Wr[a] is present in about 2 in 1000 blood samples in the White population.

Anti-Wr[a] is a frequently occurring antibody; it can be detected in 1 in 100 persons. It has even been identified in men who have never been transfused. Anti-Wr[a] is often found in the serum of patients who have formed other blood group antibodies and in the serum of patients with autoimmune hemolytic anemia.

Anti-Wr$^a$ has been reported to occur in both IgM and IgG forms. The phases of reactivity range from room temperature to AHG. Some examples react with enzyme-enhanced erythrocytes. It has been implicated in both hemolytic transfusion reactions and HDN.

## CHAPTER SUMMARY

### Lewis Blood Group System

The two common antigens of the Lewis system are Lewis$^a$ (Le$^a$) and Lewis$^b$ (Le$^b$). The Lewis blood group system is unlike the other blood group system in that genetic control of the two antigens Le$^a$ and Le$^b$ appears to reside in a single gene called Le. This system represents a complex interaction between the independent Lewis, ABO, and secretor genes and is best understood by thinking of it as a system of genetically determined water-soluble antigens present in body fluids.

The Lewis system differs from other blood group systems in three significant ways. These differences include the fact that Lewis substances are absorbed from the plasma rather than being membrane-bound antigens, the Lewis phenotype is influenced by the secretor status, and the Lewis phenotype may be modified by the ABO phenotype. In addition, the Lewis gene does not code directly for the production of Lewis antigens.

Lewis antibodies are frequently found in individuals who have never been transfused or received any other known erythrocyte antigen stimulus. Anti-Le$^a$ and anti-Le$^b$ are especially common in pregnant women. Rare cases of hemolytic disease of the newborn (HDN) have been attributed to anti-Le$^a$. Lewis antibodies have been cited as the cause of a few hemolytic transfusion reactions.

### Additional Major Blood Group Systems

The typically IgM antibody systems that are best detected at cold temperatures include MNSsU, P, and I, and Lu$^a$ antigens. The typically IgG antibody systems detectable by antiglobulin (AHG) testing include the Kell, Duffy, Kidd, and Lu$^b$ antigens.

Initially, the Lewis and Lutheran genes were believed to be linked, but it was later discovered that the Lutheran genes were actually linked to the gene-controlling secretor status. The *Lu$^a$* and *Lu$^b$* genes are codominant. The Lu(a−b+) phenotype is the most common and the Lu(a−b−) is the rarest. The Lutheran antibodies, particularly Anti-Lu$^a$, are infrequently observed but are known to occur with no known erythrocyte stimulus in most cases. Most examples of anti-Lu$^b$ are associated with known exposure to erythrocyte antigen through transfusion or pregnancy.

The M and N antigens are classically associated with paternity testing. The MNSs system includes a group of mostly low-frequency "satellite" antigens rarely of clinical significance. Several of these low-frequency antigens are considered interrelated and form the Miltenberger subsystem. Three phenotypes, MM, NN, and MN, and 10 genotypes exist in the MNSs blood group system. Antibodies of the MNSs blood group system are usually considered of minor clinical significance, but anti-S and anti-s are usually erythrocyte-stimulated IgG antibodies and can produce HDN or transfusion reactions.

In cases of paroxysmal cold hemoglobinuria, the associated antibody is usually auto-anti-P.

The Ii system appears to include only two antigens, I and i. This blood group system sometimes interacts with the ABO, I, Lewis, and P systems to form compound antibodies such as anti-IP$_1$, anti-ILe$^{bH}$, and anti-IH.

The Kell blood group system consists of Kell and its allele, Cellano (k), as well as two other major pairs of antithetic antigens, Kp$^a$ (Penney) and Kp$^b$ (Rautenberg); and Js$^a$ (Sutter) and Js$^b$ (Matthews). More than 20 antigens have been identified and incorporated into this blood group system. The Kell antigen has a strength of immunogenicity second only to the D antigen. Because of the potency of the K antigen, anti-K is one of the most common immune red blood cell antibodies and accounts for almost two thirds of non-Rh-immune red cell alloantibodies.

In the Duffy blood group system, the Fy$^a$ and Fy$^b$ genes are alleles at the same locus. Three additional antigens, (Fy3), (Fy4), and (Fy5), have been identified. Compared to the D and Kell antigens, Fy$^a$ and Fy$^b$ do not appear strongly antigenic; therefore the Duffy antibodies are seen about three times less frequently than anti-K. These antibodies are almost always stimulated by erythrocyte antigen exposure through transfusion or pregnancy. Anti-Fy$^a$ occasionally causes HDN, but has more frequently been implicated as a cause of hemolytic transfusion reactions. Fy$^b$ can cause fatal transfusion reactions.

In the Kidd blood group system, the Jk$^a$ and Jk$^b$ genes are known to be codominant alleles. Kidd antibodies are infrequently encountered. Although Kidd antibodies have been known to cause mild hemolysis, they are extremely dangerous because they disappear from the circulation rapidly and produce violent delayed hemolytic transfusion reactions.

### Other Blood Group Systems

The category of miscellaneous blood groups represents more than 300 blood group antigens, which may or may not belong to independent blood group systems such as the Xg$^a$, Wright, Diego, and Colton systems. One of the most unique blood groups is the sex-linked Xg system. Sd$^a$ is the only defined antigen in the Sid system. Rare cases have demonstrated an enhanced erythrocyte antigen, called Sd(a+ +) or "Super Sid," and another form of Sd$^a$ named Cad, was originally thought to be a form of inherited polyagglutinability. The Cartwright system consists of the high-frequency Yt$^a$ antigen and the low-frequency antigen Yt$^b$. The Colton system, like the Cartwright system, consists of two antigens, the high-frequency Co$^a$ antigen and the low-frequency Co$^b$ antigen. In the Dombrock system, Do$^a$ and Do$^b$ are the two demonstrable antigens of the system. Approximately 67% of Whites are Do(a +) and about 83% are Do(b +). The incidence of Do$^a$ is lower in Blacks, American Indians, and Orientals. The first Diego blood system antigen, Di$^a$, was identified in 1955. All Whites are Di(a −) and approximately 36% of certain South American Indians are Di(a +). Five to fifteen percent of Japanese and Chinese are Di(a +). The Di$^b$ antigen was identified in 1967 and the frequency of Di$^b$ is 100% in Whites and undetermined in other racial groups. In the Scianna blood group system, Sc1 and Sc2 are now considered antithetic antigens. The most frequent phenotype is Sc1, − 2.

## Human Leukocyte Antigens (HLA) Detectable on Erythrocytes

In 1969, the erythrocyte antigen Bg$^a$ was correlated with the leukocyte antigen HLA-B7. This was the first leukocyte antigen to be demonstrated on erythrocytes. In 1971, the identification of Bg$^b$ as HLA-B17 and Bg$^c$ as HLA-A28 was reported. Most, if not all, HLA antigens may be present on erythrocytes, but the Bg antigens, particularly Bg$^a$ and Bg$^c$, are remarkable because they give much stronger reactions than other HLA antigens. These antigens, however, cannot be detected on the erythrocytes of all individuals possessing the same antigens on their leukocytes.

## High-Incidence Antigens Unrelated to the Principal Blood Group Systems

Antigens of high frequency are defined as occurring in 99.9% of the population. Examples of high frequency antigens apparently unrelated to principal blood group systems include Augustine (At$^a$), Cromer (Cr$^a$), En$^a$, Gerbich (Ge), Gregory (Gy$^a$) and Holley (Hy), Jacobs (Jr$^a$), Joseph (Jo$^a$), Langereis (Lan), Ok$^a$, Vel (Ve). It should be noted, however, that the At(a −), Cr(a −), and Jo(a −) phenotypes are found predominantly in Blacks.

The antibodies previously referred to as high-titer, low-avidity are so-called because these antibodies exhibit reactivity at high dilutions of serum but weak agglutination at any dilution. The antibodies most frequently encountered are those directed at the high-frequency antigens, York (Yk$^a$) and Cost-Stirling (Cs$^a$), Knops-Helgeson (Kn$^a$) and McCoy (McC$^a$), Chido (Ch$^a$) and Rodgers (Rg$^a$), and John Milton Hagen (JMH).

## Low-Incidence Antigens Unrelated to the Principal Blood Group Systems

Low-incidence antigens that are unrelated to the principal blood group systems are defined as antigens with an inci-

dence of less than 1%. Examples of this type of antigen include the Wright blood group system, which is independent of all other blood group systems, and the Swann (Sw$^a$), By, Mt$^a$, and Tr$^a$ antigens.

The antigen Wr$^a$ is present in about 2 in 1000 blood samples in the White population. Anti-Wr$^a$ is a frequently occurring antibody.

## REVIEW QUESTIONS

1. Select the appropriate characteristic(s) of the Lewis blood group system:
   A. Antigens are membrane-bound lipoproteins
   B. Expression of antigens is influenced by the secretor status
   C. Antigens are adsorbed from the plasma
   D. All of the above, except **A**
2. Inheritance of sese genes and the Lewis gene produces the following phenotype:
   A. Le a + b −
   B. Le a + b +
   C. Le a − b +
   D. Le a − b −
   E. None of the above
3. Inheritance of Sese and the Lewis gene produces:
   A. Le a + b −
   B. Le a + b +
   C. Le a − b +
   D. Le a − b −
   E. None of the above
4–8. Complete the following table

| Genes | In Secretions | On Erythrocytes |
|---|---|---|
| H, Se, A, 4 | H, A, Le$^a$, Le$^b$ | H, A, Le$^b$ |
| H, Se, OO, Le | H, Le$^a$, Le$^b$ | H, 5 |
| H, Se, A, lele | H, A | H, A |
| H, sese, A, Le | 6 | H, A, 7 |
| hh, 8, A, Le | Le$^a$ | Le$^a$ |

   A. se
   B. Le
   C. Le$^a$
   D. Le$^b$ or Le$^a$, Le$^b$
   E. Se
   4. _____
   5. _____
   6. _____
   7. _____
   8. _____

Diagram for Questions 9–12

| | Lele locus | Hh locus | Sese locus | Phenotype |
|---|---|---|---|---|

Precursor Substance
Type I Chain

Le——Leᵃ + precursor substance

lele——precursor substance

```
                              ┌ H ┌ Se ——Le _ _ 9
                              │   └ sese ——Le _ _ 10
                              │
                              └ hh ┌ Se ——Le _ _ 11
                                   └ sese ——Le(a+b−)

                              ┌ H ┌ Se ——Le _ _ 12
                              │   └ sese ——Le(a−b−)
                              │
                              └ hh ┌ Se ——Le(a−b−)
                                   └ sese ——Le(a−b−)
```

**9–12.** Complete the flow diagram above. An answer can be used more than once.

- **A.** Le(a−b−)
- **B.** Le(a+b−)
- **C.** Le(a−b+)
- **D.** Le(a+b+)
- **E.** lele

9. _____
10. _____
11. _____
12. _____

**13.** The most common Lewis phenotype in Whites and Blacks is:
- **A.** Le(a+b−)
- **B.** Le(a−b+)
- **C.** Le(a+b+)
- **D.** Le(a−b−)

**14.** Select the appropriate characteristic or characteristics of the Lewis antibodies:
- **A.** Predominantly IgG and most frequently anti-Leᵇ
- **B.** Anti-Leᵃ is the most common as an individual antibody
- **C.** May demonstrate in vitro hemolysis
- **D.** Both B and C

**15–20.** Match the following:
- **A** = Typically associated with IgM type antibodies
- **B** = Typically associated with IgG type antibodies

15. Anti-Leᵃ
16. Anti-Leᵇ
17. Anti-M
18. Anti-I
19. Anti-K
20. Anti-Kidd

**21.** The most common Lutheran phenotype(s) is (are):
- **A.** Lu a+b+
- **B.** Lu a+b−
- **C.** Lu a−b+
- **D.** Lu a−b−

**22.** Fill in the blank. The allelic gene to M is _____.
- **A.** M
- **B.** N
- **C.** S
- **D.** s

**23.** P blood group antigens are:
- **A.** Proteins
- **B.** Carbohydrates
- **C.** Lipoproteins
- **D.** Glycoproteins

**24.** The most common phenotype of the P blood group system is:
- **A.** $P_1$
- **B.** $P_2$
- **C.** $P_1^k$
- **D.** $P_2^k$

**25.** The Ii antigen status of newborn cord blood erythrocytes is:
- **A.** I positive
- **B.** I negative
- **C.** i positive
- **D.** Both B and C

**26.** The allelic gene to K is:
- **A.** $J_s^a$
- **B.** $J_s^b$
- **C.** $K_p^a$
- **D.** k

**27.** The most common Kell phenotype is:
- **A.** KK
- **B.** Kk
- **C.** kk
- **D.** KJsᵃ

28. Select the most appropriate characteristic(s) of anti-K:
    - A. Usually IgM, rarely IgG
    - B. Infrequently encountered in routine blood banking
    - C. Stimulated by k antigen
    - D. Second in immunogenicity to D antigen
29. Which Duffy phenotype offers the greatest resistance to invasion by malarial parasites?
    - A. Fy a+b−
    - B. Fy a+b+
    - C. Fy a−b+
    - D. Fy a−b−
30. The most common Duffy phenotype in Whites is:
    - A. Fy a+b−
    - B. Fy a+b+
    - C. Fy a−b+
    - D. Fy a−b−
31. Which of the following statements is *not* true of the Duffy blood group system antibodies?
    - A. Mostly IgG in type
    - B. Anti-Fy$^a$ may bind complement
    - C. Almost always stimulated by RBCs
    - D. Enhanced reactivity if RBCs with corresponding antigen are treated with enzymes
32. The most common Kidd phenotype in Blacks is:
    - A. Jk(a+b−)
    - B. Jk(a+b+)
    - C. Jk(a−b+)
    - D. Jk(a−b−)
33–36. Match the following blood group system antigen or antibody with its representative characteristics.
    33. Xg$^a$
    34. Sd$^a$
    35. Anti-Yt$^a$
    36. Anti-Co$^b$
    - A. Another form of this antigen is called Cad
    - B. Has been implicated in hemolytic disease of the newborn and hemolytic transfusion reactions
    - C. Not found in the White population but found in more than one-third of the South American Indian population
    - D. Sex-linked
    - E. Has only been implicated in hemolytic disease of the newborn
37. The Scianna (SC1) antigen is _____ in frequency.
    - A. High
    - B. Low
38. A previously named HLA antigen that is not uncommonly detected on erythrocytes is:
    - A. Di$^a$
    - B. Sd$^a$
    - C. Bg$^a$
    - D. Co$^a$
39. An antigen that was previously associated with HTLA is:
    - A. Wr$^a$
    - B. Bg$^a$
    - C. York
    - D. Co$^b$

## Bibliography

Albrey, J.A., et al.: A new antibody, anti-Fy$^3$, in the Duffy blood group system. Vox Sang., *20:*29, 1971.

Allen, F.H., Jr., Diamond, K.L., and Niedziela, B.: A new blood group antigen. Nature, *167:*482, 1951.

Allen, F.H., Lewis, S.J., and Fudenberg, H.: Studies of anti-Kp$^b$, a new antibody in the Kell blood group system. Vox. Sang., *3:*1, 1958.

Allen, F.H., and Lewis, S.J.: Kp$^a$ (Penney), a new antigen in the Kell blood group system. Vox Sang., *2:*81, 1957.

Ballas, S.K., Dignam, C., Harris, M., and Marcolina, M.J.: A clinically significant anti-N in a patient whose red cells were negative for N and U antigens. Transfusion, *25*(4):377–380, 1985.

Beattie, K.M.: Perspectives on some usual and unusual ABO phenotypes. *In:* A Seminar on Antigen in Blood Cells and Body Fluids. Edited by C.A. Bell. Washington, D.C., American Association of Blood Banks, 1980, pp. 97–149.

Berlin, B.S., Chandler, R., and Green, D.: Anti-"i" antibody and hemolytic anemia associated with spontaneous cytomegalovirus mononucleosis. Am. J. Clin. Pathol., *67:*459, 1977.

Bezhad, O., et al.: A new anti-erythrocyte antibody in the Duffy system: Anti-Fy$^4$. Vox Sang., *24:*337, 1973.

Callender, S.T., and Race, R.R.: A serological and genetical study of multiple antibodies formed in response to blood transfusion by a patient with lupus erythematosus diffusus. Ann. Eugen., *13:*102, 1946.

Characteristics of Blood Group Antibodies (Product Brochure). Miami, FL, Baxter Healthcare Corporation, Dade Division, 1987.

Chown, B., Lewis, M., and Kaita, H.: The Duffy blood group in Caucasians: Evidence for a new allele. Am. J. Hum. Genet., *17:*384, 1965.

Chown, B., Lewis, M., and Kaita, H.: A "new" Kell blood group phenotype. Nature, *180:*711, 1957.

Cleghorn, T.E.: MNSs gene frequencies in English blood donors. Nature, *187:*701, 1960.

Colledge, K., Pezzulich, M., and Marsh, W.L.: Anti-Fy$^5$, an antibody disclosing a probable association between the Rhesus and Duffy blood group genes. Vox Sang., *24:*193, 1973.

Coombs, R.R.A., Mourant, A.E., and Race, R.R.: In vivo iso-sensitization of red cells in babies with haemolytic disease. Lancet, *I*(Feb. 23):264–266, 1946.

Crawford, M.N.: HLA and The Red Cell. Malvern, PA, Cooper Bio medical, 1983.

Cutbush, M., Chanarin, I.: The expected blood-group antibody, anti-Lu$^b$. Nature, *178:*855, 1956.

Cutbush, M., Mollison, P.L., and Parkin, D.M.: A new human blood group. Nature, *165:*188, 1950.

Devine, P., et al.: Serologic evidence that scianna null (SC:−1,−2) red cells lack multiple high-frquency antigens. Transfusion, *28*(4):346–349, 1988.

Diamond, L.K.: Erythroblastosis fetalis or hemolytic disease of the newborn. Proc. Roy. Soc. Med., *40:*546–550, 1947.

Furukawa, K., et al.: Examples of blood groups P and $P^k$ in Japanese families. Japanese J. Hum. Genet., *12*:137, 1974.

Giblett, E.R.: Js, a new blood group antigen found in Negroes. Nature, *181*:1221, 1958.

Giblett, E.: Blood group antibodies causing hemolytic disease of the newborn. Clin. Obstet Gynecol., *7*:1044–1055, 1964.

Graham, H.: An overview of the biochemistry of the Lewis, ABH, and P systems. *In* A Seminar on Antigens on Blood Cells and Body Fluids. 33rd Annual Meeting of the American Association of Blood Banks, 1980.

Horowitz, et al.: Cold agglutinins in infectious mononucleosis and heterophile-antibody-negative mononucleosis-like syndromes. Blood, *50*:195, 1977.

Howell, E., and Perkins, H.A.: Anti-N-like antibodies in the sera of patients undergoing chronic hemodialysis. Vox Sang., *23*: 291–299, 1972.

Ilkin, W.E., et al.: Discovery of the expected hemagglutinin, anti-$Fy^b$. Nature, *168*:1077, 1951.

Huestis, D.W., Bow, J.R., and Case, J.: *Practical Blood Transfusion.* Boston, Little, Brown and Co., 1988, pp 93–116.

Issitt, P.D.: Applied Blood Group Serology, 3rd ed. Miami, FL, Montgomery Scientific, 1985.

Jenkins, W.J., et al.: Infectious mononucleosis: An unsuspected source of anti-i. Br. J. Haematol., *11*:480, 1965.

Landsteiner, K., and Levine, P.: Proc. Soc. Exp. Biol. Med., *24*: 600, 1927.

Levine, P., et al.: A new human hereditary blood property (Cellano) present in 99.8% of all bloods. Science, *109*:464, 1949.

Marcus, D.M., and Kundu, S.: Immunochemistry of the P blood group system. *In* Immunobiology of the Erythrocyte, Progress in Clinical and Biological Research. (Edited by G. Sandler and J. Nusbacher). New York, Alan R. Liss, 1980.

Mollison, P.L.: Blood Transfusion in Clinical Medicine, 7th ed. Oxford, Blackwell Scientific Publications, 1983.

Morton, N.E., et al.: Genetic evidence confirming the localization of Sutter in the Kell blood group system. Vox Sang., *10*:608, 1965.

Naiki, M., and Marcus, D.M.: Human erythrocyte P and $P^k$ blood group antigens: Identification as glycosphingolipids. Biochem. Biophys. Res. Commun., *60*:3, 1974.

Pierce, S.R.: A review of erythrocyte antigens shared with leukocytes. *In* A seminar on Antigens on Blood Cells and Body Fluids. 33rd Annual Meeting of the American Association of Blood Banks, 1980.

Pinkerton, E.J., et al.: The phenotype Jk(a − b −) in the Kidd blood group system. Vox Sang., *4*:155, 1959.

Plant, G., et al.: A new blood group antibody, anti-$Jk^b$. Nature, *171*:431, 1953.

Rosenfield, R.E., et al.: Anti-i, a frequent cold agglutin in infectious mononucleosis. Vox Sang., *10*(5):631–634, 1965.

Schwarting, G.A., Marcus, D.A., and Metazas, M.: Identification of sialosylparagloboside as the erythrocyte receptor for an anti-p antibody. Vox Sang., *32*:257, 1977.

Shirey, R.S., et al.: The association of anti-P and early abortion. Transfusion, *27*(2):189–191, 1987.

Walker, R.A., et al.: $Js^b$ of the Sutter blood group system. Transfusion, *3*:94, 1963.

Walker, R.H. (Ed.): Technical Manual. Bethesda, Md.: American Association of Blood Banks, 259–285, 1993.

Watkins, W.M.: Blood group substances in the ABO system the genes control the arrangement of sugar residues that determine blood group specificity. Science, *152*:172, 1966.

Wimer, B.M., et al.: Haematological changes associated with the McLeod phenotype of the Kell blood group system. Br. J. Haematol., *36*:219, 1977.

# Transfusion Practices

# Pretransfusion Testing: Compatibility Testing and Antibody Detection

At the conclusion of this chapter, the reader should be able to:

- Describe the three major milestones in the development of crossmatching blood.
- Diagram and explain the constituents of the major and minor crossmatch.
- Describe the rationale of the type and screen protocol and the procedures that are included in the type and screen protocol.
- Cite the major reason for performing a pretransfusion autocontrol.
- Explain the abbreviated crossmatch procedure.
- State the primary purpose or purposes of the major crossmatch.
- Explain the purpose of screening cells in pretransfusion testing.
- Name the patient history factors that are important in the investigation of a blood bank problem and list the steps in the preliminary serologic testing of an antibody problem.
- Name the possible causes for a major crossmatch incompatibility at room temperature.
- Discuss the reasons why variable-strength reactions can be encountered in reagent screening cells or crossmatching.
- Describe the types of antibodies that can be encountered in each of the phases of testing with reagent screening cells or in a crossmatch.

- State the characteristics of cold agglutinins produced by various pathologic conditions.
- Describe the steps that can be taken if a weakly reacting antibody is encountered in the AHG phase of antibody testing.
- Discuss the advantages and disadvantages of polybrene-enhancement
- Define the terms "panagglutination," "polyagglutination," "albumin-agglutinating phenomenon," "antibody to a preservative," and "rouleaux formation."
- State the reasons why a patient could have a negative unexpected antibody screen but one or a few units of incompatible blood.
- List the potential causes of either a false positive or a false negative direct antiglobulin test.
- Name the diseases or disorders that can produce positive DAT results with polyspecific and monospecific antiseras.
- Explain the possible causes of autoimmune hemolytic anemia.
- State the four possible mechanisms that produce positive direct antiglobulin test (DAT) results due to drugs.
- Name at least five common drugs that can produce positive DAT results.
- Name at least three causes of mixed-field agglutination.

## Chapter Outline

## HISTORICAL DEVELOPMENT
## OF CROSSMATCHING

The first transfusion of human blood took place early in the nineteenth century and numerous transfusions were performed during the following 50 years. Late in the nineteenth century, adverse reactions were common. Experiments in the transfusion of presumed blood substitutes, such as human milk, electrolyte solutions, and animal blood were attempted. With Landsteiner's discovery of the ABO system at the beginning of the twentieth century, blood transfusion became established as a scientific field.

The crossmatching of blood was first described in 1907 and has been modified continually since its inception. The major milestones include the following:

1. Demonstration of the relative importance of red blood cell typing and crossmatching.
2. Development of rapid techniques for crossmatching.
3. Advent of high protein, antiglobulin (AHG), and enzyme techniques.

Many scientists have contributed to the basic theory and practice of blood transfusion. Table 7-1 lists some of the most significant events in blood transfusion history.

## THE CLASSIC CROSSMATCH: PROCEDURE
## AND RATIONALE

Although the classic crossmatch (Table 7-2) has been modified, the same basic principles are fundamental to contemporary testing. The absence of agglutination or hemolysis is essential to the safety of blood transfusion. Agglutination or hemolysis in any phase (also known as *incompatibility*) is generally an expression of the presence of an antibody and its corresponding antigen. The appearance of agglutination in vitro may be expressed as hemolysis of erythrocytes in vivo. In addition, hemolysis in vitro is considered to be a positive reaction. Although incompatibility on either the major or minor side of the crossmatch is not desired, incompatibility on the major side can produce a hemolytic transfusion reaction.

The classic crossmatch consists of a major and minor crossmatch. The major side of the crossmatch contains patient serum and donor erythrocytes; the minor crossmatch consists of the reverse combination, patient erythrocytes and donor plasma. A high-protein substance, usually 22% albumin, is added to one tube of the major and minor sides as an enhancement agent.

These tubes are centrifuged and examined immediately for hemolysis or agglutination (immediate spin-IS-room temperature phase). The set is then incubated from 15 to 60 minutes at 37° C. After incubation, the tubes are again centrifuged and examined macroscopically. All of the tubes are washed 3 times with normal physiologic saline. After the final decanting of saline, AHG antisera is added to each tube. The tubes are gently mixed, recentrifuged, and examined for agglutination. In tubes exhibiting no agglutination or hemolysis, coated erythrocytes are added,

**Table 7-1. Milestones in Blood Transfusion History**

| Year | Event |
|---|---|
| 1907 | *Ottenberg* performed ABO testing before transfusion and predicted that these tests would be important in blood transfusion therapy. |
| | *Hektoen* noted that possible danger could be avoided by selecting a donor whose erythrocytes were not agglutinated by the serum of the patient and whose serum was not agglutinated by the donor's erythrocytes. He further advocated that the recipient and donor be of the same blood group. This led laboratory scientists to consider the ABO grouping of the patient and donor as an acceptable alternative to the crossmatching tests. |
| | *Crile* advocated a 48-hour test between the serum and erythrocytes of the donor and patient. He considered that in vitro hemolysis of the patient's erythrocytes by the donor's serum was more dangerous than destruction of the erythrocytes of the donor by the patient's serum. |
| 1917 | *Bernheim and Lee* advocated the use of a matching test. Bernheim supported the use of both a major (patient's serum and donor's cells) and a minor (patient's erythrocytes and donor's serum) crossmatch and recommended testing at 37° C. Lee believed that the only important consideration was that the serum of the patient should not agglutinate or hemolyze the erythrocytes of the donor. He also proposed the use of a slide test for crossmatching, and condoned the use of group O blood for all patients. The philosophy of using group O blood without crossmatching, when facilities were unavailable, predominated throughout World War I. |
| 1918 | *Moss* noted that the hemolysis paralleled agglutination. This led to ABO blood grouping determination by agglutination rather than by the hemolysis test. All testing at this time was performed at room temperature. *Direct testing* consisted of mixing citrated drops of the patient and donor blood on glass slides and observing them microscopically for agglutination for up to 15 minutes. *Indirect testing* referred to blood grouping of patients and donors. |
| | *Vincent* advocated the use of stock test serums preserved with citrate. Direct testing using a slide technique at room temperature and Vincent's grouping procedure were the most widely used methods during the ensuing two decades. |
| 1937 | *Hoxworth and Ames* recommended that if the ABO selection of donors could be rigidly restricted to a choice of individuals from the same blood group as the patient, no further testing of compatibility would be required except as a check for possible errors in grouping and the exceptional occurrence of alloantibodies. They proposed a method whereby a 1:5 mixture of donor and patient saline-suspended, defibrinated whole blood was observed for agglutination for 15 minutes, at room temperature in a humid atmosphere. |
| | The first blood bank was established at Cook County Hospital, Chicago, Illinois. |
| 1939 | *Riddell* advocated the use of a major crossmatch. Use of the slide technique continued through the 1940s. |
| 1945 | *Diamond and Dentor* described enhancement of agglutination with bovine albumin. |
| | *Coombs, Mourant, and Race* reported a new test (Coombs or Anti-human Globulin–AHG) for the detection of weak and incomplete Rh antibodies in the *British Journal of Experimental Pathology.* |
| 1947 | *Morton and Pickles* described the effect of proteolytic enzymes as an enhancement technique. |
| 1950s | The American Association of Blood Banks requirements supported saline and high-protein phases of the crossmatch and some form of routine antibody screening. |
| | Many new blood group antigens and/or systems were described because of the antibodies discovered during compatibility testing and/or associated with hemolytic transfusion reactions. |
| | In this time period, emphasis was placed on developing tests that would detect any blood group antibodies present in a patient's serum. The reagents and basic techniques for blood grouping and crossmatching remained essentially unchanged. |

centrifuged, and examined for agglutination. Agglutination must be observed after the addition of the coated erythrocytes as a positive quality control step.

Testing at different temperatures and the addition of other agents assists in the detection of various antibodies. The detected antibodies at different phases are shown in Table 7-3.

Hemolysis, as well as agglutination, are signs of incompatibility. Cases 1 through 3 demonstrate the types of reactivity that might be detected in crossmatching patients.

## MODERN DEVELOPMENTS IN PRETRANSFUSION TESTING

Although the terms *crossmatch* and *compatibility test* are sometimes used synonymously, today the crossmatch is only part of compatibility testing in the United States. Compatibility testing now includes several tests:

1. ABO grouping and Rh typing of the donor and patient.
2. Screening of the donor's and patient's serum for unexpected antibodies.
3. Crossmatching.

**Table 7-2. Classic Crossmatch Procedure**

| Major Side | | Minor Side | |
|---|---|---|---|
| Saline | High Protein | Saline | High Protein |
| Patient's serum + donor's cells | Patient's serum + donor's cells + 22% albumin | Patient's cells + donor's plasma | Patient's cells + donor's plasma + 22% albumin |

**Table 7-3. Antibodies Detected at Various Phases**

| Phase | Antibodies Detected |
|---|---|
| Immediate spin | IgM antibodies (e.g., anti-A and anti-B, anti-Le$^a$, anti-Le$^b$, M, N) |
| 37° C | IgG antibodies–High-titered Rh antibodies (e.g., anti-D, anti-C, anti-c, anti-E, anti-e); occasionally Anti-Kell) |
| | High protein (albumin) enhances Rh antibodies. |
| AHG | IgG antibodies (e.g., anti-Fy$^a$, anti-Fy$^b$, anti-Kell, and Rh antibodies |

**Case 1: Examination at Room Temperature**

| Patient: Group O Rh Positive | Serum: Anti-A, anti-B; | RBCs: No antigens |
|---|---|---|
| + | | |
| Donor: Group A Rh Positive | Serum: Anti-B | RBCs: A antigen |

| | Major Side | Minor Side |
|---|---|---|
| Patient | Anti-A Anti-B + A antigen | No A or B antigens + Anti-B |
| | INCOMPATIBLE | COMPATIBLE |

**Case 2: Examination at 37°C**

| Patient: Group A Rh Negative with Anti-D | Serum: Anti-B, anti-D | RBCs: A antigen |
|---|---|---|
| + | | |
| Donor: Group A Rh Positive | Serum: Anti-B | RBCs: A antigen, D antigen |

| | Major Side | Minor Side |
|---|---|---|
| Patient | Anti-B Anti-D + A antigen D antigen | A antigen + Anti-B |
| | INCOMPATIBLE | COMPATIBLE |

**Case 3: Examination after Addition of AHG**

| Patient: Group A Rh Positive Kell Positive | Serum: Anti-B | RBCs: A antigen, Kell antigen |
|---|---|---|
| + | | |
| Donor: Group A Rh Positive with Anti-Kell | Serum: Anti-B, Anti-Kell | RBCs: A antigen |

| | Major Side | Minor Side |
|---|---|---|
| Patient | Anti-B | A antigen Kell antigen |
| | + | + |
| Donor | A antigen | Anti-B Anti-Kell |
| | COMPATIBLE | INCOMPATIBLE |

The developments that led to today's accepted testing are listed in Table 7-4.

## Modern Blood Banking Practices

During the last 10 years there has been a distinct change in the attitudes about pretransfusion testing. The early 1980s were a time to eliminate portions of standard testing because of the restrictive economic climate, such as DRGs and PPSs. This environment stimulated the philosophy that no testing should be done unless the results are likely to influence patient care. Protocols have been developed that are based on a balance between:

1. Patient safety
2. The number of unwanted reactions eliminated, such as cold agglutinins
3. The simplicity, sensitivity, and specificity of selected methods
4. The speed with which test procedures can be performed

**Table 7-4. Milestones in Pretransfusion Testing**

| | |
|---|---|
| 1958 | *Jennings* and *Hindman* questioned the value of the minor crossmatch. |
| 1968 | Increased acceptance of pretransfusion antibody screening with the minor crossmatch beginning to be regarded as optional. |
| 1976 | The beginning of a change in thinking about crossmatching initiated by *Giblett* in her classic Karl Landsteiner award lecture. She attacked the use of room temperature testing when screening sera from blood donors and in the more controversial area of compatibility testing. Giblett's opinions, supported by the fundamental work of *Mollison*, included the belief that antibodies reacting only at room temperature but not at 37°C were of no clinical significance. In her opinion, room-temperature testing provided no extra protection for the patient and generated extra work and problems. The exception to this opinion is that room-temperature testing should continue for the immediate spin crossmatch procedure. |
| 1976 | *Friedman et al.* and *Mintz et al.* independently advocated the use of the type and screen protocol in surgical cases that rarely required blood transfusion. The typing of the patient's erythrocytes should include ABO grouping and Rh typing and the screening of patient's serum for unexpected antibodies. Some laboratory scientists wanted to delete the AHG phase of the crossmatch for all compatibility tests, if the unexpected antibody screen was negative. |
| 1976 | *Garratty and Petz* noted that antibodies detectable only through the anti-complement activity of the AHG were very rare and that high levels of anti-C3d activity of AHG could result in many nonspecific reactions. |
| Until the mid-1970s | Tests were performed at room temperature and at 37°C, in the presence of various enhancers (e.g., albumin, enzymes). All of these approaches were designed to increase sensitivity and to detect more and more antibodies. The minor crossmatch continued to be retained as standard procedure by most blood banks. |
| 1980 | The Food and Drug Administration (FDA) and American Association of Blood Banks (AABB) required an AHG phase of the crossmatch. |
| 1980s | Testing protocols for transfusion-transmitted infectious diseases—e.g., hepatitis and human immunodeficiency virus (HIV/AIDS)—continued to be developed and expanded. |
| 1985 | AHG phase of crossmatch no longer a required procedure. |
| mid-1980s | Testing for transfusion-transmitted infectious diseases—e.g., hepatitis and acquired immunodeficiency syndrome (HIV)—was expanded and assumed new importance. |
| 1993 | *Standards* of the AABB require methods that demonstrate ABO group incompatibility, clinically significant antibodies, and shall include an AHG test. |

## Type and Screen Protocol

The type and screen procedure has emerged as an acceptable alternative to crossmatching blood. This protocol (refer to Chapter 14 for a complete description of the procedure) consists of:

1. Performing an ABO grouping and Rh typing
2. Performing an indirect antiglobulin test for unexpected antibodies

The principles of unexpected antibody screening and antibody identification are presented later in this chapter, as well as in Chapter 14, Procedures.

This protocol has been established as a safe and cost-effective measure as well as reducing the unnecessary crossmatching of blood for surgical procedures in which blood is rarely used.

Although the amount of blood needed will vary depending upon the technique used, as well as factors such as the condition of the patient, this practice is based upon observations of the amount of blood generally used in specific surgical procedures. If unusual complications produce an urgent need for blood by a patient who has had a type and screen, the patient can receive ABO group and Rh type specific blood without a preceding crossmatch.

## Streamling Compatibility Testing

In the early 1980s, the efficacy of the use of anti-A,B antisera and A₂ erythrocytes in ABO grouping, repeating

Rh typing of donor units, weak D (Dᵘ) testing, repeating antibody screening of donor units, direct antiglobulin (DAT) testing, and the preparation and testing of eluates began to be discussed. Questions were raised as to the clinical significance of antibodies reactive at room temperature or below, the usefulness of albumin in the reaction mixture, and the appropriateness of using AHG in both the antibody screening test and crossmatch.

During 1984 and 1985, the FDA and AABB allowed the AHG phase of the crossmatch to be deleted if the antibody screen was negative. Crossmatching was felt to be necessary only to confirm ABO group compatibility. By 1986, the minor crossmatch was of historic interest only.

## Current Crossmatch Requirements

The 15th edition of the American Association of Blood Banks *Standards* requires that the crossmatch shall use methods that demonstrate ABO group incompatibility and clinically significant antibodies, and shall include an antiglobulin (AHG) test. If no clinically significant unexpected antibodies were/are detected and the patient has no past record of unexpected antibodies or recent transfusion history, only serologic testing for ABO incompatibility (immediate spin crossmatch) is required.

Current requirements for the screening of patient and recipient prior to crossmatching is presented in Table 7-5. The current requirements also state that donor cells from the originally attached whole blood or component

**Table 7-5. Donor and Patient Screening Requirements**

| | ABO Grouping | | Rh Typing | Weak D (D^u) | Unexpected Antibodies |
|---|---|---|---|---|---|
| | Cells | Serum/Plasma | | | |
| Repeat testing of donor | √ | | √* | no | no |
| Testing of recipient | √ | √ | √ | no | √ |

\* If unit is labeled Rh negative

segment and serum or plasma from the recipient must be crossmatched before administration, except in cases where the need for blood is urgent. The crossmatch may be done at a facility different from the one doing the required testing for unexpected antibodies.

## Current Mandated Tests for Pretransfusion Samples

Before a specimen is used for ABO blood grouping, Rh typing or compatibility testing, a qualified person in the transfusion service must confirm that all identifying information on the request form agrees with the specimen label (see Chapter 2, page 21). In case of a discrepancy or doubt, another specimen must be obtained.

A blood sample is defined as one or more tubes of blood drawn at the same time and submitted together for testing. A blood specimen must be obtained from the patient within 3 days of the scheduled transfusion under certain circumstances. These circumstances include if the patient has been transfused in the preceding 3 months with blood or a blood component containing red blood cells, if the patient has been pregnant within the preceding 3 months, or if the patient's transfusion and/or pregnancy history is uncertain or unavailable.

Testing of patient blood for transfusion must currently include the following:

1. ABO Grouping*
   A. Anti-A and anti-B (patient red blood cells)
   B. $A_1$ and B cells (patient serum or plasma)
2. Rh Typing
   A. Anti-D by direct agglutination†
   B. Rh control‡
3. Unexpected Antibody Screen (patient serum or plasma)
   A. Methods demonstrating clinically significant antibodies
      (1) 37° C incubation
      (2) Antihuman globulin test (AHG)
   B. IgG sensitized cells to confirm negative AHG reactions (Coombs' control or check cells not pooled)**

\* Blood should not be released until any discrepancy is resolved.
† The test for weak D (D^u) is unnecessary when testing the recipient.
‡ To avoid incorrect designation of an Rh-negative recipient as Rh positive because of autoantibodies or abnormal serum proteins, a control system appropriate to the anti-D reagent in use is required.
\*\* If a licensed test system is used that does not allow for the addition of IgG-sensitized cells to each negative patient antihuman globulin test, controls must be used as recommended by the manufacturer.

4. Major Crossmatch
   A. Methods that demonstrate ABO incompatibility
   B. Methods that demonstrate clinically significant antibodies; can be eliminated in patients with:
      (1) no history of significant antibodies
      (2) a negative unexpected antibody screen

## Optional Pretransfusion Testing

In addition to the current mandated pretransfusion tests, testing of patient blood for transfusion may optionally include the following:

1. ABO Grouping
   A. Red cells with anti-A,B
   B. Serum/plasma with $A_2$ cells
2. Antibody screening (Indirect Antiglobulin Test)
   A. Room temperature incubation
   B. Additives, e.g., albumin, LISS (low ionic strength salt solution)
   C. Enzymes
   D. Polyspecific AHG in indirect antiglobulin testing
   E. Auto-control or DAT
   F. Microscopic reading of tests (only for D^u and mixed field. A magnifier viewing lamp is adequate).
3. Crossmatch
   A. 37° C and AHG testing when antibody screen is negative with no previous record of clinically significant antibodies
   B. Room-temperature incubation
   C. Enzyme tests
   D. AHG with polyspecific AHG
   E. Minor crossmatch

## In-Vivo Crossmatching

In the in-vivo crossmatch, donor red blood cells are tagged with $^{51}$Cr. The survival of these cells in the recipient's circulation is measured by counting the level of radioactivity in samples of blood from the recipient.

This procedure can be useful in a variety of circumstances. These include when (1) the patient is serologically incompatible by in-vitro crossmatch with all or most donor units and the antibody cannot be identified; (2) the antibody is known and of relatively high incidence but the clinical significance is unknown or questionable; or (3) the survival of transfused red blood cells in the recipient's circulation is markedly shortened but there is no serologic evidence of an antibody.

After injection of 1 mL of tagged donor red blood cells into the recipient's circulation, recipient samples are drawn at 1 minute, 3 minutes, 10 minutes, and 60 minutes. The 1-minute sample is considered 100%, or baseline. The 3-minute sample should exhibit no donor red blood cell destruction. If there was destruction, then the 3-minute sample would have plasma radioactivity compared to the 1-minute sample. The 10-minute and 60-minute sample counts of radioactivity are compared to the 3-minute count and expressed as a percentage. If the red blood cell survival at 1 hour is 70% or higher, and there is less than 5% activity in the plasma, then it can be assumed that a whole unit of red blood cells will not undergo rapid intravascular destruction, or cause a severe adverse effect. However, long-term survival is not guaranteed through this technique.

### Repeat Testing of Donor Blood

According to the 15th edition of the AABB *Standards,* the ABO group of all units of whole blood and red blood cell components and the Rh type of such units labeled as Rh negative must be confirmed using a sample obtained from an attached segment. This is a requirement for the transfusion service doing the crossmatch. Confirmatory testing for weak D (D^u) is not required.

Confirmatory testing must be done after the original ABO grouping and Rh typing label has been affixed to the units to permit detection of labeling errors. If a labeling discrepancy is found, the error should be reported to the collecting facility; it must be resolved before the blood is issued for transfusion. Repetition of other tests is not required.

## ANTIBODY SCREENING (INDIRECT ANTIGLOBULIN TESTING)

As the preceding sections have elucidated, screening for unexpected antibodies is essential to the safety of blood transfusion. The screening test may be conducted in lieu of an AHG crossmatch but is usually conducted in conjunction with either the crossmatch or type and screen protocols.

### Basic Screening for Unexpected Antibodies

The most common technique for screening the serum of potential transfusion recipients is a two-cell procedure. Several commercial manufacturers market the erythrocytes of individual group O donors in two- or three-vial sets, as

well as panels of 10 to 18 vials. These red cell suspensions contain a preservative and expire within a few weeks of preparation. With each set of screening cells (Table 7-6) or panel cells (Table 7-7), an analysis of the antigens present (antigen profile) is included. The lot number on the profile should correspond with the lot number on the vials.

### The Two-Cell Screening Procedure

The basic procedure for testing the patient's serum for unexpected antibodies (see Chapter 14) is identical in principle to the major crossmatch procedure. The patient's serum is combined with red cells and these combinations undergo the same phases as a crossmatch: immediate spin (room temperature) and 37° C, followed by the addition of AHG (Table 7-8).

### Preliminary Antibody Identification

If agglutination or hemolysis is observed in the screening cells, the temperature and mode of reactivity suggest which blood group systems are the most likely to be involved. It is important to remember that the cells are group O; hence, antibodies such as anti-A$_1$ will not be detected by this method of screening.

If the following reactions are observed, preliminary identification of an antibody or antibodies can be made.

**Patient Results**

| Cell No. | Room Temperature | 37° C | AHG | Control Cells |
|---|---|---|---|---|
| I | Neg | 1+ | 3+ | |
| II | Neg | 2+ | 2+ | |
| Auto | Neg | Neg | Neg | 2+ |

Using the two-cell screen antigen profile (Table 7-6), a list of possible antibodies should be developed. In this case, the temperature and mode of reactivity are characteristic of Rh antibodies. Both the D and c antigens are present on both of the reagent cells. Although these reactions could represent a mixture of two antibodies, such as anti-D and anti-c or anti-C and anti-Kell, anti-D or anti-c are the most likely choices.

### Panel Cell Identification

After agglutination has been observed in screening cells, it is necessary to test the patient's serum with more reagent cells to have a large enough variety of antigen arrangements to establish the identity of the antibody. The panel of reagent cells is treated in the same manner as the screening

**Table 7-6. Two Cell Reagent Erythrocyte Screening Set Partial Listing of Antigens Present**

| Cell No. | D | C | E | c | e | K | k | Fy^a | Fy^b | Jk^a | Jk^b | Le^a | Le^b | S | s | M | N | P$_1$ |
|---|---|---|---|---|---|---|---|---|---|---|---|---|---|---|---|---|---|---|
| I | + | + | + | + | + | 0 | + | + | 0 | + | + | + | 0 | + | + | + | 0 | + |
| II | + | 0 | 0 | + | 0 | + | + | 0 | + | + | 0 | 0 | + | 0 | + | + | 0 | + |

**Table 7-7. Panel of Reagent Erythrocyte Cells**

| Cell No. | | | Rh-Hr | | | | | | Antigens Present Kell | | | | | | Duffy | | Kidd | |
|---|---|---|---|---|---|---|---|---|---|---|---|---|---|---|---|---|---|---|
| | C | D | E | c | e | Cw | f | V | K | k | Kpa | Kpb | Jsa | Jsb | Fya | Fyb | Jka | Jkb |
| 1 | + | + | + | 0 | + | 0 | 0 | 0 | + | + | 0 | + | + | + | 0 | + | 0 | + |
| 2 | + | + | 0 | 0 | + | + | 0 | 0 | 0 | + | 0 | + | 0 | + | + | + | + | + |
| 3 | 0 | + | + | + | 0 | 0 | 0 | 0 | 0 | + | 0 | + | 0 | + | + | + | + | + |
| 4 | + | 0 | 0 | + | + | 0 | + | 0 | 0 | + | 0 | + | 0 | + | 0 | + | + | 0 |
| 5 | 0 | 0 | + | + | + | 0 | + | 0 | 0 | + | 0 | + | 0 | + | + | + | + | 0 |
| 6 | 0 | 0 | 0 | + | + | 0 | + | 0 | 0 | + | + | + | 0 | + | 0 | + | 0 | 0 |
| 7 | 0 | 0 | 0 | + | + | 0 | + | 0 | 0 | + | 0 | + | 0 | + | + | 0 | 0 | 0 |
| 8 | 0 | + | 0 | + | + | 0 | + | 0 | 0 | + | 0 | + | 0 | + | + | + | + | 0 |
| 9 | 0 | 0 | 0 | + | + | 0 | + | 0 | 0 | + | 0 | + | 0 | + | 0 | 0 | + | 0 |
| 10 | 0 | 0 | 0 | + | + | 0 | + | 0 | 0 | + | 0 | + | 0 | + | + | + | 0 | 0 |

| Antigens | Lewis | | P | MNS | | | | Lutheran | | Sex-Linked | Additional |
|---|---|---|---|---|---|---|---|---|---|---|---|
| | Lea | Leb | P1 | M | N | S | s | Lua | Lub | Xga | |
| 1 | 0 | + | + | 0 | + | + | + | 0 | + | 0 M | |
| 2 | + | 0 | + | + | + | 0 | + | 0 | + | + F | |
| 3 | 0 | + | + | 0 | + | 0 | + | 0 | + | + M | |
| 4 | 0 | + | + | + | 0 | + | 0 | + | + | + F | Co (b+) |
| 5 | 0 | + | 0 | + | + | + | + | 0 | + | + M | |
| 6 | 0 | + | 0 | + | + | 0 | + | 0 | + | 0 M | |
| 7 | 0 | + | + | + | 0 | + | + | 0 | + | 0 M | Co (b+) |
| 8 | + | 0 | + | + | + | + | 0 | 0 | + | 0 M | |
| 9 | 0 | 0 | + | + | + | + | 0 | 0 | + | + F | |
| 10 | 0 | + | 0 | 0 | 0 | 0 | + | 0 | + | + F | |
| 11 | - | - | - | - | - | - | - | - | - | - | I (neg) |

cells. The results of the patient's serum that was previously screened follow:

**Patient Results**

| Cell No. | R.T. | 37° C | AHG | Control Cells |
|---|---|---|---|---|
| 1 | Neg | 1+ | 3+ | |
| 2 | Neg | 1+ | 3+ | |
| 3 | Neg | 1+ | 3+ | |
| 4 | Neg | Neg | Neg | 2+ |
| 5 | Neg | Neg | Neg | 2+ |
| 6 | Neg | Neg | Neg | 2+ |
| 7 | Neg | Neg | Neg | 2+ |
| 8 | Neg | 1+ | 3+ | |
| 9 | Neg | Neg | Neg | 2+ |
| 10 | Neg | Neg | Neg | 2+ |
| 11 | Neg | Neg | Neg | 2+ |
| Auto | Neg | Neg | Neg | |

If the pattern of reactivity is matched against the antigens in the erythrocytes of the panel of cells (Table 7-7), the identity of the antibody or antibodies can be tentatively established. To conclusively identify an antibody, other factors, such as the absence of the antigen on the patient's erythrocytes to the probable unexpected antibody, need to be investigated.

## SOLVING ANTIBODY PROBLEMS

Most antibody-associated problems encountered in the blood bank can be resolved using a systematic approach.

Problems associated with unexpected antibodies or autoantibodies can be encountered in a variety of areas, including the following:

1. ABO grouping discrepancies, such as missing or additional antibodies or antigens (refer to Chapter 4 for additional information)
2. Rh typing, for example in the presence of a positive DAT or serum protein abnormality
3. Positive unexpected antibody screening
4. Incompatible crossmatches
5. Transfusion reactions (refer to Chapter 12)
6. Jaundice in the newborn (Refer to Chapter 11)

**Table 7-8. Two Cell Screening Procedure**

| | | Erythrocytes | | |
|---|---|---|---|---|
| | | I | II | Auto |
| Substance | Patient's serum | X | X | X |
| | Patient's cells | | | X |
| | Reagent cell I | X | | |
| | Reagent cell II | | X | |
| Tests or Examination Phase | Immediate spin | | | |
| | 22% Albumin (optinal) | X | X | |
| | 37°C Incubation | | | |
| | Saline wash 3× | | | |
| | AHG | | | |
| | Control cells (if no agglutination in previous steps) | | | |

7. Positive DAT, such as AIHA, HDN, transfusion reactions, drugs

To investigate a blood bank problem, it is important to categorize information in the areas discussed in the following sections.

### First Step—Patient History

*Age, Sex, and Race.* The race of a patient may offer a clue as to antibody specificity because specific antigens are more often lacking in individuals of certain races. For example, the Fy (a−b−) phenotype is found in 68% of the Black population and in less than 1% of the White population. By comparison, the U negative phenotype is primarily found in Blacks and the k (Cellano) negative phenotype is more prevalent in Whites.

*Blood Bank Records.* Records should be checked to confirm that the current ABO group and Rh type of the patient match the previous typing, and to alert the technologist to problems that may have been detected previously. Past records, however, only provide clues and should *not* be relied on exclusively.

*Transfusion History.* It is important to document any history of transfusion, such as the number of transfused units, the dates of transfusion, and why the units were transfused. The transfusion history should also include all blood products received in the past 3 months, such as anti-D immune globulin, plasma products, factor VIII concentrates, gamma globulin, nongroup-specific platelets, or cryoprecipitate, because a plasma product may contain an unexpected antibody of sufficient concentration to be detected in the alloantibody screen. A history of recent infusion with volume expanders, such as dextran, may explain the presence of marked rouleaux.

*Obstetric History.* A complete history should include the number of pregnancies, any stillbirths, abortions, or infants affected with hemolytic disease of the newborn or jaundice. If the patient is pregnant or postpartum, the administration of antenatal or postnatal anti-D immune globulin should be included with the transfusion history.

*Drug History.* Medications in current and long-term use by the patient should be recorded. Prescription drugs and over-the-counter medications taken presently and within the past year must be noted. Long-term effects have been noticed with some drug therapy, even after completion of treatment. Many drugs have been associated with a positive DAT and some with autoimmune hemolytic anemia. A listing of drugs that have been cited as the cause of a possible DAT is presented in Tables 7-9 and 7-10.

*Admitting Diagnosis.* The current diagnosis should include the primary diagnosis as well as a complete medical history of any other conditions that could be expected to be associated with abnormal serologic findings. Examples of serologic conditions and related disorders are presented in Table 7-11.

**Table 7-9. Substances Reported to Cause a Positive DAT**

| | |
|---|---|
| Acetaminophen* | Isoniazid |
| Aminopyrine | Levodopa |
| Amphotericin B | Mefenamic acid |
| Antihistamines | Melphalan |
| Carbromal | Mephenytoin |
| Cephalosporins | Methadone hydrochloride |
| Chlorinated hydrocarbon insecticides | Methotrexate |
| | Methyldopa |
| Chlorpropamide | Methysergide maleate |
| Chlorpromazine | Penicillin G |
| Cloxacillin | Phenacetin[1] |
| Cyclophosphamide | Phenylbutazone |
| Dexchlorpheniramine maleate | Phenytoin sodium |
| Dipyrone | Probenecid |
| Erythromycin | Procainamide |
| Ethosuximide | Quinidine |
| Fenfluramine hydrochloride | Quinine sulfate |
| Furosemide | Rifampin |
| Hydralazine hydrochloride | Streptomycin sulfate |
| Hydrochlorothiazide | Sulfonamides |
| Ibuprofen** | Tetracycline hydrochloride |
| Indomethacin | Tolbutamide |
| Insulin | Triamterene |

\* Available in over-the-counter medications.
\*\* Available in over-the-counter medications in concentrations under 200 mg.
[1] Phenacetin-containing medications have been temporarily withdrawn from distribution by most manufacturers pending FDA action.

### Second Step—Preliminary Serologic Testing

1. Obtain fresh clotted and anticoagulated specimens from the patient.
2. Centrifuge and examine the serum of the clotted specimen for hemolysis and icteric appearance.
3. Wash red blood cells from the anticoagulated specimen four times and repeat ABO grouping.
4. Perform a direct antiglobulin test (DAT) from the anticoagulated sample. If a broad-spectrum (polyspecific) AHG antiserum is used initially, additional information can be gained by repeating the DAT with anti-IgG and anticomplement antisera.
5. If the patient has a positive DAT or if the control performed with Rh modified tube and slide typing is positive, the Rh test must be repeated using saline or chemically modified anti-D antisera. If the DAT and autocontrol are negative, repeat the test with modified tube and slide anti-D antisera; the manufacturer's directions, however, must state that saline-suspended cells can be used.
6. Repeat the unexpected antibody screen. An autocontrol must be included. Two screening sets should be set up. One set should be incubated at room temperature 15° C and 4° C. The other set should be incubated at 37° C (with or without albumin) and carried through to the AHG phase. If results are positive with either or both of these screening procedures, a panel of reagent red cells can be set up and treated in the same manner as the screening sets. Note: Always grade reactions and observe for hemolysis.

**Table 7-10. Trade Names\* of Medications Containing Substances Reported to Cause a Positive DAT**

| | |
|---|---|
| Achromycin (Tetracycline hydrochloride) | Maxide (Triamterene) |
| Advil (Ibuprofen) | Mesantoin (Acetylsalicylic acid) |
| Aldoclor (Methyldopa) | Momentum (Ibuprofen) |
| Aldomet (Methyldopa) | Motrin (Ibuprofen) |
| Aldoril (Hydrochlorothiazide) | Mysteclin (Tetracycline hydrochloride) |
| Aldoril (Methyldopa) | Nuprin (Ibuprofen) |
| Alkeran (Melphalan) | Orinase (Tolbutamide) |
| Antazole (Antihistamine) | Polaramine (Dexchlorpheniramine maleate) |
| Antistin (Antihistamine) | Polycillin-PRB (Probenecid) |
| APC with codeine (Phenacetin)\*\* | Ponderax (Fenfluramine hydrochloride) |
| Apresazide (Hydrochlorothiazide) | Pondimin (Fenfluramine hydrochloride) |
| Apresoline HCl (Hydralazine hydrochloride) | Ponstel (Mefenamic acid) |
| Azolid (Phenylbutazone) | Procan SR (Procainamide) |
| Benemid (Probenecid) | Pronestyl (Procainamide) |
| Butazolidin (Phenylbutazone) | Propoxyphene (Benzenethanol) |
| Carbropent (Carbromal) | Pyradone (Aminopyrin) |
| Cephalexin (Cephalosporin) | Quinidine |
| Cloxapen (Cloxacillin) | Quinine |
| Cytoxan (Cyclophosphamide) | Rifadin (Rifampin) |
| Diabinese (Chlorpropamide) | Rifamate (Rifampin, isoniazid) |
| Dieldrin (Chlorinated hydrocarbon insecticide) | Rimactane (Rifampin) |
| Dilantin (Phenytoin sodium) | Sansert (Methysergide maleate) |
| Dolophine (Methadone) | Serpasil-Apresoline (Hydralazine hydrochloride) |
| Dyazide (Triamterene) | Sinemet (Levodopa) |
| Dyrenium (Triamterene) | Sub-Quin (Procainamide) |
| Fungizone (Amphotericin B) | Sumycin (Tetracycline hydrochloride) |
| Heptachlor (Chlorindated hydrocarbon insecticide) | Tegopen (Cloxacillin) |
| Indocin (Indomethacin) | Thorazine (Chlorpromzine) |
| INH (Isoniazid) | Topicycline (Tetracycline hydrochloride) |
| Insulin | Toxaphene (Chlorinated hydrocarbon insecticide) |
| Keflex (Cephalexin) | Tylenol (Acetaminophen) |
| Keflin (Cephalothin sodium) | Unipres (Hydralazine hydrochloride) |
| Larodopa (Levodopa) | Zarontin (Ethosuximide) |
| Lasix (Furosemide) | |

\* The trade names cited are examples. It is impractical to list the names of all products containing each drug. If any questions exist about the composition of a drug, the latest edition of a pharmaceutical index should be consulted.
\*\* Temporarily withdrawn from the market

References
Billups, N. F.: American Drug Index, 30th Ed. Philadelphia, J. B. Lippincott, 1986.
Fischbach, F. T.: A Manual of Laboratory Diagnostic Tests, 2nd Ed. Philadelphia, J. B. Lippincott Co., 1984.
Hansten, P.D.: Drug Interactions, 3rd Ed. Philadelphia, Lea & Febiger, 1975.
Kastrup, E. K. (Ed): Facts and Comparisons. Philadelphia, J. B. Lippincott, 1986.
Petz, L. D. and S. N. Swisher: Clinical Practice of Blood Transfusion. NY, Churchill Livingstone, 1981, p. 655.
Widmann, F. K. (Ed): Technical Manual, 9th Ed. Arlington, VA, Am. Assoc. of Blood Banks. 1985, p. 261.

**Table 7-11. Serologic Conditions Associated with Representative Diseases or Clinical Conditions**

| Serologic Problem | Clinical Disorder |
|---|---|
| Cold autoantibody | Autoimmune disorders (e.g., cold agglutinin disease) |
| Warm autoantibody | Hemolytic anemia, carcinoma, lymphoma, systemic lupus erythematosus |
| Anti-P | PCH, childhood viral infections |
| Anti-I, anti-IH | Pneumonia, lymphoma, viral infections |
| Anti-i | Infectious mononucleosis, cirrhosis |

## Third Step—Evaluation and Identification of an Antibody

Antibodies are often classified as "warm" or "cold," indicating the temperature at which the antibody reacts best. Another classification is IgM or IgG. IgM antibodies react best at room temperature or colder; IgG antibodies react best at 37° C and in the AHG phase.

### Investigation of Antibodies that React Best at Room Temperature

Antibodies that are representative of this category include anti-A, anti-B, anti-A,B and anti-A$_1$. Other examples include anti-Le$^a$ and anti-Le$^b$, anti-P$_1$, anti-M, and anti-N.

The auto-control (patient's serum and erythrocytes) may be positive or negative and except for unusual situations, the DAT will be negative. Problems related to this category can be divided into three types:

1. ABO grouping discrepancy or incompatible crossmatch with both a negative antibody screen and auto control
2. Positive unexpected antibody screen with a negative auto control
3. Positive unexpected antibody screen with a positive or variable auto control

***ABO Discrepancy or Incompatible Crossmatch with Both a Negative Antibody Screen and Auto-Control.*** Problems related to an ABO grouping discrepancy are usually caused by anti-$A_1$ in an $A_2$ or $A_2B$ person. Resolve this problem by testing the patient's cells with anti-$A_1$ and testing the serum with $A_1$ and $A_2$ cells.

If an ABO grouping discrepancy is not detected, other reasons for this type of problem include the presence of a weak antibody or an antibody to a low-incidence antigen. The presence of a weak antibody that reacts only with homozygous cells, such as anti-M, can create a problem. If the screening cells are MN but the reverse grouping or donor cells are MM, the antibody will not be detected with the screening cells but will react with the donor or reverse grouping cells. In other cases, such as anti-$P_1$, Lew-

is$^{a+b}$, or anti-H, the antibody may react only with those cells that have the most antigen. The presence of an antibody in the patient's serum reacting with a low incidence antigen on donor or reverse grouping cells can also create problems. In this situation, red cells from another donor or another set of reagent red cells will undoubtedly be nonreactive.

***Positive Unexpected Antibody Screen with a Negative Auto-Control.*** If the unexpected antibody screening cell reactions strengthen with colder temperatures and the autocontrol remains negative, the pattern of reactivity should be examined using two reagent screening cells followed by a panel of reagent red cells. It is important to note if the reactivity in a single test phase is variable in strength and inconsistent with a single antibody specificity. This may indicate the following:

1. A dosing antibody that may react better with cells homozygous for the antigen.
2. An antibody directed toward an antigen that has variable strength among donors, such as $P_1$, Lewis, Sd$^a$.
3. Multiple antibodies.

When examining the reagent cell antigen profile for unexpected antibodies present in the patient's serum, the temperature and mode of reactivity suggest which blood group systems are the most likely to be involved. An example follows.

**Reagent Red Blood Cell Screening Cells Partial Listing of Antigens Present**

| Cell No. | Rh-hr | | | | | Kell | | Duffy | | Kidd | | Lewis | | MNS | | | | P |
|---|---|---|---|---|---|---|---|---|---|---|---|---|---|---|---|---|---|---|
| | D | C | E | c | e | K | k | Fy$^a$ | Fy$^b$ | Jk$^a$ | Jk$^b$ | Le$^a$ | Le$^b$ | S | s | M | N | P$_1$ |
| I | + | + | 0 | + | + | + | 0 | 0 | + | + | + | 0 | + | + | + | + | + | + |
| II | + | 0 | + | + | 0 | 0 | + | + | 0 | + | 0 | 0 | + | 0 | + | + | 0 | + |

Patient Results

| Cell No. | 4° C | 15° C | Room Temperature |
|---|---|---|---|
| I | 3+ | 3+ | ± |
| II | 3+ | 3+ | ± |
| Auto | Neg | Neg | Neg |

Patient Results

| Cell No. | Room Temperature | 37° C | AHG | Control Cells |
|---|---|---|---|---|
| I | ± | Neg | ± | 2+ |
| II | ± | Neg | ± | 2+ |
| Auto | Neg | Neg | Neg | 2+ |

Based on the results obtained with the patient's sera, a list of possible antibodies should be developed. In this case, reactions in both red cells that were enhanced by cold incubation suggest an anti-M, anti-$P_1$, or anti-Le$^b$. The reaction noted in the AHG phase is suggestive of the fixation of complement at room temperature rather than

a IgG type antibody. When complement is fixed at cold or room temperatures, the reaction is typically weaker at room temperature. In addition, the reaction becomes undetectable at 37° C and reappears in the AHG phase. Further testing demonstrated the following results.

**Reagent Red Blood Cell Panel Antigen Profile Partial Listing of Antigens Present**

| Cell No. | Rh-hr | | | | | Kell | | Duffy | | Kidd | | Lewis | | MNS | | | | P |
|---|---|---|---|---|---|---|---|---|---|---|---|---|---|---|---|---|---|---|
| | D | C | E | c | e | K | k | $Fy^a$ | $Fy^b$ | $Jk^a$ | $Jk^b$ | $Le^a$ | $Le^b$ | S | s | M | N | $P_1$ |
| 1 | + | 0 | 0 | + | + | + | 0 | + | + | + | 0 | 0 | 0 | + | 0 | + | + | + |
| 2 | + | 0 | 0 | + | + | 0 | I | 0 | + | + | + | U | + | + | + | + | 0 | 0 |
| 3 | + | + | + | + | + | 0 | + | 0 | + | + | + | 0 | + | + | + | + | 0 | + |
| 4 | 0 | 0 | 0 | + | 0 | 0 | + | + | + | + | 0 | 0 | + | 0 | + | + | 0 | + |
| 5 | 0 | 0 | + | + | 0 | + | + | + | + | 0 | + | 0 | + | 0 | + | + | + | + |
| 6 | 0 | + | 0 | 0 | + | + | + | + | + | + | 0 | 0 | + | + | + | + | + | + |
| 7 | 0 | + | + | 0 | + | 0 | + | 0 | + | + | + | 0 | + | 0 | + | + | + | + |
| 8 | 0 | + | 0 | 0 | + | 0 | + | + | + | 0 | + | + | 0 | 0 | + | + | 0 | 0 |
| 9 | 0 | + | + | + | + | 0 | + | + | + | + | + | + | 0 | + | 0 | 0 | + | + |
| 10 | 0 | + | 0 | 0 | + | 0 | + | 0 | + | + | + | 0 | + | 0 | + | + | + | + |
| 11 | 0 | 0 | 0 | + | + | + | + | 0 | + | + | + | + | 0 | 0 | 0 | 0 | + | + |

Patient Results

| Cell No. | 4° C | 15° C | Room Temperature |
|---|---|---|---|
| 1 | 3+ | 3+ | ± |
| 2 | Neg | Neg | Neg |
| 3 | 3+ | 3+ | ± |
| 4 | 3+ | 3+ | ± |
| 5 | 3+ | 3+ | ± |
| 6 | 3+ | 3+ | ± |
| 7 | 3+ | 3+ | ± |
| 8 | Neg | Neg | Neg |
| 9 | 3+ | 3+ | ± |
| 10 | 3+ | 3+ | ± |
| 11 | 3+ | 3+ | ± |
| Auto | Neg | Neg | Neg |

The pattern of reactivity excludes anti-M and anti-$Le^b$ as possibilities but fits the pattern and mode of reactivity of anti-$P_1$. The autocontrol must remain negative.

MULTIPLE ANTIBODIES. In some cases, more than one antibody may be formed. Cold-reacting antibodies that may be found singly or in combination include anti-$Le^a$, anti-$Le^b$, anti-M, anti-N, and anti-$P_1$. The configuration of most panel cells is designed to provide at least one cell that is antigen-negative for similarly acting antibodies. In the preceding anti-$P_1$ example, the possibilities of anti-M and anti-$Le^b$ could be excluded because of the differential reactivity of specific cells. Cells No. 2 and 8 are positive for M antigen but negative for $P_1$ antigen. Cell No. 2 is positive for $Le^b$ antigen but negative for the $P_1$ antigen. The patient's sera did not react with cells No. 2 and 8; therefore, anti-M and anti-$Le^b$ could be excluded.

If anti-M and anti-$Le^b$ were the two possibilities, the reactivity of cells No. 1 and 8 would be important in distinguishing anti-M from anti-$Le^b$.

| Cell No. | Lewis | | MNS | | | | P |
|---|---|---|---|---|---|---|---|
| | $Le^a$ | $Le^b$ | S | s | M | N | $P_1$ |
| 1 | 0 | 0 | + | 0 | + | + | + |
| 2 | 0 | + | + | + | + | 0 | 0 |
| 3 | 0 | + | + | + | + | 0 | + |
| 4 | 0 | + | 0 | + | + | 0 | + |
| 5 | 0 | + | 0 | + | + | + | + |
| 6 | 0 | + | + | + | + | + | + |
| 7 | 0 | + | 0 | + | + | + | + |
| 8 | + | 0 | 0 | + | + | 0 | 0 |
| 9 | + | 0 | + | 0 | 0 | + | + |
| 10 | 0 | + | 0 | + | + | + | + |
| 11 | + | 0 | 0 | 0 | 0 | + | + |

FOLLOW-UP If a patient has an antibody that reacts at room temperature and the ABO grouping does not give the expected results, repeat the ABO grouping using reverse grouping cells that lack the antigen to the corresponding alloantibody. For example, if the patient has anti-M and the initial ABO grouping was as follows:

| Antisera | | | Forward Typing | Reagent Cells | | Reverse Grouping |
|---|---|---|---|---|---|---|
| Anti-A | Anti-B | Anti-A,B | | $A_1$ | B | |
| Pos | Neg | Pos | A | Pos | Pos | O |

The correct ABO grouping would be demonstrated by using M antigen negative reagent red cells for the reverse grouping.

| Antisera | | | Forward | Reagent Cells | | Reverse |
| --- | --- | --- | --- | --- | --- | --- |
| Anti-A | Anti-B | Anti-A,B | Typing | A₁ (M neg) | B (M neg) | Grouping |
| Pos | Neg | Pos | A | Neg | Pos | A |

***Positive Unexpected Antibody Screen with a Positive or Variable Autocontrol.*** Antibodies that react at room temperature or colder temperatures are referred to as *cold agglutinins*. Because nonspecific autoantibodies as well as specific cold antibodies can agglutinate a patient's own red cells as well as the reagent screening or panel cells, they may mask unexpected antibodies. When a positive DAT is found and the autoantibody is of a high titer and high thermal range, a pathologic condition such as cold-type hemolytic anemia (discussed in detail in the following section) may be present. In paroxysmal cold hemoglobinuria (PCH), the patient's serum contains a cold, complement-fixing "Donath-Landsteiner" antibody that produces both in vivo and in vitro hemolysis.

The characteristics of cold agglutinins that can be encountered in normal serum versus cold agglutinins associated with pathologic conditions are listed in Table 7-12.

LABORATORY INVESTIGATION. Several techniques can be used to differentiate harmless from pathologic cold-reacting antibodies. It is current practice to omit extensive testing (Table 7-13) to differentiate nonhemolytic, cold autoantibodies but unexpected antibodies with anti-M, anti-N, anti-P, and anti-Lewis specificities are identified.

Basic testing includes the following:

1. Determining the thermal range of the antibody by testing the patient's serum versus reagent red cells (Group O adult) at 4° C, room temperature, and 37° C.
2. Performing a DAT on the patient's red cells using polyspecific, IgG, and anti-C3 antiglobulin antisera. The IgG reaction should be negative and anti-C3 should be positive.
3. Titrating the serum (optional).

TESTING IN THE PRESENCE OF COLD AUTOAGGLUTININS. Autoantibodies can coat erythrocytes and cause spontaneous agglutination, leading to false positive results in the ABO and Rh groupings. In collecting the patient sample, a prewarmed technique can be used.

Anticoagulated red cells should be collected, kept at 37° C, and washed with 37° C saline to remove autoantibody.

These cells can be used for reliable forward cell typing and DAT testing. Specimens without anticoagulant are immediately placed in warm water, while transporting, incubated at 37° C for 10 to 15 minutes before testing, and the cells washed with prewarmed saline before alloantibody testing. Autocontrols must be performed simultaneously at each phase of testing. If the autocontrol is positive, it may be due to nondispersed agglutination caused by cancer or spontaneous agglutination produced by IgG sensitized red cells.

Autoabsorption, or absorbing the patient's serum onto his own red cells, is an alternate technique. After autoabsorption, the usual compatibility testing using the patient's auto-absorbed serum can be performed. In cases of recent transfusion, prewarmed testing techniques should be used for compatibility and antibody detection. Autoabsorption is *not* recommended.

An antibody screen with an autocontrol must be done on the absorbed serum. If the alloantibody screen is still positive, a panel must be run with the auto-absorbed serum to determine antibody specificity. If the autoantibody is very potent, the autoabsorption may have to be repeated several times before all the autoantibody is removed and the serum is used for reverse grouping, alloantibodies screening, or compatibility testing.

COMPATIBILITY TESTING. Transfusion of a patient with an urgent need for blood should not be withheld if a documented nonpathologic cold agglutinin is present and the compatibility tests are negative at 37° C. Antibodies that react optimumly at room temperature and are nonreactive when the prewarmed technique is used are usually considered clinically insignificant antibodies (anti-Leᵃ, anti-Leᵇ, anti-I, anti-IH, anti-P₁, anti-A₁, anti-M, and anti-N). Units that are crossmatch-compatible are considered suitable for transfusion, but in actual practice, antigen-negative blood is ideally chosen.

### Investigation of Antibodies that React Best at 37° C or in the AHG Phase of Testing

The types of antibodies that are representative of this category include Anti-Fyᵃ, anti-Fyᵇ, anti-S, anti-s, anti-Jkᵃ,

**Table 7-12. Characteristics of Cold Agglutinins**

| Normal Serum | Pathologic Cold Agglutinins |
| --- | --- |
| Not associated with in vivo hemolysis or occlusion | Associated with hemolytic anemia or vascular occlusion on exposure to the cold, particularly the extremities |
| Titer no greater than 1:64 | High titer, above 1:1000 |
| Thermal range (10 to 15° C) | Active in vitro up to 30° C |
| Example: Anti-H | Examples: Anti-I |

**Table 7-13. Agglutination Patterns of Typical Cold Agglutinins**

| Antibody | I | i | H | IH |
| --- | --- | --- | --- | --- |
| A₁ | 4+ | 0–1+ | 0–1+ | 0–2+ |
| A₂ | 4+ | 0–1+ | 2–3+ | 4+ |
| B | 4+ | 0 1+ | 2–3+ | 4+ |
| O (adult) | 4+ | 0–1+ | 4+ | 4+ |
| O (cord) | 0–2+ | 4+ | 3–4+ | 0–2+ |
| Auto | 0–4+ | 0–1+ | 0–2+ | 0–2+ |

anti-Jk^b, anti-K, anti-k and all of the Rh antibodies. Such antibodies are found in approximately 0.3 to 2% of the population, depending on the incidence of previous transfusions or pregnancies.

Although some of these antibodies, such as high-titered Rh antibodies, occasionally react in saline at room temperature or at 37° C, they usually react in the AHG phase. Antibodies commonly found individually or in combination are Rh, Kell, and Duffy antibodies.

After testing both reagent red blood screening cells and a panel of reagent red blood cells, the probable antibody specificity can be determined (as previously described). The final step is to test the patient's pretransfusion specimen to be certain that it lacks the corresponding antigen or antigens.

In compatibility testing, donors whose red cells have the antigen against the patient's alloantibody may demonstrate major side incompatibility. Compatible donors should *not* be selected on the basis of compatibility results alone. If the antibody is of a low titer, it may react with some but not all red cells that are antigen-positive.

If a specific antibody is present, the patient's erythrocytes should be typed for the corresponding antigen. The patient should lack the antigen that corresponds to the unexpected antibody. Red blood cell typing may not be accurate if the patient has been recently transfused. In such cases, mixed-field agglutination may be observed. The reticulocyte-rich top layers of cells can be harvested for cell typings if the patient has been transfused within the last 3 months.

## PROBLEMS IN ANTIBODY IDENTIFICATION

### Unexpected Antibody Problems

A variety of situations or conditions can present problems in antibody identification or produce pseudo-alloantibody reactions. These situations include the following:

Low-titer antibodies
High titer-low avidity antibodies
Antibodies to low-incidence antigens
Passively acquired ABO antibodies
Polyagglutination
Panagglutination
Albumin-agglutinating phenomenon
Antibody to the red cell preservative
LISS autoagglutinin
Rouleaux formation

### Low-Titer Antibodies

Low-titer antibodies can present a problem because they are difficult to detect in vitro. Certain IgG antibodies, such as anti-Kidd, anti-Duffy, and anti-Dombrock, rarely exhibit titers greater than 1:4. Antibodies to antigens of the Kidd system (anti-Jk^a, anti-Jk^b, and anti-Jk^ab) are notorious for their rapid disappearance from the blood soon after the last immunizing dose.

If weak agglutination reactions are observed, an antibody of low titer should be suspected. To investigate this type of situation, the following techniques can be used.

1. Lengthen the incubation time
2. Alter the serum/cell ratio by adding 1 or 2 extra drops of serum
3. Try different enhancement media such as enzymes, polybrene, or LISS
4. Repeat testing with a fresher specimen

### High-Incidence Antigens

High-incidence antigens include antigens that were previously referred to as antigens that could stimulate high-titer, low-avidity (HTLA) antibodies or antibodies with similar serologic characteristics that have a low antigen-binding capacity and a high titration value. Examples of antibodies to these antigens include the following: Anti-Chido, anti-Rodgers, anti-Yk^A, anti-Cs^A, anti-Kn^A, anti-McC^A and anti-SD^A.

These antibodies produce weak reactions with most red cells in AHG; agglutination is not enhanced by using enzymes. To establish the presence of one of these antibodies, the following procedures should be performed:

1. Titrate to establish "high titer"
2. Test with red cells that lack high frequency factors
3. Test with cord red blood cells
4. Test with C4-coated red cells
5. Perform neutralization studies. Anti-Chido and anti-Rodgers can be neutralized with plasma or serum from donors positive for the corresponding antigen. Anti-Sd(a) (Sid) can be neutralized with urine from most Sda+ humans and from guinea pigs.

### Antibodies to Low Incidence Antigens

Antibodies to low-incidence antigens may not be detected with reagent screening cells. However, they can become apparent because of an incompatibility with a DAT negative donor unit. The specificity of the antibody is of purely academic interest. Only the nature of the problem, which is the presence of an antibody to an occasional donor unit, should be determined.

### Passively Acquired ABO Antibodies

Passively acquired ABO antibodies can be detected after massive transfusion with blood products that are not ABO group-specific. This type of situation may manifest itself as a mixed-field reaction in forward typing or an ABO discrepancy.

Reactions are usually strongest at room temperature. A positive autocontrol or DAT may be evident, depending on the amount of transfused plasma and the patient's total blood volume.

## Polyagglutination

Polyagglutination is a condition in which erythrocytes are agglutinated by all or nearly all human sera. In testing patients or donors, a useful clue is the fact that the autocontrol is usually negative.

If polybrene enhancement is used, erythrocytes displaying polyagglutination will not agglutinate. Normal erythrocytes carry a negative charge at and near the surface, when cells are mixed with positively charged polybrene, the negative charge is overcome and the erythrocytes aggregate. In contrast, most polyagglutinable erythrocytes carry less of a negative charge because of the reduction of sialic acid at the membrane and thus fail to aggregate in polybrene.

## Panagglutination

Panagglutination is caused by an antibody that is capable of agglutinating all erythrocytes tested, including the patient's own red cells. The pattern of reactivity is nonspecific.

## Albumin Agglutinating Phenomenon

This rare phenomenon is caused by an antibody in the patient's serum that is reactive with sodium caprylate, a stabilizer, used in many commercial albumin preparations.

Initially, the serum may appear to contain an autoantibody, but further testing reveals that these reactions occur only when albumin is used. Most albumin-agglutinating phenomenon reactions are generally observed after immediate spin or 37° C incubation, although some examples have been found to be detectable only after the AHG phase. In these cases, an autocontrol in albumin is positive but the DAT is negative.

## Antibody to the Red Cell Preservative

Occasionally, a patient's serum may contain antibodies directed against a specific chemical or antibiotic in a preservative solution. Reactions with reagent erythrocytes from different diagnostic companies may vary because the compositions of the preservatives are dissimilar.

A typical example of this condition produces agglutination of reagent red cells but compatible crossmatches with all donor units. The serum usually reacts at room temperature on immediate spin with all red cells suspended in the preservative. The problem can be resolved by washing the reagent red cells to remove the preservative and retesting the serum in saline suspended cells.

## LISS Autoagglutinin

Occasionally, a patient's serum appears to contain a panagglutinin when a low ionic strength salt solution (LISS) is included as an enhancement. The phase of reactivity can be varied, but agglutination has been observed at room temperature-immediate spin and/or the AHG phase. Because it is important to rule out the possibility of a specific clinically significant antibody, testing with other enhancement media should be conducted.

## Rouleaux Formation

Rouleaux formation represents a type of pseudo-agglutination in which all erythrocytes are aggregated because of a property of the serum being tested. The appearance of the red cells, resembling stacks of coins, is often more translucent and refractile than in true agglutination.

Rouleaux produce a change in the surface charge of the red cell membrane because of an alteration in the serum or plasma. Serum alterations are caused by exogenous administration of solutions such as dextran, fibrinogen, or polyvinyl pyrolidone (PVP) or by intrinsic protein abnormalities related to a disease.

When washed cells are used for testing, no discrepancy should be noted in forward ABO grouping or Rh testing. Occasionally, rouleaux formation causes a problem in AHG testing even with washed erythrocytes. In this situation, addition of 2 drops of saline and 2 drops of albumin before addition of the patient's serum should correct the problem. Albumin corrects the abnormal albumin/globulin reaction, and saline disperses rouleaux formation.

## Problems in Compatibility Testing

Problems with incompatible crossmatches parallel most of the conditions previously discussed in solving antibody problems. The principal types of problems that can produce agglutination/incompatibility in the major crossmatch are the following:

1. Incorrect ABO grouping of patient or donor
2. An alloantibody in the patient's serum reacting with the corresponding antigen on the donor's erythrocytes
3. An autoantibody in the patient's serum reacting with the corresponding antigen on the donor's erythrocytes
4. Prior coating of the donor's erythrocytes, which produces a positive DAT
5. Abnormalities in the patient's serum
6. Contaminants in the test system (such as bacterial contamination of reagents)

Combining information from both the crossmatching observations (such as how many donor units are incompatible) and antibody screening results allows efficient resolution of many problems (Tables 7-14 and 7-15). If the crossmatch is incompatible but the reagent screening red cells are nonreactive, this may indicate one of the following:

1. Incorrect ABO grouping
2. An anti-$A_1$ in the serum of $A_2$ patient

**Table 7-14. Problem-Solving Incompatible Crossmatches (Negative Autocontrol)**

If a patient has a *negative* autocontrol, this information will aid in proceeding to the appropriate technique to solve the problem.

Temperature of Reactivity: Room Temperature—Immediate Spin

| Antibody Screen | Crossmatch | Possible Causes | Resolution |
|---|---|---|---|
| Positive | Compatible or incompatible | IgM alloantibody | Refer to section entitled investigation of antibodies that react best at room temperature |
| | Compatible or incompatible | IgM autoantibody | Refer to section entitled investigation of antibodies that react best at room temperature |
| | Compatible | Antibody to red cell preservative in screening cells | Refer to section entitled problems in serologic testing |
| Positive | All units incompatible | Passively acquired ABO antibody | |
| | One or a few units incompatible | Anti A₁ | Type patient with anti-A₁ lectin |
| | | Mistyped unit of donor blood | Quarantine unit—return to blood supplier or reprocess if an in-house unit |
| | | Dosage or variable reactivity | Test using a prewarming technique or absorbed serum |
| | | | Test with homozygous and heterozygous RBCs |
| | | Antibody to low-frequency antigen | |

Temperature of Reactivity: After incubation at 37° C or in the AHG Phase

| Antibody Screen | Crossmatch | Possible Causes | Resolution |
|---|---|---|---|
| Positive | Compatible or incompatible | IgG alloantibody | Refer to section entitled Investigation of Antibodies that React Best at 37° C or in the AHG Phase of Testing |
| Negative | All units incompatible | Passively acquired ABO antibody | |
| | One/few units incompatible | Donor has positive DAT | Return unit to blood supplier or discard |
| | | Dosage or variable reactivity | Increase ratio of serum to cells |
| | | | Use enhancement technique (e.g., enzymes) |
| | | | Retest with homozygous and heterozygous red cells |
| | | Antibody to low-frequency antigen | |

**Table 7-15. Problem-Solving Incompatible Crossmatches (Positive Autocontrol)***

If a patient has a *positive* autocontrol, this information will aid in proceeding to the appropriate technique to solve the problem.

Temperature of Reactivity: Room temperature—immediate spin

| Antibody Screen | Crossmatch | Possible Causes | Resolution |
|---|---|---|---|
| Positive | Compatible or incompatible | IgM autoantibody | Refer to section entitled investigation of antibodies that react best at room temperature |
| | Incompatible | Rouleaux | Refer to problems in antibody identification |
| | Compatible | Preservative in screening red cells | |
| | Compatible | Panagglutination caused by LISS | |
| Negative | All incompatible | Passively acquired ABO antibody | |

Temperature of Reactivity: After incubation at 37° C or in the AHG phase

| Antibody Screen | Crossmatch | Possible Causes | Resolution |
|---|---|---|---|
| Positive | All or most compatible | Rouleaux | Refer to section entitled problems in serologic testing |
| | Incompatible | Panagglutination caused by LISS | |
| | | Albumin agglutinating phenomenon (probably not present in AHG phase) | |
| Positive or Negative | Variable | Hemolytic disease of the newborn (HDN) | |
| | | Transfusion reaction | |
| | | Autoimmune disorder | |
| | | Drug-induced condition | |

* Check patient's transfusion history. If patient has received a recent transfusion (within 3 months), alloantibody may be attached to transfused cells. Antibody elution studies from the patient's red cells may be useful.

**Table 7-16. Potential Sources of Error: False Positive Direct Antiglobulin Test**

1. Improperly collected specimens, for example blood collected into tubes containing silicone gel or from an intravenous line containing 5% or 10% dextrose rather than dextrose with lactated Ringer's solution, using a large bore rather than a small bore needle, or drawing too small a volume of blood into anticoagulant.
2. Use of refrigerated clotted whole blood samples
3. Bacterial contamination due to storage of a specimen or from a septic patient
4. Contaminated saline due to leaching of colloidal silica particles from glass or metallic ions from metal containers
5. Dirty glassware, i.e., contamination with dust or detergent
6. Incomplete dispersion of red blood cells produced by overcentrifugation

**Table 7-17. Potential Sources of Error: False Negative Direct Antiglobulin Test**

1. Loss of AHG antisera potency due to factors such as bacterial contamination or improper storage
2. Inadequate or improper technique when washing red cells, which produces residual proteins, for example unbound globulins, that neutralize the AHG antisera
3. Incorrect RBC suspensions
4. Improper time or speed of centrifugation
5. Omitting AHG antisera from the test
6. Interruptions or delays in the testing process
7. Use of a saline wash solution with too low pH (less than 6.0)
8. Use of saline that has been autoclaved and stored in plastic containers.

3. An antibody against a low frequency antigen
4. A positive direct AHG test on donor red cells

The status of the patient's auto-control is also useful to know. If a patient has a positive autocontrol, it is important to check his/her transfusion history. If the patient has been transfused within the last 3 months, unexpected antibody may be attached to any remaining transfused erythrocytes. In these cases, antibody elution studies on the patient's erythrocytes may be helpful in resolving the problem. If the autocontrol agglutination results are combined with the antibody screening reactions and crossmatching results, a systematic approach to problem solving can be followed.

## THE DIRECT ANTIGLOBULIN TEST (DAT)

The direct antihuman globulin test (DAT) is used to detect erythrocyte sensitization with immunoglobulins and/or complement in vivo (refer to Chapters 3 and 13 for a full discussion of the principle of the test). If in vivo sensitization or coating of red cells does take place, a positive DAT can be detected.

The most frequent source of a false positive result is the use of refrigerated, clotted blood samples in which complement components coat erythrocytes in vitro. Any

positive DAT results obtained from a clotted blood sample should be confirmed using a freshly collected EDTA anticoagulated specimen. In vitro coating of erythrocytes and other sources of error should be excluded before further investigation of the potential causes of a positive DAT (Table 7-16). It is equally important to rule out the possibility of false negative results (Table 7-17).

### Immune Hemolysis and the DAT

Positive DAT results with polyspecific or monospecific AHG antisera (anti-IgG or anti-C3d) may be encountered in a variety of clinical conditions (Table 7-18) associated with immune hemolysis. A positive DAT, however, does *not* always indicate that the erythrocytes have a shortened survival. A small percentage of healthy donors as well as about 10% of hospital patients can have a positive DAT without clinical signs of immune hemolysis.

Conditions associated with immune hemolysis, such as HDN and delayed transfusion reactions, can be caused by alloantibodies. Conditions, such as autoimmune hemolytic anemias or drug-induced antibodies can be caused by autoantibodies. Immune hemolysis is the manifestation of an antigen-antibody reaction, which results in shortened red cell survival. Serologic findings do not determine whether or not a patient has hemolytic anemia, but they are important in establishing the immune origin and type of hemolytic anemia. This is important because each type of hemolytic anemia is treated differently.

**Table 7-18. Direct Antiglobulin Test Results Using an EDTA Speciman**

| | Type of AHG Sera | | Cells Probably Sensitized With | Possible Explanation |
|---|---|---|---|---|
| Polyspecific | Anti-IgG | Anti-C3d | | |
| Positive | Positive | Positive | IgG and C3d | Warm antibody autoimmune hemolytic anemia, including drug-induced AIHA<br>Post-transfusion of incompatible blood |
| Positive | Positive | Negative | IgG and C4 | Warm antibody autoimmune hemolytic anemia, including drug-induced AIHA<br>Post-transfusion of incompatible blood |
| Positive | Negative | Positive | C3d and/or C4 | Warm antibody autoimmune hemolytic anemia, including drug-induced AIHA<br>Cold agglutinin disease<br>Post-transfusion of incompatible blood |
| Positive | Positive | Negative | IgG | Warm antibody autoimmune hemolytic anemia, including drug-induced AIHA<br>Post-transfusion of incompatible blood<br>Drug-induced cell sensitization (Without *in vivo* hemolysis) |

**Table 7-19. Preparation of an Eluate in Cases of a Positive Direct Antiglobulin Test***
**Polyspecific Antiglobulin Test Positive**

| Anti-IgG | Anti-C3d | Recently Pregnant or Transfused | Negative Pretransfusion DAT | Hematology | Jk^a | Action |
|---|---|---|---|---|---|---|
| + | ± | Yes | Yes | | | Eluate |
| + | ± | Yes | No | | | Consult medical director |
| + | ± | No | | Abnormal | | Consult medical director |
| + | ± | No | | Normal | | No eluate |
| − | − | No | | | | No eluate |
| − | − | Yes | | | | Eluate |
| − | + | No | | | | No eluate |
| − | + | Yes | | | + | No eluate |
| − | + | Yes | | | − | Eluate |

* Johnston, M. F., and Belota, M. K.: Determination of the need for elution studies for positive direct antiglobulin tests in pretransfusion testing, Am. J. Clin. Pathol. 90 (1): p. 58–62, 1988.

The diagnosis of immune hemolysis depends on clinical findings and laboratory data. Evidence of in-vivo hemolysis includes a decreasing hemoglobin and hematocrit, reticulocytosis, hemoglobinemia, hemoglobinuria, decreased serum haptoglobin, elevated levels of lactic dehydrogence (LDH) enzyme, or increased bilirubin. It is important to note that immune hemolysis may *not* result in anemia if the bone marrow is able to compensate for the loss of erythrocytes from the circulation.

Evaluations of elution studies (see Chapter 15) have demonstrated that routine studies are nonproductive. Because most patients have serum antibody of the same specificity, it has been suggested that elutions be restricted to cases in which immune hemolysis is clinically suspected and when elutions may add clinically useful information or improve transfusion safety, such as in delayed transfusion reactions. An algorithm has recently been developed (Table 7-19) that outlines the rapid systematic evaluation of all positive direct antiglobulin tests.

**Unexpected Antibodies as the Cause of Immune Hemolysis**

The detection of antibodies has been previously discussed in this chapter. A full discussion of the mechanism and symptoms of immune hemolysis in hemolytic disease of the newborn (HDN) or transfusion reactions is presented in Chapters 11 and 12, respectively. Most patients with immune hemolysis demonstrate unexpected antibodies. In rare cases such as HDN or transfusion reactions, a positive DAT may be observed in the absence of demonstrable unexpected antibodies.

**Autoimmune Hemolytic Anemia**

Autoimmune hemolytic anemia can be classified into 4 groups:

1. Warm-reactive autoantibodies—the most common
2. Cold-reactive autoantibodies—less than 20% of cases
3. Paroxysmal cold hemoglobinuria (PCH)—rare
4. Drug-induced hemolysis—less than 20% of cases

**Warm Autoimmune Hemolytic Anemia (WAIHA)**

WAIHA is associated with antibodies reactive at warm temperatures, 37° C. In more than three fourths of cases, the red cells are coated with both IgG and complement, although some may demonstrate coating with IgG alone or more infrequently complement coating. In WAIHA, there is very little serum autoantibody because the antibody reacts optimally at 37° C and is being continuously adsorbed by erythrocytes in vivo. An elution should dem-

**Table 7-20. Serologic Characteristics in WAIHA (Patient not transfused in the last 120 days)**

| Component | Reagent Screening | Panel of Reagent RBCs | Possible Resolution | |
|---|---|---|---|---|
| Patient Serum Antibody Screen | Positive | Specific reactions | Identify auto or unexpected antibody | |
| | | Nonspecific reactions | Autoabsorption | Screen and identify underlying alloantibody |
| | | | | If serum is neg. use for X-match |
| Patient red cells | Negative Rh typing | No free antibody | | |
| | | Positive control | Saline or chemically reduced antisera | |
| | Positive DAT (IgG) Elution (optional) specificity | Pos: identify antibody; Neg: Drug + RBCs | | |

**Table 7-21. Interpretation of Direct Antiglobin Test (DAT)**

| Result | Interpretation | Cause |
|---|---|---|
| Negative | Clinically established hemolysis | Poor technique |
| | | IgA or IgM coating patient's red cells |
| | | Patient antibody has increased dissociation constant |
| | | IgG concentration on red cells too low to be detected |
| Positive | IgG positive clinical and transfusion history | |
| | Eluate positive | Transfusion reaction |
| | | Warm: AIHA |
| | | HDN |
| | | Unknown |
| | Eluate negative | ABO HDN* |
| | | Drug Antibody |
| | | Unknown |
| | C3d positive recently transfused elute positive | Transfusion reaction |
| | C3d positive recently transfused elute negative | Cold AIHA |
| | | Drug mechanism |
| | | Unknown |
| | No transfusion | Cold AIHA |
| | | Drug mechanism |
| | | Unknown |

* Eluate can be positive with A₁ and B reagent red blood cells which should be checked routinely.

onstrate an autoantibody, but testing for specificity is not routinely necessary. Serologic characteristics of WAIHA are presented in Table 7-20.

## Cold Autoimmune Hemagglutinin Disease (CHAD)

Cold autoimmune hemagglutinin disease (CHAD) in either the acute or chronic form, is the most common type of hemolytic anemia associated with cold-reactive autoantibodies. The acute form is often secondary to *Mycoplasma pneumoniae* infection or lymphoproliferative disorders, such as lymphoma. The chronic form is seen in older patients and produces a mild to moderate degree of hemolysis, with Raynaud's phenomena and hemoglobinuria occurring in cold weather.

In CHAD, a cold-reactive IgM autoantibody that reacts with erythrocytes in the peripheral circulation when the body temperature falls to 32° C or below, binds complement to red cells. Hence, complement is the only globulin detected on erythrocytes. Eluates prepared from red cells collected at 37° C will not demonstrate antibody reactivity in the eluate.

## Paroxysmal Cold Hemoglobinuria (PCH)

Paroxysmal cold hemoglobinuria (PCH) was previously associated with syphilis but is now more commonly seen as an acute transient condition secondary to viral infections, particularly in young children. PCH may also occur as an idiopathic chronic disease in older people.

The responsible autoantibody is an IgG protein that reacts with erythrocytes in colder parts of the body, causing the irreversible binding of complement components C3 and C4, to red cells. At warmer temperatures, red cells are hemolyzed and the antibody elutes from the cells. Eluates are also nonreactive. This IgG autoantibody, a biphasic hemolysin, can be demonstrated through the Donath-Landsteiner test (see Chapter 15). The autoantibody has anti-P specificity and reacts with all except the rare p or $p^K$ phenotypes. Examples of these exceptions have been described as having anti-IH specificity.

### Drug-Induced Positive DATs and Hemolysis

Positive DAT results may be drug-induced (Table 7-21) and may or may not be accompanied by hemolysis. The modes of reactivity have been described as being the result of four basic mechanisms (Table 7-22):

1. Drug adsorption
2. Immune complex
3. Membrane modification
4. Autoantibody formation

### Drug Adsorption

Penicillin is a representative example of a drug that displays drug adsorption. In this type of mechanism, the drug strongly binds to any protein, including red cell membrane proteins. This binding produces a drug-red cell-hapten

**Table 7-22. Drug-Induced Positive DAT**

| | Drug Adsorption | Immune Complex | Membrane Modification | Autoantibody Formation |
|---|---|---|---|---|
| Common cause | IgG | Complement | Nonserologic | IgG |
| Antibody Screening | Negative* | Positive† | Negative | Variable‡ |
| Eluate reactivity with reagent RBCs | Nonreactive | Nonreactive | Nonreactive | Reactive§ |
| Penicillin treated RBCs | Reactive with patient's serum and eluate | Nonreactive | Nonreactive | Nonreactive |
| Drug needed in the test system | Yes | Yes | No | No |

* Unless alloantibodies are present in the sample.
† If the drug and complement are present in the test system.
‡ If the autoantibody is high enough in titer, screening tests may be positive with all cells tested.
§ Reacts with all normal cells tested, occasionally showing Rh-like specificity.

complex that can stimulate antibody formation. The antibody is specific for this complex, and no reactions will take place unless the drug is adsorbed onto the erythrocytes. Massive doses of IV penicillin are needed to coat the red cells sufficiently for antibody attachment to occur.

Approximately 3% of affected patients demonstrate a positive DAT, and less than 5% of them develop hemolytic anemia because of the drug. The hemolysis of erythrocytes is usually extravascular and occurs slowly. It is not life-threatening and will abate when penicillin is withdrawn. There appears to be no connection between this type of antibody production and allergic penicillin sensitivity caused by IgE production.

Other drugs that display drug absorption are cephalosporin derivatives such as cefalothin sodium and quinidine.

### Immune Complex

The mechanism of immune complexing is displayed by a variety of drugs, including phenacetin, quinine, rifampin, and stibophen. In this interaction, the drug and antibody form a complex in the serum and attach nonspecifically to the erythrocytes. Once attached, this complex initiates the complement cascade, which culminates in intravascular hemolysis. The immune complex may dissociate from the red cell membrane after complement activation and attach to another red cell. This action allows a small amount of drug to produce a severe anemia. When the offending drug is discontinued, the hemolytic process disappears quickly.

### Membrane Modification

Drugs of the cephalosporin type occasionally cause a positive DAT with polyspecific and monospecific AHG antisera by membrane modification. In this type of mechanism, the drug alters the membrane so that there is a nonspecific adsorption of globulins, including IgG, IgM, IgA, and complement. Hemolysis is not a frequent complication in this type of membrane augmentation.

### Autoantibody Formation

Drugs such as methyldopa (Aldomet), L-dopa, and mefanamic acid (Ponstel) have been implicated in positive DATs because of autoantibody formation. The autoantibody formed recognizes a part of the red cell and therefore reacts with most normal erythrocytes. Some drug-induced autoantibodies have been shown to have specificities that appear to be of the Rh type, but most have no apparent specificity. Antibody production ceases with withdrawal of the drug.

### Problem-Solving in DAT Testing

Weak AHG reactions frequently cause concern in blood banking. Various conditions (summarized in Table 7-23) can produce weak reactions.

Laboratory investigation and problem-solving in DAT testing are discussed in Chapter 15, Special Blood Banking Procedures.

## CHAPTER SUMMARY

### Historical Development of Crossmatching

Although the transfusion of blood has been practiced since the nineteenth century, it was not until 1907 that the crossmatching of blood was first described. The major milestones in compatibility testing include the demonstration of the relative importance of red blood cell typing and the matching test, the development of rapid techniques for crossmatching, and the advent of high protein, antiglobulin, and enzyme techniques.

### Table 7-23. Investigation of Weak Antiglobulin Reactions

| Condition | Cause |
| --- | --- |
| Mixed-field agglutination* | Mixture of patient and donor antigens posttransfusion |
| | Interdonor incompatibility |
| | Fetomaternal hemorrhage |
| | Chimerism caused by intrauterine transfusion, dispermy or bone marrow grafts |
| | Polyagglutination caused by Tn-activation, CAD, and some acquired B-like antigens |
| Lower titer antibodies | Certain IgG antibodies rarely have titers greater than 1:4. Examples: Kidd, Duffy, Dombrock |
| High Incidence Antigens | Antibodies with low binding capacity and high titration values. Examples: Anti-Chido, anti-Rodgers, anti-Yk[a], anti-Cs[a], and anti-McC[a] |
| | Similar serologic characteristics |
| Complement fixation—cold agglutination | During incubation at room temperature or lower, red cells adsorb various complement components (e.g., C4 and C3; from fresh serum containing cold agglutinins. Adsorbed components are reactive at the AHG phase with corresponding anti-complement fragments, if present, in AHG. Positive autocontrol if cold auto antibody. Negative autocontrol if anti-$A_1$ and anti-H |

* Mixed-field agglutination appears as agglutinated erythrocytes uniformly dispersed in a background of nonagglutinated erythrocytes when viewing a microscopic field using low (10×) power.

## The Classic Crossmatch: Procedure and Rationale

Although the classic crossmatch has been modified, the same basic principles are fundamental to contemporary testing. The classic crossmatch consists of a major and a minor crossmatch. The major side of the crossmatch contains patient serum and donor's erythrocytes; the minor crossmatch consists of the reverse combination, patient erythrocytes and donor plasma. Testing at different temperatures and the addition of enhancement agents assists in the detection of various types of antibodies.

## Modern Developments in Pretransfusion Testing

Although the terms crossmatch and compatibility test are sometimes used synonymously, the crossmatch is presently only part of compatibility testing in the United States. Compatibility testing now includes ABO grouping and Rh typing of the donor and patient, screening of the donor's and patient's serum for unexpected antibodies, and crossmatching. New protocols have been developed based on a balance among patient safety; elimination of the number of unwanted transfusion reactions; the simplicity, sensitivity, and specificity of selected methods; and the speed with which test procedures can be performed.

The type and screen procedure has emerged as an acceptable alternative to crossmatching blood in many cases of elective surgery. This protocol consists of performing an ABO grouping and Rh typing, and performing an indirect antiglobulin test for unexpected antibodies.

Testing of patient blood for transfusion must currently include ABO grouping, Rh typing, unexpected antibody screening, and the major crossmatch. Optional pretransfusion testing may be included.

Current crossmatch requirements state that the crossmatch shall use methods that demonstrate ABO group incompatibility and clinically significant antibodies and shall include an antihuman globulin (AHG) test.

## Antibody Screening (Indirect Antiglobulin Testing)

Screening for unexpected antibodies is essential to the safety of blood transfusion. The screening test may be conducted in lieu of an AHG crossmatch; however, it is usually conducted in conjunction with the crossmatch, or type and screen protocol. The most common technique for screening the serum of patients is a procedure that consists of using the erythrocytes of group O donors. If agglutination or hemolysis is observed in the screening cells, the temperature and mode of reactivity suggest which blood group system antibodies are the most likely to be involved. It is important to remember that the cells are group O; hence, antibodies such as anti-$A_1$ are not detected by this method of screening. If agglutination or hemolysis is observed in the screening cells, testing the patient's serum with more reagent red cells is necessary

to establish the identity of the antibody. To conclusively identify an antibody, other factors such as the absence of the antigen on the patient's erythrocytes to the probable unexpected antibody should be investigated.

## Solving Antibody Problems

Most antibody-associated problems encountered in the blood bank can be resolved using a systematic approach. Problems associated with unexpected antibodies or autoantibodies can be encountered in situations such as ABO discrepancies, Rh typing, positive unexpected antibody screening, incompatible crossmatches, transfusion reactions, hemolytic disease of the newborn (HDN), and positive direct antiglobulin tests (DATs).

Preliminary serologic testing should consist of examining a fresh blood specimen from the patient for hemolysis and icteric appearance. Other testing should include repeating the ABO grouping and DAT. If the patient's DAT or autocontrol are positive, the Rh typing should be repeated with an appropriate antisera. If the patient's unexpected antibody screening results are positive, the serum should be additionally tested with a panel of reagent red cells.

Difficulties can be encountered involving antibodies that react best at room temperature, such as anti-$A_1$ or anti-M. Problems of this type may be demonstrated by an ABO discrepancy or incompatible crossmatch with both a negative antibody screen and autocontrol, a positive unexpected antibody screen and negative autocontrol, or a positive unexpected antibody screen with a positive or variable autocontrol. Other types of problems may involve antibodies that react best at 37° C or in the AHG phase of testing. Antibodies representative of this category include anti-$Fy^a$ (Duffy$^a$), anti-$Fy^b$ (Duffy$^b$), and anti-K (Kell).

## Problems in Serologic Testing

Various situations or conditions can present problems in serologic testing. These include low-titer antibodies; high-titer, low-avidity antibodies; antibodies to low-incidence antigens; passively acquired ABO antibodies; polyagglutination; panagglutination; albumin-agglutinating phenomenon; antibody to red cell preservative; LISS autoagglutination; and rouleaux formation.

Low-titer antibodies can be difficult to detect in vitro. If weak agglutination reactions are observed, an antibody of low titer should be suspected. To investigate a problem of this type, the incubation time can be lengthened, the serum:cell ratio can be altered, different enhancement media can be used, or testing can be repeated with a fresh specimen. High-incidence antigens that were previously called high titer, low-avidity (HTLA) antibodies have a low antigen-binding capacity and a high titration value. To establish the presence of one of these antibodies, the patient's serum can be titrated to establish "high titer," or be tested with erythrocytes that lack high frequency factors, cord blood cells, and C4-coated red cells. Neutralization studies can also be performed. Antibodies to low-incidence antigens may not be detected with reagent screening cells but may demonstrate their presence through incompatibility with a DAT-negative donor unit. Passively acquired ABO antibodies may manifest themselves as mixed-field reactions in forward typing or an ABO discrepancy.

Polyagglutination is a condition in which the patient's erythrocytes are agglutinated by all or nearly all human sera but the autocontrol is usually negative. Panagglutination is caused by an antibody that is capable of agglutinating all erythrocytes tested, including the patient's own cells. The pattern of reactivity is nonspecific. The albumin agglutinating phenomenon is a rare condition caused by an antibody in the patient's serum that is reactive with sodium caprylate, a stabilizer used in many commercial albumin preparations. Occasionally, a patient's serum may contain antibodies directed against a specific chemical or antibiotic in a preservative solution. When this condition is present, the patient's serum agglutinates reagent screening red cells but is compatible with all donor units. LISS autoagglutinin can also produce serologic problems. In this type of reaction, the patient's serum appears to contain a panagglutinin when low ionic strength salt solution (LISS) is included as an enhancement medium. Rouleaux formation represents a type of pseudo-agglutination in which all erythrocytes are aggregated because of a property of the serum being tested.

The principal types of problems that can produce agglutination or hemolysis in the major crossmatch are incorrect ABO grouping of patient or donor, an unexpected antibody in the patient's serum that reacts with the corresponding antigen on the donor's red cells, an autoantibody in the patient's serum reacting with the corresponding antigen on the donor's red cells, prior coating of the donor's red cells which produces a positive DAT, abnormalities in the patient's serum, or contaminants in the test system.

### The Direct Antiglobulin Test (DAT)

The direct antihuman globulin test (DAT) is used to detect erythrocyte sensitization with immunoglobulins and/or complement in vivo. The most frequent source of a false positive result is the use of refrigerated, clotted blood samples in which complement components coat erythrocytes in vitro. It is equally important to rule out the possibility of false negative results.

Positive DAT results with polyspecific or monospecific AHG antisera (Anti-IgG or Anti-C3d) may be encountered in a variety of clinical conditions associated with immune hemolysis, but a positive DAT does *not* always indicate shortened erythrocyte survival.

Autoimmune hemolytic anemia can be classified into four groups: warm-reactive autoantibodies, cold-reactive autoantibodies, paroxysmal cold hemoglobinuria (PCH), and drug-induced hemolysis.

Weak DAT reactions can be caused by situations such as a mixture of patient and donor antigens post-transfusion, interdonor incompatibility, low titer antibodies, or complement fixation by cold agglutinins.

## REVIEW QUESTIONS

1. Ottenberg was credited with:
   A. Encouraging the mixing of patient and donor sera and erythrocytes
   B. Performing ABO testing before transfusion
   C. A 48-hour "in vitro" hemolysis test
   D. Condoning the use of group O blood without crossmatching
2. The first blood bank for the storage of donor units was established at Cook County Hospital in Chicago in:
   A. 1906
   B. 1915
   C. 1921
   D. 1937
3. Agglutination "in vitro" may express itself as _____ "in vivo."
   A. Clumping of erythrocytes
   B. No reaction because of dilution
   C. Hemolysis
   D. Hives
4. The major crossmatch consists of a mixture of:
   A. Donor serum and patient erythrocytes
   B. Donor serum and donor erythrocytes
   C. Patient serum and donor erythrocytes
   D. Patient serum and patient erythrocytes
5–7. Select the correct answers for the crossmatch results of the following cases in questions 5, 6, and 7.
   A. Major side compatible
   B. Major side incompatible
   C. Minor side incompatible
   D. Major and minor sides compatible
5. If an $A_2$ Rh+ patient with anti-$A_1$ were crossmatched with an $A_1$ donor, the results would be:
6. If an O Rh+ patient with an anti-Kell were crossmatched with an O Rh− (Kell negative) donor with anti-D, the results would be:
7. If an O Rh− patient were crossmatched with an O Rh+ donor, the results would be:
8. The type and screen protocol consists of:
   1. ABO grouping
   2. Rh typing
   3. Unexpected antibody screening
   4. HIV screening
   5. HBsAg screening
   A. 1 only
   B. 1 and 2
   C. 1, 2, and 3
   D. 1, 4, and 5

9. The primary purpose(s) of the room temp (RT) major crossmatch is (are) to:
   1. Avoid inadvertent transfusion of ABO-incompatible blood
   2. Avoid inadvertent transfusion of Rh positive blood to an Rh negative person
   3. Demonstrate previously undetected autoantibodies
   4. Detect a drug-induced hemolytic anemia
   A. 1 only
   B. 1 and 2
   C. 1 and 3
   D. 4 only
   E. 4 and 5

10. Group O screening cells for the detection of unexpected antibodies will not detect:
    A. Anti-M
    B. Anti-N
    C. Anti-$A_1$
    D. Anti-K

11. Problems associated with unexpected antibodies or autoantibodies can be encountered in all of the following clinical conditions except:
    A. ABO discrepancies
    B. Donor reactions
    C. Transfusion reactions
    D. Hemolytic disease of the newborn

12. All of the following factors are important patient history considerations in the investigation of a blood bank problem, except:
    A. Transfusion history
    B. Obstetric history
    C. Recent history of prescriptive medications
    D. Dietary history

13–17. Arrange the steps in the preliminary serologic testing of an antibody problem in the correct sequence of performance:
    A. Perform a direct antiglobulin test
    B. Obtain a fresh specimen from the patient if more serum is needed for testing
    C. Repeat the alloantibody screen
    D. Wash the patient's erythrocytes and repeat the ABO grouping
    E. Perform a panel examination for antibody identification
    13. _____
    14. _____
    15. _____

16. _____
17. _____

18–23. Match the following antibodies with their usual optimum temperature or mode of reactivity.
    A. Room temperature or colder
    B. 37° C or antiglobulin testing
18. Anti-A
19. Anti-$Le^b$
20. Anti-K
21. Anti-S
22. Anti-$Fy^a$
23. Anti-M
    18. _____
    19. _____
    20. _____
    21. _____
    22. _____
    23. _____

24. If a major crossmatch is incompatible at room temperature but the alloantibody screen and autocontrol are both negative, the problem can be the result of:
    A. Anti-$A_1$ in an $A_2$ or $A_2B$ patient
    B. A donor with a positive direct antiglobulin test
    C. An antibody in the patient's serum reacting with a low incidence antigen on the donor's erythrocytes
    D. All of the above

25. If an antibody panel displays variable strength reactions, which of the following should be considered?
    1. Multiple antibodies
    2. Dosage effect
    3. An antibody directed toward an antigen that has variable strength among donors (e.g., $P_1$)
    4. A drug-related antibody
    5. A typical cold-reacting antibody
    A. only 1
    B. 1 and 2
    C. 1, 2, and 3
    D. 2, 3, and 4

26. If an Rh positive patient's serum produces the following reactions with the screening cells below, what are the most probable antibodies?
    A. Anti-D or anti-c
    B. Anti-K and anti-k
    C. Anti-$Le^b$ or anti-s
    D. Anti-M or anti-$P_1$

**Reagent Red Blood Cell Screening Cells Partial Listing of Antigens Present**

| Cell No. | Rh-hr | | | | | Kell | | Duffy | | Kidd | | Lewis | | MNS | | | | P |
|---|---|---|---|---|---|---|---|---|---|---|---|---|---|---|---|---|---|---|
| | D | C | E | c | e | K | k | $Fy^a$ | $Fy^b$ | $Jk^a$ | $Jk^b$ | $Le^a$ | $Le^b$ | S | s | M | N | $P_1$ |
| I | + | + | 0 | + | + | + | 0 | 0 | + | + | + | 0 | + | + | + | + | + | + |
| II | + | 0 | + | + | 0 | 0 | + | + | 0 | + | 0 | 0 | + | 0 | + | + | 0 | + |

Patient Results

| Cell No. | Room Temp. | 37° C | AHG | Coombs Check Cells |
|---|---|---|---|---|
| I | 2+ | Neg | ± | 2+ |
| II | 2+ | Neg | ± | 2+ |
| Auto | Neg | Neg | Neg | 2+ |

27. Pathologic conditions can stimulate the production of cold agglutinins with the following characteristics:
   A. A high titer and a thermal range of 10–15° C
   B. Associated with hemolytic anemia and a titer no greater than 1:64
   C. A high titer and associated with anti-H
   D. A high titer and active in vitro up to 30° C
28. If an Rh positive patient's serum produces the following reactions, what is the most probable antibody?

**Reagent Red Blood Cell Screening Cells Partial Listing of Antigens Present**

| Cell No. | Rh-hr | | | | | Kell | | Duffy | | Kidd | | Lewis | | MNS | | | | P |
|---|---|---|---|---|---|---|---|---|---|---|---|---|---|---|---|---|---|---|
| | D | C | E | c | e | K | k | Fy$^a$ | Fy$^b$ | Jk$^a$ | Jk$^b$ | Le$^a$ | Le$^b$ | S | s | M | N | P$_1$ |
| I | + | + | 0 | + | + | + | 0 | 0 | + | + | + | 0 | + | + | + | + | + | + |
| II | + | 0 | + | + | 0 | 0 | + | + | 0 | + | 0 | 0 | + | 0 | + | + | 0 | + |

Patient Results

| | RT | 37° C | AHG | CC |
|---|---|---|---|---|
| I | Neg | ± | 1+ | 2+ |
| II | Neg | ± | 1+ | 2+ |

**Red Blood Cell Panel Antigen Profile Partial Listing of Antigens Present**

| Cell No. | Rh-hr | | | | | Kell | | Duffy | | Kidd | | Lewis | | MNS | | | | P |
|---|---|---|---|---|---|---|---|---|---|---|---|---|---|---|---|---|---|---|
| | D | C | E | c | e | K | k | Fy$^a$ | Fy$^b$ | Jk$^a$ | Jk$^b$ | Le$^a$ | Le$^b$ | S | s | M | N | P$_1$ |
| 1 | + | 0 | 0 | + | + | + | 0 | + | + | + | 0 | 0 | 0 | + | 0 | + | + | + |
| 2 | + | 0 | 0 | + | + | 0 | + | 0 | + | + | + | 0 | + | + | + | + | 0 | 0 |
| 3 | + | + | + | + | + | 0 | + | 0 | + | + | + | 0 | + | + | + | + | 0 | + |
| 4 | 0 | 0 | 0 | + | 0 | 0 | + | + | 0 | + | 0 | 0 | + | 0 | + | + | 0 | + |
| 5 | 0 | 0 | + | + | 0 | + | + | + | + | 0 | + | 0 | + | 0 | + | + | + | + |
| 6 | 0 | + | 0 | 0 | + | + | + | + | + | + | 0 | 0 | + | + | + | + | + | + |
| 7 | 0 | + | + | 0 | + | 0 | + | 0 | + | + | + | 0 | + | 0 | + | + | + | + |
| 8 | 0 | + | 0 | 0 | + | 0 | + | + | 0 | 0 | + | + | 0 | 0 | + | + | 0 | 0 |
| 9 | 0 | + | + | + | + | 0 | + | + | + | + | + | + | 0 | + | 0 | 0 | + | + |
| 10 | 0 | + | 0 | 0 | + | 0 | + | 0 | + | + | + | 0 | + | 0 | + | + | + | + |
| 11 | 0 | 0 | 0 | + | + | + | + | 0 | + | + | + | + | 0 | 0 | 0 | 0 | + | + |

Patient Results

| Cell No. | 37° C | AHG* | Enzyme Enhancement |
|---|---|---|---|
| 1 | Neg | 1+ | 3+ |
| 2 | Neg | 1+ | 3+ |
| 3 | Neg | 1+ | 3+ |
| 4 | Neg | 1+ | 3+ |
| 5 | Neg | 1+ | 3+ |
| 6 | Neg | Neg | Neg |
| 7 | Neg | Neg | Neg |
| 8 | Neg | Neg | Neg |
| 9 | Neg | 1+ | 3+ |
| 10 | Neg | Neg | Neg |
| 11 | Neg | 1+ | 3+ |
| Auto | Neg | Neg | Neg |

* All negative AHG results had 2+ positive check cells

**A.** Anti-D
**B.** Anti-c
**C.** Anti-Fy$^a$ and Fy$^b$
**D.** Anti-Le$^b$

29. If a weakly reacting antibody is encountered in the AHG phase of testing, what can be done to potentially enhance the reaction?
    **A.** Extend the incubation time at 4° C
    **B.** Alter the serum:cell ratio by adding 1 or 2 additional drops of serum
    **C.** Add enzymes to the system
    **D.** Both B and C

30. The former term "high-titer—low-avidity" (HTLA) antibodies refers to:
    **A.** High-titer cold agglutinins
    **B.** Antibodies that produce strong AHG reactions
    **C.** Antibodies that react at 37° C
    **D.** Antibodies that have low antigen binding capacity

31. A mixed-field agglutination pattern of patient's serum and donor's cells can be due to:
    **A.** Cold agglutinins
    **B.** Passively acquired antibodies
    **C.** HTLA antibodies
    **D.** A type A patient crossmatched with a type B donor

32. Polybrene does *not* enhance the agglutination of
    **A.** IgG type antibodies
    **B.** Polyagglutinated erythrocytes
    **C.** Anti-D
    **D.** Anti-K

33–37. Match the following terms with their respective descriptions:

33. Panagglutination
34. Polyagglutination
35. Albumin agglutinating phenomenon
36. Antibody to a preservative
37. Rouleaux formation
    **A.** RBCs agglutinated by all or nearly all human sera; autocontrol is usually negative
    **B.** Agglutination caused by sodium caprylate
    **C.** Pseudo-agglutination caused by a serum property
    **D.** Antibody capable of agglutinating all RBCs tested, including the autocontrol

38. If a patient has a negative unexpected antibody screen but one or a few units are incompatible, the reason that would *not* be a possibility is:
    **A.** Anti-A$_1$
    **B.** Antibody to preservative
    **C.** Mistyped unit of blood
    **D.** Dosage effect

39. Which of the following is *not* a potential cause of a false positive direct antiglobulin test?
    **A.** Use of EDTA anticoagulated blood
    **B.** Use of refrigerated clotted whole blood
    **C.** Bacterial contamination of AHG anti-serum
    **D.** Dirty glassware

40. Which of the following is *not* a potential cause of a false negative direct antiglobulin test?
    **A.** Incorrect red cell suspension
    **B.** Contaminated saline
    **C.** Bacterial contamination of AHG anti-serum
    **D.** Delays in the testing process

41–43. Fill in the correct answers in the following table.

**Direct Antiglobulin Test Results**

| Polyspecific AHG | Anti-IgG | Anti-C3d | Cells Probably Sensitized with | Possible Explanation |
|---|---|---|---|---|
| Positive | Negative | Positive | 43 | Cold agglutinin disease |
| Positive | 44 | 45 | IgG | Post-transfusion of incompatible blood |

41. **A.** IgM
    **B.** C3d
    **C.** C4
    **D.** Both B and C
42. **A.** Positive
    **B.** Negative
43. **A.** Positive
    **B.** Negative
44. Autoimmune hemolytic anemia can be due to:
    **A.** Warm-reactive autoantibodies
    **B.** Cold-reactive autoantibodies
    **C.** Drugs
    **D.** All of the above
45. A positive direct antiglobulin test (DAT) result brought about by drugs can be caused by a

(an) _____ mechanism.
    **A.** Drug adsorption
    **B.** Immune complex
    **C.** Membrane modification
    **D.** All of the above
46. One of the most common drugs that can produce an IgG type of positive DAT is:
    **A.** Aldomet
    **B.** Salicylate
    **C.** Vitamin B$_6$
    **D.** Valium
47. Which of the following is *not* a cause of mixed-field agglutination?
    **A.** Interdonor incompatibility
    **B.** Fetal-maternal hemorrhage

C. Weak IgM antibodies

D. Chimerism

**48.** What can cause a negative direct antiglobulin test (DAT) in the presence of clinically established hemolysis?

A. An increased antibody dissociation constant

B. Poor technique

C. Low IgG levels on erythrocytes

D. All of the above

## Bibliography

Beck, M.L., Hicklin, B., and Pierce, S.R.: Unexpected limitations in the use of commercial antiglobulin reagents. Transfusion, 16: 71–75, 1976.

Boral, L.I., and Henry, J.B.: The Type and Screen: A safe alternative and supplement in selected surgical procedures. Transfusion, 17: 163–168, 1977.

Bruce, M., Watt, A.H., Hare, W., Blue, A., and Mitchell, R.: A serious source of error in antiglobulin testing. Transfusion, 26(2):177–181, 1986.

Chaplin, H.: Clinical usefulness of specific antiglobulin reagents in autoimmune hemolytic anemia. Prog. Hematol., 8:25–49, 1973.

Cordle, D., et al.: Safety and cost containment data advocate abbreviated crossmatching. Abstract of paper at 39th Annual Meeting of the American Association of Blood Banks, Transfusion, 26(6): 1986.

Dzik, W.H., and Darling, C.A.: Positive Direct antiglobulin Test (DAT) due to anti-formaldehyde antibodies. Transfusion, 26(6): 578, 1986.

Freedman, J., Wright, J., Lim, F.C., and Garvey, M.B.: Hemolytic warm IgM autoagglutinins in autoimmune hemolytic anemia. Transfusion, 27(6):464–467, 1987.

Garratty, G., and Petz, L.D.: The significance of red cell bond complement components in the development of standards and quality control for the anticomplement, components of antiglobulin sera. Transfusion, 16:297–306, 1976.

Garratty, G.: Abbreviated pretransfusion testing. Transfusion, 26(3):217–219, 1986.

Geisland, J.R., Milam, J.D.: Spuriously positive direct antigloblin tests caused by silicone gel. Transfusion, 20:711–713, 1980.

Giblett, E.R.: Blood group alloantibodies: An assessment of some laboratory practices. Transfusion, 17:299–307, 1977.

Gilliland, B.C., Leddy, J.P., and Baughn, J.H.: The detection of cell-bound antibody on complement coated human red cells. J. Clin. Invest., 49:898–906, 1970.

Grindon, A.J., and Wilson, M.J.: False-Positive DAT caused by variables in sample procurement. Transfusion, 21:313–314, 1981.

Issitt, P.D.: Applied Blood Group Serology. 3rd Ed. Miami, Montgomery Scientific, 1985. pp. 478–495.

Judd, W.J.: Streamlining Serological Testing: Scientific Considerations. Blood Banking in a Changing Environment. Edited by D.M. Smith. Arlington, Va., American Association of Blood Banking, 1984, pp. 15–40.

Kim, B., and Anderson, H.: Correspondence from American Red Cross, Blood Services, Rochester, New York, December, 1985.

Moscow, J.A., Casper, A.J., Kodis, C., and Fricke, W.A.: Positive direct antiglobulin test results after intravenous immune globulin administration. Transfusion, 27(3):248–249, 1987.

Noto, T.A.: How to interpret a positive DAT. Diagn. Med. Sept/Oct.: 59–61, 64–67, 70, 1982.

Ortho Diagnostics Product Brochure, Results of Parallel Tests Using an EDTA Specimen. Raritan, NJ, Ortho Diagnostics, Inc., 1977.

Oberman, H.A.: The crossmatch-A brief historical perspective. Transfusion, 21(6):645–651, 1981.

Oberman, H.A., et al.: Role of the crossmatch in testing for serologic incompatibility. Transfusion. 22:12–16, 1982.

Park, H.: Limitations of the immediate-spin crossmatch. Transfusion, 25(6):588, 1985.

Pliska, C.: Low ionic strength solution (LISS). Lab. Med., 11(3): 159–164, 1980.

Pohl, B.A.: Immediate-spin crossmatch: How serious are the problems? Transfusion, 25(6):589, 1985.

Proujan, B. (Ed.): Changes to 12th edition of Standards Announced—Testing of Recipient Blood. AABB News Briefs, 11(6):3, 1988.

Robertson, V.M., Dickson, L.G., Romond, E.H., and Ash, R.C.: Positive antiglobulin tests due to intravenous immunoglobulin in patients who received bone marrow transplant. Transfusion, 27(1):28–31, 1987.

Salama, A., Gottsche, B., Schleiffer, T., and Mueller-Eckhardt, C.: Immune complex mediated intravascular hemolysis due to IgM cephalosporin-dependent antibody. Transfusion, 27(6): 460–463, 1987.

Schmidt, P.J., Samia, C.T., Gregory, K.R., and Leparc, G.F.: Rational reduction in pretransfusion testing. Lab. Med., 17(8): 467–470, 1986.

Sererat, Surapong, et al.: Why not antiglobulin compatibility testing? Transfusion, 25(6):589, 1985.

Shirley, R.S., et al.: The efficacy of performing red cell elutions in pretransfusion testing of patients with positive antiglobulin tests. Transfusion, 24:417, 1984.

Shulman, I.A., et al.: Unreliability of the immediate-spin crossmatch to detect ABO incompatibility. Transfusion, 25(6):589, 1985.

Steane, E.A., et al.: A proposal for compatibility testing incorporating the manual hexadimethrine bromide (Polybrene) Test. Transfusion, 25(6):540–544, 1975.

Steane, S.: Drug-Induced Red Blood Cell Sensitization and Destruction. In Pittiglio, D.H. (Ed.): Modern Blood Banking and Transfusion Practices. Philadelphia, F.A. Davis, pp. 447–458, 1985.

Widmann, F.K. (Ed.): Standards for blood banks and transfusion services, 15th edition. Bethesda, MD, American Association of Blood Banks: pp. 24–25, 1993.

# Clinical Problems in Blood Banking

At the conclusion of this chapter, the reader should be able to:

■ Analyze and solve serologic problems related to blood group systems, drugs, and hemolytic disease of the newborn.

## Chapter Outline

Basic-Level Case Studies Cases 1–20
Advanced-Level Case Studies Cases 21–26

In this chapter, typical examples of serologic problems encountered in the blood bank are presented. The first group of case studies integrate the concepts and practices presented in preceding chapters at a basic level. The last grouping of cases is at the advanced level of competency.

## ABO DISCREPANCY

### Case 1

Submitted by Polly F. Kay, MT(ASCP), MHS
School of Medical Technology
Anderson Memorial Hospital
Anderson, South Carolina

### History and Laboratory Data

A unit of blood from a healthy homologous donor yielded the following results on processing:

|  | Anti-A | Anti-B | Anti-A, B | Anti-D | Rh control | $A_1$ cells | B cells |
|---|---|---|---|---|---|---|---|
| Forward RBC typing | 1+ | 3+ | 3+ | 3+ | Neg |  |  |
| Serum reverse typing |  |  |  |  |  | 3+ | Neg |

### Questions

1. What blood type does the forward typing indicate?
2. What blood type does the reverse serum typing indicate?
3. What additional tests should be done to confirm this donor's phenotype?

### Discussion

1. The forward typing indicates group AB.
2. The reverse serum grouping indicates group B.
3. To resolve this discrepancy, the donor's serum was tested with three $A_1$ cells, three $A_2$ cells, and three O cells. The donor's red cells were additionally tested with anti-$A_1$ lectin, and no agglutination was observed. The following reactions were observed with the donor's serum and the panel of known cells.

### Laboratory Data (Case 1)

**Patient Results**

| Reagent Cell No. and Type | Reaction |
|---|---|
| 1 $A_1$ | 3+ |
| 2 $A_1$ | 3+ |
| 3 $A_1$ | 3+ |
| 4 $A_2$ | Neg |
| 5 $A_2$ | Neg |
| 6 $A_2$ | Neg |
| 7 O | Neg |
| 8 O | Neg |
| 9 O | Neg |

The serum antibody was identified as anti-$A_1$. Because the donor's cells failed to agglutinate the anti-$A_1$ lectin, the cells were classified as $A_2$. Other subgroups of A were excluded because of the original reaction observed with the anti-A reagent. Anti-A reagent agglutinates $A_1$ and $A_2$ red cells. Refer to Chapter 4 for a full discussion of discrepancies in the ABO system.

## Conclusion

This donor is of the $A_2B$ phenotype with an anti-$A_1$ antibody.

# Rh ANTIBODIES

## Case 2

### History and Laboratory Data

A 24-year-old White woman, group AB RhD negative, weak D ($D^u$) positive, received 2 units of AB Rh positive blood when her first child was delivered. Three years later, she received another 2 units of AB Rh positive blood at the same hospital. This patient's husband is Rh negative as were her first two children. She never received antenatal or postpartum immune globulin D (IgG). One year later, she had the following test results when a prenatal screen was performed during her third pregnancy.

### Laboratory Data (Case 2)

**Reagent Red Blood Cell Screening Cells**
**Partial Listing of Antigens Present**

| Cell No. | Rh-hr | | | | | Kell | | Duffy | | Kidd | | Lewis | | MNS | | | | P |
|---|---|---|---|---|---|---|---|---|---|---|---|---|---|---|---|---|---|---|
| | D | C | E | c | e | K | k | Fy$^a$ | Fy$^b$ | Jk$^a$ | Jk$^b$ | Le$^a$ | Le$^b$ | S | s | M | N | P$_1$ |
| I | + | 0 | + | + | + | 0 | + | + | 0 | + | + | 0 | + | + | + | + | 0 | + |
| II | 0 | + | 0 | + | 0 | 0 | + | 0 | + | + | 0 | 0 | + | 0 | + | + | 0 | + |

**Patient Results**

| Cell No. | Immediate Spin | 37° C | AHG | Coombs Control |
|---|---|---|---|---|
| I | Neg | Neg | 2+ | |
| II | Neg | Neg | Neg | 2+ |

**Reagent Red Blood Cell Panel Antigen Profile**
**Partial Listing of Antigens Present**

| Cell No. | Rh-hr | | | | | Kell | | Duffy | | Kidd | | Lewis | | MNS | | | | P |
|---|---|---|---|---|---|---|---|---|---|---|---|---|---|---|---|---|---|---|
| | D | C | E | c | e | K | k | Fy$^a$ | Fy$^b$ | Jk$^a$ | Jk$^b$ | Le$^a$ | Le$^b$ | S | s | M | N | P$_1$ |
| 1 | 0 | 0 | 0 | + | + | 0 | + | + | + | + | 0 | 0 | 0 | + | 0 | + | + | + |
| 2 | 0 | 0 | 0 | + | + | 0 | + | 0 | + | + | + | 0 | + | + | + | + | 0 | 0 |
| 3 | 0 | + | + | + | + | 0 | + | 0 | + | + | + | 0 | + | + | + | + | 0 | + |
| 4 | + | 0 | + | + | 0 | 0 | + | + | 0 | + | 0 | 0 | + | 0 | + | + | 0 | + |
| 5 | + | 0 | + | + | 0 | 0 | + | + | + | 0 | + | 0 | + | 0 | + | + | + | + |
| 6 | + | + | 0 | 0 | + | + | + | + | + | + | 0 | 0 | + | + | + | + | + | + |
| 7 | + | + | 0 | 0 | + | 0 | + | 0 | + | + | + | 0 | + | 0 | + | + | + | + |
| 8 | + | + | + | 0 | + | 0 | + | + | 0 | 0 | + | + | 0 | 0 | + | + | 0 | 0 |
| 9 | + | + | 0 | 0 | + | 0 | + | + | + | + | + | + | 0 | + | 0 | + | + | + |
| 10 | + | + | 0 | 0 | + | + | 0 | 0 | + | + | + | 0 | + | 0 | + | + | + | + |
| 11 | + | 0 | 0 | + | + | 0 | + | 0 | + | + | + | + | 0 | 0 | 0 | 0 | + | + |

**Patient Results**

| Cell No. | Immediate Spin | 37° C | AHG | Coombs Control |
|---|---|---|---|---|
| 1 | Neg | Neg | Neg | 2+ |
| 2 | Neg | Neg | Neg | 2+ |
| 3 | Neg | Neg | Neg | 2+ |
| 4 | Neg | Neg | 2+ | |
| 5 | Neg | Neg | 2+ | |
| 6 | Neg | Neg | 2+ | |
| 7 | Neg | Neg | 3+ | |
| 8 | Neg | Neg | 2+ | |
| 9 | Neg | Neg | 1+ | |
| 10 | Neg | Neg | 1+ | |
| 11 | Neg | Neg | 2+ | |

## Questions

1. Based on the antigen profile of the two screening cells and the phase of reactivity, name all the possible unexpected antibodies that could be present in this patient's serum.

2. Based on the possible unexpected antibodies identified in answer No. 1 and the antigen profile of the panel of reagent red cells, what is the identity of the antibody?

3. Could other techniques be used to enhance the reactivity of this antibody?

4. Why would a weak D ($D^u$) positive person develop an unexpected antibody to a related Rh antigen?

5. What type of blood should this patient have received in the past and what type must she receive if future transfusions are necessary?

## Discussion

1. Reactivity in the AHG phase suggests either an Rh antibody or an AHG reactive antibody. Based on the major antigens cited in two cell antigen profiles, several antibodies are possible: anti-D, anti-E, anti-e, anti-Fy$^a$, and anti-Jk$^b$, and anti-S.

2. The patient's antibody-containing serum does not react with any of the red cell antigens expressed on panel cells 1, 2, or 3. She is also known to be e antigen-positive. Therefore, the pattern and mode of reactivity of the antibody or antibodies exclude all the possible antibodies cited in Answer 1, but are consistent with anti-D.

3. Yes, enzyme treatment of reagent screening and/or panel cells is an excellent method of strengthening the reactivity of Rh antibodies. Such treatment usually produces reactions at 37° C.

4. The expression of a positive test for weak D (D$^u$) when the results of D antigen testing are negative may be caused by several factors. Refer to Chapter 5 for a full discussion of weak D (D$^u$). In this case, the patient was a genetic weak D (D$^u$) and the introduction of D antigen by transfusion was recognized by her immune system as foreign. A secondary anamnestic response occurred when the D antigen was reintroduced following the delivery of her second child.

5. This patient should have received D and weak D (D$^u$) negative blood. She *must* receive D and weak D (D$^u$) negative blood if future transfusions are needed.

## Conclusion

Transfusion-induced anti-D unexpected antibody.

## Case 3

### History and Laboratory Data

A 43-year-old Black woman was admitted for a cholecystectomy. The patient had 4 living children; the youngest was 15 years old. She had no history of prior transfusions. An unexpected antibody was discovered on the routing preoperative blood bank workup.

### *Laboratory Data (Case 3)*

| | |
|---|---|
| Blood grouping | B Positive |
| Indirect antiglobulin test (Coombs') | Positive |
| Reactive phases | AHG and 37° C with ficin-treated reagent cells |
| DAT | Negative |

The results of the two-cell screening and the panel of reagent red cells follow:

**Reagent Red Blood Cell Screening Cells**
**Partial Listing of Antigens Present**

| Cell No. | Rh-hr | | | | | Kell | | Duffy | | Kidd | | Lewis | | MNS | | | | P |
|---|---|---|---|---|---|---|---|---|---|---|---|---|---|---|---|---|---|---|
| | D | C | E | c | e | K | k | Fy$^a$ | Fy$^b$ | Jk$^a$ | Jk$^b$ | Le$^a$ | Le$^b$ | S | s | M | N | P$_1$ |
| I | 0 | + | 0 | + | + | 0 | + | 0 | + | + | + | 0 | + | + | + | + | 0 | + |
| II | + | 0 | + | + | 0 | 0 | + | + | 0 | + | 0 | 0 | + | 0 | + | + | 0 | + |

**Patient Results**

| Cell No. | Immediate Spin | 37° C | AHG | Coombs Control | 37° C Enzyme-Treated |
|---|---|---|---|---|---|
| I | Neg | Neg | Neg | 2+ | Neg |
| II | Neg | Neg | 2+ | | 3+ |
| Auto | Neg | Neg | Neg | 2+ | Neg |

**Reagent Red Blood Cell Panel Antigen Profile**
**Partial Listing of Antigens Present**

| Cell No. | Rh-hr | | | | | Kell | | Duffy | | Kidd | | Lewis | | MNS | | | | P |
|---|---|---|---|---|---|---|---|---|---|---|---|---|---|---|---|---|---|---|
| | D | C | E | c | e | K | k | Fy$^a$ | Fy$^b$ | Jk$^a$ | Jk$^b$ | Le$^a$ | Le$^b$ | S | s | M | N | P$_1$ |
| 1 | 0 | 0 | 0 | + | + | 0 | + | + | + | + | 0 | 0 | 0 | + | 0 | + | + | + |
| 2 | 0 | 0 | 0 | + | + | 0 | + | 0 | + | + | + | 0 | + | + | + | + | 0 | 0 |
| 3 | 0 | + | 0 | + | + | 0 | + | 0 | + | + | + | 0 | + | + | + | + | 0 | + |
| 4 | + | 0 | + | + | 0 | 0 | + | + | 0 | + | 0 | 0 | + | 0 | + | + | 0 | + |
| 5 | + | 0 | + | + | 0 | 0 | + | + | + | 0 | + | 0 | + | 0 | + | + | + | + |
| 6 | + | + | 0 | 0 | + | + | + | + | + | + | 0 | 0 | + | + | + | + | + | + |
| 7 | + | + | 0 | 0 | + | 0 | + | 0 | + | + | + | 0 | + | 0 | + | + | + | + |
| 8 | + | + | + | 0 | + | 0 | + | 0 | 0 | 0 | I | + | 0 | 0 | + | + | 0 | 0 |
| 9 | + | + | 0 | + | + | 0 | + | + | + | + | + | 0 | + | 0 | 0 | 0 | + | + |
| 10 | + | + | 0 | 0 | + | + | 0 | 0 | + | + | + | 0 | + | 0 | + | + | + | + |
| 11 | + | 0 | 0 | + | + | 0 | + | 0 | + | + | + | + | 0 | 0 | 0 | 0 | + | + |

**Patient Results**

| Cell No. | Immediate Spin | 37° C | AHG | Coombs Control |
|---|---|---|---|---|
| 1 | Neg | Neg | Neg | 2+ |
| 2 | Neg | Neg | Neg | 2+ |
| 3 | Neg | Neg | Neg | 2+ |
| 4 | Neg | Neg | 2+ | |
| 5 | Neg | Neg | 2+ | |
| 6 | Neg | Neg | Neg | 2+ |
| 7 | Neg | Neg | Neg | 3+ |
| 8 | Neg | Neg | 2+ | |
| 9 | Neg | Neg | Neg | 1+ |
| 10 | Neg | Neg | Neg | 1+ |
| 11 | Neg | Neg | Neg | 2+ |

## Questions

1. Based on the antigen profile of the two screening cells and the phase of reactivity, name all the possible unexpected antibodies that could be present in this patient's serum.
2. Based on the possible unexpected antibodies identified in answer No. 1 and the antigen profile of the panel of reagent red cells, what is the identity of this unexpected antibody?
3. What additional testing should be conducted to confirm the identity of the antibody?
4. Briefly describe some of the characteristics of the antigen-antibody system to which this antibody belongs.
5. What was the source of this patient's antigen exposure?

## Discussion

1. Reactivity in the AHG phase suggests either an Rh antibody or an AHG reactive antibody. The major antigens reacting in the two-cell antigen screening test suggest the presence of one or more of several unexpected antibodies: anti-D, anti-E, anti-Fyᵃ, and anti-Jkᵃ. The known presence of the D antigen, however, excludes the possibility of anti-D.

2. The pattern of reactivity in AHG distinguishes the antibody as anti-E.
3. If possible, the patient's red cells should be tested for the presence of the corresponding antigen. In this case, it was possible to test the patient's red cells accurately because she had not been transfused within the last 3 months. Her red cells were E negative.
4. The E antigen is part of the Rhesus (Rh) blood group system described in Chapter 5. Anti-E is usually an IgG (sometimes IgM) antibody and does not bind complement. Seventy percent of White persons are E negative. This antibody has been implicated in hemolytic reactions and HDN.
5. Most cases of anti-E represent unexpected antibodies formed in response to E positive erythrocyte transfusions or pregnancies, although a few are believed to be secondary to naturally occurring antigens. In this case, the patient had had four pregnancies, which were probably the source of the antigenic exposure.

## Conclusion

Anti-E unexpected antibody, probably resulting from previous pregnancies.

## Case 4

### History and Laboratory Data

A 20-year-old woman was a prenatal outpatient (8 weeks gestation). She had no history of prior transfusions but had had one previous pregnancy. The patient was group A, Rh positive and demonstrated a positive unexpected antibody screening test. During the patient's last pregnancy, another blood bank had identified the antibody Fyᵃ in the patient's serum. Her past records did not include any additional antigen testing.

*Laboratory Data (Case 4)*

**Reagent Red Blood Cell Screening Cells**
**Partial Listing of Antigens Present**

| Cell No. | Rh-hr D | C | E | c | e | Kell K | k | Duffy Fyᵃ | Fyᵇ | Kidd Jkᵃ | Jkᵇ | Lewis Leᵃ | Leᵇ | MNS S | s | M | N | P P₁ |
|---|---|---|---|---|---|---|---|---|---|---|---|---|---|---|---|---|---|---|
| I | + | 0 | + | + | + | 0 | + | + | 0 | + | + | 0 | + | + | + | + | 0 | + |
| II | 0 | + | 0 | + | 0 | + | 0 | 0 | + | + | 0 | 0 | + | 0 | + | + | + | + |

**Patient Results**

| Cell No. | Immediate Spin | 37° C | AHG |
|---|---|---|---|
| I | 3+ | 1+ | + |
| II | ± | Neg | ± |

**Reagent Red Blood Cell Panel Antigen Profile**
**Partial Listing of Antigens Present**

| Cell No. | Rh-hr | | | | | Kell | | Duffy | | Kidd | | Lewis | | MNS | | | | P |
|---|---|---|---|---|---|---|---|---|---|---|---|---|---|---|---|---|---|---|
| | D | C | E | c | e | K | k | Fy$^a$ | Fy$^b$ | Jk$^a$ | Jk$^b$ | Le$^a$ | Le$^b$ | S | s | M | N | P$_1$ |
| 1 | 0 | 0 | 0 | + | + | 0 | + | + | + | + | 0 | 0 | 0 | + | 0 | + | + | + |
| 2 | 0 | + | 0 | + | + | 0 | + | 0 | + | + | + | 0 | + | + | + | + | + | 0 |
| 3 | 0 | + | 0 | + | + | 0 | + | + | + | + | + | 0 | + | + | + | 0 | + | + |
| 4 | + | + | + | + | 0 | 0 | + | + | 0 | + | 0 | 0 | + | 0 | + | + | + | + |
| 5 | + | 0 | + | + | 0 | 0 | + | + | + | 0 | + | 0 | + | 0 | + | + | 0 | + |
| 6 | + | + | 0 | 0 | + | + | + | + | + | + | 0 | 0 | + | + | + | + | 0 | + |
| 7 | 0 | + | 0 | 0 | + | 0 | + | 0 | + | + | + | 0 | + | 0 | + | + | 0 | + |
| 8 | 0 | 0 | + | + | + | 0 | + | + | 0 | 0 | + | + | 0 | 0 | + | + | 0 | 0 |
| 9 | 0 | 0 | 0 | + | + | 0 | + | 0 | + | + | + | + | 0 | + | 0 | + | 0 | + |
| 10 | 0 | + | 0 | 0 | + | + | 0 | + | + | + | + | 0 | + | 0 | + | 0 | + | + |

**Patient Results**

| Cell No. | Immediate Spin | 37° C | AHG | Coombs Control |
|---|---|---|---|---|
| 1 | ± | Neg | ± micro | |
| 2 | ± | Neg | ± micro | |
| 3 | Neg | Neg | Neg | 2+ |
| 4 | ± | Neg | ± micro | |
| 5 | 2+ | 1+ | ± micro | |
| 6 | 2+ | 1+ | ± micro | |
| 7 | 2+ | 1+ | ± micro | |
| 8 | 2+ | 1+ | ± micro | |
| 9 | 2+ | 1+ | 1+ | |
| 10 | Neg | Neg | Neg | 2+ |
| Auto | Neg | Neg | Neg | 2+ |

## Questions

1. Based on the pattern of reactivity, does this patient have only the previously identified anti-Fy$^a$?
2. What antibody (antibodies) is (are) suggested by the screening and panel cells?
3. Why are the reactions of the I screening cell as well as the panel cells No. 5 through No. 9 stronger than those of the other reactive cells?
4. Would additional tests be of value?
5. Was this patient immunized as the result of her previous pregnancy?

## Discussion

1. No. The pattern of reactivity and the specific cells demonstrating agglutination in both the screening cells and panel of cells do *not* suggest the presence of a Fy$^a$ unexpected antibody. The screening cells suggest an antibody that has an optimal thermal range of 4 to 20° C. The specific blood group antigens present on the group O reagent cells that exhibit this behavior are Lewis, MNS, and P.
2. The agglutination pattern, graded by strength as well as specificity, is typical of the reactivity demonstrated by anti-M. Most examples of anti-M have a definite affinity for cooler temperatures. Anti-M is usually an IgM antibody, although it may occasionally be an IgG antibody,

and it usually does not bind complement. It typically reacts in the saline phase, but it may occasionally react in the AHG phase. Refer to Chapter 6 for a full discussion of the MNS system.
3. Examination of the MN phenotypes of the reagent cells demonstrates that the stronger-reacting cells are homozygous MM cells rather than heterozygous MN cells. The difference in strength of agglutination is caused by the "dosage effect."

Almost all anti-M antibodies show some dosage effect. Anti-M displays dosage at 4 to 20° C. This means that it reacts more strongly with MM cells than with MN cells. Additionally, if an anti-M reacts at 37° C, it generally will do so only with type MM cells.
4. In this case, it was important to exclude an underlying anti-Fy$^a$ because of the previously identified antibody in the patient's history. The patient's red cells were typed for Fy$^a$ antigen and found to be positive. Therefore, the previous identification of the antibody as anti-Fy$^a$, was an error. The patient's red cells were also typed for the M and N antigen. She was found to be M (negative) and N (positive).
5. No. Testing of both the patient's husband and their first baby revealed that both were M (negative) and N (positive). Anti-M is a fairly frequent environmentally stimulated antibody. The usual mode of stimulation is through exposure to antigenically similar, naturally occurring substances by either ingestion or inhalation.

## Conclusion

Anti-M.

---

# COLD-REACTING ANTIBODIES

## Case 5

### History and Laboratory Data

A 6-year-old Black boy had a diagnosis of congenital spherocytosis with acute hemolytic anemia. On admission, his hematocrit was 16% and one unit of packed red cells was ordered for transfusion. According to the patient's pediatrician, the child had never been transfused. The patient was group A, Rh positive. All units crossmatched were weakly incompatible at room temperature, 37° C and AHG.

The patient's DAT was negative with polyspecific, IgG,

and C3d antisera. Although the DAT was negative, an elution technique was performed. The elution studies, however, failed to demonstrate a specific antibody. The results of his two-cell reagent screening cells and an accompanying panel of reagent red cells follows.

*Laboratory Data (Case 5)*

**Reagent Red Blood Cell Screening Cells**
**Partial Listing of Antigens Present**

| Cell No. | _____ Rh-hr _____ | | | | | Kell | | Duffy | | Kidd | | Lewis | | MNS | | | | P |
|---|---|---|---|---|---|---|---|---|---|---|---|---|---|---|---|---|---|---|
| | D | C | E | c | e | K | k | Fy$^a$ | Fy$^b$ | Jk$^a$ | Jk$^b$ | Le$^a$ | Le$^b$ | S | s | M | N | P$_1$ |
| I | + | 0 | + | + | + | 0 | + | + | 0 | + | + | 0 | + | + | + | + | 0 | + |
| II | 0 | + | 0 | + | 0 | + | 0 | 0 | + | + | 0 | 0 | + | 0 | + | + | 0 | + |

**Patient Results**

| Cell No. | Immediate Spin | 37° C | AHG |
|---|---|---|---|
| I | ± | ± | ± |
| II | ± | ± | ± |

**Reagent Red Blood Cell Panel Antigen Profile**
**Partial Listing of Antigens Present**

| Cell No. | _____ Rh-hr _____ | | | | | Kell | | Duffy | | Kidd | | Lewis | | MNS | | | | P |
|---|---|---|---|---|---|---|---|---|---|---|---|---|---|---|---|---|---|---|
| | D | C | E | c | e | K | k | Fy$^a$ | Fy$^b$ | Jk$^a$ | Jk$^b$ | Le$^a$ | Le$^b$ | S | s | M | N | P$_1$ |
| 1 | 0 | 0 | 0 | + | + | 0 | + | + | + | + | 0 | 0 | 0 | + | 0 | + | + | + |
| 2 | 0 | + | 0 | + | + | 0 | + | 0 | + | + | + | 0 | + | + | + | + | 0 | 0 |
| 3 | 0 | + | 0 | + | + | 0 | + | 0 | + | + | + | 0 | + | + | + | + | 0 | + |
| 4 | + | + | + | + | 0 | 0 | + | + | 0 | + | 0 | 0 | + | 0 | + | + | 0 | + |
| 5 | + | 0 | + | + | 0 | 0 | + | + | + | 0 | + | 0 | + | 0 | + | + | + | + |
| 6 | + | + | 0 | 0 | + | + | + | + | + | + | 0 | 0 | + | + | + | + | + | + |
| 7 | + | + | 0 | 0 | + | 0 | + | 0 | + | + | + | 0 | + | 0 | + | + | + | + |
| 8 | + | 0 | + | + | + | 0 | + | + | 0 | 0 | + | + | 0 | 0 | + | 0 | + | 0 |
| 9 | + | 0 | 0 | + | + | 0 | + | + | + | + | + | + | 0 | + | 0 | 0 | + | + |
| 10 | + | + | 0 | 0 | + | + | 0 | 0 | + | + | + | 0 | + | 0 | + | + | + | + |
| 11 | + | 0 | 0 | + | + | 0 | + | 0 | + | + | + | + | 0 | 0 | 0 | 0 | + | + |

**Patient Results**

| Cell No. | Immediate Spin | 37° C | AHG |
|---|---|---|---|
| 1 | ± | ± | ± |
| 2 | ± | ± | ± |
| 3 | ± | ± | ± |
| 4 | ± | ± | ± |
| 5 | ± | ± | ± |
| 6 | ± | ± | ± |
| 7 | ± | ± | ± |
| 8 | ± | ± | ± |
| 9 | ± | ± | ± |
| 10 | ± | ± | ± |
| 11 | ± | ± | ± |
| Auto | ± | ± | ± |

## Questions

1. What is the cause of hemolysis if the DAT is negative?
2. What does the reactivity pattern of the Group O reagent red cells indicate?

3. What technique can be used to crossmatch units for transfusion?

## Discussion

1. With a negative DAT, the cause of the hemolysis is more likely to be related to the spherocytosis and a superimposed infection than a cold autoagglutinin.
2. The reactivity observed in the screening and panel cells, and the autocontrol is typical of a nonspecific cold agglutinin. Because the patient had no history of transfusion, it is unlikely that he has an unexpected antibody.
3. Compatible blood should not be difficult to find, especially if a pre-warmed crossmatch is performed.

## Conclusion

Nonspecific cold autoagglutinin.

## AHG-REACTING ANTIBODIES

### Case 6

#### History and Laboratory Data

A 90-year-old White woman with chronic renal failure was admitted to the hospital to be transfused with 3 units of packed red cells. Her hemoglobin was 6.0 g/dL. She had received numerous past transfusions, but had not been transfused for the past 3 months. Her history also included one pregnancy.

She was group O, Rh positive, and one of the 3 units crossmatched was incompatible. Her unexpected antibody screen was also positive. However, her DAT was negative. Results of the screening and a panel of reagent red cells are presented below. Investigation of her past medical records indicated that anti-Kell had been identified in her serum at another hospital 14 months earlier and anti-S had been eluted from her red cells during the same hospitalization.

**Patient Results**

| Cell No. | Immediate Spin | 37° C | AHG | Coombs Control Cells |
|---|---|---|---|---|
| 1 | Neg | 1+ | 2+ | |
| 2 | Neg | Neg | Neg | 2+ |
| 3 | Neg | Neg | Neg | 2+ |
| 4 | Neg | Neg | Neg | 2+ |
| 5 | Neg | Neg | Neg | 2+ |
| 6 | Neg | Neg | Neg | 2+ |
| 7 | Neg | Neg | Neg | 1+ |
| 8 | Neg | Neg | Neg | 2+ |
| 9 | Neg | Neg | Neg | 1+ |
| 10 | Neg | Neg | Neg | 2+ |
| 11 | Neg | Neg | Neg | 2+ |
| Auto | Neg | Neg | Neg | 2+ |

*Laboratory Data (Case 6)*

**Reagent Red Blood Cell Screening Cells**
**Partial Listing of Antigens Present**

| Cell No. | Rh-hr | | | | | Kell | | Duffy | | Kidd | | Lewis | | MNS | | | | P |
|---|---|---|---|---|---|---|---|---|---|---|---|---|---|---|---|---|---|---|
| | D | C | E | c | e | K | k | Fy$^a$ | Fy$^b$ | Jk$^a$ | Jk$^b$ | Le$^a$ | Le$^b$ | S | s | M | N | P$_1$ |
| I | + | 0 | + | + | + | 0 | + | + | 0 | + | + | 0 | + | + | + | + | 0 | + |
| II | 0 | + | 0 | + | 0 | + | 0 | 0 | + | + | 0 | 0 | + | 0 | + | + | 0 | + |

**Patient Results**

| Cell No. | Immediate Spin | 37° C | AHG | Coombs Control Cells |
|---|---|---|---|---|
| I | Neg | Neg | Neg | 2+ |
| II | Neg | Neg | 2+ | |

**Reagent Red Blood Cell Panel Antigen Profile**
**Listing of Antigens Present**

| Cell No. | Rh-Hr | | | | | | | | Kell | | | | | | Duffy | | Kidd | |
|---|---|---|---|---|---|---|---|---|---|---|---|---|---|---|---|---|---|---|
| | C | D | E | c | e | C$^w$ | f | V | K | k | Kp$^a$ | Kp$^b$ | Js$^a$ | Js$^b$ | Fy$^a$ | Fy$^b$ | Jk$^a$ | Jk$^b$ |
| 1 | + | + | + | 0 | + | 0 | 0 | 0 | + | + | 0 | + | 0 | + | 0 | + | 0 | + |
| 2 | + | + | 0 | 0 | + | + | 0 | 0 | 0 | + | 0 | + | 0 | + | + | + | + | 0 |
| 3 | 0 | + | + | + | 0 | 0 | 0 | 0 | 0 | + | 0 | + | 0 | + | + | + | + | 0 |
| 4 | + | 0 | 0 | + | + | 0 | + | 0 | 0 | + | 0 | + | 0 | + | 0 | + | + | + |
| 5 | 0 | 0 | + | + | + | 0 | + | 0 | 0 | + | 0 | + | 0 | + | + | + | + | 0 |
| 6 | 0 | 0 | 0 | + | + | 0 | + | 0 | 0 | + | 0 | + | 0 | + | 0 | + | 0 | + |
| 7 | 0 | 0 | 0 | + | + | 0 | + | 0 | 0 | + | 0 | + | 0 | + | + | 0 | 0 | + |
| 8 | 0 | + | 0 | + | + | 0 | + | 0 | 0 | + | 0 | + | 0 | + | 0 | 0 | + | 0 |
| 9 | 0 | 0 | 0 | + | + | 0 | + | 0 | 0 | + | 0 | + | 0 | + | + | + | + | + |
| 10 | 0 | 0 | 0 | + | + | 0 | + | 0 | 0 | + | 0 | + | 0 | + | + | + | + | + |

**Antigens Present (continued)**

| Cell No. | Lewis | | P | MNS | | | | Lutheran | | Sex-Linked | | Additional |
|---|---|---|---|---|---|---|---|---|---|---|---|---|
| | Le^a | Le^b | P_1 | M | N | S | s | Lu^a | Lu^b | Xg^a | | |
| 1 | 0 | + | + | 0 | + | + | + | 0 | I | 0 | M | |
| 2 | I | 0 | + | + | + | 0 | + | 0 | + | + | M | Co (b+) |
| 3 | 0 | + | + | 0 | + | 0 | + | 0 | + | + | M | |
| 4 | 0 | + | + | + | 0 | + | 0 | + | + | + | F | Co (b+) |
| 5 | 0 | + | 0 | + | + | + | + | 0 | + | + | M | |
| 6 | 0 | + | 0 | + | + | 0 | + | 0 | + | 0 | M | |
| 7 | 0 | + | + | + | 0 | + | + | 0 | + | 0 | M | Co (b+) |
| 8 | + | 0 | + | + | + | + | 0 | 0 | + | 0 | M | |
| 9 | 0 | 0 | + | + | + | + | 0 | 0 | + | + | F | |
| 10 | 0 | + | 0 | 0 | 0 | 0 | + | 0 | + | + | F | |
| 11 | | | | | | | | | | | | I (neg) |

**Patient Results**

| Cell No. | Immediate Spin | 37° C | AHG | Coombs Control Cells |
|---|---|---|---|---|
| 1 | Neg | 1+ | 2+ | |
| 2 | Neg | Neg | Neg | 2+ |
| 3 | Neg | Neg | Neg | 2+ |
| 4 | Neg | Neg | Neg | 2+ |
| 5 | Neg | Neg | Neg | 2+ |
| 6 | Neg | Neg | Neg | 2+ |
| 7 | Neg | Neg | Neg | 1+ |
| 8 | Neg | Neg | Neg | 2+ |
| 9 | Neg | Neg | Neg | 1+ |
| 10 | Neg | Neg | Neg | 2+ |
| 11 | Neg | Neg | Neg | 2+ |
| Auto | Neg | Neg | Neg | 2+ |

## Questions

1. Based on the reactions of the two screening cells and the panel of reagent red cells, what antibody (antibodies) is (are) present?
2. What antibody is producing the incompatible crossmatch?
3. Why was a second antibody not demonstrated?
4. Briefly describe some of the characteristics of the undetectable antibody.
5. What type blood should this woman receive?

## Discussion

1. The pattern of reactivity is consistent only with anti-K.
2. The anti-K was reacting with one of the crossmatched units, which was found to be K (positive).
3. The titer of the anti-S was undoubtedly too low to be clinically detectable.
4. Anti-S usually occurs as an immune antibody in the sera of multiparous women or multitransfused patients. Rare examples of environmentally stimulated anti-S which react best in saline at room temperature have been observed. This antibody is capable of causing HDN. Hemolytic transfusion reactions attributable to it have also occurred. The antibody is most often found in conjunction with other antibodies, except anti-A and anti-B.

Anti-S is not a commonly detected unexpected antibody despite the frequency of the S antigen in the general population. This suggests that the S antigen is capable of initiating an immune response only in very susceptible individuals. A full discussion of the MNS system is presented in Chapter 6.

5. Because anti-S was reported from a previous eluate, this patient should be transfused only with K-neg, S-neg units even though the anti-S is not demonstrable at present.

## Conclusion

Anti-K with a history of anti-S.

## Case 7

### History and Laboratory Data

A 70-year-old White woman was hospitalized for a below-the-knee amputation. She had received 3 units of packed red cells during a surgical procedure 7 months earlier. She had also received 2 units of packed red cells to correct a mild anemia one week earlier. Her obstetrical history included two living children and one miscarriage.

Her blood type was group B_1 Rh negative. She had had a negative unexpected antibody screen one week earlier. A repeat antibody screen performed while cross-matching the preoperative units of blood revealed a positive unexpected antibody screen. She also exhibited a positive DAT. An eluate of the patient's red cells and serum revealed the following pattern of reactivity using two screening cells and a red cell reagent panel.

***Laboratory Data (Case 7)***

**Direct Antiglobulin Profile**

| | Polyspecific Anti-Human Serum (Rabbit) | Control Pts Washed RBCs + Normal Saline | Anti-Human Serum Anti-IgG (Rabbit) | Anti-Human Serum Anti-C3d Serum (Rabbit) |
|---|---|---|---|---|
| Red cell test results | 1+ micro | Negative | 1+ micro | Negative |

**Reagent Red Blood Cell Screening Cells (Using an eluate from the patient's red cells)**
**Partial Listing of Antigens Present**

| Cell No. | Rh-hr D | C | E | c | e | Kell K | k | Duffy Fy$^a$ | Fy$^b$ | Kidd Jk$^a$ | Jk$^b$ | Lewis Le$^a$ | Le$^b$ | MNS S | s | M | N | P P$_1$ |
|---|---|---|---|---|---|---|---|---|---|---|---|---|---|---|---|---|---|---|
| I | + | 0 | + | + | + | 0 | + | + | 0 | + | + | 0 | + | + | + | + | 0 | + |
| II | 0 | + | 0 | + | 0 | 0 | + | 0 | + | + | 0 | 0 | + | 0 | + | + | 0 | + |

**Patient Results**

| Cell No. | Immediate Spin | 37° C | AHG | Coombs Control Cells |
|---|---|---|---|---|
| I | Neg | Neg | 1+ | |
| II | Neg | Neg | Neg | 2+ |

**Reagent Red Blood Cell Panel Antigen Profile**
**Partial Listing of Antigens Present**

| Cell No. | Rh-hr D | C | E | c | e | Kell K | k | Duffy Fy$^a$ | Fy$^b$ | Kidd Jk$^a$ | Jk$^b$ | Lewis Le$^a$ | Le$^b$ | MNS S | s | M | N | P P$_1$ |
|---|---|---|---|---|---|---|---|---|---|---|---|---|---|---|---|---|---|---|
| 1 | 0 | 0 | 0 | + | + | 0 | + | + | + | + | 0 | 0 | 0 | + | 0 | + | + | + |
| 2 | 0 | 0 | 0 | + | + | 0 | + | 0 | + | + | + | 0 | + | + | + | + | 0 | 0 |
| 3 | 0 | + | 0 | + | + | 0 | + | 0 | + | + | + | 0 | + | + | + | + | 0 | + |
| 4 | + | 0 | + | + | 0 | 0 | + | + | 0 | + | 0 | 0 | + | 0 | + | + | 0 | + |
| 5 | + | 0 | + | + | 0 | 0 | + | + | + | 0 | + | 0 | + | 0 | + | + | + | + |
| 6 | + | + | 0 | 0 | + | + | + | + | + | + | 0 | 0 | + | + | + | + | + | + |
| 7 | + | + | 0 | 0 | + | 0 | + | 0 | + | + | + | 0 | + | 0 | + | + | + | + |
| 8 | + | + | + | 0 | + | 0 | + | + | 0 | 0 | + | + | 0 | 0 | + | + | 0 | 0 |
| 9 | + | + | 0 | + | + | 0 | + | + | + | + | + | + | 0 | + | 0 | 0 | + | + |
| 10 | + | + | 0 | 0 | + | + | 0 | 0 | + | + | + | 0 | + | 0 | + | + | + | + |
| 11 | + | 0 | 0 | + | + | 0 | + | 0 | + | + | + | + | 0 | 0 | 0 | 0 | + | + |

**Patient Results**

| Cell No. | 37° C | AHG | Coombs Control Cells |
|---|---|---|---|
| 1 | Neg | 2+ | |
| 2 | Neg | Neg | 2+ |
| 3 | Neg | Neg | 2+ |
| 4 | Neg | 2+ | |
| 5 | Neg | 2+ | |
| 6 | Neg | 2+ | |
| 7 | Neg | Neg | 1+ |
| 8 | Neg | 2+ | |
| 9 | Neg | 1+ | |
| 10 | Neg | Neg | 1+ |

## Questions

1. What is the identity of the unexpected antibody?
2. Why was the patient's antibody screen negative before and positive at the time of this crossmatch?
3. Should additional tests be performed?
4. Why was the DAT positive?
5. Briefly discuss the characteristics of the blood group system involved in this case.

## Discussion

1. The patient's serum and elution both demonstrated anti-Fy$^a$ reactivity.

2. Post-transfusion sensitization against Fy$^a$ antigen, consistent with a delayed hemolytic transfusion reaction, caused the differences in the test observations. The original antigenic exposure probably occurred as the result of the pregnancy or the packed red cells administered 7 months previously. The anti-Fy$^a$ was not detected on the unexpected antibody screen one week earlier or when the specimen was retested. However, the most recent transfusion undoubtedly produced a secondary anamnestic response.
3. Yes. When the two units transfused one week earlier were typed for the Fy$^a$ antigen, both were found to be Fy$^a$ positive.
4. The positive DAT resulted from the transfused Fy$^a$ positive red cells being coated with the patient's Fy$^a$ unexpected antibody.
5. The Fy$^a$ antigen belongs to the Duffy blood group system. Anti-Fy$^a$ is usually an IgG antibody, sometimes capable of binding complement. This antibody has been implicated in hemolytic transfusion reactions and HDN. It usually develops in response to antigenic exposure through transfusion or pregnancy to Fy$^a$ positive red cells. A complete discussion of this blood group system can be found in Chapter 6.

## Conclusion

Anti-Fy$^a$ associated with delayed hemolytic transfusion reaction.

## Case 8

### History and Laboratory Data

A 33-year-old man was admitted for a perforated ulcer. He had a history of multiple transfusions. A stat crossmatch for 8 units of packed cells was ordered while the patient was in surgery.

The man was group A, Rh positive. He had a positive unexpected antibody screen and negative DAT. The results of the two cell screening and subsequent reagent red cell panel follow.

### *Laboratory Data (Case 8)*

**Reagent Red Blood Cell Screening Cells**
**Partial Listing of Antigens Present**

| Cell | Rh-hr | | | | | Kell | | Duffy | | Kidd | | Lewis | | MNS | | | | P |
|------|---|---|---|---|---|---|---|---|---|---|---|---|---|---|---|---|---|---|
| No. | D | C | E | c | e | K | k | Fy$^a$ | Fy$^b$ | Jk$^a$ | Jk$^b$ | Le$^a$ | Le$^b$ | S | s | M | N | P$_1$ |
| I | + | + | 0 | + | + | + | 0 | 0 | + | + | + | 0 | + | + | + | + | 0 | + |
| II | + | 0 | + | + | 0 | 0 | + | + | 0 | + | 0 | 0 | + | 0 | + | + | 0 | + |

**Patient Results**

| Cell No. | Immediate Spin | 37° C | AHG | Coombs Control |
|------|------|------|------|------|
| I | Neg | Neg | 2+ | |
| II | Neg | Neg | Neg | 2+ |

**Reagent Red Blood Cell Panel Antigen Profile**
**Partial Listing of Antigens Present**

| Cell | Rh-hr | | | | | Kell | | Duffy | | Kidd | | Lewis | | MNS | | | | P |
|------|---|---|---|---|---|---|---|---|---|---|---|---|---|---|---|---|---|---|
| No. | D | C | E | c | e | K | k | Fy$^a$ | Fy$^b$ | Jk$^a$ | Jk$^b$ | Le$^a$ | Le$^b$ | S | s | M | N | P$_1$ |
| 1 | + | 0 | 0 | + | + | + | 0 | + | + | + | 0 | 0 | 0 | + | 0 | + | + | + |
| 2 | + | 0 | 0 | + | + | 0 | + | 0 | + | + | + | 0 | + | + | + | + | 0 | 0 |
| 3 | + | + | + | + | + | 0 | + | 0 | + | + | + | 0 | + | + | + | + | 0 | + |
| 4 | 0 | 0 | 0 | + | 0 | 0 | + | + | 0 | + | 0 | 0 | + | 0 | + | + | 0 | + |
| 5 | 0 | 0 | + | + | 0 | + | + | + | + | 0 | + | 0 | + | 0 | + | + | + | + |
| 6 | 0 | + | 0 | 0 | + | + | + | + | + | + | 0 | 0 | + | + | + | + | + | + |
| 7 | 0 | + | + | 0 | + | 0 | + | 0 | + | + | + | 0 | + | 0 | + | + | + | + |
| 8 | 0 | + | 0 | 0 | + | 0 | + | + | 0 | 0 | + | + | 0 | 0 | + | + | 0 | 0 |
| 9 | 0 | + | + | + | + | 0 | + | + | + | + | + | + | 0 | + | 0 | 0 | + | + |
| 10 | 0 | + | 0 | 0 | + | 0 | + | 0 | + | + | + | 0 | + | 0 | + | + | + | + |
| 11 | 0 | 0 | 0 | + | + | + | + | 0 | + | + | + | + | 0 | 0 | 0 | 0 | + | + |

**Patient Results**

| Cell No. | Immediate Spin | 37° C | AHG | Coombs Control |
|------|------|------|------|------|
| 1 | Neg | Neg | 2+ | |
| 2 | Neg | Neg | Neg | 2+ |
| 3 | Neg | Neg | Neg | 1+ |
| 4 | Neg | Neg | Neg | 2+ |
| 5 | Neg | Neg | 2+ | |
| 6 | Neg | Neg | 2+ | |
| 7 | Neg | Neg | Neg | 2+ |
| 8 | Neg | Neg | Neg | 3+ |
| 9 | Neg | Neg | Neg | 2+ |
| 10 | Neg | Neg | Neg | 2+ |
| 11 | Neg | Neg | 1+ | |
| Auto | Neg | Neg | Neg | 2+ |

### Questions

1. Based on the two-cell screening, what are the possible unexpected antibodies in this patient's serum?

2. What is the identity of the unexpected antibody or antibodies?
3. Briefly discuss the characteristics of the blood group system involved in this case.
4. How is the antibody formed?

### Discussion

1. The results of the two-cell screening suggest the presence of either an Rh or AHG reactive unexpected antibody. The antigens present in the I cell but not in the II cell are C, K, Fy$^b$, Jk$^b$, and S.
2. The reaction in the AHG phase of the 1, 5, 6, and 11 cell indicates that one unexpected antibody is present: anti-K.
3. The K antigen is part of the Kell system and is present in 9% of the White population. Anti-K is usually an IgG antibody but may rarely be observed as an IgM antibody. Typically, it reacts in the antiglobulin phase, although it

may be observed at 37° C in albumin. It may bind complement. This antibody has been implicated in HDN and hemolytic transfusion reactions. A complete discussion of this blood group system can be found in Chapter 16.
4. Antibody formation usually results from erythrocyte antigen exposure, either during pregnancy or through transfusions. In this case, prior blood transfusions had exposed the patient to the Kell antigen.

## Conclusion

Anti-Kell induced through prior blood transfusions.

## Case 9

### History and Laboratory Data

An 18-year-old White woman (group O, Rh positive) was 24 hours post-partum. Because of a low hematocrit, 2 units of packed red cells were ordered. The patient had no known history of pregnancy or prior transfusions.

Two of 4 units crossmatched produced incompatible results. The patient's indirect antiglobulin unexpected antibody screening test was also positive. The results of these tests follow.

*Laboratory Data (Case 9)*

**Reagent Red Blood Cell Screening Cells**
**Partial Listing of Antigens Present**

| Cell No. | D | C | E | c | e | K | k | Fy$^a$ | Fy$^b$ | Jk$^a$ | Jk$^b$ | Le$^a$ | Le$^b$ | S | s | M | N | P$_1$ |
|---|---|---|---|---|---|---|---|---|---|---|---|---|---|---|---|---|---|---|
| I | + | 0 | + | + | + | 0 | + | + | 0 | + | + | 0 | + | + | + | + | 0 | + |
| II | 0 | + | 0 | + | 0 | 0 | + | 0 | + | + | 0 | + | + | 0 | + | + | 0 | + |

(Rh-hr: D C E c e; Kell: K k; Duffy: Fy$^a$ Fy$^b$; Kidd: Jk$^a$ Jk$^b$; Lewis: Le$^a$ Le$^b$; MNS: S s M N; P: P$_1$)

**Patient Results**

| Cell No. | Immediate Spin | 37° C | AHG | Coombs Control Cells |
|---|---|---|---|---|
| I | Neg | Neg | Neg | 2+ |
| II | ± | ± | 1+ | 2+ |

**Reagent Red Blood Cell Panel Antigen Profile**
**Partial Listing of Antigens Present**

| Cell No. | D | C | E | c | e | K | k | Fy$^a$ | Fy$^b$ | Jk$^a$ | Jk$^b$ | Le$^a$ | Le$^b$ | S | s | M | N | P$_1$ |
|---|---|---|---|---|---|---|---|---|---|---|---|---|---|---|---|---|---|---|
| 1 | + | 0 | 0 | + | + | + | 0 | + | + | + | 0 | 0 | 0 | + | 0 | + | + | + |
| 2 | + | 0 | 0 | + | + | 0 | + | 0 | + | + | + | 0 | + | + | + | + | 0 | 0 |
| 3 | + | + | + | + | + | 0 | + | 0 | + | + | + | 0 | + | + | + | + | 0 | + |
| 4 | 0 | 0 | 0 | + | 0 | 0 | + | + | 0 | + | 0 | 0 | + | 0 | + | + | 0 | + |
| 5 | 0 | 0 | + | + | 0 | + | + | + | + | 0 | + | 0 | + | 0 | + | + | + | + |
| 6 | 0 | + | 0 | 0 | + | + | + | + | + | + | 0 | 0 | + | + | + | + | + | + |
| 7 | 0 | + | + | 0 | + | 0 | + | 0 | + | + | + | 0 | + | 0 | + | + | + | + |
| 8 | 0 | + | 0 | 0 | + | 0 | + | + | 0 | 0 | + | + | 0 | 0 | + | + | 0 | 0 |
| 9 | 0 | + | + | + | + | 0 | + | + | + | + | + | + | 0 | + | 0 | 0 | + | + |
| 10 | 0 | + | 0 | 0 | + | 0 | + | 0 | + | + | + | 0 | + | 0 | + | + | + | + |
| 11 | 0 | 0 | 0 | + | + | + | + | 0 | + | + | + | + | 0 | 0 | 0 | + | + | + |

**Patient Results**

| Cell No. | Immediate Spin | 37° C | AHG | Coombs Control Cells |
|---|---|---|---|---|
| 1 | Neg | Neg | Neg | 2+ |
| 2 | Neg | Neg | Neg | 2+ |
| 3 | Neg | Neg | Neg | 2+ |
| 4 | Neg | Neg | Neg | 2+ |
| 5 | Neg | Neg | Neg | 2+ |
| 6 | Neg | Neg | Neg | 2+ |
| 7 | Neg | Neg | Neg | 1+ |
| 8 | 1+ | ± | 2+ | |
| 9 | 1+ | ± | 2+ | |
| 10 | Neg | Neg | Neg | 1+ |
| 11 | ± | Neg | 1+ | |

### Questions

1. Based on the reactions in the two-cell screening panel, what antibodies are probably in this serum?
2. What is the identity of the unexpected antibody or antibodies?
3. Briefly discuss the characteristics of the blood group system involved in this case.
4. How is the antibody formed?

### Discussion

1. The II cell of the screening cells was the only reactive cell. The following antigens are present on this cell but not on the I cell: C, Fy$^b$, and Le$^a$.

2. The pattern of reactivity of the panel of reagent red cells is consistent with the pattern and type or reactivity seen with anti-Le$^a$.

3. The Le(a) antigen is part of the Lewis blood group system. Anti-Le$^a$ is an IgM antibody, known to fix complement, and is capable of producing hemolytic transfusion reactions. HDN has not been reported due to anti-Le$^a$. A full discussion of the Lewis blood group system is presented in Chapter 6.

4. Patients develop anti-Le$^a$ through inhalation or ingestion of Le$^a$-like antigenic determinants. Transient anti-Le$^a$ is not uncommon during pregnancy.

## Conclusion

Anti-Le$^a$ related to pregnancy.

## Case 10

### History and Laboratory Data

A 76-year-old Black man was admitted for sepsis and kidney failure. He was group AB, Rh negative. His history included receiving two units of packed cells 5 years before. The patient had also been recently transfused; therefore, mixed field agglutination patterns were observed when other Rh antigens were tested.

Rh(D) Neg; weak D (D$^u$) neg; rh$'$(C)1 + MF; rh$''$(E)1 + MF; hr$'$(c)2 + MF; hr$''$(e)2 + MF

During the preparation of several units of packed red cells for transfusion, a negative unexpected antibody screen was observed and a weakly positive DAT was detected. No unexpected antibodies were detected using multiple testing techniques.

### *Laboratory Data (Case 10)*

**Direct Antiglobulin Profile**

|  | Polyspecific AHG (Rabbit) | Control Pts washed RBCs + Normal Saline | AHG Anti-IgG (Rabbit) | AHG Anti-C3d serum (rabbit) |
| --- | --- | --- | --- | --- |
| Red cell test results | Positive ± weak microscopic | Negative | Positive ± strong microscopic | Negative |

Heat ether elevate of the patient's red cells revealed the following pattern of reactivity using two screening cells and a red cell reagent panel.

**Reagent Red Blood Cell Screening Cells**
**Antigens Present**

| Cell No. | Rh-hr | | | | | Kell | | | | | | Duffy | |
| --- | --- | --- | --- | --- | --- | --- | --- | --- | --- | --- | --- | --- | --- |
|  | D | C | E | c | e | K | k | Kp$^a$ | Kp$^b$ | Js$^a$ | Js$^b$ | Fy$^a$ | Fy$^b$ |
| I | + | 0 | + | + | + | + | + | 0 | + | 0 | + | 0 | + |
| II | 0 | + | 0 | + | 0 | 0 | + | 0 | + | 0 | + | 0 | + |

**Antigens Present (continued)**

| Cell No. | Kidd | | Lewis | | MNS | | | | P |
| --- | --- | --- | --- | --- | --- | --- | --- | --- | --- |
|  | Jk$^a$ | Jk$^b$ | Le$^a$ | Le$^b$ | S | s | M | N | P$_1$ |
| I | + | + | 0 | + | + | + | + | 0 | + |
| II | + | + | + | 0 | + | 0 | + | + | 0 |

**Patient Results**

| Cell No. | Immediate Spin | 37° C | AHG | Coombs Control Cells |
| --- | --- | --- | --- | --- |
| I | Neg | Neg | Neg | 2+ |
| II | Neg | Neg | Neg | 2+ |

**Reagent Red Blood Cell Panel Antigen Profile**
**Antigens Present**

| Cell. No. | C | D | E | c | e | Cw | f | V | K | k | Kpa | Kpb | Jsa | Jsb | Fya | Fyb | Jka | Jkb |
|---|---|---|---|---|---|---|---|---|---|---|---|---|---|---|---|---|---|---|
| | | | Rh-Hr | | | | | | | | Kell | | | | Duffy | | Kidd | |
| 1 | + | + | + | 0 | + | 0 | 0 | 0 | + | + | 0 | + | + | + | 0 | + | 0 | + |
| 2 | + | + | 0 | 0 | + | + | 0 | 0 | 0 | + | 0 | + | 0 | + | + | + | + | 0 |
| 3 | 0 | + | + | + | 0 | 0 | 0 | 0 | 0 | + | 0 | + | 0 | + | + | + | + | 0 |
| 4 | + | 0 | 0 | + | + | 0 | + | 0 | 0 | + | 0 | + | 0 | + | 0 | + | + | + |
| 5 | 0 | 0 | + | + | + | 0 | + | 0 | 0 | + | 0 | + | 0 | + | + | + | + | 0 |
| 6 | 0 | 0 | 0 | + | + | 0 | + | 0 | 0 | + | + | + | 0 | + | 0 | + | 0 | + |
| 7 | 0 | 0 | 0 | + | + | 0 | + | 0 | 0 | + | 0 | + | 0 | + | + | 0 | 0 | + |
| 8 | 0 | + | 0 | + | + | 0 | + | 0 | 0 | + | 0 | + | 0 | + | + | + | + | 0 |
| 9 | 0 | 0 | 0 | + | + | 0 | + | 0 | 0 | + | 0 | + | 0 | + | 0 | 0 | + | + |
| 10 | 0 | 0 | 0 | + | + | 0 | + | 0 | 0 | + | 0 | + | 0 | + | + | + | 0 | 0 |

**Antigens Present (continued)**

| Cell No. | Lea | Leb | P1 | M | N | S | s | Lua | Lub | Xga | | Additional |
|---|---|---|---|---|---|---|---|---|---|---|---|---|
| | Lewis | | P | | MNS | | | Lutheran | | Sex-Linked | | |
| 1 | 0 | + | + | 0 | + | + | + | 0 | + | 0 | M | |
| 2 | + | 0 | + | + | + | 0 | + | 0 | + | + | F | |
| 3 | 0 | + | + | 0 | + | 0 | + | 0 | + | + | M | |
| 4 | 0 | + | + | + | 0 | + | 0 | + | + | + | F | Co (b+) |
| 5 | 0 | + | 0 | + | + | + | + | 0 | + | + | M | |
| 6 | 0 | + | 0 | + | + | 0 | + | 0 | + | 0 | M | |
| 7 | 0 | + | + | + | 0 | + | + | 0 | + | 0 | M | Co (b+) |
| 8 | + | 0 | + | + | + | + | 0 | 0 | + | 0 | M | |
| 9 | 0 | 0 | + | + | + | + | 0 | 0 | + | + | F | |
| 10 | 0 | + | 0 | 0 | 0 | 0 | + | 0 | + | + | F | |
| 11 | — | — | — | — | — | — | — | — | — | — | | I (neg) |

**Patient Results**

| Cell No. | Immediate Spin | 37° C | AHG | Coombs Control |
|---|---|---|---|---|
| 1 | Neg | Neg | 2+ | |
| 2 | Neg | Neg | Neg | 2+ |
| 3 | Neg | Neg | Neg | 2+ |
| 4 | Neg | Neg | Neg | 2+ |
| 5 | Neg | Neg | Neg | 2+ |
| 6 | Neg | Neg | Neg | 2+ |
| 7 | Neg | Neg | Neg | 2+ |
| 8 | Neg | Neg | Neg | 2+ |
| 9 | Neg | Neg | Neg | 2+ |
| 10 | Neg | Neg | Neg | 2+ |
| 11 | Neg | Neg | Neg | 2+ |
| Auto | Neg | Neg | Neg | 2+ |

## Questions

1. Based on the results of the screening and reagent panel cells, what is the identity of the antibody in the eluate?
2. Why was the patient's serum unexpected antibody screen negative?
3. What further tests should be done?
4. Briefly describe the blood group system involved in this case.

## Discussion

1. The heat ether eluate prepared from the patient's red cells was positive with one cell tested. This cell is positive for Jsa antigen.
2. The patient had an extremely low titer of unexpected antibody. The presence of Jsa antibody, however, was enough to coat the Jsa positive transfused cells. It was suspected that the patient had an anti-Jsa, but samples of the previously transfused units were unavailable to confirm whether or not a positive Jsa unit of blood was transfused.
3. The patient's DAT should be monitored to detect increases in its strength.
4. The Jsa antigen is one of the Kell blood group antigens. Anti-Jsa was discovered in 1958 during routine compatibility tests in the serum of a previously transfused White man. The Jsa (Sutter) antibody is typically an AHG reacting antibody. The Jsa antigen is present in about 20% of Blacks but is apparently absent in Whites. The Kell blood group system is fully described in Chapter 6.

## Conclusion

Anti-Jsa.

## MULTIPLE ANTIBODIES

### Case 11

History and Laboratory Data

A 72-year-old White woman with degenerative osteoarthritis was admitted for elective total knee replacement surgery. She was group O, Rh negative. Her transfusion and obstetric histories were unavailable. In preparation of the two units of packed red cells preoperatively, both units were incompatible; however, the autocontrol was negative. The two-cell screening test was also positive. The results of the two-cell screening procedure and a reagent panel of red cells follow.

*Laboratory Data (Case 11)*

**Reagent Red Blood Cell Screening Cells**
**Partial Listing of Antigens Present**

| Cell No. | Rh-hr | | | | | Kell | | Duffy | | Kidd | | Lewis | | MNS | | | | P |
|---|---|---|---|---|---|---|---|---|---|---|---|---|---|---|---|---|---|---|
| | D | C | E | c | e | K | k | Fy$^a$ | Fy$^b$ | Jk$^a$ | Jk$^b$ | Le$^a$ | Le$^b$ | S | s | M | N | P$_1$ |
| I | 0 | + | 0 | 0 | + | 0 | + | 0 | + | + | + | 0 | + | + | + | + | 0 | + |
| II | + | 0 | + | + | 0 | + | 0 | + | 0 | + | 0 | 0 | + | 0 | + | + | 0 | + |

**Patient Results**

| Cell No. | Immediate Spin | 37° C | AHG |
|---|---|---|---|
| I | Neg | Neg | 2+ |
| II | Neg | 1+ | 3+ |

**Reagent Red Blood Cell Panel Antigen Profile**
**Partial Listing of Antigens Present**

| Cell No. | Rh-hr | | | | | Kell | | Duffy | | Kidd | | Lewis | | MNS | | | | P |
|---|---|---|---|---|---|---|---|---|---|---|---|---|---|---|---|---|---|---|
| | D | C | E | c | e | K | k | Fy$^a$ | Fy$^b$ | Jk$^a$ | Jk$^b$ | Le$^a$ | Le$^b$ | S | s | M | N | P$_1$ |
| 1 | 0 | 0 | 0 | + | + | 0 | + | + | + | + | 0 | 0 | 0 | + | 0 | + | + | + |
| 2 | 0 | 0 | 0 | + | + | 0 | + | 0 | + | + | + | 0 | + | + | + | + | 0 | 0 |
| 3 | 0 | + | 0 | + | + | 0 | + | 0 | + | + | + | 0 | + | + | + | + | 0 | + |
| 4 | + | 0 | + | + | 0 | 0 | + | + | 0 | + | 0 | 0 | + | 0 | + | + | 0 | + |
| 5 | + | 0 | + | + | 0 | 0 | + | + | + | 0 | + | 0 | + | 0 | + | + | + | + |
| 6 | + | + | 0 | 0 | + | + | + | + | + | + | 0 | 0 | + | + | + | + | + | + |
| 7 | + | + | 0 | 0 | + | 0 | + | 0 | + | + | + | 0 | + | 0 | + | + | + | + |
| 8 | + | + | + | 0 | + | 0 | + | + | 0 | 0 | + | + | 0 | 0 | + | + | 0 | 0 |
| 9 | + | + | 0 | + | + | 0 | + | + | + | + | + | + | 0 | + | 0 | 0 | + | + |
| 10 | + | + | 0 | 0 | + | + | 0 | 0 | + | + | + | 0 | + | 0 | + | + | + | + |
| 11 | + | 0 | 0 | + | + | 0 | + | 0 | + | + | + | + | 0 | 0 | 0 | 0 | + | + |

**Patient Results**

| Cell No. | Immediate Spin | 37° C | AHG | Control Check Cells |
|---|---|---|---|---|
| 1 | Neg | Neg | Neg | 2+ |
| 2 | Neg | Neg | Neg | 2+ |
| 3 | Neg | Neg | 1+ | |
| 4 | Neg | 1+ | 2+ | |
| 5 | Neg | 1+ | 2+ | |
| 6 | Neg | 1+ | 2+ | |
| 7 | Neg | 1+ | 2+ | |
| 8 | Neg | 1+ | 2+ | |
| 9 | Neg | 1+ | 2+ | |
| 10 | Neg | 1+ | 2+ | |
| 11 | Neg | 1+ | 2+ | |

Questions

1. Based on the two cell screening test, what is (are) the possible unexpected antibody or antibodies?

2. Is the pattern of cell reactivity in the panel of reagent red cells consistent with any specific unexpected antibody?
3. What other tests would support the agglutination results?
4. Briefly discuss the antigen-antibody systems involved in this case.

Discussion

1. The reaction with screening cell I in only the antiglobulin phase implies either a low titer Rh antibody or an AHG reactive antibody. Possible antigens present on the I cell that would fit into one of these categories include: C, e, k, Fy$^b$, or Jk$^b$.

The reaction of the II cell with albumin at 37° C suggests the presence of high-titered Rh antibody (the D, E, and c antigens are present on this cell) or a high titered anti-K which can exhibit reactivity at 37° C in albumin.
2. The patient's serum demonstrated agglutination in

cells 3 through 11. The AHG pattern of the panel cells excludes most of the antibodies identified as possibilities for the I screening cell (anti-e, anti-k, anti-Fy$^b$, and anti-Jk$^b$). The pattern of anti-C, however, would not be excluded if a second antibody existed in the serum.

Cells 4 through 11 exhibited agglutination at the 37° C phase, which is similar to the activity displayed in screening cell II. This pattern of reactivity excludes the other probable antibodies (anti-E, anti-c, or anti-K) identified in question 2 but is consistent with the presence of the alloantibody, anti-D.

3. Testing of the patient's red cells for the absence of D and C antigens would confirm the patient's ability to produce corresponding antibodies, if she had been antigenically stimulated by antigenic exposure and had the capability of mounting an immune response.

The patient is already known to lack the D antigen; therefore, anti-D is one of the probable unexpected antibodies. Results of additional antigen testing of her red cells were C-Negative, E-Positive, e-Positive, K-Positive, k-Positive, Fy$^b$-Negative, JK$^b$-Negative.

4. The D and C antigens belong to the Rhesus (Rh) blood group system. Most anti-D and anti-C antibodies are of the IgG type, although anti-D is occasionally demonstrated in the IgM form and rarely as IgA. The formation of anti-D is usually stimulated by antigenic exposure during pregnancy or through transfusion to D positive RBCs. Anti-C is produced in response to the transfusion of C positive erythrocytes.

Anti-D is a well-known cause of HDN and can produce a hemolytic transfusion reaction, if the corresponding D antigen is introduced into the circulation of a patient with the unexpected antibody. Anti-C has also been implicated in hemolytic transfusion reactions, if the antigen and corresponding antibody are united.

Anti-C is a rare antibody in Rh positive persons, and is rarely the only unexpected antibody, if it occurs, in Rh negative subjects. The combination of anti-D and anti-C in Rh negative subjects is more common.

### Conclusion

Anti-D and anti-C unexpected antibodies, cause unknown.

## Case 12

### History and Laboratory Data

An 83-year-old White man was suffering from anemia (hematocrit 22%) and congestive heart failure. He was receiving two types of medication, Bumex and Demerol. He was group O, Rh positive (most probable genotype $R_2r$) and had been transfused with 6 units of packed cells over the last 2½ to 4½ months.

A weakly positive DAT and positive unexpected antibody screen were discovered on the pretransfusion workup. An initial serum antibody panel and elution studies using conventional techniques were nonspecific. The specimen was referred to a reference laboratory for further studies. His phenotype was performed using autologous red cells obtained by using simplified reticulocyte-rich cell separation techniques. Additional antigen typings: M+N+S−s+; P1+; Le(a−b+); K−; Fy(a+b−); Jk(a−b+). DAT: IgG−1+, C3-neg.

### *Laboratory Data (Case 12)*

**Direct Antiglobulin Profile**

| | Polyspecific AHG (Rabbit) | Control (Pts Washed Red Cells + Normal Saline) | AHG Anti-IgG (Rabbit) | AHG Anti-C3d (Rabbit) |
|---|---|---|---|---|
| Red cell negative results | Positive ± Micro | Negative | Positive 1+ | Negative |

**Enzyme-Treated Reagent Red Blood Cell Screening Cells**
**Partial Listing of Antigens Present**

| Cell No. | Rh-hr | | | | | Kell | | Duffy | | Kidd | | Lewis | | MNS | | | | P |
|---|---|---|---|---|---|---|---|---|---|---|---|---|---|---|---|---|---|---|
| | D | C | E | c | e | K | k | Fy$^a$ | Fy$^b$ | Jk$^a$ | Jk$^b$ | Le$^a$ | Le$^b$ | S | s | M | N | P$_1$ |
| I | 0 | + | + | + | + | 0 | + | + | 0 | + | 0 | 0 | + | 0 | + | + | 0 | + |
| II | + | 0 | + | + | 0 | 0 | + | 0 | + | + | + | 0 | + | + | + | + | 0 | + |

**Patient's Serum Results**

| Cell No. | Immediate Spin | 37° C | AHG | Coombs Control |
|---|---|---|---|---|
| I | Neg | ± | 1+ | |
| II | Neg | Neg | Neg | 2+ |

**Enzyme-Treated Red Blood Cell Panel Antigen Profile**
**Partial Listing of Antigens Present**

| Cell | Rh-hr | | | | | Kell | | Duffy | | Kidd | | Lewis | | MNS | | | | P |
| No. | D | C | E | c | e | K | k | Fy$^a$ | Fy$^b$ | Jk$^a$ | Jk$^b$ | Le$^a$ | Le$^b$ | S | s | M | N | P$_1$ |
|---|---|---|---|---|---|---|---|---|---|---|---|---|---|---|---|---|---|---|
| 1 | 0 | 0 | 0 | + | + | 0 | + | + | + | + | 0 | 0 | 0 | + | 0 | + | + | + |
| 2 | 0 | 0 | 0 | + | + | 0 | + | 0 | + | + | + | 0 | + | + | + | + | 0 | 0 |
| 3 | 0 | + | + | + | + | 0 | + | 0 | + | + | + | 0 | + | + | + | + | 0 | + |
| 4 | + | 0 | 0 | + | 0 | 0 | + | + | 0 | + | 0 | + | + | 0 | + | + | 0 | + |
| 5 | + | 0 | + | + | 0 | 0 | + | + | + | 0 | + | 0 | + | + | + | + | + | + |
| 6 | + | + | 0 | 0 | + | + | + | + | + | + | 0 | 0 | + | + | + | + | + | + |
| 7 | + | + | + | 0 | + | 0 | + | 0 | + | + | + | 0 | + | 0 | + | + | + | + |
| 8 | + | + | 0 | 0 | + | 0 | + | + | 0 | 0 | + | + | 0 | 0 | + | + | 0 | 0 |
| 9 | + | + | + | + | + | 0 | + | + | + | + | + | + | 0 | + | 0 | 0 | + | + |
| 10 | + | + | 0 | 0 | + | + | 0 | 0 | + | + | + | 0 | + | 0 | + | + | + | + |
| 11 | + | 0 | 0 | + | + | 0 | + | 0 | + | + | + | + | 0 | 0 | 0 | 0 | + | + |

**Patient's Serum Results**

| Cell No. | Immediate Spin | 37° C | AHG | Coombs Control |
|---|---|---|---|---|
| 1 | Neg | Neg | 1+ | |
| 2 | Neg | Neg | 1+ | |
| 3 | Neg | ± | 2+ | |
| 4 | Neg | Neg | Neg | 2+ |
| 5 | Neg | Neg | Neg | 2+ |
| 6 | Neg | ± | 2+ | |
| 7 | Neg | ± | 2+ | |
| 8 | Neg | ± | 2+ | |
| 9 | Neg | ± | 2+ | |
| 10 | Neg | ± | 2+ | |
| 11 | Neg | ± | 1+ | |
| Auto | Neg | Neg | Neg | 2+ |

## Questions

1. What does the positive DAT profile suggest?
2. Why was an enhancement technique used to further study the patient's serum?
3. What antibody (antibodies) does (do) the results of the two enzyme-treated screening cells suggest?
4. Can this patient have an antibody to a self-antigen?
5. Would an elution prepared from the patient's positive DAT cells be of value?

## Discussion

1. Positive reactions with both polyspecific and IgG AHG suggest the presence of an IgG type antibody. Refer to Chapter 3 for a full discussion of the causes of a positive DAT.
2. Enhancement techniques such as enzyme treatment or polybrene frequently strengthen the reactions of certain antigen-antibody systems, e.g., Rh. Techniques such as enzyme treatment, however, can also destroy antigen receptor sites. For example, the treatment of Fy$^a$ positive cells with trypsin or papain makes them nonreactive with anti-Fy$^a$ sera.*
3. The antigens present on the I screening cell but not

* Zmijewski, Fletcher: *Immunohematology* (2nd ed.), New York, Appleton Century Crofts, 1972, p. 166.

on the II cell are C, e, and Fy$^a$. The enzyme-treated panel reactions at 37° C are consistent with anti-C activity. The additional reactions in the AHG phase suggest the presence of another unexpected antibody.

A negative autocontrol excludes the possibility that a nonspecific autoantibody is clouding the picture. Enzyme treatment should have destroyed the Fy$^a$ receptor sites; therefore, anti-Fy$^a$ should be excluded for this reason and also because the patient is Fy$^a$ positive. The only other possibility based upon the reagent screening cell reactivity is anti-e. The patient, however, is also positive for the e antigen.

4. Yes. The detection of a possible anti-e in this patient's serum is somewhat unexpected because the patient's own reticulocyte-rich red cells are e positive. However, an adsorption using R2R2 red cells on the serum was performed and there was no significant reduction in the strength of this antibody after adsorption.

Like the D antigen, the e antigen is a structure with many different components. It is probable that this patient is an e "mosaic." In this mosaic, the e antigen lacks one or more of the normal components. Just like individuals with the weak D (D$^u$) mosaic, these individuals can produce antibodies to that portion of the antigen which they lack. In this case, the patient was undoubtedly transfused with normal e positive red cells, which elicited the observed antibody response. Refer to Chapter 5 for a full discussion of the Rh blood group system.

5. In this case, elution of the red cells and analysis of the eluate did not yield any specific reactions.

## Conclusion

Anti-C and anti-e.

## Case 13

### History and Laboratory Data

A 94-year-old White woman was admitted to the hospital because of gastrointestinal (GI) hemorrhage. She was group A, Rh positive. Her transfusion history included 4 units of packed red cells 1 month prior to admission and another 4 units of packed red cells 10 days previously. Her medications included alpha-methyldopa, cephalo-thin, penicillin, Persantine, Feosol, and Lasix. In preparing 4 units for transfusion, a positive unexpected antibody screen and a weakly positive DAT were detected.

### Laboratory Data (Case 13)

**Direct Antiglobulin Profile**

|  | Polyspecific AHG (Rabbit) | Control Pts Washed RBCs + Normal Saline | AHG Anti-IgG (Rabbit) | AHG Anti-C3d Serum (Rabbit) |
|---|---|---|---|---|
| Red cell test results | Positive ± micro | Negative | Positive ± micro | Negative |

**Reagent Red Blood Cell Screening Cells**
**Partial Listing of Antigens Present**

| Cell No. | Rh-hr D | C | E | c | e | Kell K | k | Duffy Fy$^a$ | Fy$^b$ | Kidd Jk$^a$ | Jk$^b$ | Lewis Le$^a$ | Le$^b$ | MNS S | s | M | N | P P$_1$ |
|---|---|---|---|---|---|---|---|---|---|---|---|---|---|---|---|---|---|---|
| I | + | 0 | + | + | + | 0 | + | + | 0 | + | + | 0 | + | + | + | + | 0 | + |
| II | 0 | + | 0 | + | 0 | + | 0 | 0 | + | + | 0 | 0 | + | 0 | + | + | 0 | + |

**Patient Results**

| Cell No. | Immediate Spin | 37° C | AHG | Coombs Control Cells |
|---|---|---|---|---|
| I | Neg | 1+ | 2+ | |
| II | Neg | Neg | Neg | 3+ |

**Reagent Red Blood Cell Panel Antigen Profile**
**Partial Listing of Antigens Present**

| Cell No. | Rh-hr D | C | E | c | e | Kell K | k | Duffy Fy$^a$ | Fy$^b$ | Kidd Jk$^a$ | Jk$^b$ | Lewis Le$^a$ | Le$^b$ | MNS S | s | M | N | P P$_1$ |
|---|---|---|---|---|---|---|---|---|---|---|---|---|---|---|---|---|---|---|
| 1 | 0 | 0 | 0 | + | + | 0 | + | + | + | + | 0 | 0 | 0 | + | 0 | + | + | + |
| 2 | 0 | + | 0 | + | + | 0 | + | 0 | + | + | + | 0 | + | + | + | + | 0 | 0 |
| 3 | 0 | + | 0 | + | + | 0 | + | 0 | + | + | + | 0 | + | + | + | + | 0 | + |
| 4 | + | + | + | + | 0 | 0 | + | + | 0 | + | 0 | 0 | + | 0 | + | + | 0 | + |
| 5 | + | 0 | + | + | 0 | 0 | + | + | + | 0 | + | 0 | + | 0 | + | + | + | + |
| 6 | + | + | 0 | 0 | + | + | + | + | + | + | 0 | 0 | + | + | + | + | + | + |
| 7 | + | + | 0 | 0 | + | 0 | + | 0 | + | + | + | 0 | + | 0 | + | + | + | + |
| 8 | + | 0 | + | + | + | 0 | + | + | 0 | 0 | + | + | 0 | 0 | + | + | 0 | 0 |
| 9 | + | 0 | 0 | + | + | 0 | + | + | + | + | + | + | 0 | + | 0 | 0 | + | + |
| 10 | + | + | 0 | 0 | + | + | 0 | 0 | + | + | + | 0 | + | 0 | + | + | + | + |
| 11 | + | 0 | 0 | + | + | 0 | + | 0 | + | + | + | + | 0 | 0 | 0 | 0 | + | + |

**Patient Results**

| Cell No. | Immediate Spin | 37° C | AHG | Coombs Control Cells |
|---|---|---|---|---|
| 1 | Neg | Neg | Neg | 2+ |
| 2 | Neg | Neg | Neg | 2+ |
| 3 | Neg | Neg | Neg | 3+ |
| 4 | Neg | 2+ | 3+ | |
| 5 | Neg | Neg | 2+ | |
| 6 | Neg | Neg | Neg | 2+ |
| 7 | Neg | Neg | Neg | 1+ |
| 8 | Neg | 2+ | 3+ | |
| 9 | Neg | Neg | Neg | 1+ |
| 10 | Neg | Neg | Neg | 2+ |
| 11 | Neg | Neg | Neg | 2+ |
| Auto | Neg | Neg | Neg | 2+ |

**Reagent Red Blood Cell Screening Cells**
**Partial Listing of Antigens Present**

| Cell No. | Rh-hr | | | | | Kell | | Duffy | | Kidd | | Lewis | | MNS | | | | P |
|---|---|---|---|---|---|---|---|---|---|---|---|---|---|---|---|---|---|---|
| | D | C | E | c | e | K | k | Fyᵃ | Fyᵇ | Jkᵃ | Jkᵇ | Leᵃ | Leᵇ | S | s | M | N | P₁ |
| I | + | 0 | + | + | + | 0 | + | + | 0 | + | + | 0 | + | + | + | + | 0 | + |
| II | 0 | + | 0 | + | 0 | + | 0 | 0 | 0 | + | + | 0 | + | 0 | + | + | 0 | + |

**Patient Results Using an Eluate from the Patient's Red Cells**

| Cell No. | Immediate Spin | 37° C | AHG | Coombs Control Cells |
|---|---|---|---|---|
| I | Neg | Neg | Neg | 2+ |
| II | Neg | Neg | 2+ | |

**Reagent Red Blood Cell Panel Antigen Profile**
**Partial Listing of Antigens Present**

| Cell No. | Rh-hr | | | | | Kell | | Duffy | | Kidd | | Lewis | | MNS | | | | P |
|---|---|---|---|---|---|---|---|---|---|---|---|---|---|---|---|---|---|---|
| | D | C | E | c | e | K | k | Fyᵃ | Fyᵇ | Jkᵃ | Jkᵇ | Leᵃ | Leᵇ | S | s | M | N | P₁ |
| 1 | 0 | 0 | 0 | + | + | 0 | + | + | + | + | 0 | 0 | 0 | + | 0 | + | + | + |
| 2 | 0 | + | 0 | + | + | 0 | + | 0 | + | + | + | 0 | + | + | + | + | 0 | 0 |
| 3 | 0 | + | 0 | + | + | 0 | + | 0 | + | + | + | 0 | + | + | + | + | 0 | + |
| 4 | + | + | + | + | 0 | 0 | + | + | 0 | + | 0 | 0 | + | 0 | + | + | 0 | + |
| 5 | + | 0 | + | + | 0 | 0 | + | + | + | 0 | + | 0 | + | 0 | + | + | + | + |
| 6 | + | + | 0 | 0 | + | + | + | + | + | + | 0 | 0 | + | + | + | + | + | + |
| 7 | + | + | 0 | 0 | + | 0 | + | 0 | + | + | + | 0 | + | 0 | + | + | + | + |
| 8 | + | 0 | + | + | + | 0 | + | + | 0 | 0 | + | + | 0 | 0 | + | + | 0 | 0 |
| 9 | + | 0 | 0 | + | + | 0 | + | + | + | + | + | + | 0 | + | 0 | 0 | + | + |
| 10 | + | + | 0 | 0 | + | + | 0 | 0 | + | + | + | 0 | + | 0 | + | + | + | + |
| 11 | + | 0 | 0 | + | + | 0 | + | 0 | + | + | + | + | 0 | 0 | 0 | 0 | + | + |

**Patient Results Using an Eluate from the Patient's Red Cells**

| Cell No. | Immediate Spin | 37° C | AHG | Coombs Control Cells |
|---|---|---|---|---|
| 1 | Neg | Neg | 2+ | |
| 2 | Neg | Neg | Neg | 2+ |
| 3 | Neg | Neg | Neg | 2+ |
| 4 | Neg | Neg | 2+ | 3+ |
| 5 | Neg | Neg | 2+ | |
| 6 | Neg | Neg | 2+ | |
| 7 | Neg | Neg | Neg | 1+ |
| 8 | Neg | Neg | 2+ | |
| 9 | Neg | Neg | 1+ | |
| 10 | Neg | Neg | Neg | 2+ |
| 11 | Neg | Neg | Neg | 2+ |
| Auto | Neg | Neg | Neg | 2+ |

## Questions

1. What is the identity of the antibody or antibodies in the patient's serum?
2. What is the identity of the antibody or antibodies from the eluate?
3. Explain the inconsistency between the serum and eluate.
4. What further tests should be conducted?
5. Explain the mechanism of the involved reaction.

## Discussion

1. The pattern of reactivity of the patient's serum is consistent with the reactions of an anti-E.
2. The elution from the patient's red cells produced the reactivity pattern of an anti-Fyᵃ.
3. The inconsistency between the serum and elution unexpected antibodies may be related to recent transfusions of Fyᵃ positive blood. A delayed hemolytic transfusion reaction cannot be excluded with the available data.

The absence of anti-Fyᵃ in the serum may be explained by its adsorption onto transfused Fyᵃ positive cells. Alternatively, passive infusion of anti-Fyᵃ in donor blood plasma could explain this set of circumstances if the patient received whole blood. In units of packed cells, the little donor plasma that remains is unlikely to be detectable.

4. The patient's E and Fyᵃ antigen status should be determined. If possible, the antigen status of the transfused units should also be determined. In this case, the patient was both E and Fyᵃ antigen negative. Several of the previously transfused units of blood were either E or Fyᵃ antigen-positive.
5. Based on the positive DAT, the eluate specificity, and the patient's and donor's phenotype, there is serologic evidence of a transfusion reaction. This type of reaction can occur when the patient has produced an antibody through

previous exposure to a blood group antigen but has no demonstrable level of antibody at the time of transfusion.

The transfused red cells act as a secondary antigenic stimulus. The corresponding antibody is produced while the transfused red cells are still circulating, thus resulting in a positive DAT. When a previously negative DAT becomes positive or a positive DAT increases in strength after transfusion, this type of reaction should be investigated and further transfusions delayed until an eluate prepared from the patient's red cells can be tested.

In this case, if additional units are required for transfusion therapy, they should be negative for both the E and $Fy^a$ antigens. Approximately 25% of A, Rh positive units should be E neg and $Fy^a$ neg.

## Conclusion

Anti-E and anti-$Fy^a$.

## Case 14

### History and Laboratory Data

An 85-year-old Black woman had a history of chronic GI bleeding. She had received multiple transfusions over the last decade. Her last transfusion of 2 units of packed red cells had been 6 months previously. She was admitted to the hospital for anemia, and 4 units of packed red cells were ordered for administration. Her blood type was group A, Rh positive.

A weakly reacting unexpected antibody, anti-$Fy^a$, had been demonstrated in her serum 6 months previously. Her unexpected antibody screen was positive again on this admission. The results of the two-cell screening procedure and reagent cell panel follow.

### *Laboratory Data (Case 14)*

**Reagent Red Blood Cell Screening Cells**
**Partial Listing of Antigens Present**

| Cell No. | D | C | E | c | e | K | k | $Fy^a$ | $Fy^b$ | $Jk^a$ | $Jk^b$ | $Le^a$ | $Le^b$ | S | s | M | N | $P_1$ |
|---|---|---|---|---|---|---|---|---|---|---|---|---|---|---|---|---|---|---|
| I | + | 0 | + | + | + | 0 | + | + | 0 | + | 0 | 0 | + | 0 | + | + | 0 | + |
| II | 0 | + | 0 | + | 0 | 0 | + | 0 | + | 0 | + | 0 | + | + | + | + | 0 | + |

**Patient Results**

| Cell No. | Immediate Spin | 37° C | AHG | AHG Check Cells |
|---|---|---|---|---|
| I | Neg | Neg | ± | 2+ |
| II | Neg | Neg | Neg | 2+ |

**Reagent Red Blood Cell Panel Antigen Profile**
**Partial Listing of Antigens Present**

| Cell No. | D | C | E | c | e | K | k | $Fy^a$ | $Fy^b$ | $Jk^a$ | $Jk^b$ | $Le^a$ | $Le^b$ | S | s | M | N | $P_1$ |
|---|---|---|---|---|---|---|---|---|---|---|---|---|---|---|---|---|---|---|
| 1 | + | 0 | 0 | + | + | 0 | + | + | + | + | 0 | 0 | 0 | + | 0 | + | + | + |
| 2 | + | 0 | 0 | + | + | 0 | + | 0 | + | + | + | 0 | + | + | + | + | 0 | 0 |
| 3 | + | + | 0 | + | + | 0 | + | 0 | + | + | + | 0 | + | + | + | + | 0 | + |
| 4 | 0 | 0 | + | + | 0 | 0 | + | + | 0 | + | 0 | 0 | + | 0 | + | + | 0 | + |
| 5 | 0 | 0 | + | + | 0 | 0 | + | + | + | 0 | + | 0 | + | 0 | + | + | + | + |
| 6 | 0 | + | 0 | 0 | + | + | + | + | + | + | 0 | 0 | + | + | + | + | + | + |
| 7 | 0 | + | 0 | 0 | + | 0 | l | 0 | + | + | + | 0 | + | 0 | + | + | + | + |
| 8 | 0 | + | + | 0 | + | 0 | + | 0 | 0 | 0 | + | + | 0 | 0 | + | + | 0 | 0 |
| 9 | 0 | + | 0 | + | + | 0 | + | + | + | + | + | + | 0 | + | 0 | 0 | + | + |
| 10 | 0 | + | 0 | 0 | + | + | 0 | 0 | + | + | + | 0 | + | 0 | + | + | + | + |

**Patient Results**

| Cell No. | Immediate Spin | 37° C | AHG | AHG Check Cells |
|---|---|---|---|---|
| 1 | Neg | Neg | ⊥ | |
| 2 | Neg | Neg | ± | |
| 3 | Neg | Neg | ± | |
| 4 | Neg | Neg | ± | |
| 5 | Neg | Neg | ± | |
| 6 | Neg | Neg | ± | |
| 7 | Neg | Neg | ± | |
| 8 | Neg | Neg | Neg | 2+ |
| 9 | Neg | Neg | ± | |
| 10 | Neg | Neg | ± | |
| Auto | Neg | Neg | Neg | 2+ |

## Questions

1. Based on the reactions of the I screening cell, what is (are) the possible unexpected antibody or antibodies?
2. Is anti-Fy$^a$ the only unexpected antibody present?
3. What additional testing could confirm the identity of the unexpected antibody or antibodies exhibited by the reagent red cells?

**Additional Patient Antigens**

Rh$_0$ (D) 4+; rh' (C) neg; rh'' (E) 3+; hr' (c) 3+; hr'' (e) 3+; Rh cont neg.

| Le$^a$ | Le$^b$ | M | N | S | s | Fy$^a$ | Fy$^b$ | Jk$^a$ | Jk$^b$ | K | k |
|---|---|---|---|---|---|---|---|---|---|---|---|
| 0 | + | + | + | + | + | 0 | + | 0 | + | 0 | + |

4. Obviously, this patient should receive ABO-compatible blood. Because anti-Jk$^a$ and anti-Fy$^a$ often cause shortened red cell survival, she should receive only blood typed as negative for Jk$^a$ and Fy$^a$ antigens.
5. Approximately 8% of A positive units should be suitable for this patient. The Duffy and Kidd blood group systems are fully discussed in Chapter 6.

## Conclusion

Anti-Fy$^a$ and anti-Jk$^a$, probably transfusion-induced.

*Laboratory Data (Case 15)*

**Reagent Red Blood Cell Screening Cells**
**Partial Listing of Antigens Present**

| Cell No. | Rh-hr | | | | | Kell | | Duffy | | Kidd | | Lewis | | MNS | | | | P |
|---|---|---|---|---|---|---|---|---|---|---|---|---|---|---|---|---|---|---|
| | D | C | E | c | e | K | k | Fy$^a$ | Fy$^b$ | Jk$^a$ | Jk$^b$ | Le$^a$ | Le$^b$ | S | s | M | N | P$_1$ |
| I | + | + | + | + | + | 0 | + | + | 0 | + | + | + | 0 | + | + | + | 0 | + |
| II | 0 | 0 | 0 | + | 0 | + | + | 0 | + | + | 0 | 0 | + | 0 | + | + | 0 | + |

4. What type blood should this patient receive?
5. What percentage of blood would be appropriate for this patient?

## Discussion

1. The antigens that are present only in the I screening cell are: D, E, e, Fy$^a$, and Jk$^a$.
2. No. The reactions in cells 1, 4, 5, 6, and 9 are consistent with the pattern of anti-Fy$^a$; however, additional reactions in cells 2, 3, 7, and 10 suggest the presence of another unexpected antibody. Anti-D is excluded because the patient is known to be Rh positive. Both anti-E and anti-e can be excluded because the No. 8 cell did not react; it has both the E and e antigens. All the reactive cells, however, possess either the Fy$^a$ antigen and/or the Jk$^a$ antigen. Therefore, anti-Jk$^a$ is the second unexpected antibody present in this serum.
3. Additional antigens can be tested for on the patient's red blood cells. In this case, an antigen profile was performed. It demonstrated the following:

## Case 15

### History and Laboratory Data

A 22-year-old Black woman with polycystic ovaries was admitted for bilateral ovarian wedge resections. She had no history of prior transfusion or pregnancy. Her preoperative crossmatch for 2 units of packed red cells demonstrated incompatibilities with both units and a positive unexpected antibody screen. Reactions were at both 37° C and AHG. Her blood type was a group A, Rh positive and her DAT was negative. The results of her serum tested with two screening cells and a panel of reagent red cells follow.

**Patient Results**

| Cell No. | Immediate Spin | 37° C | AHG |
|---|---|---|---|
| I | 1+ | ± | 2+ |
| II | 1+ | ± | 2+ |

**Reagent Red Blood Cell Panel Antigen Profile**
**Antigens Present**

| Cell No. | \multicolumn{8}{c}{Rh-Hr} | | | | | | | | \multicolumn{6}{c}{Kell} | | | | | | \multicolumn{2}{c}{Duffy} | | \multicolumn{2}{c}{Kidd} | |
|---|---|---|---|---|---|---|---|---|---|---|---|---|---|---|---|---|---|---|---|
| | C | D | E | c | e | Cw | f | V | K | k | Kpa | Kpb | Jsa | Jsb | Fya | Fyb | Jka | Jkb |
| 1 | + | + | + | 0 | + | 0 | 0 | 0 | + | + | 0 | + | + | + | 0 | + | 0 | + |
| 2 | + | + | 0 | 0 | + | + | 0 | 0 | 0 | + | 0 | + | 0 | + | + | + | + | 0 |
| 3 | 0 | + | + | + | 0 | 0 | 0 | 0 | 0 | + | 0 | + | 0 | + | + | + | + | 0 |
| 4 | + | 0 | 0 | + | + | 0 | + | 0 | 0 | + | 0 | + | 0 | + | 0 | + | + | + |
| 5 | 0 | 0 | + | + | + | 0 | + | 0 | 0 | + | 0 | + | 0 | + | + | + | + | 0 |
| 6 | 0 | 0 | 0 | + | + | 0 | + | 0 | 0 | + | + | + | 0 | + | 0 | + | 0 | + |
| 7 | 0 | 0 | 0 | + | + | 0 | + | 0 | 0 | + | 0 | + | 0 | + | + | 0 | 0 | + |
| 8 | 0 | + | 0 | + | + | 0 | + | 0 | 0 | + | 0 | + | 0 | + | + | + | + | 0 |
| 9 | 0 | 0 | 0 | + | + | 0 | + | 0 | 0 | + | 0 | + | 0 | + | 0 | 0 | + | + |
| 10 | 0 | 0 | 0 | + | + | 0 | + | 0 | 0 | + | 0 | + | 0 | + | + | + | 0 | 0 |

**Antigens Present (continued)**

| Cell No. | \multicolumn{2}{c}{Lewis} | | P | \multicolumn{4}{c}{MNS} | | | | \multicolumn{2}{c}{Lutheran} | | Sex-Linked | | Additional |
|---|---|---|---|---|---|---|---|---|---|---|---|---|
| | Lea | Leb | P1 | M | N | S | s | Lua | Lub | Xga | | Additional |
| 1 | 0 | + | + | 0 | + | + | + | 0 | + | 0 | M | |
| 2 | + | 0 | + | + | + | 0 | + | 0 | + | + | F | |
| 3 | 0 | + | + | 0 | + | 0 | + | 0 | + | + | M | |
| 4 | 0 | + | + | + | 0 | + | 0 | + | + | + | F | Co (b+) |
| 5 | 0 | + | 0 | + | + | + | + | 0 | + | + | M | |
| 6 | 0 | + | 0 | + | + | 0 | + | 0 | + | 0 | M | |
| 7 | 0 | + | + | + | 0 | + | + | 0 | + | 0 | M | Co (b+) |
| 8 | + | 0 | + | + | + | + | 0 | 0 | + | 0 | M | |
| 9 | 0 | 0 | + | + | + | + | 0 | 0 | + | + | F | |
| 10 | 0 | + | 0 | 0 | 0 | 0 | + | 0 | + | + | F | |
| 11 | | | | | | | | | | | | I (neg) |

**Patient Results**

| Cell No. | Immediate Spin | 37° C | AHG | Coombs Control Cells |
|---|---|---|---|---|
| 1 | 1+ | ± | 2+ | |
| 2 | 1+ | ± | 2+ | |
| 3 | 1+ | ± | 2+ | |
| 4 | 1+ | ± | 2+ | |
| 5 | 1+ | ± | 2+ | |
| 6 | 1+ | ± | 3+ | |
| 7 | 1+ | ± | 1+ | |
| 8 | 1+ | ± | 2+ | |
| 9 | Neg | Neg | Neg | 2+ |
| 10 | 1+ | ± | 2+ | |
| 11 | 1+ | ± | 2+ | |
| Auto | Neg | Neg | Neg | 2+ |

## Questions

1. Based on the reactions of the screening cells, what is (are) the possible unexpected antibody (unexpected antibodies)?

2. Based on the reactions of the screening cells combined with the panel cell reactions, what is (are) the possible unexpected antibody (unexpected antibodies)?

3. What additional testing could confirm the identity of the suspected unexpected antibody or antibodies?

4. Briefly discuss the characteristics of this woman's genotype.

5. What type blood should this patient receive?

## Discussion

1. The type of reaction exhibited by the screening cells is typical of Lewis antibodies. Reactions at room temperature with the fixation of complement becoming apparent during the AHG phase of testing are a common observation.

2. Each of the two screening cells is positive for one of the Lewis antigens. The panel cell reactions also display reactivity with cells that are positive for either the Lea or Leb antigens.

3. Testing the patient's RBCs for the presence of Lea and Leb antigens would validate the possibility of the suspected unexpected antibodies. If the patient lacks the Lea and Leb antigens, she could theoretically form antibodies to these nonself-antigens. This patient was subsequently typed and found to be Lea negative and Leb negative.

4. The genotype Le(a−b−) occurs in 22% of Blacks and 6% of Whites. Persons with this genotype may produce anti-Lea and/or anti-Leb. Development of Lea and/or Leb antibodies is usually due to exposure to some agent other than red blood cells.

5. It is common practice to select Lea and Leb negative blood if the corresponding unexpected antibodies are identified in the patient's circulation. However, Mollison* believes that transfusing across the anti-Lea, Leb barrier can be done without any serious reactions.

* Mollison, P.L.: Blood Transfusion in Clinical Medicine, 5th ed., pp. 489 and 512–514.

Conclusion

Anti-Le$^a$ and anti-Le$^b$.

## POSITIVE DIRECT ANTIGLOBULIN TESTS

### Case 16

#### History and Laboratory Data

A 65-year-old White woman had carcinoma of the breast and was currently receiving chemotherapy. She was group A, Rh negative (rr). Her medications included Nitro-Dur, Lasix, Solu-Medrol, cefoxitin, and Zantac. She had received two units of packed red cells three days before. The patient had no other history of transfusion, but was the mother of three children.

Two units of packed red cells were ordered to correct her anemia. As a result of crossmatching, a weakly positive autocontrol was demonstrated. A direct antiglobulin profile was performed on the current specimen and on a specimen that had been used for crossmatching 3 days earlier. The results of these tests follow. Further tests of the patient's serum and an eluate, all prepared from the patient's red cells with reagent red cells, were nonreactive.

*Laboratory Data (Case 16)*

**Direct Antiglobulin Profile**

|  | Polyspecific AHG (Rabbit) | Control Pts Washed RBCs + Normal Saline | AHG Anti-IgG (Rabbit) | AHG Anti-C3d Serum (Rabbit) |
|---|---|---|---|---|
| Red cell test results |  |  |  |  |
| Fresh specimen | Positive 1+ micro | Negative | Positive 1+ micro | Negative |
| 72-hr-old specimen | Negative | Negative | negative | Negative |

#### Questions

1. What is the most probable cause of this patient's positive DAT?
2. What medications could be responsible for this positive DAT?
3. Are the laboratory findings clinically significant?

#### Discussion

1. Reactivity to IgG antisera suggests the possibility of immunization; however, only a short interval has elapsed since any known red cell antigenic exposure. Therefore, the possibility of a drug-related cause of the positive AHG is more likely.
2. This patient's positive AHG may be associated with cefoxitin and/or Lasix therapy. This drug has been reported to cause a positive DAT with a nonreactive eluate in 3% or less of patients receiving this medication.
3. No. If this patient is not hemolyzing her erythrocytes, the DAT findings are clinically insignificant.

#### Conclusion

Positive DAT, probably drug-induced.

### Case 17

#### History and Laboratory Data

A 71-year-old White man was admitted to the hospital because of fatigue. He had an established diagnosis of lymphoma and was presently receiving five different medications: prednisone, Leukovorin, Lasix, Clotrimasol, and Allopurinol. He had received several units of packed red cells over the last 3 months.

Because his hematocrit was low, 4 units of packed red cells were ordered. A positive autocontrol was demonstrated during the crossmatch procedure. He had a weakly positive DAT, but no unexpected antibodies were detected in his serum.

*Laboratory Data (Case 17)*

**Direct Antiglobulin Profile**

|  | Polyspecific AHG (Rabbit) | Control Pts Washed RBCs + Normal Saline | AHG Anti-IgG (Rabbit) | AHG Anti-C3d Serum (Rabbit) |
|---|---|---|---|---|
| Red cell test results | Positive 1+ micro | Positive 1+ micro | Positive 1+ micro | Positive 1+ micro |

## Questions

1. Do the DAT reactions suggest the possible cause of the positive DAT?
2. What procedure or procedures should be performed next?
3. Can the causative agent be identified?

## Discussion

1. No. The cause of the positive DAT is difficult to identify specifically from the DAT reactions. The control test is positive, which demonstrates that an autoantibody is present; however, another underlying reaction could also be present.
2. In the case of a positive DAT, an elution should be prepared from the patient's red cells. The eluate and a serum sample should be tested simultaneously. In this case, an eluate was prepared from the patient's red cells. The eluate and serum were tested, but no reactions were demonstrated with the reagent red cells.

*Laboratory Data (Case 18)*

**Direct Antiglobulin Test Profile**

| | Polyspecific AHG (Rabbit) | Control Pts Washed RBCs + Normal Saline | AHG Anti-IgG (Rabbit) | AHG Anti-C3d Serum (Rabbit) |
|---|---|---|---|---|
| Cell test results | 1+ | Negative | Negative | ± |
| Repeat testing (2 days later) | 1+ | Negative | Negative | ± |

## Questions

1. What do the results of the DAT suggest?
2. Should the patient's unexpected antibody screen be positive?
3. What is the most probable reason for this patient's positive DAT?
4. Can drugs, such as the one the patient is receiving, produce a positive DAT?
5. What additional tests should be performed?

## Discussion

1. A positive DAT with polyspecific and anti-C3d antisera suggests the possibility of a drug-related reaction. A full discussion of drug-induced positive DATs is presented in Chapter 7.
2. No. If the positive DAT were related only to drug therapy, the unexpected antibody screening test would be negative.
3. Several significant facts suggest the cause of the positive DAT. The patient has no history of prior transfusions or pregnancy. Additionally, the DAT did not react with IgG sera and the alloantibody screen was negative. Because the patient was receiving intravenous penicillin, the positive DAT is probably related to this therapy.

3. In this case, the agent responsible for the positive DAT was considered to be a nonspecific weak autoantibody, possibly related to the patient's lymphoproliferative disorder.

## Conclusion

Positive DAT, possibly related to the patient's lymphoproliferative disorder.

## Case 18

### History and Laboratory Data

A 52-year-old Black woman was admitted to the hospital following a motor vehicle accident. She was started on penicillin intravenously upon admission. She had no previous history of transfusion or pregnancy.

Laboratory tests performed several days after admission revealed evidence of hemolytic anemia (slightly elevated bilirubin, increased reticulocyte count, and decreased hemoglobin and hematocrit). A DAT profile was ordered. The results follow.

4. Yes. Penicillin has been reported to cause a positive DAT in 3% of patients receiving large doses of the drug intravenously. However, hemolytic anemia associated with penicillin therapy is rare. If the patient is hemolyzing his or her own red cells, penicillin-induced immune hemolysis should be suspected.
5. The patient's serum and an eluate prepared from the DAT-positive RBCs should be tested against penicillin-treated red cells (see Chapter 15). In this case, the serum and eluate reacted strongly against penicillin-treated red cells. However, the serum and eluate continued to be negative with red cells not treated with the drug.

## Conclusion

Drug-induced positive DAT due to penicillin antibodies.

## Case 19

### History and Laboratory Data

An 84-year-old Black man was admitted to the hospital because of a seizure disorder and gastrointestinal (GI) bleeding. The patient had no history of prior transfusions. He was receiving several medications: Dilantin, Cimetidine, and alpha-methyldopa (Aldomet). The Aldomet had been administered for the last 24 hours. He had no evidence, either clinically or by laboratory studies, of hemolysis.

Because of the GI bleeding, a type and crossmatch for 6 units of packed cells was ordered. The patient was group B, Rh positive and demonstrated a positive autocontrol during the crossmatch procedure. His serum unexpected antibody screening cells were nonreactive. Subsequent testing revealed the following DAT profile.

### *Laboratory Data (Case 19)*

**Direct Antiglobulin Profile**

|  | Polyspecific AHG (Rabbit) | Control Pts Washed RBCs + Normal Saline | AHG Anti-IgG (Rabbit) | AHG Anti-C3d Serum (Rabbit) |
|---|---|---|---|---|
| Red cell test results | 1+ | Negative | 1+ | Negative |

### Questions

1. What is the most probable reason for the patient's positive DAT?
2. Should an elution of the positive DAT red cells be performed?
3. What conclusions can be drawn from the laboratory data?
4. Discuss the consequences of the observed reaction in vivo.

### Discussion

1. Because the patient had no history of prior transfusions, it is unlikely that the positive DAT is due to a specific blood group system antibody. However, the accuracy of a patient's history may be questionable, particularly with elderly or disoriented patients.
2. Yes, an elution of the DAT positive red cells should be performed. In this case, elution of the patient's red cells revealed the presence of non-specific reactivity against all panel cells. The results of this procedure follow.

**Reagent Red Blood Cell Screening Cells**
**Partial Listing of Antigens Present**

| Cell No. | Rh-hr | | | | | Kell | | Duffy | | Kidd | | Lewis | | MNS | | | | P |
|---|---|---|---|---|---|---|---|---|---|---|---|---|---|---|---|---|---|---|
| | D | C | E | c | e | K | k | Fy$^a$ | Fy$^b$ | Jk$^a$ | Jk$^b$ | Le$^a$ | Le$^b$ | S | s | M | N | P$_1$ |
| I | + | + | 0 | 0 | + | + | 0 | 0 | + | 0 | + | + | 0 | + | + | 0 | + | + |
| II | + | 0 | + | + | 0 | 0 | + | + | 0 | + | 0 | 0 | + | 0 | + | + | 0 | + |

**Patient Results (using an elution from patient's RBCs)**

| Cell No. | Immediate Spin | 37° C | AHG |
|---|---|---|---|
| I | Neg | Neg | 1+ |
| II | Neg | Neg | ± |

**Reagent Red Blood Cell Panel Antigen Profile**
**Partial Listing of Antigens Present**

| Cell No. | Rh-hr | | | | | Kell | | Duffy | | Kidd | | Lewis | | MNS | | | | P |
|---|---|---|---|---|---|---|---|---|---|---|---|---|---|---|---|---|---|---|
| | D | C | E | c | e | K | k | Fy$^a$ | Fy$^b$ | Jk$^a$ | Jk$^b$ | Le$^a$ | Le$^b$ | S | s | M | N | P$_1$ |
| 1 | + | 0 | 0 | + | + | 0 | + | + | + | + | 0 | 0 | 0 | + | 0 | + | + | 0 |
| 2 | + | 0 | 0 | + | + | 0 | + | 0 | + | + | + | 0 | + | + | + | + | 0 | + |
| 3 | + | + | + | + | + | 0 | + | 0 | + | + | 0 | 0 | + | + | + | + | 0 | + |
| 4 | 0 | 0 | 0 | + | 0 | 0 | + | + | 0 | + | 0 | 0 | + | 0 | + | + | 0 | 0 |
| 5 | 0 | 0 | + | + | 0 | + | + | + | + | 0 | + | 0 | + | 0 | + | + | + | + |
| 6 | 0 | + | 0 | 0 | + | 0 | + | + | + | + | 0 | 0 | + | + | + | + | + | + |
| 7 | 0 | + | + | 0 | + | 0 | + | 0 | + | + | + | 0 | + | 0 | + | + | + | + |
| 8 | 0 | + | 0 | 0 | + | 0 | + | + | 0 | 0 | + | + | 0 | 0 | + | + | 0 | 0 |
| 9 | 0 | + | + | + | + | 0 | + | + | + | + | + | + | 0 | + | 0 | 0 | + | + |
| 10 | 0 | + | 0 | 0 | + | + | 0 | 0 | + | + | + | 0 | + | 0 | + | + | + | + |
| 11 | 0 | 0 | 0 | + | + | 0 | + | 0 | + | + | + | + | 0 | 0 | 0 | 0 | + | + |

**Patient Results**

| Cell No. | Immediate Spin | 37° C | AHG |
|---|---|---|---|
| 1 | Neg | Neg | ± |
| 2 | Neg | Neg | 1+ |
| 3 | Neg | Neg | 1+ |
| 4 | Neg | Neg | 2+ |
| 5 | Neg | Neg | ± |
| 6 | Neg | Neg | 2+ |
| 7 | Neg | Neg | 2+ |
| 8 | Neg | Neg | 1+ |
| 9 | Neg | Neg | ± |
| 10 | Neg | Neg | 2+ |
| 11 | Neg | Neg | 1+ |
| Auto | Neg | Neg | ± |

3. The pattern of reactivity observed in the DAT and reagent red cells is consistent with an alpha-methyldopa-induced autoantibody. The eluate prepared from red cells of patients taking this drug usually reacts with all cells without the presence of the drug in the test system, indicating the development of a warm-reactive autoantibody. The in vitro tests for compatibility cannot be used to predict the cell survival of transfused red cells because all units may appear incompatible when unadsorbed serum is used. A full discussion of drug-induced positive DATs is presented in Chapter 7.

4. Approximately 10 to 30% of patients taking Aldomet have a positive DAT while less than 1% develop hemolytic anemia. Because the treatments of AIHA and drug-induced anemia are different, it is important that the cause of the anemia be determined. In patients who do experience a hemolytic anemia caused by the drug therapy, the hemoly-

sis usually regresses within a few weeks after cessation of the drug.

Transfusion may be of some benefit to patients showing signs of erythrocyte hemolysis, but the benefit is usually only temporary. The transfused red cells are eliminated at the same accelerated rate as the patient's own red cells. If the patient is not hemolyzing, the autoantibody is probably not clinically significant.

### Conclusion

Drug-induced positive DAT caused by antibody to alpha-methyldopa (Aldomet).

## Case 20

### History and Laboratory Data

A 75-year-old White man was diagnosed as having idiopathic (autoimmune) thrombocytopenia. He also had concurrent anemia and was admitted for transfusion therapy. Two years previously, the patient had exhibited a strongly positive DAT (IgG and C3d). Nonspecific warm and cold autoantibodies were also reported at that time, but no unexpected antibodies were detected.

On this admission, this group A, Rh positive patient had both a positive DAT and a positive indirect antiglobulin reaction in the AHG phase. Reactions were also observed at 5° C. He had not received any transfusions within the last 3 months and was not receiving any medications.

Results of any elution studies or cold agglutinin titers were not available.

### *Laboratory Data (Case 20)*

**Direct Antiglobulin Profile**

| | Polyspecific AHG (Rabbit) | Control Pts Washed RBCs + Normal Saline | AHG Anti-IgG (Rabbit) | AHG Anti-C3d Serum (Rabbit) |
|---|---|---|---|---|
| Red cell test results | Positive 4+ | Negative | Positive 3+ | Positive |

**Reagent Red Blood Cell Screening Cells**
**Partial Listing of Antigens Present**

| Cell No. | Rh-hr | | | | | Kell | | Duffy | | Kidd | | Lewis | | MNS | | | | P |
|---|---|---|---|---|---|---|---|---|---|---|---|---|---|---|---|---|---|---|
| | D | C | E | c | e | K | k | Fyª | Fyᵇ | Jkª | Jkᵇ | Leª | Leᵇ | S | s | M | N | P₁ |
| I | + | 0 | + | + | + | 0 | + | + | 0 | + | + | 0 | + | + | + | + | 0 | + |
| II | 0 | + | 0 | + | 0 | 0 | + | 0 | + | + | 0 | 0 | + | 0 | + | + | 0 | + |

**Patient Results**

| Cell No. | Immediate Spin | 37° C | AHG |
|---|---|---|---|
| I | ± | Neg | 4+ |
| II | ± | Neg | 3+ |

**Reagent Red Blood Cell Panel Antigen Profile**
**Partial Listing of Antigens Present**

| Cell No. | D | C | E | c | e | K | k | Fy^a | Fy^b | Jk^a | Jk^b | Le^a | Le^b | S | s | M | N | P_1 |
|---|---|---|---|---|---|---|---|---|---|---|---|---|---|---|---|---|---|---|
| 1 | 0 | 0 | 0 | + | + | 0 | + | + | + | + | 0 | 0 | 0 | + | 0 | + | + | + |
| 2 | 0 | 0 | 0 | + | + | 0 | + | 0 | + | + | + | 0 | + | + | + | + | 0 | 0 |
| 3 | 0 | + | 0 | + | + | 0 | + | 0 | + | + | + | 0 | + | + | + | + | 0 | + |
| 4 | + | 0 | + | + | 0 | 0 | + | + | 0 | + | 0 | 0 | + | 0 | + | + | 0 | + |
| 5 | + | 0 | + | + | 0 | 0 | + | + | + | 0 | + | 0 | + | 0 | + | + | + | + |
| 6 | + | + | 0 | 0 | + | + | + | + | + | + | 0 | 0 | + | + | + | + | + | + |
| 7 | + | + | 0 | 0 | + | 0 | + | 0 | + | + | + | 0 | + | 0 | + | + | + | + |
| 8 | + | + | + | 0 | + | 0 | + | + | 0 | 0 | + | + | 0 | 0 | + | + | 0 | 0 |
| 9 | + | + | 0 | + | + | 0 | + | + | + | + | + | + | 0 | + | 0 | 0 | + | + |
| 10 | + | + | 0 | 0 | + | + | 0 | 0 | + | + | + | 0 | + | 0 | + | + | + | + |
| 11 | + | 0 | 0 | + | + | 0 | + | 0 | + | + | + | + | 0 | 0 | 0 | 0 | + | + |

**Patient Results**

| Cell No. | Immediate Spin | 37° C | AHG | 5° C |
|---|---|---|---|---|
| 1 | ± | Neg | 4+ | 4+ |
| 2 | ± | Neg | 3+ | 4+ |
| 3 | ± | Neg | 3+ | 4+ |
| 4 | ± | Neg | 3+ | 4+ |
| 5 | ± | Neg | 4+ | 4+ |
| 6 | ± | Neg | 4+ | 4+ |
| 7 | ± | Neg | 4+ | 4+ |
| 8 | ± | Neg | 4+ | 4+ |
| 9 | ± | Neg | 4+ | 4+ |
| 10 | ± | Neg | 3+ | 4+ |
| Auto | ± | Neg | 4+ | 4+ |

## Questions

1. What does the reactivity pattern suggest?
2. What additional tests can be performed?
3. Should any precautions be taken when transfusing this patient?

## Discussion

1. The serum demonstrates a nonspecific cold autoantibody strongly reactive in the AHG phase and at 5° C.
2. In this case, an autoabsorption with formaldehyde-treated rabbit red cell eliminated the antibody reactions. This confirmed the presence of a nonspecific cold agglutinin. No unexpected antibody was detected.
3. A warming coil is suggested for future transfusions.

*Laboratory Data (Case 21)*

## Conclusion

Persistently strong positive DAT, idiopathic nonspecific cold agglutinin (cold-agglutinin disease).

## ADVANCED-LEVEL CASE STUDIES

### Case 21

#### History and Laboratory Data

A 20-year-old Black man with a known diagnosis of mild hemophilia was admitted to the hospital because of injuries sustained in a motor vehicle accident. A crossmatch for 6 units of blood was ordered. The patient was currently receiving AHF and had been transfused with packed red cells within the last 3 months. He was also receiving Colace medication.

At the time of crossmatching the currently requested units of blood, both a positive unexpected antibody screen and a weakly positive DAT were discovered. All of the crossmatches were incompatible. The patient was group A, Rh positive with the most probable genotype $R_2R_2$. The results of the DAT profile and patient's serum with a two-cell screening set and a panel of reagent red cells follow. An eluate prepared from the DAT positive cells was negative with the two screening cells (I and II) and the panel of reagent red cells.

**Direct Antiglobulin Profile**

| | Polyspecific AHG (Rabbit) | Control Pts Washed RBCs + Normal Saline | AHG Anti-IgG (Rabbit) | AHG Anti-C3d Serum (Rabbit) |
|---|---|---|---|---|
| Red cell test results | Positive 1+ weak | Negative | Positive ± | Negative |

**Reagent Red Blood Cell Screening Cells**
**Partial Listing of Antigens Present**

| Cell No. | D | C | E | c | e | K | k | Fy^a | Fy^b | Jk^a | Jk^b | Le^a | Le^b | S | s | M | N | P_1 |
|---|---|---|---|---|---|---|---|---|---|---|---|---|---|---|---|---|---|---|
| I | + | 0 | + | + | + | 0 | + | + | 0 | + | + | 0 | + | + | + | + | 0 | + |
| II | 0 | + | 0 | + | 0 | + | 0 | 0 | + | + | 0 | 0 | + | 0 | + | + | 0 | + |

**Patient Results**

| Cell No. | Immediate Spin | 37° C | AHG | Coombs Control Cells |
|---|---|---|---|---|
| I | Neg | ± | 1+ | |
| II | Neg | Neg | Neg | 2+ |

## Reagent Red Blood Cell Panel Antigen Profile
## Antigens Present

| Cell No. | Rh-Hr | | | | | | | | Kell | | | | | | Duffy | | Kidd | |
|---|---|---|---|---|---|---|---|---|---|---|---|---|---|---|---|---|---|---|
| | C | D | E | c | e | Cʷ | f | V | K | k | Kpᵃ | Kpᵇ | Jsᵃ | Jsᵇ | Fyᵃ | Fyᵇ | Jkᵃ | Jkᵇ |
| 1 | + | + | + | 0 | + | 0 | 0 | 0 | + | + | 0 | + | 0 | + | 0 | + | 0 | + |
| 2 | + | + | 0 | 0 | + | + | 0 | 0 | 0 | + | 0 | + | 0 | + | + | + | + | 0 |
| 3 | 0 | + | + | + | 0 | 0 | 0 | 0 | 0 | + | 0 | + | 0 | + | + | + | + | 0 |
| 4 | + | 0 | 0 | + | + | 0 | + | 0 | 0 | + | 0 | + | 0 | + | 0 | + | + | + |
| 5 | 0 | 0 | + | + | + | 0 | + | 0 | 0 | + | 0 | + | 0 | + | + | + | + | 0 |
| 6 | 0 | 0 | 0 | + | + | 0 | + | 0 | 0 | + | 0 | + | 0 | + | 0 | + | 0 | + |
| 7 | 0 | 0 | 0 | + | + | 0 | + | 0 | 0 | + | 0 | + | 0 | + | 0 | 0 | 0 | + |
| 8 | 0 | + | 0 | + | + | 0 | + | 0 | 0 | + | 0 | + | 0 | + | 0 | 0 | + | 0 |
| 9 | 0 | 0 | 0 | + | + | 0 | + | 0 | 0 | + | 0 | + | 0 | + | + | + | + | + |
| 10 | 0 | 0 | 0 | + | + | 0 | + | 0 | 0 | + | 0 | + | 0 | + | + | + | + | + |

## Antigens Present (continued)

| Cell No. | Lewis | | P | MNS | | | | Lutheran | | Sex-Linked | | Additional |
|---|---|---|---|---|---|---|---|---|---|---|---|---|
| | Leᵃ | Leᵇ | P₁ | M | N | S | s | Luᵃ | Luᵇ | Xgᵃ | | |
| 1 | 0 | + | + | 0 | + | + | + | 0 | + | 0 | M | |
| 2 | + | 0 | + | + | + | 0 | + | 0 | + | + | M | Co (b+) |
| 3 | 0 | + | + | 0 | + | 0 | + | 0 | + | + | M | |
| 4 | 0 | + | + | + | 0 | + | 0 | + | + | + | F | Co (b+) |
| 5 | 0 | + | 0 | + | + | + | + | 0 | + | + | M | |
| 6 | 0 | + | 0 | + | + | 0 | + | 0 | + | 0 | M | |
| 7 | 0 | + | + | + | 0 | + | + | 0 | + | 0 | M | Co (b+) |
| 8 | + | 0 | + | + | + | + | 0 | 0 | + | 0 | M | |
| 9 | 0 | 0 | + | + | + | + | 0 | 0 | + | + | F | |
| 10 | 0 | + | 0 | 0 | 0 | 0 | + | 0 | + | + | F | |
| 11 | | | | | | | | | | | | I (neg) |

**Patient Results**

| Cell No. | Immediate Spin | 37° C | AHG | Coombs Control Cells |
|---|---|---|---|---|
| 1 | Neg | ± | 1+ weak | |
| 2 | Neg | ± | 1+ weak | |
| 3 | Neg | Neg | Neg | 2+ |
| 4 | Neg | ± | 1+ weak | |
| 5 | Neg | ± | 1+ weak | |
| 6 | Neg | ± | 1+ weak | |
| 7 | Neg | ± | 1+ weak | |
| 8 | Neg | ± | 1+ weak | |
| 9 | Neg | ± | 1+ weak | |
| 10 | Neg | ± | 1+ weak | |
| 11 | Neg | ± | 1+ weak | |
| Auto | Neg | Neg | Neg | 2+ |

**Enzyme-Enhanced Reagent Red Blood Cells + Patient's Serum**

| Cell No. | 37° C |
|---|---|
| 1 | 2+ |
| 2 | 2+ |
| 3 | Neg |
| 4 | 2+ |
| 5 | 2+ |
| 6 | 2+ |
| 7 | 2+ |
| 8 | 2+ |
| 9 | 2+ |
| 10 | 2+ |
| 11 | 2+ |
| Auto | Neg |

## Questions

1. What antibody or antibodies are present in the patient's serum?
2. Why was the eluate negative? What further tests can be performed?
3. Would crossmatching only units negative for the antigen(s) to the corresponding antibody (antibodies) identified in questions No. 1 and 2 yield compatible results?
4. What further steps should be taken?
5. Briefly discuss the characteristics of the last antibody identified.

## Discussion

1. The weak pattern of AHG reactivity was further enhanced with enzymes, and both patterns were consistent with anti-e.
2. The eluate did not contain an antibody to any of the antigens present on the screening or panel cells. Medications could be ruled out as the source of a drug-induced DAT because the patient was receiving no medications implicated in producing a positive DAT. The patient, however, had been and was receiving AHF.

The eluate was tested against three $A_1$ and three $A_2$ cells. Although the eluate was nonreactive with group O cells, agglutination was observed with $A_1$ reagent cells. Demonstration of the presence of anti-A is consistent with passive acquisition of anti-A by way of AHF concentrate.
3. No. In this case, when the patient was crossmatched with six units of O positive, e-negative packed red cells, one unit was incompatible.
4. In this case, the hospital blood bank was unable to

identify any additional unexpected antibodies and sent a specimen of the patient's blood as well as segments from the incompatible unit to a reference laboratory. The reference laboratory identified another unexpected antibody, anti-$Kp^a$. Additional antigen typings were also performed: $M-N+S-s+$; $P_1-$; $Le(a-b+)$; $K-k+$; $Fy(a-b+)$; $Jk(a-b+)$; $Kp^a-$.
5. Anti-$Kp^a$ is an antibody to a low-frequency antigen. This antibody has been implicated in HDN. It has also been implicated in transfusion reactions and often causes shortened red cell survival. The frequency of the antigen in the random population is 2%. For a full discussion of the Kell blood group system, refer to Chapter 6.

## Conclusion

Anti-e, anti-$A_1$, and anti-$Kp^a$.

## Case 22

### History and Laboratory Data

A 71-year-old White woman is group $A_2$, Rh positive ($R_1R_1$). She has an established diagnosis of multiple myeloma and has received numerous transfusions over the last 10 years. Her most recent transfusion was 4 months ago. She was admitted for anemia and fatigue secondary to multiple myeloma. She has been receiving two medications, Keflex and Tolinase.

Four units of packed cells were ordered for transfusion. All of the 4 units crossmatched were incompatible microscopically. Her unexpected antibody screen was weakly positive, as was the autocontrol. A DAT profile was also performed.

### *Laboratory Data (Case 22)*

**Direct Antiglobulin Profile**

|  | Polyspecific AHG (Rabbit) | Control Pts Washed RBCs + Normal Saline | AHG Anti-IgG (Rabbit) | AHG Anti-C3d Serum (Rabbit) |
|---|---|---|---|---|
| Red cell test results | Positive ± weak | Negative | Positive ± weak | Negative |

**Reagent Red Blood Cell Screening Cells**
**Partial Listing of Antigens Present**

| Cell No. | Rh-hr |  |  |  |  | Kell |  | Duffy |  | Kidd |  | Lewis |  | MNS |  |  |  | P |
|---|---|---|---|---|---|---|---|---|---|---|---|---|---|---|---|---|---|---|
|  | D | C | E | c | e | K | k | $Fy^a$ | $Fy^b$ | $Jk^a$ | $Jk^b$ | $Le^a$ | $Le^b$ | S | s | M | N | $P_1$ |
| I | + | 0 | + | + | + | + | + | + | 0 | + | 0 | 0 | + | + | + | + | 0 | + |
| II | 0 | + | 0 | + | 0 | 0 | + | 0 | + | 0 | + | 0 | + | 0 | + | + | 0 | + |

**Patient Results**

| Cell No. | Immediate Spin | 37° C | AHG | Coombs Control Cells |
|---|---|---|---|---|
| I | Neg | Neg | ± | 3+ |
| II | Neg | Neg | ± | 3+ |

**Reagent Red Blood Cell Panel Antigen Profile**
**Partial Listing of Antigens Present**

| Cell No. | Rh-hr | | | | | Kell | | Duffy | | Kidd | | Lewis | | MNS | | | | P |
|---|---|---|---|---|---|---|---|---|---|---|---|---|---|---|---|---|---|---|
| | D | C | E | c | e | K | k | Fy$^a$ | Fy$^b$ | Jk$^a$ | Jk$^b$ | Le$^a$ | Le$^b$ | S | s | M | N | P$_1$ |
| 1 | 0 | 0 | 0 | + | + | 0 | + | + | + | + | 0 | 0 | 0 | + | 0 | + | + | + |
| 2 | 0 | 0 | 0 | + | + | 0 | + | 0 | + | + | + | 0 | + | + | + | + | 0 | 0 |
| 3 | 0 | + | 0 | + | + | 0 | + | 0 | + | + | + | 0 | + | + | 0 | + | 0 | + |
| 4 | + | 0 | + | + | 0 | 0 | + | + | 0 | + | 0 | 0 | + | 0 | + | + | 0 | + |
| 5 | + | 0 | + | + | 0 | 0 | + | + | + | 0 | + | 0 | + | + | 0 | + | + | + |
| 6 | + | + | 0 | 0 | + | + | + | + | + | + | 0 | 0 | + | + | + | + | + | + |
| 7 | + | + | 0 | 0 | + | 0 | + | 0 | + | + | + | 0 | + | 0 | + | + | + | + |
| 8 | + | + | + | 0 | + | 0 | + | 0 | 0 | 0 | + | + | 0 | 0 | + | + | 0 | 0 |
| 9 | + | + | 0 | + | + | 0 | + | + | + | + | + | + | 0 | + | 0 | 0 | + | + |
| 10 | + | + | 0 | 0 | + | + | 0 | 0 | + | + | + | 0 | + | 0 | + | + | + | + |

**Patient Results**
**Elution of DAT Positive Cells**

| Cell No. | Immediate Spin | 37° C | AHG | Coombs Control |
|---|---|---|---|---|
| 1 | Neg | Neg | ± | 2+ |
| 2 | Neg | Neg | ± | 2+ |
| 3 | Neg | Neg | ± | 2+ |
| 4 | Neg | Neg | ± | 2+ |
| 5 | Neg | Neg | ± | 2+ |
| 6 | Neg | Neg | ± | 2+ |
| 7 | Neg | Neg | ± | 2+ |
| 8 | Neg | Neg | ± | 2+ |
| 9 | Neg | Neg | ± | 2+ |
| 10 | Neg | Neg | ± | 2+ |
| Auto Control | Neg | Neg | ± | 2+ |

**Patient Results**
**Serum (Using Prewarming Technique)**

| Cell No. | Immediate Spin | 37° C | AHG | Coombs Control |
|---|---|---|---|---|
| 1 | Neg | ± | 1+ | |
| 2 | Neg | ± | 1+ | |
| 3 | Neg | ± | 1+ | |
| 4 | Neg | ± | 1+ | |
| 5 | Neg | ± | 1+ | |
| 6 | Neg | Neg | ± | 2+ |
| 7 | Neg | Neg | ± | 2+ |
| 8 | Neg | Neg | ± | 2+ |
| 9 | Neg | ± | 1+ | |
| 10 | Neg | Neg | ± | 2+ |
| Auto Control | Neg | Neg | Neg | 2+ |

## Questions

1. What is the cause of the positive DAT?
2. Can other crossmatch techniques be attempted?
3. What do the results of the serum unexpected antibody tests suggest?
4. What is the explanation for the weakly reacting reagent cells and the continuing incompatible units?

## Discussion

1. A heat ether eluate prepared from the patient's red cells was inconclusive because it reacted with all panel cells tested (panagglutinin). Two of the medications presently being given to the patient (Keflex and Tolinase) have been implicated in producing a positive DAT. Screening the eluate for cephalosporin antibodies (Chapter 15) could rule out Keflex as the source of the positive DAT. If this procedure yields negative results, the patient's disorder or her medication, Tolinase, may be the cause.

2. Yes. Consistent with the diagnosis of multiple myeloma, the patient's serum and cells are exhibiting very strong rouleaux formation. The rouleaux seem only to interfere with testing at extended incubations at room temperature and below. Saline replacement technique did produce a negative autocontrol; however, the crossmatched units continued to be incompatible.

3. The prewarmed serum reactivity was consistent with the activity of anti-c. The patient's genotype would also support the possibility of this unexpected antibody. The weak reactions in the c negative cells could not be explained. When c negative units were crossmatched using a prewarming technique, 3 out of 4 units continued to be incompatible.

4. This patient's specimen and segments from the c (negative)-incompatible units were forwarded to a reference laboratory for further study. The reference laboratory confirmed the findings of the blood bank and identified the cause of the weakly reacting cells and incompatible crossmatches.

The report stated that this specimen exhibited anti-York. This antibody generally causes agglutination reactions at the AHG phase. Reactions range from weakly macroscopic to microscopic positives. The corresponding Yk$^a$ antigen is present on 92 to 98% of the red cells of the random population; therefore, the major problem this antibody causes is the incompatibility of nearly all donor units when crossmatching. Anti-Yk$^a$ has not been implicated in hemolytic transfusion reactions or in increased red cell destruction. Anti-Yk$^a$ is often found in the presence of other unexpected antibodies. If transfusions are needed, this patient should receive c negative crossmatch-compatible units.

## Conclusion

Cold autoagglutinin, anti-York, and anti-c.

## Case 23

### History and Laboratory Data

An 86-year-old White woman was admitted for a fractured hip and anemia. She had received 13 units of packed red cells over the last 4 months. Her blood type was group O, Rh positive (genotype R²r, cDE/cde).

During the preparation of 2 units of packed cells preoperatively, one of the units was weakly incompatible. The unexpected antibody screening cells were very weakly positive (microscopically). The DAT was positive.

***Laboratory Data (Case 23)***

**Direct Antiglobulin Profile**

|  | Polyspecific Anti-Human Serum (Rabbit) | Control Pts Washed RBCs + Normal Saline | Anti-Human Serum Anti-IgG (Rabbit) | Anti-Human Serum Anti-C3d Serum (Rabbit) |
|---|---|---|---|---|
| Red cell test results | Positive 1+ | Negative | Positive 1+ | Negative |

**Reagent Red Blood Cell Screening Cells**

**Partial Listing of Antigens Present**

| Cell No. | Rh-hr | | | | | Kell | | Duffy | | Kidd | | Lewis | | MNS | | | | P |
|---|---|---|---|---|---|---|---|---|---|---|---|---|---|---|---|---|---|---|
|  | D | C | E | c | e | K | k | Fyᵃ | Fyᵇ | Jkᵃ | Jkᵇ | Leᵃ | Leᵇ | S | s | M | N | P₁ |
| I | + | 0 | + | + | + | 0 | + | + | 0 | + | + | 0 | + | + | + | + | 0 | + |
| II | 0 | + | 0 | + | 0 | + | 0 | 0 | + | + | 0 | 0 | + | 0 | + | + | 0 | + |

**Patient Results Using an Eluate from the DAT Positive RBCs**

| Cell No. | Immediate Spin | 37° C | AHG | Coombs Control Cells |
|---|---|---|---|---|
| I | Neg | Neg | Neg | 2+ |
| II | Neg | Neg | 2+ |  |

**Reagent Red Blood Cell Panel Antigen Profile**
**Partial Listing of Antigens Present**

| Cell No. | Rh-hr | | | | | Kell | | Duffy | | Kidd | | Lewis | | MNS | | | | P |
|---|---|---|---|---|---|---|---|---|---|---|---|---|---|---|---|---|---|---|
|  | D | C | E | c | e | K | k | Fyᵃ | Fyᵇ | Jkᵃ | Jkᵇ | Leᵃ | Leᵇ | S | s | M | N | P₁ |
| 1 | 0 | 0 | 0 | + | + | 0 | + | + | + | + | 0 | 0 | 0 | + | 0 | + | + | + |
| 2 | 0 | + | 0 | + | + | 0 | + | 0 | + | + | + | 0 | + | + | + | + | 0 | 0 |
| 3 | 0 | + | 0 | + | + | 0 | + | 0 | + | + | + | 0 | + | + | + | + | 0 | + |
| 4 | + | + | + | + | 0 | 0 | + | + | 0 | + | 0 | 0 | + | 0 | + | + | 0 | + |
| 5 | + | 0 | + | + | 0 | 0 | + | + | + | 0 | + | 0 | + | 0 | + | + | + | + |
| 6 | + | + | 0 | 0 | + | + | + | + | + | + | 0 | 0 | + | + | + | + | + | + |
| 7 | + | + | 0 | 0 | + | 0 | + | 0 | + | + | + | 0 | + | 0 | + | + | + | + |
| 8 | + | 0 | + | + | + | 0 | + | + | 0 | 0 | + | + | 0 | 0 | + | + | 0 | 0 |
| 9 | + | 0 | 0 | + | + | 0 | + | + | + | + | + | + | 0 | 0 | 0 | + | + | + |
| 10 | + | + | 0 | 0 | + | + | 0 | 0 | + | + | + | 0 | + | 0 | + | + | + | + |
| 11 | + | 0 | 0 | + | + | 0 | + | 0 | + | + | + | + | 0 | 0 | 0 | 0 | + | + |

## Patient Results Using an Eluate from the DAT Positive RBCs

| Cell No. | Immediate Spin | 37° C | AHG |
|---|---|---|---|
| 1 | Neg | Neg | 1+ |
| 2 | Neg | Neg | 2+ |
| 3 | Neg | Neg | 2+ |
| 4 | Neg | Neg | 3+ |
| 5 | Neg | Neg | 2+ |
| 6 | Neg | Neg | 2+ |
| 7 | Neg | Neg | 1+ |
| 8 | Neg | Neg | 2+ |
| 9 | Neg | Neg | 2+ |
| 10 | Neg | Neg | 1+ |
| 11 | Neg | Neg | 2+ |
| Auto | Neg | Neg | ± |

## Adsorbed Eluate

| Cell No. | Immediate Spin | 37° C | AHG | Coombs Control Cells |
|---|---|---|---|---|
| I | Neg | Neg | Neg | 2+ |
| II | Neg | Neg | 2+ | |

## Adsorbed Eluate

| Cell No. | Immediate Spin | 37° C | AHG | Coombs Control |
|---|---|---|---|---|
| 1 | Neg | Neg | ± micro | 2+ |
| 2 | Neg | Neg | Neg | 2+ |
| 3 | Neg | Neg | Neg | 3+ |
| 4 | Neg | Neg | Neg | 2+ |
| 5 | Neg | Neg | Neg | 2+ |
| 6 | Neg | Neg | 2+ | |
| 7 | Neg | Neg | Neg | 1+ |
| 8 | Neg | Neg | Neg | 2+ |
| 9 | Neg | Neg | Neg | 1+ |
| 10 | Neg | Neg | 2+ | |
| 11 | Neg | Neg | Neg | 2+ |
| Auto | Neg | Neg | Neg | 2+ |

## Patient Results
## Enzyme-Treated RBCs + Patient Serum

| Cell No. | Immediate Spin | 37° C |
|---|---|---|
| I | Neg | ± micro |
| II | Neg | 2+ |

## Enzyme Treated RBCs + Patient Serum

| Cell No. | Immediate Spin | 37° C |
|---|---|---|
| 1 | Neg | ± |
| 2 | Neg | 2+ |
| 3 | Neg | 2+ |
| 4 | Neg | 3+ |
| 5 | Neg | ± micro |
| 6 | Neg | 2+ |
| 7 | Neg | 2+ |
| 8 | Neg | ± micro |
| 9 | Neg | ± micro |
| 10 | Neg | 2+ |
| 11 | Neg | ± micro |
| Auto | Neg | Neg |

## Questions

1. What is the most probable cause of the positive DAT?
2. What procedure should be done next?
3. What is the significance of the positive DAT reaction?
4. If the unexpected antibody screening cells are negative or weakly nonspecific, does this indicate that no unexpected antibodies are present in the patient's serum?
5. What is the cause of the persistent weakly positive reactions?

## Discussion

1. The reactivity with both polyspecific and IgG antisera suggests a warm antibody.
2. An elution of the positive DAT cells was prepared. Although it demonstrated warm autoantibody activity, it was reactive with all cells (1+ to 3+). An adsorbed eluate was subsequently prepared to remove autoantibody reactivity. When testing the adsorbed eluate, an underlying anti-K was demonstrated.

Additional antigens were tested. A phenotype was performed on the top layer harvested from simplified cell separation. These results are as follows:

## Antigen Profile

| | Le$^a$ | Le$^b$ | M | N | S* | s* | P$_1$ | Fy$^a$* | Fy$^b$* | Jk$^a$* | Jk$^b$* | K* | k* |
|---|---|---|---|---|---|---|---|---|---|---|---|---|---|
| Patient's Cells | 0 | + | + | + | + | + | + | + | 0 | 0 | + | 0 | + |

\* Chloroquine-treated cells

3. Based on the positive DAT, the eluate specificity, and the patient's phenotype, there is serologic evidence of a delayed transfusion reaction because of anti-K. This type of reaction can occur when the patient has been previously exposed to a blood group antigen but has no demonstrable level of antibody at the time of transfusion and compatible crossmatches. If the transfused cells are positive for the antigen, in this case Kell, the transfused red cells act as a secondary antigenic stimulus and the antibody is produced while the transfused red cells are still in the circulation.

4. No. A negative unexpected antibody screen does not unequivocally mean that unexpected antibodies are absent

in the patient's serum. Antibodies may be present that are not represented on the group O screening cells, such as low frequency antigens or immune anti-A. Low-titer antibodies can also be missed.

In this case, the weakly reactive nonspecific cell reactions with screening cells needed to be explained. An enzyme-enhanced technique was tried. The reactions using this technique demonstrated another antibody, anti-C. However, some of the cells continued to be weakly reactive. Additional crossmatches with K (neg) and C (neg) demonstrated weakly incompatible (microscopic) agglutination. The specimen was sent to a reference laboratory for further study.

5. In the hands of the reference laboratory, weak, nonspecific reactions were observed at the indirect antiglobulin phase with 75% of K and C negative red cells tested. High incidence antigens were suspected because of the weak, nonspecific, and stringy agglutination observed in this multiply transfused patient.

In an attempt to determine if these reactions were due to these antibodies, the patient's serum was adsorbed with pooled platelets. Platelets have white cell (HLA) antigens

as well as ABO and unique platelet antigens and can be used to adsorb HLA antibodies.

After adsorption, the patient's serum was nonreactive with the previously positive red cells. Thus, it appears likely that the nonspecific reactivity at the AHG phase is caused by HLA antibody production.

Conclusion

Anti-K, anti-C, and HLA antibodies.

## Case 24

### History and Laboratory Data

A 78-year-old White woman was diagnosed as having an evolving myeloproliferative disorder. Her blood type was group A, Rh positive. She had been receiving folic acid, potassium, and Apresoline. She had received 5 units of packed RBCs one month before the detection and identification of an anti-Kell unexpected antibody in her serum. She also had a positive DAT with K specificity demonstrated from an eluate. The anti-C3d results were unexplained.

**Direct Antiglobulin Profile**

| | Polyspecific Anti-Human Serum (Rabbit) | Control Pts Washed RBCs + Normal Saline | Anti-Human Serum Anti-IgG (Rabbit) | Anti-Human Serum Anti-C3d Serum (Rabbit) |
|---|---|---|---|---|
| Red cell test results | Positive 1+ | Negative | Positive 1+ | Positive ± micro |

During the next 3-month period, she received an additional 4 units of Kell negative packed red cells. At the time of her next admission, a positive DAT was observed. The results of these tests follow.

*Laboratory Data (Case 24)*

**Reagent Red Blood Cell Screening Cells**
**Partial Listing of Antigens Present**

| Cell No. | D | C | E | c | e | K | k | Fyᵃ | Fyᵇ | Jkᵃ | Jkᵇ | Leᵃ | Leᵇ | S | s | M | N | P₁ |
|---|---|---|---|---|---|---|---|---|---|---|---|---|---|---|---|---|---|---|
| I | + | 0 | + | + | + | 0 | + | + | 0 | + | + | 0 | + | + | + | + | 0 | + |
| II | 0 | + | 0 | + | 0 | + | 0 | 0 | + | + | 0 | 0 | + | 0 | + | + | 0 | + |

**Patient Results**
**Eluate of DAT Positive RBCs**

| Cell No. | Immediate Spin | 37° C | AHG | Coombs Control Cells |
|---|---|---|---|---|
| I | Neg | Neg | ± | 1+ |
| II | Neg | 1+ | 2+ | |

**Reagent Red Blood Cell Panel Antigen Profile**
**Antigens Present**

| Cell No. | C | D | E | c | e | Cʷ | f | V | K | k | Kpᵃ | Kpᵇ | Jsᵃ | Jsᵇ | Fyᵃ | Fyᵇ | Jkᵃ | Jkᵇ |
|---|---|---|---|---|---|---|---|---|---|---|---|---|---|---|---|---|---|---|
| | | | Rh-Hr | | | | | | | | Kell | | | | Duffy | | Kidd | |
| 1 | + | + | + | 0 | + | 0 | 0 | 0 | + | + | 0 | + | 0 | + | 0 | + | 0 | + |
| 2 | + | + | 0 | 0 | + | + | 0 | 0 | 0 | + | 0 | + | 0 | + | + | + | + | 0 |
| 3 | 0 | + | + | + | 0 | 0 | 0 | 0 | 0 | + | 0 | + | 0 | + | + | + | + | 0 |
| 4 | + | 0 | 0 | + | + | 0 | + | 0 | 0 | + | 0 | + | 0 | + | 0 | + | + | + |
| 5 | 0 | 0 | + | + | + | 0 | + | 0 | 0 | + | 0 | + | 0 | + | + | + | + | 0 |
| 6 | 0 | 0 | 0 | + | + | 0 | + | 0 | 0 | + | 0 | + | 0 | + | 0 | + | 0 | + |
| 7 | 0 | 0 | 0 | + | + | 0 | + | 0 | 0 | + | 0 | + | 0 | + | + | 0 | 0 | + |
| 8 | 0 | + | 0 | + | + | 0 | + | 0 | 0 | + | 0 | + | 0 | + | 0 | 0 | + | 0 |
| 9 | 0 | 0 | 0 | + | + | 0 | + | 0 | 0 | + | 0 | + | 0 | + | + | + | + | + |
| 10 | 0 | 0 | 0 | + | + | 0 | + | 0 | 0 | + | 0 | + | 0 | + | + | + | + | + |

**Antigens Present (continued)**

| Cell No. | Leᵃ | Leᵇ | P₁ | M | N | S | s | Luᵃ | Luᵇ | Xgᵃ | | Additional Antigen |
|---|---|---|---|---|---|---|---|---|---|---|---|---|
| | Lewis | | P | | MNS | | | Lutheran | | Sex-Linked | | |
| 1 | 0 | + | + | 0 | + | + | + | 0 | + | 0 | M | |
| 2 | + | 0 | + | + | + | 0 | + | 0 | + | + | M | Co (b+) |
| 3 | 0 | + | + | 0 | + | 0 | + | 0 | + | + | M | |
| 4 | 0 | + | + | + | 0 | + | 0 | + | + | + | F | Co (b+) |
| 5 | 0 | + | 0 | + | + | + | + | 0 | + | + | M | |
| 6 | 0 | + | 0 | + | + | 0 | + | 0 | + | 0 | M | |
| 7 | 0 | + | + | + | 0 | + | + | 0 | + | 0 | M | Co (b+) |
| 8 | + | 0 | + | + | + | + | 0 | 0 | + | 0 | M | |
| 9 | 0 | 0 | + | + | + | + | 0 | 0 | + | + | F | |
| 10 | 0 | + | 0 | 0 | 0 | 0 | + | 0 | + | + | F | |
| 11 | | | | | | | | | | | | I (neg) |

**Patient Results**
**Eluate of DAT Positive RBCs**

| Cell No. | Immediate Spin | 37° C | AHG | Coombs Control Cells |
|---|---|---|---|---|
| 1 | Neg | 1+ | 2+ | |
| 2 | Neg | Neg | ± | 2+ |
| 3 | Neg | Neg | ± | 2+ |
| 4 | Neg | Neg | ± | 2+ |
| 5 | Neg | Neg | ± | 2+ |
| 6 | Neg | Neg | ± | 2+ |
| 7 | Neg | Neg | ± | 2+ |
| 8 | Neg | Neg | ± | 2+ |
| 9 | Neg | Neg | ± | 2+ |
| 10 | Neg | Neg | ± | 2+ |
| 11 | Neg | Neg | Neg | 2+ |
| Auto | Neg | Neg | Neg | 2+ |

**Patient Results—Serum**

| Cell No. | Immediate Spin | 37° C | AHG | Coombs Control Cells |
|---|---|---|---|---|
| I | Neg | Neg | ± | 1+ |
| II | Neg | 1+ | 2+ | |

**Patient Results—Serum**

| Cell No. | Immediate Spin | 37° C | AHG | Coombs Control Cells |
|---|---|---|---|---|
| 1 | Neg | 1+ | 2+ | |
| 2 | Neg | Neg | 2+ | |
| 3 | Neg | Neg | ± | 2+ |
| 4 | Neg | Neg | ± | 2+ |
| 5 | Neg | Neg | ± | 2+ |
| 6 | Neg | Neg | ± | 2+ |
| 7 | Neg | Neg | ± | 2+ |
| 8 | Neg | Neg | ± | 2+ |
| 9 | Neg | Neg | ± | 2+ |
| 10 | Neg | Neg | ± | 2+ |
| 11 | Neg | Neg | Neg | 2+ |
| Auto | Neg | Neg | Neg | 2+ |

## Questions

1. What is the identity of the antibody in the eluate?
2. What is the explanation for the weakly reactive agglutination pattern in the reagent cells within the patient's serum?
3. Does the reaction pattern of the reagent cells suggest the presence of any other unexpected antibodies?
4. Briefly describe the characteristics of the most recently discovered antibody in this patient's serum.

## Discussion

1. The patient's heat eluate was weakly reactive with all panel cells tested. She is not receiving any medications known to cause a positive DAT. Anti-K specificity was demonstrated in the eluate. Because this patient has been recently transfused, with K negative units only, the presence of anti-K in her eluate is probably caused by the Matuhasi-Ogato Phenomenon. This phenomenon occurs when a specific antigen-antibody complex forms and another antibody that is not directed against an antigen on the red cells involved in the specific complex is unable to bind to the complex and can be recovered in eluates subsequently made.

2. Weak, nonspecific reactions were observed at the AHG phase with most of the K negative red cells tested. In an attempt to determine if these reactions were caused by high incidence antigens, the patient's serum was adsorbed with pooled platelets. After adsorption, the patient's serum was nonreactive with the previously positive (K negative) red cells. Thus, it appears likely that the nonspecific reactivity at the AHG phase was due to HLA antibody production.

3. Yes. The strongly reacting No. 2 cell is consistent with anti-$C^w$ reactivity.

4. The $C^w$ antigen is part of the Rhesus blood group system. It is present in about 1% of the population. Anti-$C^w$ is formed either through previous transfusions or pregnancies, or more rarely through inhalation or ingestion of similar antigens. Anti-$C^w$ has been implicated in hemolytic transfusion reactions and HDN.

## Conclusion

Anti-K, anti-$C^w$, and HLA antibodies.

## Case 25

### History and Laboratory Data

A 67-year-old White woman received 1 unit of fresh frozen plasma and 6 units of packed RBCs 1 month earlier for injuries sustained in a motor vehicle accident. Four units of packed red cells were ordered preoperatively for orthopedic repair of injuries sustained in that accident. She was the mother of eight children and reported that all pregnancies had been normal and all of her children were healthy at birth. Her blood type was group O, Rh positive.

All of the crossmatches were incompatible and the unexpected antibody screen was also positive. Agglutination occurred in all phases of the crossmatches and antibody screening (RT, 37° C, AHG). Additionally, the patient's auto control was positive.

*Issit, P.D.: *Spectra Biological Applied Blood Group Serology*, ed. 2, p. 346.

### *Laboratory Data (Case 25)*

**Reagent Red Blood Cell Screening Cells**
**Partial Listing of Antigens Present**

| Cell No. | Rh-hr D | C | E | c | e | Kell K | k | Duffy Fy$^a$ | Fy$^b$ | Kidd Jk$^a$ | Jk$^b$ | Lewis Le$^a$ | Le$^b$ | MNS S | s | M | N | P P$_1$ |
|---|---|---|---|---|---|---|---|---|---|---|---|---|---|---|---|---|---|---|
| I | + | 0 | + | + | + | + | + | + | 0 | + | 0 | 0 | + | + | + | + | 0 | + |
| II | 0 | + | 0 | + | 0 | 0 | + | 0 | + | 0 | + | 0 | + | 0 | + | + | 0 | + |

**Reagent Red Blood Cell Panel Antigen Profile**
**Partial Listing of Antigens Present**

| Cell No. | Rh-hr D | C | E | c | e | Kell K | k | Duffy Fy$^a$ | Fy$^b$ | Kidd Jk$^a$ | Jk$^b$ | Lewis Le$^a$ | Le$^b$ | MNS S | s | M | N | P P$_1$ |
|---|---|---|---|---|---|---|---|---|---|---|---|---|---|---|---|---|---|---|
| 1 | 0 | 0 | 0 | + | + | 0 | + | + | + | + | 0 | 0 | 0 | + | 0 | + | + | + |
| 2 | 0 | 0 | 0 | + | + | 0 | + | 0 | + | + | + | 0 | + | + | + | + | 0 | 0 |
| 3 | 0 | + | 0 | + | + | 0 | + | 0 | + | + | + | 0 | + | + | + | + | 0 | + |
| 4 | + | 0 | + | + | 0 | 0 | + | + | 0 | + | 0 | 0 | + | 0 | + | + | 0 | + |
| 5 | + | 0 | + | + | 0 | 0 | + | + | + | 0 | + | 0 | + | 0 | + | + | + | + |
| 6 | + | + | 0 | 0 | + | + | + | + | + | + | 0 | 0 | + | + | + | + | + | + |
| 7 | + | + | 0 | 0 | + | 0 | + | 0 | + | + | + | 0 | + | 0 | + | + | + | + |
| 8 | + | + | + | 0 | + | 0 | + | 0 | 0 | 0 | + | + | 0 | 0 | + | + | 0 | 0 |
| 9 | + | + | 0 | + | + | 0 | + | + | + | + | + | + | 0 | + | 0 | 0 | + | + |
| 10 | + | + | 0 | 0 | + | + | 0 | 0 | + | + | + | 0 | + | 0 | + | + | + | + |

**Initial Patient Results**

| Cell No. | Immediate Spin | 37° C | AHG |
|---|---|---|---|
| I | 2+ | 2+ | 3+ |
| II | 1+ | ± | 4+ |

**Initial Patient Results**

| Cell No. | Immediate Spin | 37° C | AHG |
|---|---|---|---|
| 1 | ± | Neg | 3+ |
| 2 | 1+ | ± | 4+ |
| 3 | 1+ | 1+ | 4+ |
| 4 | 2+ | 3+ | 3+ |
| 5 | 2+ | 3+ | 3+ |
| 6 | 2+ | 3+ | 3+ |
| 7 | 1+ | 1+ | 2+ |
| 8 | 2+ | 3+ | 3+ |
| 9 | 2+ | 3+ | ± |
| 10 | 2+ | 3+ | 3+ |
| Auto Control | 1+ | 3+ | 4+ |

## Questions

1. What is the most probable explanation for the reactions observed in the initial reagent red cell screening?
2. What procedures can be performed to investigate the presence of any other antibodies?
3. Are any additional unexpected antibodies present in the patient's serum?
4. Can all of the weakly reactive agglutinations be attributed to the presence of the cold antibody?
5. What is the appropriate type of blood for transfusing this patient?

## Discussion

1. The initial reagent red cell panel demonstrated agglutination of all cells (panagglutination) and a positive (4+) autocontrol. This is the type of pattern that is typical of a cold autoagglutinin.
2. Because of the strong cold autoagglutinin, the patient's serum was subjected to a double autoabsorption of the patient's papain-treated cells. The strength of the auto control decreased to ±.

Repeat testing was conducted with absorbed serum. The results of this testing follow.

**Patient Results—Absorbed Patient's Serum**

| Cell No. | Immediate Spin | 37° C | AHG |
|---|---|---|---|
| I | Neg | 2+ | 3+ |
| II | Neg | Neg | ± |

**Patient Results—Absorbed Patient's Serum**

| Cell No. | Immediate Spin | 37° C | AHG | Coombs Control |
|---|---|---|---|---|
| 1 | Neg | Neg | ± | 2+ |
| 2 | Neg | Neg | ± | 2+ |
| 3 | Neg | Neg | ± | 2+ |
| 4 | Neg | 1+ | 3+ | |
| 5 | Neg | ± | 3+ | |
| 6 | Neg | Neg | 3+ | |
| 7 | Neg | Neg | ± | 2+ |
| 8 | Neg | ± | 3+ | |
| 9 | Neg | Neg | ± | |
| 10 | Neg | Neg | 3+ | |
| Auto Control | ± | ± | ± | 2+ |

3. Yes. Removal of the strong reactivity due to the cold agglutinin unmasked a pattern of reactivity that was consistent with other unexpected antibodies. The I screening cell suggests antibodies to any of the following antigens: E, K, Fyᵃ, Jkᵃ, and S. However, the panel of reagent cell agglutination excludes anti-Fyᵃ, -Jkᵃ, and -S. It is consistent with anti-E and anti-K in addition to the cold autoagglutinin.

The patient's red cells were phenotyped and found to be negative for both the E and K antigens.
4. No. Subsequent testing by a reference laboratory disclosed that the patient also had anti-Knopps (Knᵃ)/McCoy (McCᵃ). The Knopps (Knᵃ) and McCoy (McCᵃ) antigens are of high frequency and are present on more than 98% of the red cells of the random population. These antigens have often been found to be phenotypically related. Neither anti-Knᵃ or anti-McCᵃ is known to cause reduced red cell survival following transfusion of antigen positive units.
5. The patient should receive O positive, E negative, Kell negative crossmatch-compatible (or least incompatible) donor units for transfusion. Prewarming or cold auto absorption should be considered if the cold agglutinin causes crossmatching difficulties.

## Conclusion

Anti-E, anti-K, anti-Knᵃ/McCᵃ, and a cold agglutinin.

## Case 26

Submitted by Polly F. Kay, MT(ASCP), MHS, and Marion Hursey
School of Medical Technology
Anderson Memorial Hospital
Anderson, South Carolina

### History and Laboratory Data

A 62-year-old Black man was admitted to the hospital with a 5.6 g/dL hemoglobin. He had a long history of atherosclerotic coronary heart disease and severe end-stage renal disease. The patient was on maintenance chronic hemodialysis and had a history of previous transfusions 1 and 5 years before admission.

On an earlier admission the same year, this serum demonstrated an antibody (or antibodies) which reacted with all cells of a reagent panel. Randomly crossmatched blood was incompatible with 72 units of blood in the blood bank. A specimen was submitted to a reference laboratory for antibody identification. The results indicated that the serum contained an Rh antibody of "broad specificity" and that his red cells lacked one or more high frequency Rh antigens; the serum was compatible only with Rh null cells.

Additional samples were referred to an AABB reference laboratory for confirmation of the antibody identification and help in obtaining blood for transfusion. The only positive reactions during Rh phenotyping were with anti-D and anti-c antisera. Exact specificity of the antibody could not be confirmed as either anti-hr$^s$ or anti-hr$^B$.

Family members were located and their samples were also sent to the AABB reference laboratory for testing. Three children were incompatible with the patient's serum. A sister was compatible and appeared to have the same Rh phenotype as the patient. The sister donated blood, three times to date. These units were frozen until transfused. One other rare donor, who is hr$^s$ (−), hr$^B$ (−), Hr$_o$ (−), was located. This donor is participating in an autologous frozen blood program for herself; however, she released two of her frozen units for this patient. These units were stored frozen until needed.

On admission in June of that year, the patient was admitted to Coronary Care with a 6.1 g/dL hemoglobin and a possible myocardial infarction. Two units of the frozen blood were successfully crossmatched and transfused. The patient left the hospital against medical advice. In August, he was again admitted with severe anemia. Another frozen unit was crossmatched and transfused. Colonic polyps were discovered at this time, but surgery was postponed until more compatible blood could be located.

Blood samples were sent to the National Red Cross Rare Donor Center in Washington, D.C. and to the Atlanta Red Cross for mass random crossmatching by capillary technique with predominantly Black donors. To date, approximately 3000 donors have been tested. One additional donor appears to be compatible and three are microscopically incompatible. The Rh phenotypes of these donors have not yet been determined. All 4 units have been frozen and are available for an emergency.

The patient later underwent surgery, successfully, for the colonic polyps after receiving the last two originally identified compatible units from his sister and the rare donor. A system has evolved in which his sister will continue to donate blood on a periodic basis. These units will be frozen for future use. In the meantime, the Red Cross continues to screen donors for other sources of blood for this patient.

## Questions

1. When a patient's unexpected antibody screen is positive and an extraordinary number of donors is incompatible, what could some of the reasons be?
2. Why would a patient develop unexpected antibodies of this type?
3. Is it harmful to transfuse a patient with this type of problem?
4. Why was it important to locate suitable donors in this situation?

## Discussion

1. It is important in cases of positive unexpected antibody screens and panagglutination that the pattern of reactivity be investigated. If activity is strong at room temperature or colder, a cold agglutinin must be excluded. Assuming that the patient's DAT and autocontrol are negative, other facts can be excluded. In this case, significant reactivity of the patient's serum in the AHG phase with all donors tested suggests an unexpected antibody to a high-incidence antigen.
2. Unexpected antibodies to high incidence antigens occur because the patient lacks the corresponding antigen. Hence, transfusion of almost all units of donor blood could stimulate antibody production against the corresponding antigen.
3. Not always. Transfusion of antigen-positive blood that is not known to reduce red survival, such as Knopps/McCoy, presented in the previous case, can generally be given without a transfusion reaction. However, the attending physician should decide if transfusing least incompatible blood is in the best interest of the patient.
4. Antibodies of the Rh system are known to cause hemolytic transfusion reactions when antigen-positive blood is transfused to a patient with the corresponding antibody. In this case, the exact specificity of the antibody could not be confirmed as either anti-hr$^s$ or anti-hr$^B$. Therefore, it was important that hr$^s$ (−), hr$^B$ (−), and Hr$_o$ (−) donors be located. Refer to Chapter 5 for a full discussion of the Rh system.

## Conclusion

Probable anti-hr$^s$ or anti-hr$^B$.

# 9

# Transfusion Policies and Practices

At the conclusion of this chapter, the reader should be able to:

- Describe the requirements for the selection of blood for transfusion to a patient and discuss the risk of immunization when transfusing a patient.
- Name at least six common surgical procedures for which the type and screen protocol is appropriate.
- Explain the steps that must be followed in transfusion emergency situations.
- Name the first sign of immunization in a patient who has received blood possessing a foreign antigen.
- Define the term "massive transfusion."
- List the clinical priorities in massive transfusion situations.
- Name and describe six adverse conditions associated with the rapid infusion of massive amounts of blood.
- Explain the purpose of an exchange transfusion of a newborn infant and discuss the selection of donor blood for exchange transfusion of a newborn infant.
- Describe the special blood requirements of patients with cold-reacting unexpected antibodies or a warm autoantibody.

## Chapter Outline

## ROUTINE TRANSFUSION REQUESTS

Most of the blood provided by a blood bank is used by patients undergoing surgical procedures or with acute unexpected blood loss. The balance is used for correction of chronic anemias not treatable by surgery or other means and for patients with special needs, such as oncology or dialysis patients.

In the early 1980s, the need to eliminate the time and expense of unnecessary crossmatching was recognized. Based on the established prospective need for blood in specific surgical procedures, the type and screen protocol (discussed in Chapter 7) was developed. Blood banks have now established what types of cases are most likely to use blood and the average number of units of blood usually required. The prospective use of blood varies from one hospital to another, depending on factors such as the patient's presurgical condition and age, and the type of surgi-

## Table 9-1. Typical Surgical Blood Order Schedule

| Type of Surgery | Maximum Standard Crossmatch Order (Units) | Type of Surgery | Maximum Standard Crossmatch Order (Units) |
|---|---|---|---|
| *Dental Surgery* | | *Pulmonary and Vascular Surgery* | |
| Full mouth extraction | 0 | Abdominal aortic aneurysm resection | 4 WB and 2 PC |
| Extraction, impacted molars | 0 | Aortofemoral bypass graft | 4 WB and 2 PC |
| *General Surgery* | | Aortiliac bypass graft | 4 WB and 2 PC |
| Abdominal-perineal resection | 4 PC | Bronchoscopy | 0 |
| Amputation | T&S | Endarterectomy: femoral or carotid | 2 PC |
| Anal fistula excision | T&S | Femoral–femoral bypass graft | 2 PC |
| Appendectomy | T&S | Femoral–popliteal bypass graft | 2 PC |
| Breast biopsy | T&S | Thoracotomy | 4 PC |
| Cholecystectomy | T&S | *Gynecologic and Obstetric Surgery* | |
| Colon resection | 2 PC | Cesarean section | T&S |
| Colostomy or closure | T&S | Dilatation, curettage, and conization | 0 |
| Esophageal resection | 4 PC | Hysterectomy, radical and pelvic | 4 PC |
| Excision of anal fissure or fistula/sphincterotomy | 0 | lymphadenectomy | |
| Excision of skin lesions | 0 | Hysterectomy, simple (including TAH/BSO) | T&S |
| Exploratory laparotomy | T&S | Hysterectomy and anterior-posterior repair | 1 PC |
| Gastrectomy | 4 PC | Laparoscopic tubal ligation | T&S |
| Gastroscopy | 0 | Marshall-Marchetti procedure | 0 |
| Hemicolectomy | 2 PC | Ovarian wedge resection, ovarian cystectomy | T&S |
| Hemorrhoidectomy | 0 | Stamey procedure | T&S |
| Hernia repair, hiatal | 2 PC | Tuboplasty | T&S |
| Hernia repair, inguinal or femoral | 0 | Uterine suspension, fulguration of endometrial | T&S |
| Hernia repair, ventral | T&S | implants | |
| Lymph node biopsy | 0 | Vaginal plastic procedures | T&S |
| Mastectomy, modified radical | 2 PC | *Neurosurgery* | |
| Mastectomy, simple | T&S | Carpal tunnel release | T&S |
| Parathyroidectomy | T&S | Craniotomy for aneurysm | T&S |
| Sigmoidectomy | 2 PC | Craniotomy for tumor | T&S |
| Splenectomy | T&S | Craniotomy for traumatic hematoma (acute) | T&S |
| Thyroid lobectomy | T&S | Craniotomy for chronic subdural hematoma | T&S |
| Vagotomy and antrectomy | T&S | Craniotomy for AVM | T&S |
| Vein stripping | T&S | Cranio for rhizotomy | T&S |
| *Ear, Nose and Throat* | | Craniotomy for EC-IC | T&S |
| Caldwell-LUC | T&S | Depressive laminectomy (cervical, thoracic, or | T&S |
| Excision of submandibular gland | 0 | lumbar) | |
| Myringotomy | 0 | Laminectomy for disc removal (lumbar) | T&S |
| Laryngectomy | 1 PC | Laminectomy for rhizotomy | 2 WB + 2 PC |
| Mastoidectomy | 0 | Bilateral $T_{2-3}$ sympathectomy | 0 |
| Neck dissection (radical) | 4 PC | Laminectomy for spinal tumor | 2 WB + 2 PC |
| Parotidectomy | 0 | Shunts, VP and VA, (if an alloantibody is detected | T&S |
| Septoplasty | 0 | 2 WB should be available) | |
| Tonsillectomy and adenoidectomy | T&S | Laminectomy for chordotomy | 2 WB + 2 PC |
| Transantral ethmoidectomy | T&S | Percutaneous chordotomy | T&S |
| Tympanoplasty | 0 | Craniotomy for excision of abscess | 2 WB |
| *Orthopedic Surgery* | | Burr hole for tapping of cyst or abscess | T&S |
| Amputation, toe | 0 | Carotid endarterectomy | T&S |
| Arthroscopy | 0 | *Ophthalmologic Surgery* | |
| Arthrotomy–removel of loose body | 0 | Cataract removal | 0 |
| Carpal tunnel repair | 0 | Recession, eye | 0 |
| Excision, Morton's neuroma | 0 | Entropion or extropion repair | 0 |
| Fracture, closed reduction | 0 | *Urologic Surgery* | |
| Fracture, open reduction, internal fixation | 2 PC | Cystectomy, radical | 4 WB |
| Hip nailing/hip screw | 3 PC | Cystectomy, segmental | T&S |
| Leg amputation | 0 | Cystoscopy | 0 |
| Meniscectomy | 0 | Cystourethropexy | 0 |
| Minor hand or foot surgery | 0 | Fulguration of bleeding bladder tumor | 1 PC |
| Open reduction | T&S | Hydrocelectomy | 0 |
| Osteotomy | 1 PC | Ileal conduit–colon conduit | 1 PC |
| Removal of hip pin | T&S | Needle biopsy, prostate | 0 |
| Shoulder reconstruction | T&S | Nephrectomy, radical | 4 WB |
| Spinal fusion | 2 PC | Nephrectomy, simple | T&S |
| Synovectomy | 0 | Orchiectomy | T&S |
| Total hip replacement | 4 PC | Orchiopexy | T&S |
| Total knee replacement | T&S | Penile prosthesis | T&S |
| *Plastic Surgery* | | Perineal prostatectomy | 2 PC |
| Augmentation mammoplasty | T&S | Prostate biopsy | 0 |
| Facelift | 0 | Pyelolithotomy | T&S |
| Reduction mammoplasty | T&S | Suprapubic prostatectomy | 2 PC |
| Rhinoplasty | 0 | Transurethral resection of bladder tumor | T&S |
| Skin flap | T&S | Ureteral dilatation | 0 |
| Skin graft, minor | T&S | Ureteral reimplantation | T&S |
| Skin graft, major (severe burns) | T&S | Ureterolithotomy | T&S |

Key:  T&S = Type and Screen
     WB = Whole Blood
     PC = Packed Red Blood Cells

**Table 9-2. Selection of Donor Blood According to ABO Group**

| Patient's Type | Donor Blood 1st Choice | Donor Blood 2nd Choice* | Donor Blood 3rd Choice* |
|---|---|---|---|
| O | O | None | |
| A | A | O (RBCs) | |
| $A_1$ with anti-H | $A_1$ | None | |
| $A_2$ with anti-$A_1$ | $A_2$ | O (RBCs) | |
| B | B | O (RBCs) | |
| AB | AB | A or B RBCs† | O RBCs |
| $A_1$B with anti-H | $A_1$B | $A_1$ or B RBCs† | |
| $A_2$B with anti-$A_2$ | $A_2$B | $A_2$ or B RBC† | O RBC |

* When donor blood of recipient's group is not available.
† It does not make much difference which of these is chosen. Because they are mutually incompatible, both must not be given concurrently. Type B has the advantage of avoiding possible complications due to the presence of anti-$A_1$ or anti-H in the recipient serum.
(From Huestis, D.W., Bove, J.R., and Busch, S.: Practical Blood Transfusion. (3rd ed.). Boston, Little, Brown and Co., 1982, p. 206.)

cal technique used. Table 9-1 presents a summary of a typical blood order schedule.

## Selection of Blood for Crossmatching

The *first requirement* for blood selection is the ABO group of the patient (Table 9-2). Recipients must receive the ABO group-specific whole blood or ABO compatible red blood cell components. This requirement is absolute in the case of group O recipients. If volume replacement is needed, red blood cells can be resuspended in saline or volume expanders can be infused. The subgroups A and AB are unimportant unless the patient has potent anti-$A_1$ or anti-H, in which case donor blood group $A_2$ or $A_2$B, or $A_1$ or $A_1$B, respectively, would be selected.

When blood of the same ABO group is not available, the next choice is red blood cells of a group that are compatible by major crossmatch. The most important consideration is that the donor red blood cells must be compatible with both the recipient's anti-A or anti-B and any other clinically significant antibody the prospective recipient may have. This is because every foreign red blood cell transfused becomes instantly and totally surrounded by the recipient's plasma, which provides complete contact between antigens on the donor's red blood cells and the patient's plasma antibodies. If the patient's plasma contains an antibody to the corresponding antigen on the foreign red blood cells the two will combine and a serious reaction may take place. The reverse situation, in which the donor's plasma has the antibody and the recipient's red blood cells have the antigen, is not as dangerous. The incoming donor antibody is instantly diluted by the recipient's much larger volume of plasma before the antibody has an opportunity to interact with the recipient's red blood cells.

## The Universal Donor

The term "universal donor" often has been applied to group O, Rh negative blood products. There is no such thing as a universal donor! The use of this term for group O individuals is based on the lack of A, B, and D antigen on the red blood cells. The plasma of group O persons, however, does contain anti-A and anti-B, which is able to react with recipient red blood cells of other blood groups. The extraction of plasma from whole blood units removes about 80% of the antibody from the unit. If the residual antibody is high in titer, a considerable amount of activity remains. If a significant amount of anti-A and anti-B accumulates in the patient's circulation, it prevents reverting to transfusing blood of the patient's own blood type. Washed or deglycerolized red blood cells contain little or no residual plasma with accompanying antibodies.

The use of group O blood does not prevent sensitization of the patient to other blood group antigens that may be missing from their own red blood cells. Indiscriminate use of group O Rh negative blood may also produce a shortage of this type and could have serious consequences if a group O Rh negative person needed to be transfused.

## The Universal Recipient

A group AB recipient lacks both anti-A and anti-B and may safely receive red blood cells from donors of other blood groups. Group O, however, is the poorest choice because it contains some anti-A, anti-B, and cross-reacting anti-A,B.

## Other Requirements

The *second requirement* in the selection of blood is the Rh type of the patient. Rh negative recipients should receive Rh negative whole blood or red blood cell components, except for reasonable qualifying circumstances. Rh positive recipients may receive either Rh positive or Rh negative whole blood or red blood cell components.

Testing for D is considered sufficient. The risk of immunization depends on factors such as the immunogenicity of a specific antigen, the frequency of the antigen in the donor population and an individual's capacity to form antibodies.

The D antigen is an important antigen because of its immunogenicity (potency) and the fact that a person has an 85% chance of receiving Rh positive blood. Although weak D ($D^u$) is less immunogenic than D, weak D ($D^u$) positive individuals can produce anti-D. Therefore, the weak D ($D^u$) status of a recipient does not need to be determined; they should receive Rh negative blood. Weak D ($D^u$) positive donors are regarded as Rh positive donors. The comparative risk of immunization to antigens other than A, B, and D, based on the number of antibodies encountered and the frequencies of the antigens in the population in descending order are: K, c, E, k, e, Fy$^a$, C, Jk$^a$, S, Jk$^b$, and s.

The *third requirement* is the use of antigen negative blood in patients in whom an unexpected antibody is detected. When clinically significant unexpected antibodies are found during testing, or if the recipient has a past history of such antibodies, whole blood or red blood cell components lacking in the corresponding antigen should be selected for transfusion. The unexpected antibody should be identified before blood is selected for transfusion. In addition, the blood product should be crossmatch-compatible.

If a situation is clinically urgent, it is sometimes necessary to issue blood which is crossmatch-incompatible. The crossmatch technique by which the antibody reactivity is strongest should be used and recorded. When clinical circumstances warrant deviation from the standard protocol, the deviation must be approved by the physician responsible for the transfusion service.

### Blood Shortages

Inability of a blood bank to meet patient needs for blood and blood products may result from a shortage of blood within the regional system or depletion of certain types in the blood bank inventory because of massive transfusion needs.

A shortage of blood may be due to:

1. Increased general demand, e.g., major disaster.
2. Insufficient blood collections, e.g., seasonal variation.
3. Disproportionate collection and need of specific blood types, e.g., group O Rh negative, group B Rh positive.
4. Inability to provide antigen-negative blood for a patient with an antibody to a high incidence antigen or in cases of multiple alloantibodies.

In addition to increased donor recruitment efforts for all blood or specific types of blood, donation of autologous blood (see Chapter 2) may alleviate the problems.

---

## EMERGENCY TRANSFUSION SITUATIONS

---

Orderly management of a patient requiring urgent blood transfusions requires communication of the severity of the need and the extent of the emergency to the blood bank by the attending physician. This allows a determination of the anticipated blood use and the extent of pretransfusion testing that can be completed before issuing the blood.

### Emergency Processing and Issuing of Blood

When there is a desperate need for blood, uncrossmatched or partially crossmatched blood might be requested by a physician. When blood is released before the crossmatch is completed, an Emergency Release Form (Fig. 9-1A,B) must be completed. This form, which must be signed by the ordering physician, indicates that the patient's life will be in jeopardy without an emergency transfusion. Such a statement does not absolve the blood bank from its responsibility to issue properly labelled donor blood or to complete typing and compatibility testing as soon as possible.

Other requirements in the event of an urgent request for blood are described below.

### Steps To Follow in an Emergency

When an urgent request for blood is received:

1. Immediately obtain a blood specimen from the patient and attach a numbered bracelet on the patient's arm. Both the specimen and the patient should be minimally identifiable by number if time does not permit additional information or if other information about the patient, for example, name, is unknown. Blood specimens *must* be collected before any blood is administered.
2. Promptly determine the ABO group and Rh type of the patient, and begin compatibility testing. Determination of the ABO group and Rh type should take less than 5 minutes. Most patients can receive volume support during this brief interval. Any blood that is released before pretransfusion testing is fully completed should be group and type compatible. The blood typing must be from the patient's current specimen. Previous blood bank records must *not* be used to determine the recipient's blood group and the blood group must not be taken from other records. If group O blood is to be used in a patient of an unknown type, it should be in the form of packed red blood cells and the patient should be switched to his or her own type as soon as possible (see Table 9-3).
3. Indicate, in a conspicuous fashion on the tag or label attached to the donor units, that compatibility testing has not been completed at the time of issue.
4. Complete compatibility tests promptly (stat), even though the transfusion has already been started. If an incompatibility is detected at any stage of testing, immediately notify the patient's physician and the blood bank medical director, and, if possible, retrieve the donor units at once.
5. Complete all records and forms as in a routine situation.

### Compatibility Testing in the Emergency Situation

The hazard of transfusing blood to a patient whose serum has not been screened for unexpected antibodies must balance the risk of an unfavorable outcome, such as a hemolytic transfusion reaction, against the danger to the patient of postponing transfusion. An increased possibility of error exists when the haste and disruption created by an emergency upset routine procedures.

I request the release of blood for _____,

Patient's Name or Identification

_____ , _____ , _____ , _____ ,

Hospital ID Number      Location           Age         Sex

_____ , at _____ on _____ .

Race                    Time                   Date

Nature of the Emergency: _____

    I believe this patient's life will be in jeopardy *without* an emergency transfusion; therefore, I accept the responsibility for, and release the Blood Bank Medical Director and Blood Bank personnel of the responsibility for, any adverse patient reaction resulting from this transfusion, which might have been prevented if time had allowed for complete pretransfusion testing.

    I further understand that the Blood Bank personnel will complete routine compatibility testing as soon as possible and that they will report the results immediately to me.

Signed: _____ , M.D.

**A**

FOR BLOOD BANK USE:

The patient's AB and RH groups (if known) are _____ .

Patient Unexpected Antibody Screen
- A. Not performed
- B. Immediate spin only
- C. Centrifuged post-incubation
- D. Completed

Donor Unit Number

1. _____   Stage of crossmatch when released;
- A. No pretransfusion testing performed
- B. Immediate spin only
- C. Centrifuged post-incubation

2. _____
- A. No pretransfusion testing performed
- B. Immediate spin only
- C. Centrifuged post-incubation

3. _____
- A. No pretransfusion testing performed
- B. Immediate spin only
- C. Centrifuged post-incubation

_____          _____
Blood Bank Technologist                                Date

**B**

**Figure 9-1.** Example of an emergency release of blood form. A, Physician's release form; B, Form for blood bank use.

The most important function of the major crossmatch is confirmation of ABO compatibility. In general, IgG antibodies causing incompatible crossmatches result in decreased red blood cell survival of transfused cells but usually do not cause life-threatening intravascular hemolysis.

**Changing Blood Groups**

The blood bank policy manual should contain established guidelines for switching to a different blood group during an urgent situation, such as massive transfusion. At times of blood shortage, the medical director of the blood bank and the patient's physician should not feel constrained to transfuse only ABO and Rh specific blood. When deciding on the appropriateness of switching blood types, it is essential that the patient's clinical condition be assessed to anticipate the extent of the prospective blood requirement. A plan for switching blood types should maintain the greatest flexibility in meeting the patient's total requirements.

The age and sex of a patient are an important consideration in selecting and switching blood types. For example, it would be well to avoid transfusing Rh positive blood

**Table 9-3. Principles to be Followed When Switching Blood Types Because of Shortages**

| Patient's Blood Type and Rh Type | Principle |
|---|---|
| O negative | 1. Use only group O, Rh negative blood if patient is sensitized to D antigen.<br>2. Use group O, D, and weak D (Dᵘ) negative, C negative and/or E positive blood in preference to D positive blood.<br>3. Avoid transfusing anything but group O, Rh negative blood to patients (especially women) under 45.<br>4. Restrict the use of group O, Rh positive blood for group O, Rh negative patients to acute emergency situations, and then use only if the patient either has a negative antibody screen for anti-D or definitely lacks Rh antibodies.<br>5. If massive volumes of bood are required and switching to Rh positive blood is inevitable, avoid wasting group O, Rh negative blood by switching D antigen as early as possible. |
| A negative or B negative | 1. Use only Rh negative blood if patient is sensitized to D antigen i.e., group specific, Rh negative or group O, Rh negative packed RBCs.<br>2. Use D and weak D (Dᵘ) negative, C negative and /or E positive in preference to D positive.<br>3. Avoid transfusing anything but Rh negative blood to patients (especially women) under 45.<br>4. Restrict use of Rh positive blood to acute emergency situations, and then use only if the patient has a negative alloantibody screen for anti-D or definitely lacks Rh antibodies.<br>5. If massive volumes of blood are required and switching to Rh positive blood is inevitable, avoid wasting Rh negative blood by switching as early as possible.<br>6. Conserve group O blood. Only group O blood can be given to a group O recipient. |
| AB negative | 1. Use only Rh negative blood if the patient is sensitized to D antigen.<br>2. Use D and weak D (Dᵘ) negative, C negative and/or E positive in preference to D positive.<br>3. Group A blood may be used (as packed RBCs) unless the patient has anti-A₁.<br>4. The patient should initially be switched to group A blood and then, secondarily, may be switched to group O blood. Always do this before switching Rh types.<br>5. Avoid transfusing anything but Rh negative blood to patient (especially women) under age 45.<br>6. Restrict the use of Rh positive blood to acute emergency situations and then use only if the patient has a negative unexpected antibody screen or definitely lacks Rh antibodies.<br>7. If massive volumes of blood are required and switching to Rh positive blood is inevitable, avoid wasting Rh negative by switching as early as possible.<br>8. Conserve group O blood. Only group O blood can be given to a group O recipient. |
| O positive | 1. A group O patient may receive only group O blood.<br>2. Rh negative blood may be used, but this should be avoided due to supply problems. |
| A positive or B positive | 1. Group O blood may be given as packed red cells.<br>2. Rh negative blood may be used, but this should be avoided because of supply problems. |
| AB positive | 1. Group A blood may be used (as packed red cells, unless the patient has anti-A₁).<br>2. Switch initially to group A blood and then, secondarily, to group O blood.<br>3. Conserve group O blood. Only group O blood can be given to a group O recipient.<br>4. Rh negative blood may be used, but this should be avoided because of supply problems. |

to an Rh negative woman of childbearing age. In such cases, it is usually preferable to switch ABO groups before switching from Rh negative to Rh positive blood.

If the estimated total transfusion requirements of an actively bleeding Rh negative patient (without anti-D) exceed the available amount of appropriate Rh negative blood, the change to Rh positive should be done immediately to conserve this relatively scarce blood type. In such situations, the blood bank medical director should be consulted. If Rh positive blood must be given to an Rh negative patient, Rh negative blood should be given as soon as possible if additional transfusions are needed because immunization to the D antigen is likely to occur. The first evidence of immunization is usually the development of a positive DAT preceding detectable antibody in the patient's serum.

The principles of switching blood (Table 9-3) detail the strategy to be used in overcoming a shortage. When this is done, the transfused red blood cells should *always* be in the form of packed red blood cells rather than whole blood.

## MASSIVE TRANSFUSION

Massive transfusion is defined as the administration of enough blood or components within less than 24 hours to constitute a complete volume replacement. In an infant, this would be slightly more than half a unit and in an adult it would be 8 to 10 or more units. Situations associated with massive transfusion include treatment of acute bleeding associated with traumatic injury or surgery, and exchange transfusion subsequent to hemolytic disease of the newborn (HDN).

### Physiologic Results of Hemorrhage

The various changes brought about by acute hemorrhage, e.g., decreased blood pressure, rapid and thready pulse, increased respiratory rate, and constriction of the peripheral blood vessels which produces cold, clammy-feeling skin, can be referred to as hypovolemic shock syndrome. Many factors affect the amount of hemorrhage that will cause shock, but a rapid loss of 15 to 20% of blood volume leads to shock symptoms in most individuals. Almost all patients with hemorrhagic or hypovolemic shock have lost 35 to 40% of their blood volume; an average adult in severe hypovolemic shock has probably lost about 2 liters of blood. In many cases, for example, internal injuries and fractures, not all of the lost blood is visible.

One of the first responses to severe, acute bleeding is the body's physiologic attempt to restore the circulating blood volume to normal by shifting fluid from extravascular to intravascular spaces. Although this fluid does not have the oxygen-carrying capabilities of red blood cells nor the osmotic properties of plasma, it does stabilize the circulation. The effect of this shift in fluid to the intravascular spaces is that the remaining circulating red blood cells will be diluted and produce the characteristic drop in red blood cell parameters: hemoglobin, hematocrit, and red blood cell count. Dilution begins almost as soon as the onset of hemorrhage and continues for as long as 72 hours after all bleeding has stopped. During this 3-day period, the hemoglobin and hematocrit values are unreliable because they do not reflect the total amount of bleeding during this period. In the first few hours of active bleeding, hemoglobin and hematocrit values may be misleadingly high despite obvious and substantial amounts of blood loss.

**Initial Treatment of a Hemorrhaging Patient**

Problems associated with massive transfusion may arise from one or more conditions including:

1. The primary state for which the blood is administered
2. Complications of the initial malady
3. Underlying secondary disorders
4. Abnormalities in the transfused blood.

It is *vital* that a blood specimen for blood bank use be obtained before transfusion is initiated. Identification of the patient with a wristband is essential to the safety of the impending blood transfusion (see Fig. 2-1). Errors such as misidentification of either the patient or the specimen are more likely to occur in this type of nonroutine situation.

The first priority in the treatment of a patient for massive transfusion is the restoration of blood volume. This allows the body to regain an acceptable blood pressure to enable oxygen and nutrients to be delivered to essential organs and to prevent or halt disseminated intravascular coagulation (DIC). Blood volume can be expanded with electrolytes, plasma substitutes, blood, or blood components. Electrolytes, for example, normal saline, are usually the first solutions to be administered to the critically injured patient. Emergency volume replacement solutions,

for example, normal saline or lactated Ringer's, do not replace the oxygen-carrying capacity of the blood. If the circulation is effective, an increased rate of blood flow delivers an adequate quantity of oxygen to the tissues that will compensate for the lower level of hemoglobin. Following expansion of volume, the next priority is the restoration of an adequate level of hemoglobin to ensure that the patient's oxygen-carrying capacity does not drop below the level at which compensation is possible and to remove the strain on the heart caused by the increased demand for cardiac output.

**Adverse Conditions Associated with Massive Transfusion**

Many adverse situations have been associated with the rapid infusion of massive amounts of blood. These situations include:

1. Citrate toxicity
2. Hypocalcemia
3. Hypothermia
4. 2,3 DPG depletion
5. Depletion of coagulation factors and platelets
6. Accumulation of biochemicals and microaggregates

Citrate Toxicity

In most transfusion situations, the infusion of blood mixed with anticoagulant-preservative and changes associated with storage (see Chapter 2) can be corrected by the patient's physiology shortly after infusion. After the administration of blood under usual circumstances, the patient's pH may initially reflect excess acid, but the subsequent metabolism of citrate results in a net excess of base. In cases of massive transfusion where the volume of transfusion is high and the rate is rapid, the patient's ability to compensate cannot keep up. This produces a need to correct disturbances in acid-base balance.

Hypocalcemia

Ionized calcium, the physiologically active form of calcium, has been demonstrated to be lowered because of the massive transfusion of citrated blood, but this is rarely of clinical importance. This depression of ionized calcium is because the citrate concentration in a donor unit is sufficient to bind with the ionized calcium of the unit itself, with excess citrate remaining available to complex with calcium in the recipient.

Hypocalcemia is almost never witnessed because the body is able to mobilize additional calcium from bones as needed. Additionally, body cells rapidly metabolize infused citrate. Citrate is first converted to bicarbonate and ultimately to carbon dioxide and water. The general attitude is that a warm adult with a normally functioning liver can tolerate a unit of blood every 5 minutes without needing supplemental calcium. If this rate is exceeded or if hypothermia or severe liver disease exists, calcium infusion may be indicated, but calcium-containing solutions should not be administered through the same infusion lines as the blood because clotting in the line can result.

## Hypothermia

Hypothermia can result from the rapid (more than 100 mL/minute for 30 minutes) transfusion of refrigerated blood. Large volumes of rapidly infused cold blood can lower the temperature of the sino-atrial node to below 30° C, at which point ventricular arrhythmias occur.

Warming blood during massive transfusion can avoid the adverse effects of hypothermia, such as cardiac arrhythmia, and enhance the body's homeostatic mechanism, which is being stressed. Warming of blood must be carefully controlled and should not slow the rate of infusion significantly.

## 2,3 DPG Deletion

If the oxygen-carrying capacity of the blood does decrease as a result of DPG depletion, the recipient may compensate by increasing the rate of blood flow to the tissues. The patient will be able to restore DPG biochemically to normal levels within a few hours. In most cases of massive transfusion, the level of DPG in the transfused blood is of no significance. However, DPG depletion can be potentially dangerous under the following circumstances:

1. When the volume of transfused blood results in an almost complete exchange within a few hours.
2. When all or most of the transfused blood has been stored for more than 1 or 2 weeks.
3. When the recipient lacks the ability to increase his/her cardiac output.

## Depletion of Coagulation Factors

Massive transfusion is sometimes associated with coagulation abnormalities that have been attributed to dilution or the "washout" of coagulation factors or platelets. It has been established that massive transfusion with stored blood or plasma will not by itself reduce the activity of any plasma coagulation factors to a level at which hemostasis is compromised.

The occurrence of abnormal bleeding during massive transfusion indicates that simple dilution is *not* the only problem. Large amounts of plasma substitutes may aggravate a bleeding tendency. The bleeding time of an adult can be prolonged if more than one liter of dextran is rapidly transfused, presumably because dextran coats the platelets and impairs their function; however, coagulation function is not impaired by albumin, plasma protein fractions, or electrolytes except for their dilutional effect.

Although the patient's plasma maintains adequate levels

of coagulation factors in uncomplicated situations where there is no increased rate of consumption, the major complication impairing hemostasis during massive transfusion is disseminated intravascular coagulation (DIC). DIC is almost inevitable when extensive tissue damage is accompanied by prolonged shock and the resultant poor perfusion. It leads to the loss of platelets as well as the consumption of plasma coagulation factors V, VIII, II (prothrombin), and factor I (fibrinogen). Secondary fibrinolysis complicates the situation by releasing fibrin breakdown products which, in turn, inhibit coagulation and platelet plug formation. If the circulation is improved by restoring blood volume to normal, this enhances the removal of activated clotting factors by the mononuclear phagocytic system or neutralization by normal circulatory inhibitors. As the patient's blood volume is being restored, it may be necessary to replace coagulation factors and platelets. If fibrinogen is low, cryoprecipitate should be transfused. Cryoprecipitate contains 250 mg of fibrinogen and the transfusion of 16 bags should raise fibrinogen level of the average adult by more than 100 mg/dL (see Chapter 9 for a complete discussion of blood components).

Although abnormal test results do not always correlate with clinical problems, a massively transfused patient should be monitored after or during transfusion. A platelet count, prothrombin time, and activated partial thromboplastin time should be performed. If abnormal bleeding occurs, platelet concentrates or fresh frozen plasma should be administered based on the laboratory test results and the patient's clinical symptoms. Additional tests may be indicated to evaluate the possibility of DIC.

## Depletion of Platelets

Platelet counts do decline in massively transfused patients and can fall below $100 \times 10^9/L$ after infusion of 15 to 20 units of whole blood. Dilution of the patient's circulating platelets occurs as soon as the splenic pool reserves have been exhausted. Once the platelet reserves are exhausted, it takes 4 to 5 days for the synthesis of new platelets to restore the normal quantity.

At 1 to 6° C the microtubules in the platelets are disrupted; therefore, the lifespan of platelets in donated blood is limited. Recovery of viable platelets in whole blood is about 20% of normal after 72 hours. Platelet concentrates are the most effective method of preventing or correcting the dilutional thrombocytopenia of uncomplicated massive blood transfusion as well as augmenting the thrombocytopenia caused by DIC. Because platelet concentrates stored at room temperature for 72 hours have substantial quantities of the labile coagulation factors, a pool of eight platelet concentrates, with a volume of about 400 mL, should be considered the therapeutic equivalent of 1 to 2 units of fresh frozen plasma. Therefore, platelet concentrates can help to correct coagulation factor deficiencies and thrombocytopenia.

## Accumulation of Biochemicals and Microaggregates

Plasma potassium which accumulates in stored blood is of no significance in the massive transfusion of adult patients. Ammonia is also not significant, except for patients with severe liver failure. There is also no evidence of plasticizers leaching from blood containers.

Microaggregates composed of platelets, granulocytes, and fibrin increase progressively in stored blood but these aggregates are larger if red cells have been prepared by centrifugation. Microaggregate filters have been suggested after more than 5 to 10 units of blood have been transfused in rapid succession.

## Compatibility Testing in Cases of Massive Transfusion

Following the infusion of many units of blood over a short period of time, the composition of circulating blood changes and the proportion of the patient's own red blood cells and plasma to the total blood volume decreases. Consequently, the pretransfusion specimen ceases to represent the patient's current status and crossmatches using the initial specimen have limited validity.

According to the 15th edition of the American Association of Blood Banks (AABB) *Standards,* when a patient has received an amount of blood approximating the total blood volume within 24 hours, compatibility testing may be abbreviated. This deviation from usual practice must be at the discretion of the physician responsible for the transfusion service. In addition, the abbreviated crossmatch must follow written policy guidelines.

If the pretransfusion specimen contained no unexpected antibodies, it is permissible to perform a saline immediate-spin crossmatch for confirmation of ABO compatibility. This is particularly applicable if ten or more units of blood have been transfused. However, if unexpected antibodies were initially present in the patient specimen, the same policy of confirmation of ABO group compatibility is permissible, provided that the donor blood has been screened for the corresponding antigen. This policy must be set forth in the laboratory procedures manual.

## Exchange Transfusion

Exchange transfusion of a newborn infant is used in the treatment of both the anemia and hyperbilirubinemia that characterize hemolytic disease of the newborn (HDN; refer to Chapter 11 for a full discussion of HDN). Small amounts of blood are removed from the baby and replaced with donor blood until a one or two total blood volume exchange is accomplished. It is necessary to both maintain blood volume and prevent circulatory overload during the procedure.

Exchange transfusion replaces the antibody-coated red blood cells with compatible donor cells and removes bilirubin and circulating maternal antibody from the baby's plasma. A two-volume exchange achieves an 80 to 90% removal of red blood cells and 25 to 35% removal of bilirubin. The small amount of bilirubin removed is due to *extravascular* bilirubin, which is not removed by the procedure and is released into the plasma following the exchange transfusion.

Criteria for performing an exchange include:

1. The degree of anemia
2. The cord blood and plasma bilirubin level
3. The rate of the rise of bilirubin
4. The maturity of the baby

Performing an initial exchange transfusion or subsequent exchanges is based on restoring an adequate red cell volume and removing the product of red blood cell hemolysis, bilirubin. Generally, a bilirubin increase greater than 0.5 mg/dL per hour or a rise of 10 mg/dL in the first 24 hours is an indication for an exchange transfusion. Accumulation of bilirubin in nervous tissue, i.e., the brain, can result in *kernicterus,* which may occur at bilirubin levels of 20 mg/dL or greater in a full-term infant and lower levels in a premature infant. A 3- or 4-day old baby may be able to tolerate much higher levels than a premature infant.

## SELECTION OF BLOOD IN SPECIAL CASES

### Blood Requirements for Exchange Transfusion

Blood for the exchange transfusion of a newborn infant must be negative for the red blood cell antigen to which the mother has the corresponding antibody. It must also be ABO group and RH type compatible with the infant's blood group (Table 9-4). If the mother's specimen is not available, group O red blood cells must be selected. Rh positive blood may be given to an Rh positive infant whenever the mother lacks anti-D. Donor blood should also be negative for hemoglobin S and cytomegalovirus (CMV).

### Blood Needed for Intrauterine Transfusion

Blood for intrauterine transfusion must be as fresh as possible and group O Rh negative. In addition, the red blood cells must be compatible with the mother's specimen. Because viable lymphocytes in the donated blood are capable of causing graft-versus-host disease, irradiated blood should be used (see Chapter 10 for a full discussion of blood products).

**Table 9-4. Selection of ABO Group Compatible for Exchange Transfusion**

| Mother's Group | Infant's Group | Donor Group |
|---|---|---|
| O, A, or B | O | O |
| O or B | A | O |
| A or AB | A | A or O |
| O or A | B | O |
| B or AB | B | B or O |
| A | AB | A or O |
| B | AB | B or O |
| AB | AB | AB, A, B, or O |

## Blood Component Selection in Neonates

### Red Blood Cell Transfusion

Very small premature newborns are among the most heavily transfused patients. Eighty percent of neonates weighing less than 1,500 g born annually in the United States require multiple red blood cell transfusions. Specific indications for red blood cell transfusion include blood replacement, when 5–10% of the estimated total blood volume has been removed for laboratory testing, particularly if hematocrit values have dropped rapidly and/or if mechanical ventilation is required. Neonates with severe respiratory disease requiring oxygen and/or ventilator support are usually maintained at a hematocrit value above 40% and hemoglobin level above 13.0 g/dL. Other clinical indications for red blood cell transfusion include problems presumed to be related to anemia (e.g., tachycardia or failure to thrive).

### Platelet Transfusion

The platelet count of healthy neonates should be 150 × $10^9$/L or greater. Lower platelet counts suggest potential clinical problems (e.g., intracranial hemorrhage); high-risk infants frequently exhibit thrombocytopenia. If the platelet count falls below 50 × $10^9$/L in stable, or below 100 × $10^9$/L in sick, premature neonates, some neonatologists order platelet transfusions. A usual indication is the maintenance of the platelet count above 50 × $10^9$/L in infants with active bleeding, or in those undergoing invasive procedures. Thrombocytopenia is usually caused by accelerated platelet destruction.

### Granulocyte Transfusions

Neonates are susceptible to severe bacterial infections due to quantitative and qualitative abnormalities of neutrophils (PMNs). The absolute blood PMN count is abnormal if it falls below 3.0 × $10^9$/L during the first week of life. The mechanisms responsible for neutropenia during septicemia are believed to be partly attributable to the collective effects of three abnormalities of the bone marrow: decreased PMN production, a small PMN storage pool, and PMN reserves released at an excessively rapid and maybe poorly regulated rate from the marrow storage pool during stress.

### Other Transfusion Considerations

The occurrence of cytomegalovirus (CMV) infection associated with transfusion in neonates is of extreme importance. This blood-borne pathogen (see Chapter 13 for a full discussion) should be a consideration when deciding to transfuse a neonate. The use of special precautions (e.g., CMV seronegative blood or irradiated blood products) in neonates remains controversial.

## Transfusion of Newborn Infants

Newborn infants and recipients under 4 months of age, particularly premature babies, often present problems when transfusion is required. There are important physiologic differences between the newborn and older children or adults. In the newborn infant, it is reasonable, on an immunologic basis, to provide sequential transfusions from the same donor who is antigen-compatible for some of the most immunogenic factors. In general, repeating the crossmatch with the same donor blood is unnecessary for the first 6 weeks of life. Although fresh heparinized blood provides the benefits of high 2,3 DPG levels, clotting factors, platelets, and a more physiologic pH, conventional blood bank units that are less than 1 week old have adequate 2,3 DPG and clotting factors. Clotting and platelets are not needed unless the baby has a bleeding tendency, in which case they can be administered as blood component concentrates.

## Compatibility Testing in Infants under 4 Months

### Screening Protocol

An initial pretransfusion specimen must be tested to determine an infant's ABO group and Rh type. ABO grouping requires testing the infant's red cells with anti-A and anti-B reagents only. The method of testing must include an antiglobulin phase using either reagent or donor red blood cells. Tests for anti-A must use $A_1$ cells. Subsequent testing of an infant's serum or plasma for anti-A and/or anti-B must be conducted under certain conditions. These conditions include the following:

1. If the cells selected for transfusion are not group O
2. If a nongroup-O infant has received blood components containing agglutinins directed against his or her own A and/or B antigens, and if subsequent donor red blood cells selected for transfusion are not group O

The Rh type shall be determined with anti-D typing reagents. Testing for weak D($D^u$) is unnecessary in Rh negative infants.

Repeat testing of infant's ABO grouping and Rh typing may be omitted for the remainder of the infant's hospital admission under specific circumstances. These circumstances include the situation in which all of the red blood cells transfused during that period of time are ABO compatible and are either Rh negative or of the infant's original Rh type.

An infant's initial pretransfusion specimen must be tested for unexpected antibodies. If the initial unexpected antibody screen is negative, repeat testing may be omitted for an infant less than 4 months of age during any one hospital admission. The method of testing for unexpected antibodies in the serum or plasma of either the infant or mother must be able to demonstrate clinically significant antibodies. The method must include 37° C incubation preceding an antiglobulin test using reagent red blood cells that are not pooled. Alternate testing methods may be substituted if appropriate documentation is available.

## Compatibility Protocol

Crossmatching is unnecessary during the remainder of an infant's hospital admission, if certain conditions are met. The list of these conditions include:

1. If no anti-A or anti-B is detected in the infant's serum or plasma
2. If ABO compatible red blood cells are to be transfused even if anti-A or anti-B has been detected
3. If an infant's initial unexpected antibody screen is negative, it is unnecessary to perform an initial or subsequent crossmatches

If an infant's initial antibody screen demonstrates clinically significant unexpected red blood cell antibodies, units must be prepared for transfusion that do not contain the corresponding antigen until antibody is no longer demonstrable in the infant's serum.

## Transfusion Products

Infant recipients must not be transfused with whole blood, plasma, or other blood components that contain clinically significant unexpected antibodies. In the case of infant recipient, several other factors are of importance in the selection of blood products. These factors include:

1. If a recipient of massive or exchange transfusion is hypoxic or acidotic, it may be desirable to transfuse only blood known to lack hemoglobin S.
2. If an infant recipient weighs less than 1200 g at birth, and either the infant or the mother is CMV-antibody negative or the cytomegalovirus (CMV) status is unknown, cellular components should be selected or processed to reduce the risk of transfusion-associated CMV disease.

## Blood Needs of Patients with Cold Antibodies

Antibodies that are inactive below 37° C are of little clinical significance. When the crossmatches are incubated at 37° C (using the prewarming technique), red blood cells containing the antigen will not be agglutinated. If the patient's cold antibody is of a specific type, such as anti-M, antigen negative blood may be selected but is not mandatory.

## Blood Needs of Patients with Warm Autoantibodies

When a patient with a warm autoantibody has to be transfused, the attending physician and blood bank medical director must decide jointly to administer blood that is not truly compatible in vitro. If autoabsorption is used to

decrease the degree of agglutination, the crossmatch report should include the techniques used and the observed results.

## Blood Needs of Patients with a Positive DAT

If a patient has a positive DAT, the following protocol is suggested for deciding whether or not the patient can be transfused.

A patient *can* be transfused if:

1. The unexpected antibody screening test is negative *and*
2. The crossmatched units are compatible *and*
3. There is no history of whole blood or packed red blood cell transfusion in the last three months

Note: The attending physician should be notified. One lavender-top (EDTA) and one red-top tube should be stored in the refrigerator prior to transfusion.

A patient *cannot* be transfused without further consultation if:

1. There is a history of transfusion of whole blood or packed red cells within the last 3 months *or*
2. The unexpected antibody screen is positive *or*
3. The crossmatched units are incompatible

Further steps should be taken as follows:

1. Notify the attending physician to determine the need for transfusion.
   A. If the patient's physician determines that a transfusion is needed as soon as possible (urgently), use the following guidelines:

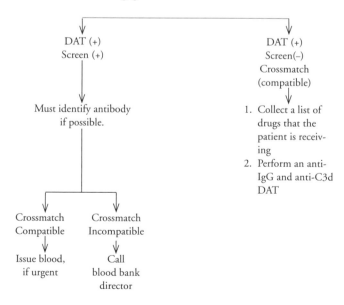

B. Perform an eluate if the patient is hemolyzing red cells and requires a transfusion. Signs of hemolysis include an elevated lactic dehydrogenase (LDH), an elevated bilirubin, and an increased reticulocyte count. Another sign of hemolysis is a decreasing hematocrit over a period of time without overt blood loss. Other guidelines for performing an elution procedure can be found in Table 6-19.

## CHAPTER SUMMARY

### Routine Transfusion Requests

Blood provided by a blood bank is for patients undergoing surgical procedures or for those with acute unexpected blood loss. Other patients may need transfusions to correct anemias. Because the need to eliminate unnecessary crossmatching has been recognized, the type and screen protocol has been developed for specific surgical procedures.

The first requirement for blood selection is the ABO group of the patient. The term "universal donor" often has been applied to group O, Rh negative blood products. There is no such thing as a universal donor. The use of this term for group O individuals is based on the lack of A, B, and D antigen on the erythrocytes. The use of group O does not prevent sensitization of the patient to other blood group antigens that may be missing from their own red cells. The second requirement in the selection of blood is the Rh type of the patient. D is an important antigen because of its immunogenicity and the fact that a person has an 85% chance of receiving Rh positive blood. Although weak D ($D^u$) is less immunogenic than D, $D^u$ positive individuals can produce anti-D. The third requirement is the use of antigen-negative blood in patients in whom an unexpected antibody is detected.

### Emergency Transfusion Situations

Orderly management of a patient requiring urgent blood transfusion requires communication of the severity of the need and the extent of the emergency to the blood bank by the attending physician. When there is a desperate need for blood, uncrossmatched or partially crossmatched blood might be requested by a physician. In these situations, an emergency release form must be completed.

### Massive Transfusion

Massive transfusion is defined as the administration of enough blood or components within less than 24 hours to constitute a complete volume replacement. In an infant, this is slightly more than half a unit and in an adult 8 to 10 or more units.

The first priority in the treatment of candidates for massive transfusion is restoration of blood volume to regain an acceptable blood pressure to enable oxygen and nutrients to be delivered to essential organs and to prevent or halt disseminated intravascular coagulation (DIC). Following expansion of volume, the next priority is the restoration of an adequate level of hemoglobin to ensure that the patient's oxygen-carrying capacity does not drop below the level at which compensation is possible and to remove the strain from the heart caused by the increased demand for cardiac output.

Various adverse situations have been associated with rapid infusion of massive amounts of blood.

Exchange transfusion of a newborn infant is used in treatment of both the anemia and hyperbilirubinemia that characterize hemolytic disease of the newborn. Exchange transfusion replaces the antibody-coated erythrocytes with compatible donor cells as well as removing bilirubin and circulating maternal antibody from the baby's plasma.

### Selection of Blood in Special Cases

Blood for exchange transfusion must be negative for the erythrocyte antigen to which the mother has the corresponding antibody. It must also be ABO and Rh compatible with the infant's blood group. If the mother's specimen is not available, group O erythrocytes must be selected.

Blood for intrauterine transfusion must be as fresh as possible; it must also be group O, Rh negative. The donor unit must be compatible with the mother's specimen. Because viable lymphocytes in the donated blood are capable of causing graft-versus-host disease, irradiated blood should be used.

Newborn infants, particularly premature ones, often present problems when a transfusion is required. It is reasonable, on an immunologic basis, to provide sequential transfusions from the same donor who is antigen-compatible for some of the most immunogenic factors.

Patients with cold-reacting unexpected antibodies may present special problems. Although this type of antibody is considered of no clinical significance, in vitro agglutination can be avoided when a prewarming technique is used. If the patient's cold antibody is a specific type such as anti-M, antigen-negative blood may be selected but is not mandatory.

When a patient with a warm autoantibody has to be transfused, the attending physician and blood bank medical director must jointly decide whether to administer blood that is not truly compatible *in vitro*.

## REVIEW QUESTIONS

**1–4.** Arrange the following requirements in the correct sequence of priority for the selection of blood for a patient.

    **A.** Rh specific

    **B.** ABO group specific

    **C.** Antigen negative blood in patients with an unexpected clinically significant antibody

    **D.** Group O whole blood

    **E.** Major crossmatch ABO-compatible erythrocytes

    **1.** _____

    **2.** _____

    **3.** _____

    **4.** _____

5. Group O, Rh negative blood has several disadvantages when used as "universal donor" blood for a patient of a different blood type. Which of the following is *not* a disadvantage?
   A. Anti-A and anti-B can react with the recipient's erythrocytes
   B. It can prevent switching back to the patient's own blood type
   C. It can provide for the immediate emergency needs of a patient until his/her ABO group is determined
   D. It can produce a shortage of this type of blood

6. The poorest ABO choice of blood for an AB recipient is:
   A. Group A
   B. Group B
   C. Group AB
   D. Group O

7. If a patient is group O and donor blood of the recipient's own type is not available, what other type (or types) can be used as packed erythrocytes?
   A. Group A
   B. Group B
   C. Group AB
   D. None of the above

8. If a patient is group $A_2$ with anti-$A_1$ and donor blood of the recipient's own group is not available, what other type (or types) can be used as packed erythrocytes?
   A. $A_1$
   B. B
   C. $A_1B$
   D. O

9. If a patient is group $A_2B$ with anti-$A_1$ and donor blood of the recipient's own group is not available, what other type (or types) can be used as packed erythrocytes?
   A. $A_2$ or B
   B. $A_1$
   C. $A_2$
   D. B

10. The risk of immunization in the selection of Rh type when transfusing a patient depends on all of the following factors except:
    A. The patient's antigen status
    B. The ABO group of the patient
    C. The immunogenicity of the antigen
    D. The frequency of the antigen in the donor population

11–15. When an urgent request for blood is received, certain procedural steps should be followed. Arrange the following procedural steps in their proper sequence.

A. Determine the patient's ABO and Rh group
B. Complete compatibility testing
C. Identify units of blood that have been partially crossmatched
D. Identify the patient and draw a blood specimen
E. Complete all records and forms

11. _____
12. _____
13. _____
14. _____
15. _____

16. The first evidence of immunization in a patient who has received blood possessing an antigen is:
    A. In vivo hemolysis
    B. Detectable antibody in the patient's serum
    C. A positive direct antiglobulin test
    D. Hemoglobinuria

17. If a group AB, Rh negative patient is admitted with massive bleeding, which of the following units of packed cells would be the *least* desirable to transfuse?
    A. Group O Rh Negative
    B. Group O (D Negative, C Negative, E Positive)
    C. Group O Rh Positive
    D. Group A Rh Negative

18. In an adult, a massive transfusion is defined as the administration of more than _____ units of blood in less than 24 hours.
    A. 2–4
    B. 4–6
    C. 6–8
    D. 8–10

19. Shock symptoms can be caused by the rapid loss of _____% or more blood volume.
    A. 5–10
    B. 10–15
    C. 15–20
    D. 20–25

20. From the list of adverse reactions associated with massive transfusion which of the following does *not* belong on the list?
    A. Citrate toxicity
    B. Permanent change in blood type
    C. Hypocalcemia
    D. Hypothermia

21. The depletion of 2,3 DPG is usually *not* of concern unless one or more of the following is true:
    1. The volume of transfused blood results in an almost complete exchange within a few hours
    2. All or most of the blood has been refrigerated for 1 or 2 weeks

3. All of the units of blood are frozen deglycerolized RBCs
4. The patient lacks the ability to increase cardiac output
   A. Only 1
   B. 1 and 2
   C. Only 3
   D. 1, 2 and 4

22. Bleeding due to impaired platelet function can occur in a massively transfused patient if _____ is rapidly administered.
    A. Albumin
    B. Whole blood
    C. Dextran
    D. Plasma protein fractions

23. The major complication that impairs hemostasis in an uncomplicated case of massive transfusion is:
    A. Thrombosis
    B. Primary fibrinolysis
    C. Accumulation of calcium
    D. Disseminated intravascular coagulation

24. In an exchange transfusion of an infant, a one or two total blood volume exchange is accomplished. How much blood does this represent?
    A. ½ to 1 pint
    B. 1 to 2 pints
    C. 2 to 4 pints
    D. 4 to 8 pints

25. The decision to perform an exchange transfusion in an infant is based on two or more of the following criteria:
    1. The degree of anemia
    2. The maturity of the baby
    3. The cord blood bilirubin level
    4. The infant's circulating plasma bilirubin level
    5. The rate of rise of the circulating plasma bilirubin
    A. 1 and 2
    B. 1, 2, and 3
    C. 3 and 4
    D. All of the above

26. In the selection of blood for exchange transfusion, what characteristic or characteristics apply?
    A. It must be negative for the RBC antigen to which the mother has the circulating antibody
    B. It must be ABO and Rh compatible with the infant's blood group
    C. It can be Group O
    D. All of the above

27. In the case of an exchange transfusion, if the mother is group O or A and the baby is group B, what donor type or types should be selected?
    A. Group A
    B. Group B
    C. Group O
    D. Group O or Group A

28. Blood selected for intrauterine transfusion should be two or more of the following:
    1. Compatible with the mother's blood
    2. As fresh as possible
    3. Group O Rh negative
    4. Irradiated
    5. Enriched with fresh frozen plasma
    A. 1 and 2
    B. 2 and 3
    C. 3 and 4
    D. All of the above, except 5

29. If a newborn infant requires transfusions, which of the following factors is (are) important?
    1. Sequential transfusions from the same donor
    2. Repeating the crossmatch with each transfusion
    3. The use of fresh heparinized blood
    4. The use of bank blood that is less than 1 week old
    5. All of the above
    A. 1 and 2
    B. 1, 3 and 4
    C. Only 3
    D. 3 and 4

30. If a patient has a cold antibody, what consideration or considerations is/are mandatory?
    A. The antibody specificity should be determined
    B. A prewarming technique should be used
    C. The attending physician and blood bank director should decide to administer the blood
    D. The patient's serum should be absorbed with group O cells

## Bibliography

Bordin, G.M.: Transfusion of racially unmatched blood. New Eng. J. of Med., *323*(20):1420, 1990.

Boyd, P.R., Sheedy, K.C., and Henry, J.B.: Type and screen: Use and effectiveness in elective surgery. Am. J. Clin. Path., *73*(5): 694–699, 1980.

Cooper, E.S., and Rodrigue, J.E.: Legal issues in transfusion medicine. Lab. Med., *23*(12):794–796, 1992.

Dodsworth, H. and Dudley, H.A.F.: Increased efficiency of transfusion practice in routine surgery using pre-operative antibody screening and selective ordering with an abbreviated crossmatch. Br. J. Surg., *72*:102–104, 1985.

Huestis, D.W., Bove, J.R., and Busch, S.: Practical blood transfusion, 4th ed. Boston: Little, Brown, 1988, 169–210.

Insalaco, S.J., and Potter, A.R.: Neonatal transfusion therapy. Lab. Med., *16*(3):149–156, 1985.

Kitchens, C.S.: Are transfusions overrated? Surgical outcomes of Jehovah's Witnesses. Am. J. Med., *94*:117–124, 1993.

Kuriyan, M., and Kim, D.U.: The maximum surgical blood order schedule: Choice of methods used in its development. Lab. Med., *19*(3):156–159, 1988.

McMican, A.: Neonatal transfusion therapy. Lab. Med., *19*(6): 353–356, 1988.

Mollison, P.: *Blood transfusion in clinical medicine,* 6th ed. Oxford: Blackwell Scientific Publication, 1979.

Murphy, R.J.C., Malhotra, C., and Sweet, A.Y.: Death following an exchange transfusion with hemoglobin SC blood. J. Ped., *96:* 110, 1980.

Nelson, C.C., Otteson, S.P., and Johnson, R. Massive transfusion. Lab. Med., *22*(2):94–98, 1991.

Oberman, H.A.: Surgical blood ordering, blood shortage situations, and emergency transfusion. *In Clinical Practice of Blood Transfusion.* Edited by L.D. Petz and S.N. Swisher. New York: Churchill-Livingstone, 1981, pp. 393–404.

Perkins, H.A.: Strategies for Massive Transfusion. *In Clinical Practice of Blood Transfusion.* Edited by L.D. Petz and S.N. Swisher. New York: Churchill-Livingstone, 1981, pp. 485–491.

Petz, L., and Swisher, S.N. Blood transfusion in acquired hemolytic anemias. *In Clinical Practice of Blood Transfusion.* Edited by L.D. Petz and S.N. Swisher. New York: Churchill-Livingstone, 1981, pp. 623–661.

Schmidt, P.J.: Rh negative blood. Med. Lab. Observer, February 1990, pp. 84–85.

Shulman, I.A., Morales, J., Nelson, J.M., and Saxena, S.: Emergency blood transfusion protocols. Lab. Med., *20*(3):166–168, 1989.

Strauss, R.G.: Case analysis approach to neonatal transfusions. Lab. Med., *23*(4):239–244, 1992.

Widmann, F.: *Standards for blood banks and transfusion services.* Bethesda, MD. American Association of Blood Banks, 1993.

# 10

# Transfusion Therapy: Blood and Blood Components

At the conclusion of this chapter, the reader should be able to:

- List the components that can be prepared from one unit of whole blood.
- Explain the advantages of whole blood.
- Compare the advantages of red blood cells to whole blood.
- Describe the advantages and disadvantages, the most appropriate clinical applications for whole blood, red blood cells, washed red cells, frozen/deglycerolized, leukocyte-poor red cells, and neocyte-enriched cells.
- State the currently approved FDA approved shelf-life of whole blood drawn into CPDA-1 anticoagulant.
- State the expiration time of packed red blood cells prepared in an open system.
- List at least three techniques for preparing leukocyte-poor blood.
- State the proper storage conditions for platelet concentrates and the maximum pH of stored platelet concentrates.
- State the required minimum percentage and concentration of platelets in random donor platelets.

- Describe the clinically appropriate condition or conditions for granulocyte transfusions.
- Define the term "graft-versus-host disease (GHVD)" and explain the mechanism of this disorder.
- Name at least three blood products that can cause GVHD and describe how GVHD can be prevented.
- Compare the uses and differences between single-donor plasma, fresh-frozen single-donor plasma, and cryoprecipitate.
- Calculate the number of bags of cryoprecipitate needed, given the desired level of factor VIII activity and the patient's plasma volume.
- State the length of time in which a defrosted unit of cryoprecipitate must be given.
- State the major disadvantage of Factor IX complex.
- Compare and contrast the synthetic red blood cell substitutes, and discuss the role of recombinant DNA technology in the production of blood components.

## INTRODUCTION

The collection and refrigerated preservation of whole human blood has been a well-established practice for more than 50 years in the United States. Although it was previously possible to enter glass bottles and remove the plasma from sedimented units, the introduction of plastic bags with attached multiple collection units and high speed

**Table 10-1. Guidelines for Shelf Life, Storage, and Clinical Appropriateness**

| Blood Product | Shelf Life | Storage Temperature | Appropriate Use |
|---|---|---|---|
| Whole Blood | CPDA-1 = 35 days | 1–6° C (storage)<br>1–10° C (transport) | Treatment of cardiopulmonary bypass patients either intraoperatively or up to 6 hours postoperatively |
| Packed Red Blood Cells | CPDA-1 = 35 days | 1–6° C (storage)<br>1–10° C (transport) | Treatment of symptomatic anemia<br>Anemia requiring correction prior to anesthesia |
| Washed Red Blood Cells | CPDA-1 = 35 days (closed system) = 24 hours (open system) | 1–6° C (storage)<br>1–10° C (transport) | Prevention of clinically severe allergic reactions to plasma-containing products in sensitized patients |
| Neocyte-Enriched Red Cells | CPDA-1 = 35 days (closed system) = 24 hours (open system) | 1–6° C (storage)<br>1–10° C (transport) | Treatment of patients who are chronically transfusion dependent (e.g., sickle cell anemia) |
| Leukocyte-Poor* Blood | Not applicable | Not applicable | Treatment of febrile reactions not controlled by anti-pyretic premedication<br>Prevention or to delay the onset of HLA sensitization in chemotherapy patients<br>Lowering the risk of cytomegalovirus infection in neonates who weigh <1200 g or immunosuppressed patients*<br>IgA-deficient recipients |
| Frozen/Deglycerolized Red Blood Cells | Up to 10 years | −80° C | Prevention of nonhemolytic febrile transfusion reactions due to platelets or leukocytes; or plasma allergy; prevention of cytomegalovirus exposures; autologous transfusion |
| Irradiated Blood Components | Same as original blood product | Same as original blood product | Prevention of graft-versus-host disease in patients such as those undergoing ablative chemotherapy (e.g., bone marrow transplant candidates or patients with congenital or acquired cell-mediated immunodeficiencies) |
| Granulocytes | Up to 24 hours | 20–24° C without agitation | Treatment of patients with absolute neutropenia, evidence of progressive infection with hematologic disorders or lack of clinical response to antibiotics with concurrent granulocytopenia |
| Platelets | Up to 7 days | 20–24° C with continuous gentle agitation | Treatment of patients with thrombocytopenia having active bleeding or at risk of bleeding |
| Single-Donor Plasma | CPDA-1 = 40 days<br>Up to 5 years | 1–6° C, if not frozen<br>If −18° C | Treatment of severe burns or hypovolemic shock |
| Fresh Frozen Plasma | 12 months | −18 to −30° C or colder (optimal) | Treatment of some patients with deficiencies for which no concentrates are available; cases of massive transfusion; multiple coagulation factors deficiency |
| Cryoprecipitate | 12 months | −18° C or colder | |

Other human plasma products (see Table 10-3)

* Prepared with a blood filter

temperature-controlled centrifuges made the current practice of blood component therapy a reality.

It is now possible to harvest a variety of blood components from a single unit of whole blood (Table 10-1). The separation of a single unit of whole blood into multiple components has increased the effectiveness of blood utilization from each individual blood donation. The cellular components of whole blood are erythrocytes, leukocytes, and platelets (thrombocytes). The three major classes of whole blood plasma derivatives currently licensed in the United States are coagulation products, such as anti-hemophilic factor (AHF), immune globulins, and plasma volume expanders.

## WHOLE BLOOD

The use of anticoagulated whole blood has been drastically reduced over the past two decades in favor of component therapy. In certain situations, however, all the constituents of whole blood are needed by a patient. Because of the extensive effort to utilize blood components, hospital blood banks may receive up to 99% of red cell units as packed cells rather than whole blood. Under these circumstances, whole blood is frequently not available when needed. Combining components to meet a patient's need for whole blood increases both the risk and cost of transfusion therapy to the patient.

## Clinical Indications

Whole blood is appropriate for use if *both* enhanced oxygen-carrying capacity and blood volume replacement are needed concurrently. Appropriate patients include those with cardiopulmonary bypass, either intraoperatively or up to 6 hours postoperatively. Whole blood is indicated for actively bleeding patients who have lost over 25% of their blood volume i.e., acute massive blood loss. Fresh (less than 24-hour-old) whole blood is now considered unnecessary for the correction of coagulation deficiencies because coagulation Factors V and VIII rapidly deteriorate. Specific components are the more appropriate and safer choice.

## Methods

The collection of blood for use as whole blood or later separation into components is discussed in detail in Chapter 2. The quantity of anticoagulant (63 mL) such as citrate phosphate dextrose (CPD) is appropriate for 450 mL of whole blood. A 10% leeway is permitted in the volume of whole blood; therefore, a unit is considered satisfactory if it contains between 405 and 495 mL of whole blood. Less than 405 mL is unsatisfactory.

## Storage Requirements

Whole blood must be refrigerated *as soon as possible* after collection. The temperature must be maintained at 1 to 6° C during storage and between 1 and 10° C if transported. The length of storage (shelf-life) varies with the type of anticoagulant used. Citrate phosphate dextrose adenine-1 (CPDA-1) has an approved shelf-life of 35 days in most states.

## Advantages

Whole blood carries less risk, particularly of blood-borne diseases, and is more cost-effective than combined component therapy if a bona fide need exists. The administration of packed red blood cells and fresh frozen plasma doubles the patient's risk of exposure to infectious agents and is more costly.

## Disadvantages

Indiscriminate use of whole blood can reduce the availability of components to multiple patients. Additionally, congestive heart failure produced by hypervolemia can occur in patients who are not actively bleeding.

## Special Notes

Whole blood (less than 4 or 5 days old) is the component of choice for exchange transfusion in newborn infants. This ensures plasma electrolyte concentrations that are tolerable for infants and also ensures adequate levels of 2,3 diphosphoglycerate (2,3 DPG).

## RED BLOOD CELL PRODUCTS

### Red Blood Cells

The proper name of this component is (name of anticoagulant) red blood cells. In the interest of better patient care, the use of red cells has actively and effectively replaced whole blood for transfusion. Replacement of whole blood with red cells has been stimulated by the economic benefits of using blood products as components and has been successful.

### Clinical Indications

Patients in need of the oxygen-carrying capabilities of the hemoglobin within red blood cells are candidates for packed red blood cells. Patients with chronic blood loss who cannot compensate for this loss through normal bone marrow replacement mechanisms or erythropoietin therapy and patients who lack normal bone marrow activity are examples of transfusion candidates. Red blood cells are the component of choice for patients who cannot tolerate an increased blood volume (e.g., patients with congestive heart failure).

### Methods

The desirable method of collection of blood for the preparation of packed red blood cells is to use blood collection units with an attached satellite bag. Collection of blood from the donor using this method is the same as collecting an individual unit of whole blood. The unit of whole blood may be allowed to sediment during refrigerated storage or centrifuged at any time up to the expiration date of the whole blood. The separation of plasma from the unit is usually performed during initial processing of the donor unit and must be done within 8 hours of blood collection if fresh frozen plasma containing coagulation factors is desired.

Separation of plasma from the initial collection bag is performed by transferring the plasma from the top of the unit to a satellite bag with the aid of a plasma expressor or plasma separator. The amount of plasma transferred to the satellite bag can be weighed with a scale. Under most circumstances, approximately 225 mL 250 (232–258 g) of plasma are harvested. The red cells remaining in the original collection bag have a packed cell volume (hematocrit) of about 70%. The final packed cell volume must *not* exceed 80%. If units are collected in CPDA-1, the hematocrit should be measured each month on a representative sample to assure a final hematocrit of no more than

80%. Further processing of red cells to produce washed red cells or frozen/deglycerolized red cells may take place.

## Storage Requirements

After the plasma has been harvested, red cells must be stored and transported under the same conditions as whole blood. If the whole blood was collected in CPDA-1, the allowable length of storage is 35 days. Red cells collected and separated in a closed system using integral tubing between the primary and satellite bag and properly refrigerated have the same expiration date as the whole blood from which they were separated, if the hematocrit does not exceed 80%. If the primary container is entered to remove the plasma or the sterility of the system is disrupted, the red cells have a 24-hour expiration. The new date and time of expiration must be noted on the label and in the records.

Storage temperature must be maintained between 1° C and 6° C (1° C–10° C if transported).

## Advantages

Packed red cells minimize circulatory overload because of the reduced volume of the component compared to whole blood. Additionally, the volumes of anticoagulant and electrolytes are reduced.

## Disadvantages

The transfusion of red cells when whole blood is required necessitates additional transfusion of fresh-frozen plasma, resulting in a doubled rate of exposure to blood-borne diseases, such as hepatitis, and foreign antigens. The actual transfusion of packed red cells is slower than whole blood because of the increased viscosity of the component. Additionally, charges to the patient are increased. In this situation, optimal medical care is compromised.

## Special Notes

Rejuvenating depleted 2,3 DPG and ATP to normal levels can be accomplished by incubating stored red cells with a rejuvenating solution. Several types of additive solutions are licensed for use with packed red cells. Some restore or increase red cell levels of 2,3 DPG and/or ATP to normal levels or above by adding substances such as adenine or pyruvate to red blood cells. To date, red cells stored in the anticoagulant preservative additive solutions Adsol (AS-1) or Nutricel (As-3) have not been studied or licensed for use with rejuvenation solutions. Rejuvenation may be performed up to 3 days after the red cells expire, provided they have been stored continuously at 1 to 6° C. One of the major advantages of rejuvenation is that it extends the use of outdated units of autologous blood which are still needed by their donors without incurring the additional cost associated with freezing and deglycerolization of red cells.

Rejuvenated red cells regain normal oxygen transport and delivery characteristics as well as improve post-transfusion survival. After rejuvenation, the red cells may be washed, reconcentrated, and transfused within 24 hours or glycerolized and frozen for later use. Labels must indicate the use of rejuvenating solutions. When additive solutions approved by the FDA are used, storage times and temperatures shall be those approved by the FDA.

## Washed Red Blood Cells

Washed red blood cells are the red blood cells remaining after washing with a volume of comparable solution using a method known to remove almost all of the plasma.

The use of washed red blood cells has declined with the increased availability of deglycerolized red blood cells. This type of component, however, may be requested in special circumstances.

### Clinical Indications

Disorders requiring saline-washed red blood cells are rare. Patients with paroxysmal nocturnal hemoglobinuria or hypersensitivity to plasma protein need red cells devoid of plasma protein. Patients who experience severe allergic reactions to plasma-containing products not controlled by antihistamine premedication are appropriate candidates. Emergency transfusion of group O red cells to a patient of another ABO group may also benefit from the removal of antibodies from the plasma.

### Methods

Packed red cells can be washed by multiple batch processing through centrifugation and decanting of the supernatant saline. It is generally more convenient to use equipment designed for deglycerolization of frozen red cells. The efficiency of washing depends on the amount of saline and the method used.

### Storage Requirements

Washed cells should be stored or transported in the same manner as whole blood. Storage times shall be those approved by the FDA. This preparation must be used within 24 hours if prepared in an open system.

### Advantages

Transfusing washed red cells reduces the incidence of febrile reactions due to leukocytes and platelets. The reduced number of microaggregates because of washing is advantageous to patients with pulmonary dysfunction, cardiopulmonary bypass patients, or recipients of massive transfusion.

Because of the trace amounts of residual protein in washed red cells, the product is almost devoid of plasma proteins, including regular and unexpected antibodies.

This may reduce the incidence of anaphylactic reactions due to plasma proteins or soluble substances in the plasma. Washing also eliminates anticoagulants, unwanted metabolites such as ammonia and accumulated lactic acid (lactate), and electrolytes.

## Disadvantages

Preparation of washed red cells is a time-consuming and labor-intensive process. The additional cost to the patient may not be warranted. Although transfusion reactions associated with leukocytes and platelets may be reduced through the use of washed red cells, the use of this product is not the most efficient way to remove leukocytes. An expanded discussion of leukocyte-poor blood is presented later in this chapter.

### Neocyte-Enriched Blood

In 1978, it was first demonstrated that young red blood cells (*neocytes*) had a longer in vivo survival than unfractionated cells from the same donor population. Neocytes have a significantly longer survival time than transfused mature red cells and pyruvate kinase, an age-dependent red cell enzyme activity that is 1.3 times greater than that of mature red cells.

## Clinical Indications

Because neocytes have an extended in vivo survival time, infusion of these red cells could reduce blood requirements in transfusion-dependent patients, such as those with thalassemia and chronic anemias.

## Methods

Neocytes can be prepared by apheresis or from an ordinary unit of blood. Techniques for isolating neocytes rely on the differences in density between neocytes and more mature red cells. Separation of neocytes with automated equipment from a unit of whole blood is based on the buoyant density of neocytes during centrifugation. When an automated cell processor is used, the larger, less dense red cells are expressed earlier than the older, heavier cells during deglycerolization and/or washing. The first half of the processed unit produces a uniformly younger cell population. The remaining half of the unit consists of older red cells. Units of anticoagulated whole blood must be processed within 24 hours of collection.

## Storage Requirements

Neocyte-rich units of red blood cells must be stored and transported in the same manner as whole blood. This type of product must be used within 24 hours if an open system is used in preparation.

## Advantages

Each mL of erythrocytes theoretically deposits approximately 1 mg of iron in the tissue. A condition referred to as *hemochromatosis* is likely to develop in chronically transfused patients. Transfusion of neocytes with a mean cell age of 30 days and a potential transfused survival of 90 days could reduce the needs of patients with chronic transfusion requirements, thereby reducing the subsequent deposition of iron in the tissues.

With some techniques it is possible to retain platelets, residual red cells, and plasma as transfusion products. This makes the processing of neocytes more economical. The residual fraction of older red cells may be transfused to patients for whom chronic red cell transfusion therapy is not indicated. If leukocytes are initially removed by sedimentation followed by filtration, the resulting product has $99.3 \pm 0.5\%$ of the leukocytes removed.

## Disadvantages

Some investigators suggest that neocyte transfusion does not significantly reduce transfusion requirements; however, considerable interest in this approach remains. Current techniques for neocyte preparation are technically difficult, time-consuming, and expensive. Automated techniques require costly equipment such as a continuous-flow cell separator or cell washer.

### Leukocyte-Poor Blood

The standards for leukocyte reduction in leukocyte-poor blood have been based in the past on the percentage of reduction of leukocytes in a red cell product. From the standpoint of the recipient, the total number of leukocytes received is more significant than the percentage of reduction of the initial leukocyte count. Current AABB standards require retention of 80% of the original red cell mass.

When leukocyte-reduced red blood cells are requested for prevention of febrile, nonhemolytic transfusion reactions, the component should be prepared by a method known to reduce the leukocyte number in the final component to less than $5 \times 10^8$. When intended for other purposes, the component should be prepared by a method known to reduce the leukocyte number in the final component to less than $5 \times 10^6$.

### Clinical Indications

Leukocyte-reduced red blood cell and platelet transfusions are indicated for selected patients who are likely to receive long-term transfusion support, to prevent recurrent febrile reactions in patients whose reactions are not controlled by anti-pyretic premedication, and to prevent or delay HLA sensitization to leukocyte antigens in chemotherapy patients. Leukocyte-depleted transfusions may also be indicated to delay or prevent refractoriness to platelet transfusion and acute lung injury in chemotherapy patients. In addition, transfusions to neonates < 1200 g or to cytomegalovirus may not be transmitted by blood components containing fewer than $10^7$ leukocytes per transfusion.

## Methods

The historical method of buffy coat removal of centrifuged red blood cells by the use of adhesion filters yielded about an 80% reduction in leukocytes. Various strategies have been used to reduce the number of leukocytes in cellular blood components. Components prepared by techniques that are only of historical interest, either because of lack of efficacy or excessive cost, include double-spun, buffy-coat-poor units; saline-washed red blood cells; frozen, deglycerolized red blood cells, and centrifuged red blood cells followed by microaggregate filtration.

Recent technologic advances in leukocyte removal have made it possible to achieve up to a 99.9% reduction in the number of leukocytes in cellular blood components. Third-generation filtration technology (Table 10-2) for leukocyte reduction has demonstrated the superiority of modern blood filters with respect to leukocyte removal and the prevention of alloimmunization. Third-generation filters remove leukocytes by adherence. Most of these filter types are designed for bedside use. Many third-generation filters are not interchangeable for red blood cells and platelets—therefore, each type of filter needs to be reviewed before use to obtain optimal transfusion support.

### Storage Requirements

Leukocyte-poor red cells are stored and transported under the same conditions as whole blood except where the protocol specifies other conditions.

**Table 10-2. Blood Transfusion Filters for Blood Components**

| Generation | Pore Size (microns) | Filter Mechanism | Comments |
|---|---|---|---|
| First | 170–260 | Screen filter | A standard blood filter—removes gross debris; used for all blood components |
| Second | 20–40 | Micropore screen filter | Microaggregate or micropore filter; removes 75–90% of leukocytes; used only for red blood cells |
| Third | Not applicable | Adhesion | An adsorption filter; removes 99–99.9% of leukocytes; used for both red blood cells and platelets |

Adapted from Lane, T. A. et al. Leukocyte reduction in blood component therapy. Annals of Internal Medicine *117*(2):151–162, 1992.

### Advantages

Leukocyte removal is adequate for all but the most highly alloimmunized patients. It is estimated that units of blood containing less than $0.5 \times 10^9$/L leukocytes generally do not cause febrile reactions in alloimmunized patients, but a comparison of the total number of leukocytes remaining in red blood cell preparations processed by various methods can be misleading as an indication of effectiveness in preventing nonhemolytic, febrile transfusion reactions.

### Disadvantages

In patients who have not previously experienced nonhemolytic, febrile reactions due to leukocyte immunization, the cost of product processing is not warranted. Other reasons for using leukocyte-poor blood, such as the prevention of HLA immunization in renal allograft patients or possible reduction in leukocyte-transmitted diseases such as cytomegalovirus, are not warranted in most patients.

## Red Blood Cells Frozen; Red Blood Cells Deglycerolized

The science of cryobiology delves into the events which occur when cells are taken from their normal environmental temperature to temperatures below their freezing point. It is the phase transition of water to ice, when subfreezing temperatures are induced, possibly bringing death to cells. The relationship between low temperature and life remained largely unexplained until 1941, when Luyet and Gehenio published their classic, "Life and Death at Low Temperature." Since that time, great interest has flourished in preservation of cells by freezing. The major contribution brought on by this interest has been frozen red blood cells.

Glycerol, by virtue of its powerful water-binding properties, reduces the degree to which solvent water in biologic systems enters the nonsolvent crystalline ice phase. Glycerolization allows the preservation and extended storage of red cells. The in vivo survival and oxygen-carrying capabilities of the red cells are related to the length of time they are kept in the refrigerator between donation and freezing, not the length of storage at low temperatures. After thawing and deglycerolization, the end product results in the recovery of more than 85% of initial donor's red blood cells, which are largely free of the original plasma, leukocytes, and other formed elements.

### Clinical Indications

Frozen/deglycerolized red cells are advocated in a variety of clinical situations, including:

1. Alloimmunized patients who have previously experienced nonhemolytic febrile transfusion reactions due to leukocytes or platelets.

2. Patients who are allergic to constituents of plasma proteins, such as those with IgA deficiencies.
3. Neonates or immunocompromised patients in whom the threat of exposure to cytomegalovirus exists.
4. Patients who need or desire autologous transfusions.

## Methods

While a protein solution such as plasma does not require control of the freezing rate or a cryoprotective additive, the cellular constituents of blood will not withstand the rigors of freezing and thawing unless a cryoprotective agent is added to the cells. Although many compounds have some cryoprotective capacity, only those which are nontoxic and biologically acceptable were used for the preservation of blood. Some typical cryoprotective additives are glycerol and dimethylsulfoxide (DMSO), which are intracellular additives that penetrate the cell, and glucose and polyvinylpyrrolidone (PVP), which function extracellularly.

The most popular method in current clinical use for freezing human red blood cells requires the intracellular additive glycerol at room temperature in either high or low concentration. The high-concentration method uses a glycerol solution of approximately 45% with the slow freeze-thaw technique. The low-concentration method uses a glycerol solution of approximately 18% for the rapid freeze-thaw technique.

*Freezing Technique.* A unit of anticoagulated whole blood less than 6 days old, except when rejuvenated, is centrifuged. Glycerol is added as a cryoprotectant. The thoroughly mixed, glycerolized red cells are then transferred to a suitable freezer-adapted plastic bag. The entire unit is then placed in a −80° C storage freezer, where cooling takes place over a period of several hours.

*Thawing Technique.* Frozen cells are thawed by agitation in a 35° C water bath for 10 minutes. The protocol for deglycerolization of high glycerol frozen blood is based on Dr. Meryman's concept of using diluent and wash solutions containing sodium chloride in successively decreasing concentrations to control the osmotic stress on the cells.

During the deglycerolization process, the red cells perform a series of gymnastics. In their transition from glycerol to the first saline solution, which is hypertonic, the red cells shrink into tight balls. The cells are then gradually expanded by the introduction of serially weaker salt solutions. The thawed glycerolized cells are continuously exposed to a decreasing gradient hypertonic wash of saline until isotonic conditions are reached using either a batch-wash technique or continuous-flow instrumentation.

The end product will have a final residual glycerol concentration of less than 1% and a supernatant hemoglobin concentration within acceptable range.

This meets the current standard for adequate removal of cryoprotective agents and minimal free hemoglobin in the supernatant solution. In addition, recovery of at least 80% of the original red blood cells following the deglycerolization process and viability of at least 70% of the transfused cells 24 hours after transfusion fulfill regulatory requirements. At the time of preparation of the final component intended for transfusion, the integrally connected tubing must be filled with an aliquot of the component and sealed in such a manner that it will be available for subsequent compatibility testing.

### Storage Requirements

Following deglycerolization, the red cells can be stored and transported under the same conditions as whole blood, but a 24-hour dating restriction must be observed because the bag has been entered.

The expiration date for frozen red blood cells for routine transfusion is 10 years from the date of phlebotomy if stored at −65° C or colder. Shipping frozen blood is possible with use of a suitable styrofoam container containing dry ice that will maintain the proper temperature.

### Advantages

*Reduction of Leukocytes and Platelets.* Nonhemolytic febrile transfusion reactions are most frequently caused by leukocyte antibodies; hence, the administration of a product with a minimal number of leukocytes is the most common application of deglycerolized red cells. Leukocytes given to a sensitive recipient can produce diffuse capillary and endothelial damage, impair function of vital organs, and cause necrosis in tumors. These reactions can be prevented in a direct way by removing leukocytes from the blood to be transfused. The average total leukocyte count in a unit of frozen, deglycerolized red cells washed by continuous flow technique is $0.3 \times 10^9$/L, compared to batch-washed red blood cells with an average total leukocyte count of $8.8 \times 10^9$/L.

In addition to the prevention of nonhemolytic, febrile transfusion reactions, the intentional transfusion of 5 units of deglycerolized red cells prior to cadaver renal allografting provides the optimum benefit for graft survival and renal function. Intentional transfusions of previously frozen cells are given, even if the hemoglobin level of the transplant candidate would not otherwise warrant transfusion in these cases at Massachusetts General Hospital, Boston. There is also a very low incidence of HLA antibody formation, a complication that could significantly reduce the number of potentially compatible kidney donors.

Because platelets are also reduced in deglycerolized red cells, the prevention of nonhemolytic, febrile transfusion reactions in patients with platelet antibodies is another advantage of this blood product. Platelet antigen sensitization may also be decreased. Transfusing red cells that have a very low risk of subsequent HLA antibody formation is the optimum initial therapy for patients who need red cells earlier in their illness and who may later need platelets, for example, leukemia patients.

***Plasma Protein Removal.*** The removal of plasma proteins is another one of the assets of deglycerolized red cells. The incidence of febrile transfusion reactions may be reduced or eliminated in patients who exhibit sensitivity to plasma proteins. Plasma removal is particularly important to IgA-deficient patients who have been previously immunized to IgA. In patients with classical hemophilia with anti-factor VIII antibodies, an anamnestic increase in antibody titers can occur if they are given whole blood or conventional red cells. Additionally, patients with paroxysmal nocturnal hemoglobinuria can experience hemolytic episodes if they are transfused with complement contained in the plasma of whole blood or packed cells.

Through the removal of plasma proteins which contain naturally occurring isoagglutinins and may include alloantibodies, a twofold benefit is gained. The passive transmission of antibodies is reduced by removing most of the plasma protein. In special circumstances, the transfusion of group O cells to patients of other ABO blood groups is safer.

### Reduction or Removal of Viruses

HEPATITIS. Although post-transfusion hepatitis was previously reported following the transfusion of deglycerolized red cells from unscreened donors, it appears that the rates of incidence and severity of post-transfusion hepatitis were considerably lower than the rates observed following the administration of conventional whole blood or red cells.

The mechanism by which the hepatitis virus was eluted or inactivated was unknown. It is presumed that the virus was physically displaced from within and without the red cell membrane through the washing process.

CYTOMEGALOVIRUS (CMV). CMV infections can be transmitted by blood transfusion. In one study, 52% of 72 patients with a history of multiple transfusions demonstrated CMV antibodies (seroconversion) in an average of 8 weeks after transfusion. Attempts to grow CMV from deglycerolized red cells have been unsuccessful.

A very low incidence of CMV infections has been observed in the newborn nursery among babies with respiratory distress syndrome who have been transfused with only deglycerolized group O, Rh-compatible red cells on a routine basis to prevent iatrogenic anemia. In evaluating the prevention of transfusion-acquired CMV and its severity in neonates, it was found that no infant in either group receiving seronegative (CMV antibody negative) blood developed a transfusion-acquired CMV infection. The incidence of transfusion-associated CMV infections among infants receiving CMV antibody positive blood was 32.4%. This data supports the concept that the use of deglycerolized red cells or CMV antibody negative blood prevents transfusion-acquired CMV infections. The use of deglycerolized red cells is preferred to screening donors for CMV antibody in an effort to prevent transfusion-acquired CMV infection.

***Autologous Transfusion.*** Frozen red cells make autologous transfusion more practical. Receiving one's own blood is the only sure method of eliminating the possibility of antigenic exposure and acquisition of a blood-borne infectious disease, such as hepatitis or HIV.

Long-term preservation is useful for patients who have previously experienced major problems in crossmatching their blood, such as those with antibodies to high-incidence, red cell antigens or those with extremely rare blood types. Storage of 5 units is generally recommended because the amount is great enough to be useful but not enough to occupy excessive freezer space. Frozen autologous blood storage is recommended for patients who are not expected to have crossmatching problems but who have an elective surgical procedure with predictable blood usage planned in the future. If a person's red cell status is normal, any amount of blood can be donated for frozen storage.

Autologous donation programs have been initiated for pregnant women, children, and adolescents but must be conducted with extreme care under a physician's supervision. The concept of autologous frozen blood has been applied to patients with sickle cell anemia. Long-term cryopreservation of sickle (HbSS) red cells opens the possibility of exploring autologous transfusion to treat sickle cell disease patients during anemic episodes that are not due to sickling. Cryopreserved hemoglobin SS-containing red cells retain their capacity to sickle and therefore are not expected to be of benefit in treating vascular complications of sickling. In vitro red cell losses due to freezing, thawing and deglycerolization are greater than in normal (HbA) red cells; however, the remaining thawed red cells have metabolic characteristics and intravascular survival similar to those of fresh hemoglobin S red cells. Because of the elimination of antigenic exposure and blood-borne infectious disease, deglycerolized red cells could prove useful for autologous transfusion of selected sickle cell anemia patients when they are severely anemic due to a complication not directly related to sickling.

***Maintenance of 2,3 DPG and ATP levels.*** Freezing successfully prevents depletion of both the oxygen-carrying capabilities and energy levels of red cells. This is demonstrated by the fact that 2,3 DPG and ATP levels in red cells are not significantly lowered when measured after freezer storage. Red cell survival in deglycerolized units stored for 48 hours averages 87.8%, and at 72 hours it averages 81.4%. Rejuvenated units have an average survival of 82.5% at 72 hours. The average DPG at 72 hours is 7.2 $\mu$mol/g Hgb for nonrejuvenated blood and 13.7 $\mu$mol/g Hgb for rejuvenated blood. This characteristic is an advantage when considering long-term storage of rare types and surplus blood because of seasonal fluctuation in blood donations.

***Elimination of Anticoagulants and Metabolites.*** Another benefit of frozen deglycerolized red cells is the elimination of anticoagulants and lactic acid. The potassium content of the resuspended cells is consistently low. These characteristics are helpful in the clinical care of patients with uremia, congestive heart failure, and the metabolic derangements that take place during multi-unit transfusions.

## Disadvantages

The high cost of a unit of deglycerolized red cells is the most frequently cited disadvantage; another is the limited 24-hour expiration time.

## Special Notes

It may be desirable to refreeze thawed units. The current AABB standards do not address refreezing thawed units because this should not be considered routinely desirable practice. However, if a high-priority blood unit is inadvertently thawed and/or deglycerolized, the physician responsible for the blood bank may sanction the refreezing of the unit. In cases of refreezing, documentation of the valuable nature of the unit and the reasons for refreezing must be recorded.

# PLATELETS

## Fresh Random Donor or Pooled Platelets

The introduction of blood platelets as a blood component became possible when plastic whole-blood donor collection bags with multiple satellite containers became available in the late 1960s. This technology permitted the separation, storage, and transport of platelet concentrates to be used as readily available blood bank components. Collection by cytopheresis is also possible.

## Clinical Indications

Patients with severe thrombocytopenia or platelet dysfunction with symptoms of bleeding are candidates for platelet concentrate transfusions to induce hemostasis or prevent intracranial bleeding and catastrophic hemorrhage in other organ systems. Severe thrombocytopenia is defined quantitatively as a platelet count less than $20 \times 10^9$/L. Conditions associated with severely decreased platelet counts include:

1. Bone marrow failure in conditions such as aplastic anemia.
2. Bone marrow suppression in patients receiving chemotherapy or radiation therapy.
3. Bone marrow replacement by malignant cells, as in acute leukemia or myeloid metaplasia.
4. Platelet consumption disorders.
5. Massive volume replacement for severe traumatic bleeding.
6. Abnormal platelet function.

Leukemia patients are frequent recipients of platelet concentrate transfusions. The Platelet Transfusion Subcommittee of the Acute Leukemia Task Force suggests platelet transfusion under the following circumstances:

1. Treatment of hemorrhage, including any overt bleeding such as epistaxis or hematuria.
2. Suspected or proven internal bleeding (intracranial, intracutaneous, or intramuscular).
3. If the risk of hemorrhage is high because the platelet counts falls below $10 \times 10^9$/L.

However, platelet transfusion therapy should be tailored to the individual patient, and rigid thresholds for transfusion mistakenly assume that all patients carry the same risk of bleeding at all times.

Contraindications for this form of therapy include conditions in which the likelihood of benefit is remote (e.g., patients with demonstrated platelet refractoriness); other examples include stable patients with thrombotic thrombocytopenic purpura and patients with heparin-induced thrombocytopenia.

## Methods

Platelets survive poorly in stored refrigerated blood, therefore, whole blood is kept at room temperature (20 to 24° C) before separation. Platelets must be separated from whole blood within 8 hours after collection in an anticoagulated, primary donor unit with two satellite bags. Platelet-rich plasma (PRP) must be separated from whole blood by centrifugation within 8 hours after phlebotomy.

The unit of whole blood is first centrifuged at a low speed to separate PRP into the upper portion and red cells into the lower portion of the initial collection bag. The PRP is then expressed with a manual plasma extractor into an attached satellite bag, leaving the red cells in the original primary bag. This unit is usually separated from the satellite bags and labeled as packed red cells.

The remaining attached bags are recentrifuged at a high speed to produce an aggregated platelet button from the PRP. With a plasma extractor, approximately 200 mL of platelet-poor plasma is removed, leaving 50 mL of platelet-poor plasma with the platelet button. The 200 mL of plasma may be used as a single-donor unit of recovered plasma or fresh frozen plasma. The bag containing the platelet button and 50 mL of plasma is separated and allowed to rest undisturbed for an hour at room temperature to enhance platelet disaggregation. The platelets are then placed on a mechanical rotator to gently resuspend the platelet button. Most of the platelets from the whole blood unit are present in the platelet concentrate, which must be continuously agitated until used.

In addition to the labor-intensive process of recovering platelets from single units of anticoagulated blood, platelets may be collected by hemapheresis. Individual units of platelets from a unit of whole blood, also referred to as *random-donor platelets,* usually contain from 6 to 8 $\times$ $10^{10}$ platelets per bag. Regulations, however, require that 75% of the sampled units contain a minimum of 5.5 $\times$ $10^{10}$ platelets per bag at the maximal storage time or at the time of use. Units of random-donor platelets are normally suspended in about 50 mL of plasma to maintain a pH of 6.0 or greater throughout the storage period. Platelets harvested from a single donor by pheresis must contain a minimum of 3 $\times$ $10^{11}$ platelets in at least 75% of the units tested. These platelets are suspended in about 200 mL of plasma per bag.

Platelets prepared from individual units of whole blood are generally pooled in batches of 6–10 units prior to transfusion to adult patients (1 unit/10 kg). The disadvantage of pooled platelets compared to platelets from a single-donor source is the exposure of the patient to more donors. This increase of exposure increases the risk to the patient of antigen sensitization and development of infectious diseases.

In facilities that regularly prepare platelets, quality assurance procedures must include measurement of the platelet count, pH, and plasma volume of 4 units per month. These measurements should be conducted at the end of the allowable storage period or at the time of use. The pH must be 6.0 or greater in all units tested at the end of the storage period. In addition, units with grossly visible platelet aggregates after storage must not be used.

## Storage Requirements

*Length of Time.* The introduction of new types of plastic collection bags has produced extensive testing of platelet storage. Guidelines for testing platelets for transfusion indicate that platelets stored or processed with experimental techniques should be tested by a battery of laboratory procedures, observation of the hemostatic efficacy in patients, and determination of circulating survival time. These guidelines expedited approval by the FDA of second-generation platelet containers, which extended storage time from 3 to 5 days.

These new plastic bags optimize oxygen and carbon dioxide exchange and can be stored for as long as 7 days. The most important concern is maintenance of the pH at greater than 6.0 to prevent loss of viability, which signals an irreversible change in the shape of platelets from a normal disc to spiny spheres. The pH at maximum platelet storage depends on many factors:

1. The anticoagulant in which the initial whole blood is collected.
2. The method of preparation.
3. The surface area and thickness of the storage container.
4. The type of plastic used.
5. The concentration of platelets and volume of plasma.
6. The adequacy of agitation.
7. The storage temperature.

It has become possible to lengthen platelet storage time from 3 to 5 days because increased oxygen permeability of 25% was produced by decreasing the thickness of the plastic film or increasing the size of the second-generation bags. However, if the platelets do not get enough oxygen, oxidative phosphorylation is blocked and the platelets accelerate their production of lactic acid threefold through glycolysis. Under low oxygen conditions, there is complete utilization of glucose, the pH is less than 6.0, and all the platelets assume the nonviable spiny sphere form. If the pH of the platelet concentrate rises above 7.3, there may be some loss of viability.

*Temperature.* Differences in pH, platelet count, morphology score, osmotic recovery, and release of lactic dehydrogenase (LDH) during storage have all been shown to be related to storage time, temperature, type of plastic storage bag, and type of agitation. Ideally, platelets should be stored at the lowest temperature compatible with normal survival to reduce metabolic requirements. Few studies of the viability of platelet concentrates stored at temperatures other than room temperature (20–24° C) and 4° C have been performed.

Present practice is to store platelet concentrates at room temperature with continuous gentle agitation. When platelet concentrates were stored for 3 days in conventional plastic bags, the difference in the mean life span after storage at 21° C was significantly different from that after storage at 18° C. Platelet viability is compromised after storage for 3 days at 18° C and possibly at 19.5° C, and this illustrates the need for quality control of temperature during short-term platelet storage. Reduction in viability after storage at lower temperature is correlated with a reduction in the number of normal discoid platelets. Cold storage of platelets (1 to 6° C) is allowed by the FDA and has been observed to provide immediate hemostasis. However, after 48 hours they irreversibly lose their discoid shape and cannot reassemble their microtubules.

Because no studies have evaluated the effectiveness of platelet storage at temperatures other than room temperature in second-generation plastic bags, it would be prudent to store platelets collected in these containers at a temperature close to 22° C. This is particularly true for blood banks that store platelets in an open room where "room temperature" may be poorly controlled and exposure to temperatures below 20 or 21° C may occur.

AABB standards requires that the temperature be recorded at least every 4 hours during platelet storage. The most desirable platelet storage temperature is 20 to 24° C, but core temperatures during shipping vary. Studies have demonstrated that single styrofoam containers with a coolant maintain the core temperature best.

*Agitation.* Agitation of cold-stored platelets causes clumping and rapid loss of cellular viability. Units with grossly visible platelet aggregates after storage should not be issued for transfusion. The optimum method of storing platelet concentrates for transfusion is not known; therefore, they are stored in various types of plastic bags and on different types of agitators at 20 to 24° C. Although platelet storage requires some form of continuous gentle agitation, the best type of agitation is unknown. There is little in vivo data showing that a particular mode of agitation is better when used with one type of plastic bag than with another.

The storage of platelet concentrates for 5 days on a 6 rpm elliptical rotator is the least desirable method of storage; all other combinations gave acceptable and similar results. These modes of agitation were a 1 rpm elliptical rotator and 2 or 6 rpm circular rotators.

## Advantages

A platelet concentrate prepared from a single unit of whole blood can elevate a patient's platelet count by 5 to 12 $\times$ $10^9$/L in 1 to 2 hours after infusion. The total dose of platelets required for a patient depends not only on the degree of thrombocytopenia but also on the patient's size and factors such as the presence of fever, sepsis, splenomegaly, and platelet antibodies.

A guideline for the effectiveness of the transfusion of platelets is to calculate a *corrected count increment* 1 hour after infusion. The following formula is used:

$$\text{Corrected count increment} = \frac{\left(\begin{array}{c}\text{Post-} \\ \text{transfusion} \\ \text{platelet count}\end{array} - \begin{array}{c}\text{Pretransfusion} \\ \text{platelet count}\end{array}\right) \times \begin{array}{c}\text{Body Surface} \\ \text{Area}\end{array} (m^2)}{\begin{array}{c}\text{Approximate total number of platelets infused} \\ \text{or number of units transfused} \\ \text{(multiple of } 10^{11})\end{array}}$$

A CCI of >4000–5000 if the number of units transfused is used or >7000–10,000 if the total number of platelets used are the reference values.

Another system for calculating transfusion effectiveness is the *percent recovery*. This formula, which takes splenic pooling into account by using the factor of 2/3, is:

$$\text{Percent recovery} = \frac{\left(\begin{array}{c}\text{Post-} \\ \text{transfusion} \\ \text{platelet count}\end{array} - \begin{array}{c}\text{Pretransfusion} \\ \text{platelet count}\end{array}\right) \times \text{Blood Volume}}{\text{Approximate total number of platelets infused} \times \frac{2}{3}}$$

The expected recovery of platelets is 60% at 1 hour and 40% at 24 hours. If a patient fails to demonstrate the expected platelet response, a refractory state should be suspected.

## Disadvantages

Various adverse reactions can result from the transfusion of platelet concentrates, including:

1. Bacterial contamination.
2. Transmission of viral blood-borne diseases such as hepatitis or AIDS.
3. Transmission of parasitic diseases, such as malaria, due to red blood cell contamination.
4. Pulmonary edema caused by plasma volume if more than 10 units are administered to a patient with poor cardiac status.
5. Febrile or allergic reactions caused by plasma proteins.
6. Anaphylaxis in IgA-deficient recipients.
7. Febrile reactions caused by leukocyte contamination.
8. Graft-versus-host disease in immunocompromised recipients if many viable lymphocytes are present in the concentrate.

## Special Notes

The donor plasma in platelets should be ABO compatible with the recipient's red blood cells, especially when the component is to be transfused to infants. The crossmatch requirement can be waived if the component is prepared by a method that is expected to result in a component containing less than 5 mL of red blood cells.

Platelets prepared by cytapheresis must be crossmatched with a major crossmatch that demonstrates ABO incompatibility and unexpected clinically significant antibodies, and an anti human globulin (AHG) test, unless previous testing demonstrated no such antibodies. In such a case, only ABO compatibility needs to be demonstrated. Donor red blood cells for crossmatching may be obtained from a properly identified sample collected at the time of phlebotomy.

Platelet transfusions from donors mismatched for crossreactive HLA antigens provide hemostasis and platelet survival equivalent to HLA-matched platelets in patients without platelet-specific antibodies. If HLA-matched platelets are unavailable from a family member, most hemapheresis programs choose donors for immunized patients with alloantibodies based on the recipient's HLA typing. However, even with fully HLA-matched platelets, 6 to 39% of platelet transfusions are unsuccessful. Patients negative for HLA-A2 antigens, however, have a better response to single-donor platelets with major mismatches than those who possess the HLA-A2 antigen.

In addition to HLA typing, many programs include a screening test for lymphocytotoxicity (HLA) antibody to determine the degree of sensitization to the general population. Donor selection does not usually include a crossmatch, which uses patient serum against donor lymphocytes because the crossmatch procedure is believed to be a poor predictor of platelet survival giving high false positive and high false negative results (accuracy ranges from 30 to 75%).

## Frozen Platelets

### Clinical Indications

Patients with severe thrombocytopenia and bleeding or who are at a high risk of hemorrhage are candidates for platelet transfusions. Frozen units of platelets may be useful as autologous units or when fresh units are unavailable.

### Methods

Platelets have been frozen using the cryoprotective agent, DMSO, and stored in the vapor phase of liquid nitrogen ($-120°$ C) for as long as 3 years before inducing effective hemostasis. However, the freeze-thaw process causes a loss of 30 to 40% of the platelets, and about 50% of the platelets infused are in the nonviable form. Additionally, frozen platelets showed considerable structural damage, with 33% balloon forms counted after thawing as compared to less than 1% before freezing.

### Advantages

Frozen autologous platelet concentrates have been used to support leukemic platelets during thrombocytopenic periods, and in patients undergoing intensive chemotherapy for solid tumors. The use of frozen autologous platelets reduces alloimmunization and transfusion-related infections and provides platelets when needed. Frozen allogeneic platelets are also potentially useful. Freezing platelets from HLA-matched donors for alloimmunized patients would minimize the inconvenience to the donors, and frozen platelets from healthy donors could be used during emergencies.

### Disadvantages

Fresh platelets provide significantly better 1- and 24-hour corrected increments than frozen autologous platelets. To achieve the same effect as 1 unit of fresh, single-donor platelet pheresis product, 2 frozen units are necessary.

## GRANULOCYTES

### Clinical Indications

Leukocyte concentrates, primarily neutrophils, may be of value to patients with severe neutropenia who have a life-threatening systemic infection uncontrolled by antibiotics. Patients who would most frequently be considered appropriate candidates are those with neutropenia induced by chemotherapy or radiation therapy.

### Methods

Granulocyte concentrations are prepared by leukapheresis. Preparation of granulocyte concentrations from single units of whole blood does not produce a sufficient quantity to be of therapeutic value. The component shall contain a minimum of $1.0 \times 10^{10}$ granulocytes in at least 75% of the units tested.

### Storage Requirements

The present AABB standards specify that granulocytes be stored at 20 to 24° C without agitation for up to 24 hours. Although granulocytes may be stored for up to 24 hours, it is best to transfuse them as soon as possible after collection.

#### Factors Related to the Storage of Leukocytes

Recent studies have shown that after 8 hours of storage, granulocytes have a reduced ability to circulate, and migrate to a site of inflammation. When neutrophilic granulocytes (PMNs) are stored for 24 hours, several changes take place:

1. Decreased receptor affinity for chemotactic substances, associated with excessive hydrogen ion accumulation, particularly in units with a high concentration of leukocytes.
2. Decreased adherence properties.
3. Defective energy metabolism and glycogenolysis.

Storage of neutrophils produces a reduction in intracellular ATP levels, especially if the units are stored at 6° C. Because glycogen is the chief metabolic fuel source for phagocytosis and a facultative source for chemotaxis, alterations in the content or metabolism of glycogen in stored PMNs might cause impaired ATP maintenance and functional defects observed in the cells. Neutrophils (PMNs) stored at high concentration are particularly susceptible to depletion of ATP. Maintaining the intracellular ATP levels in stored leukocytes by adding bicarbonate buffer prevents reduction of ATP and aids maintenance of chemotactic function. Chemotactic impairment, observed in neutrophils stored for 24 hours in high concentrations, may be partially due to proteolytic autolysis.

PMNs stored for 48 hours, regardless of concentration, have defective degranulation of both primary and secondary granule contents. These cells have a defective capacity to degranulate in response to inflammatory stimuli.

### Advantages

In patients at high risk of death due to an overwhelming bacterial infection that is uncontrollable through drug therapy, leukocyte transfusions may be of value.

### Disadvantages

The major impediment to storage of granulocyte concentrates for transfusion is rapid impairment in the ability of the neutrophilic granulocytes to migrate toward inflammatory stimuli, both in vitro and in vivo. Although storage at room temperature is preferable to 6° C storage for the maintenance of chemotactic function, and maintaining pH may optimize chemotactic function, efforts to maintain chemotaxis of PMNs after storage have been largely unsuccessful. The major reason for impaired chemotaxis of stored granulocytes is still unknown and requires further investigation.

## Special Notes

Although lymphocytes freeze well when glycerolized, granulocytes are extremely sensitive to the freezing/thawing process. This property of granulocytes restricts the freezing of these cells with present technologies. Only a few centers still advocate the therapeutic use of granulocyte concentrates obtained from patients with CML. All white cell units derived from CML donors should be irradiated to prevent GVHD. However, if the goal is transient myeloid engraftment, CML leukocytes that are *not* irradiated should be used.

In the administration of granulocytes, micro-aggregate filters of the depth type should not be used in the administration set.

The red blood cells in granulocytes shall be ABO compatible with the recipient's plasma. Granulocytes must be crossmatched unless the method is expected to result in a component containing less than 5 mL of red blood cells. The donor red blood cells for the crossmatch may be obtained from a properly identified sample.

## IRRADIATED BLOOD AND BLOOD COMPONENTS

Since animal experiments in the mid-1950s, it has been known that the infusion of immunocompetent lymphocytes into animals with impaired immunity can lead to engraftment of donor cells, with an intense and frequently fatal immunologic reaction of engrafted cells against the host, or graft-versus-host disease. A similar graft-versus-host reaction was subsequently described in susceptible human recipients.

Graft-versus-host disease (see Chapter 12, Transfusion Reactions, for a full discussion of graft-versus-host disease) is caused by the proliferation of mature donor-derived T lymphocytes in response to major and minor histocompatibility antigens in the host. The time needed for the disease to develop and the clinical manifestations of acute post-transfusion graft-versus-host disease are nearly identical to those of severe acute post-transplantation graft-versus-host disease, and their etiology has been assumed to be the same.

Graft-versus-host disease can occur after the transfusion of blood or various blood products, including:

1. Fresh and stored whole blood.
2. Packed red cells stored for as long as 12 days.
3. Buffy coat—poor or washed red cells.
4. Platelet concentrates.
5. Granulocyte concentrates.
6. Single units of fresh plasma.

Although graft-versus-host disease has not been reported after transfusion of frozen/deglycerolized red cells, a small number of viable lymphocytes may remain after deglycerolization and washing. Although processing frozen blood removes up to 95% of leukocytes, the remaining mononuclear cells can undergo normal blast transformation and mitotic activity in vitro.

The occurrence of graft-versus-host disease after transfusion of noncellular frozen blood products such as fresh frozen plasma (FFP) or cryoprecipitate has not been documented. Because no cryoprotective agent is used with these components, the final product is not expected to contain viable leukocytes; therefore, a graft-versus-host response is not expected in susceptible hosts.

The risk of graft-versus-host disease can be minimized by irradiating whole and various other components immediately before infusion. Studies are currently being conducted to evaluate the efficacy of irradiating blood and components before storage. Prophylactic irradiation of whole blood products and components before transfusion is presently the most efficient way to prevent post-transfusion graft-versus-host disease. In patients with post-transfusion graft-versus-host disease, approximately 90% die of acute complications of the disease, usually infection.

## Clinical Indications

The infusion of lymphocyte-containing whole blood or blood components presents the risk of inducing graft-versus-host disease from the infused lymphocytes to patients who are immunosuppressed or have severe immunodeficiency disorders. Irradiation of these components can reduce this risk.

### High-Risk Patients

Patients at the highest risk, with an absolute need for irradiated blood products, include:

1. Recipients of autologous or allogeneic bone marrow grafts. Recipients of autologous bone marrow may be expected to have the same risk of post-transfusion graft-versus-host disease as patients receiving allogeneic bone marrow.
2. Children with severe congenital immunodeficiency syndromes involving T lymphocytes. The degree of immunodeficiency in the host, rather than the number of transfused immunocompetent cells, determines whether graft-versus-host disease will occur.
3. Donations to immunocompetent first-degree relatives.

## Intermediate-Risk Patients

Patients considered to be at less risk of developing graft-versus-host disease include:

1. Infants receiving intrauterine transfusions followed by exchange transfusions and possibly infants receiving only exchange transfusions. The immune mechanism of the fetus and newborn infant may not be sufficiently mature to reject foreign lymphocytes, and previous transfusions may induce a state of immune tolerance in the newborn. Transfused lymphocytes may continue to circulate for a prolonged time in some immunologically tolerant hosts without the development of graft-versus-host disease. There is insufficient evidence to recommend irradiation of transfused blood in all premature infants.

2. Patients receiving total body radiation or immunosuppressive therapy for disorders such as lymphoma and acute leukemia. Although routine irradiation of blood products given to these patients can be justified, it cannot be regarded as absolutely indicated because the risk of developing graft-versus-host disease is so small. However, blood product irradiation is advised for selected patients with hematologic malignancies, especially when transfusions are given at or near the time of sustained and severe therapy-induced immunosuppression.

## Lowest-Risk Patients

Patients who are also at risk but are considered to be the least susceptible are:

1. Patients with solid tumors. The incidence of the development of graft-versus-host disease is difficult to determine. However, in nonhematologic malignancies such as neuroblastoma, the disease has developed. In one case, it developed after the infusion of a single unit of packed red cells.

2. Patients with aplastic anemia receiving anti-thymocyte globulin may theoretically be at increased risk of post-transfusion graft-versus-host disease during therapy-induced periods of lymphocytopenia.

3. AIDS patients. Although a theoretic risk of post-transfusion graft-versus-host disease may exist in patients with AIDS, the disease has not actually been observed in this disorder, and routine use of irradiated blood is not recommended.

4. Recipients of donor units known to be from a blood relative.

## Methods

A self-contained commercially available cesium[137] source is the most commonly used method of irradiating blood components. Quality control of irradiation equipment is essential to monitor the decay of the cesium source, which influences the length of time a unit is exposed to radiation.

Once a unit has been exposed to a certain radiation dose and then removed from the source, it is not radioactive. Irradiated blood does not pose a threat of potential radiation exposure to staff members manipulating it or to patients to whom it is administered. If an irradiated unit is no longer needed for the intended recipient, it may be transfused safely to another patient who does not necessarily require such a special component. Blood and cellular components should be irradiated with a minimum of 25 Gy (2500 cGy) in order to reduce the risk of graft-versus-host disease.

An alternate solution to providing quantities of irradiated blood is irradiating the units before storage. This requires packing red blood cells drawn into CPDA-1 to a hematocrit of 75 ± 1% and irradiating at 4000 cGy on the day of donation. Analysis was conducted every 7 days. Irradiation caused a slight decrease in red cell ATP and 2,3 DPG and a slight increase in plasma hemoglobin compared to the controls. Methemoglobin, pH, and glucose consumption were identical to those of the nonirradiated controls. The evidence indicates that irradiation did not cause biochemical or metabolic changes in the red cells or differences between irradiated and nonirradiated stored red cells in function or viability.

## Storage Requirements

Whole blood or blood components should be stored in the manner required for each specific component, whether or not the product is irradiated.

## Effects of Radiation on Specific Cellular Components

### Lymphocytes

Ionizing radiation is known to inhibit lymphocyte mitotic activity and blast transformation. Irradiation of normal donor lymphocytes with 1500 cGy from a cesium[137] source causes a 90% reduction in mitogen-stimulated [14]C-thymidine incorporation. An 85% reduction in mitogen-induced blast transformation after exposure to 1500 rad and a 97 to 98.5% reduction in mitogenic response were noted after exposure to 5000 cGy.

### Granulocytes

Ionizing radiation may impair granulocyte function, and this impairment is dose-dependent. The degree of actual damage to granulocytes is controversial. Chemotactic activity decreased linearly with increasing doses of irradiation, from 500 to 120,000 cGy, but the reduction only reached statistical significance at 10,000 cGy. A linear dose-response curve demonstrates that granulocyte locomotion is affected by very small doses of irradiation. A dose of 2000 cGy is likely to eliminate lymphocytic mitotic activity and prevent graft-versus-host disease without causing significant damage to granulocytes or altering their chemotactic or bactericidal ability. Irradiation prior to transfusion has been demonstrated to contribute to defective oxidative metabolism, but this effect is highly variable.

### Mature Red Blood Cells

Mature red cells appear to be highly resistant to radiation damage. After exposure to 10,000 cGy, $^{52}$Cr-labeled in vivo red cell survival was the same as that of untreated controls. In 1981, Button showed that stored red cells could be treated with up to 20,000 cGy without changing their viability or in vitro properties, including ATP and 2,3 DPG levels, plasma hemoglobin, and potassium ions.

### Platelets

Ionizing radiation may impair platelet function. Although this impairment is dose-dependent, the effect of irradiation on platelets has been difficult to characterize. Several studies have demonstrated unchanged in vivo platelet survival after exposure to 5000 to 75,000 cGy. A 33% decrease in the expected platelet count increase was noted after transfusion of platelets exposed to 5000 cGy, and similarly irradiated autologous platelets had a diminished ability to correct the bleeding times in a small number of volunteers who had consumed aspirin. In one study, platelet aggregation was not affected by exposure to 5000 cGy, but an impaired response to collagen was noted.

## Advantages

Blood product irradiation is believed to be the most efficient and probably the most economical method available to prevent post-transfusion graft-versus-host disease.

In addition, irradiation prior to storage may be of value in mass casualty situations in which a large number of patients may be suddenly immunosuppressed from inadvertent exposure to toxic chemical or nuclear radiation. In a disaster situation of this type, irradiation of blood immediately before transfusion may be impractical due to the lack of equipment or shortage of time.

## Disadvantages

The cost of the equipment and additional labor requirements may be perceived as a disadvantage in a cost-benefit assessment.

## PLASMA

Plasma is the noncellular, straw-colored fluid portion of anticoagulated whole blood that can be observed after whole blood is allowed to settle or is centrifuged. Chemically, plasma is comprised of water, electrolyte ions such as sodium ($Na^+$) and ($K^+$) potassium ions, and proteins. The soluble plasma proteins are primarily albumin, globulin, and coagulation factors.

At the present time, human donor plasma is the raw material for the production of numerous diagnostic and therapeutic products, in addition to those described in this section (Table 10 3). The requirements for plasma cannot be met with the plasma byproducts of whole-blood collection; therefore, plasmapheresis techniques can be used to collect large quantities of donor plasma. Plasma can be separated from units of whole blood and stored as single-donor plasma or fresh-frozen plasma.

Plasma separated from outdated whole blood is somewhat different in chemical composition from plasma ex-

**Table 10-3. Human Plasma Products**

| Plasma Product | Possible Uses |
| --- | --- |
| Albumin (5%) | Treatment of patients with hypovolemic shock; cases of hypoalbuminemia and decreased oncotic pressure; hemodialysis patients with fluid overload, hypotension, or unstable cardiovascular status; replace-fluid during therapeutic plasma exchange; patients with labile pulmonary-cardiovascular status of unknown cause. |
| Anti-Inhibitor Coagulant Complex | Treatment of bleeding associated with the presence of Factor VIII inhibitor |
| Anti-Thrombin III | Treatment of bleeding associated with anti-thrombin III (AT III) deficiency and thromboembolism or liver disease |
| Factor VIII Concentrate | Treatment of Hemophilia A |
| Factor IX Complex | Prophylaxis and treatment of Factor IX deficiency (hemophilia B) bleeding episodes |
| Factor XIII | Treatment of bleeding and disorders of wound healing due to Factor XIII deficiency |
| Haptoglobin | Intravascular clot lysis defects; therapeutic plasma exchange in case of thrombotic thrombocytopenic purpura; in infants with protein-losing enteropathy; selected patients with immune deficiencies |
| Cryoprecipitate | Treatment of patients with von Willebrand's disease, Hemophilia A, or deficiencies of factor XIII or fibrinogen. |
| IgM-enriched Immune Globulin | Treatment and prevention of septicemia and septic shock due to the liberation of toxins during antibiotic therapy |
| Immune Globulin to Specific Infectious Diseases | Passive immunization subsequent to Rabies, Rubella, Varicella-Zoster. |
| Plasma Protein Fraction | Treatment of hypovolemia due to shock, trauma, surgery or burns |
| Prothrombin complex | Treatment of patients with hereditary disease (history and laboratory evidence) of Factor II, VII, IX, or X. |

* It is preferable to use cytomegalovirus (CMV) antibody–negative products.

tracted from whole blood shortly after blood donation. The major change in plasma that has been in contact with red blood cells for an extended period of time is that it has higher levels of potassium ions and ammonia. Either form of plasma can be used for temporary volume replacement in patients who are depleted of whole blood or protein. Plasma may also be appropriate for coagulation factor replacement. However, when plasma which was immediately separated from whole blood originally collected in acid citrate dextrose (ACD) or citrate phosphate dextrose adenine (CPD) was stored at 6° C for 35 days, it was observed that activation of the coagulation, fibrinolytic, and kallikrein systems and decrease in coagulation inhibitors occurred. These conditions of storage had no significant effect on the levels of the main thrombin inhibitor, antithrombin III.

Components such as cryoprecipitate or antihemophilic factor (AHF) can be prepared from human plasma. Fractionation of human plasma can be into albumin or immune globulins. As the result of biotechnology, recombinant DNA-produced blood components such as factor VIII are available.

**Single-Donor Plasma**

Clinical Indications

Patients with severe burns or hypovolemic shock are appropriate candidates for this blood component. Depending on the type of coagulation deficiency as well as the method of storage, patients with coagulation defects may also be suitable transfusion candidates.

Methods

Single-donor plasma may be separated from a unit of whole blood using a plasma extractor. The original unit of whole blood should have been collected into an integral satellite bag system which allows for uncontaminated separation into the satellite bag. The separation must occur before the fifth day after the expiration date of the unit of whole blood.

Storage Requirements

If the unit is *not* frozen, single-donor plasma must be stored at 1 to 6° C and may be kept for *no more* than 40 days from the date of whole blood collection if the anticoagulant CPDA-1 anticoagulant was used. When stored frozen at −18° C or lower, single-donor plasma has a shelf-life of up to 5 years.

Advantages

Specifically using plasma when colloid volume expansion or most coagulation factors are needed rather than whole blood reduces the risk of sensitization to cellular antigens and is cost-effective.

Disadvantages

Single-donor plasma has the same risks of infectious disease due to blood-borne agents as a unit of whole blood. Transfusion reactions caused by plasma proteins and, to a lesser degree, cellular components are a possibility.

Special Notes

Plasma from which cryoprecipitate has been removed must be so designated.

**Fresh-Frozen Plasma**

According to the National Institutes of Health (NIH), fresh-frozen plasma is defined as the fluid portion of 1 unit of human blood that has been centrifuged, separated, and frozen at −18° C or colder within 8 hours of collection from the donor. Fresh-frozen plasma contains:

1. Labile and stable components of the coagulation, fibrinolytic, and complement systems.
2. Proteins that maintain osmotic pressure and immunity.
3. Other proteins which have diverse activities.
4. Fats, carbohydrates, and minerals in concentrations similar to those in the circulation.

The use of fresh-frozen plasma has increased tenfold within the past 10 years and has reached almost 2 million units annually. Much of this increase over the last decade is related to decreases in whole blood availability rather than to use for labile coagulation factor replacement. Recent estimates are that fresh-frozen plasma is definitely or possibly indicated in 54 to 58% of patients. Educational efforts addressing the appropriate use of fresh-frozen plasma should be initiated.

Clinical Indications

Few specific indications for the use of fresh-frozen plasma exist. Indications are generally limited to the treatment of deficiencies of coagulation proteins for which specific factor concentrates are unavailable or undesirable. Appropriate use of fresh-frozen plasma belongs in the following categories according to the NIH:

1. Massive transfusion. Hemorrhage in patients receiving massive transfusions is caused more frequently by thrombocytopenia than by depletion of coagulation factors. Use of fresh-frozen plasma should be confined to patients in whom factor deficiencies are presumed to be the sole or primary problem. There is no evidence that the prophylactic administration of fresh-frozen plasma decreases transfusion requirements in patients receiving multiple transfusions who do not have documented coagulation defects.
2. Single or multiple coagulation protein deficiencies, either prophylactically or in the treatment of bleeding.

Fresh-frozen plasma can be used to replace factor deficiencies of factors II, V, VII, IX, X, and XI if unacceptable or inappropriate specific component therapy is neither available nor appropriate.

3. Warfarin reversal. Patients who have been given the anticoagulant warfarin sodium are deficient in the functional vitamin K-dependent coagulation factors II, VII, IX and X, as well as proteins C and S. These functional deficiencies can be reversed by the administration of vitamin K. When such patients are actively bleeding or require emergency surgery, fresh-frozen plasma or single-donor plasma can be used to achieve immediate hemostasis.

4. Use in antithrombin III deficiency. Fresh-frozen plasma can be used as a source of antithrombin III in patients who are deficient in this inhibitor and are undergoing surgery, or who require heparin for treatment of thrombosis.

5. In conjunction with therapeutic plasma exchange for the treatment of thrombotic thrombocytopenic purpura (TTP).

6. Treatment of immunodeficiencies. Fresh-frozen plasma can serve as a source of immunoglobulin for children and adults with immunoglobulin deficiencies as an alternate to intravenous purified immune globulin. Fresh-frozen plasma is indicated in infants with secondary immunodeficiencies associated with severe protein loss caused by enteropathy and in patients in whom total parenteral nutrition is ineffective.

Inappropriate use of FFP includes use to expand blood volume and use as a source of immunoglobulins. In addition, administration of FFP to prevent surgical bleeding complications because of a mild to moderate prolongation of the prothrombin (PT) or activated partial thromboplastin time (aPTT) is inappropriate.

## Methods

After the collection of non-heparinized anticoagulated whole blood, fresh-frozen plasma can be prepared from a single heavy spin or from a double centrifugation to prepare a platelet concentrate at the same time. Each unit contains about 225 mL of plasma. The plasma should be frozen in a protective container within 8 hours after collection by placing it in a dry ice alcohol bath or in a freezer at −30° C or below. The bag should be frozen in a horizontal position and stored in a vertical position so that inadvertent thawing will be noticed on visual inspection. If a liquid freezing bath is used, the plastic container must be protected from chemical altuation.

## Storage Requirements

Fresh-frozen plasma should be stored at −18° C or below within 8 hours of collection from the donor and separation from the donor red blood cells. To maintain adequate

levels of factors V and VIII, plasma must be stored frozen. The optimal storage is at −30° C or colder with a dating period of 12 months after donation of the original unit of whole blood. If fresh-frozen plasma has been maintained constantly in the frozen state of −18° C or below, it shall be stored for no longer than 12 months from the date of phlebotomy.

When requested, the unit of fresh-frozen plasma must be thawed inside a clean plastic bag with agitation in a waterbath at temperatures between 30 and 37° C. It is important to prevent water contamination. If the intended use of the plasma is for the correction of labile coagulation factor deficiencies, it must be stored at 1 to 6° C after thawing. If the plasma is intended for correcting coagulation deficiencies, it must be stored at 1 to 6° C and transfused within 24 hours after thawing.

Microwave thawing of fresh-frozen plasma is still considered an experimental technique. One of the major concerns of using this method of thawing is the leaching of plasticizer from the storage bag. Microwave-thawed plasma contains precipitated denatured protein (mainly albumin and fibrinogen), and a significant reduction of coagulation factors IX, X, XI and fibrinogen has been demonstrated with microwave-thawed plasma as compared to fresh plasma. A recent modification of the microwave-thawing method is the specially designed rotating temperature-controlled oven. With this equipment, no statistically significant differences in measured proteins compared with 37° C waterbath thawing were noted.

## Advantages

The major advantage of fresh-frozen plasma is that, if appropriately used, it provides effective use of whole blood through component therapy. Through the use of plasma alone, the risk of alloimmunization to erythrocyte, leukocyte, and platelet antigens is reduced compared to the risk with use of whole blood.

## Disadvantages

The combined use of fresh-frozen plasma and packed red cells as a substitute for whole blood can have significant adverse effects in terms of the cost and safety of blood transfusion. The risks of fresh-frozen plasma include the same risks as whole blood: disease transmission, allergic and anaphylactoid reactions, and excessive intravascular volume. The incidence of nonicteric and icteric hepatitis following multiple transfusions of fresh-frozen plasma probably ranges between 3 and 10%. Although the risk is less than with whole blood or packed red cells, the potential for alloimmunization is present, as has been demonstrated by the infrequent formation of Rh antibodies.

## Special Notes

Fresh frozen plasma should be ABO compatible with the recipient's red blood cells, especially when the component is to be transfused to infants. Crossmatching is not required. Inappropriate use of fresh-frozen plasma could be avoided by the increased use of whole blood or safer, cheaper volume expanders. No justification exists for the use of fresh frozen plasma as a volume expander, nutritional source (NIH), or as a source of immunoglobulins. Administration of FFP to patients with mild to moderate prolongations of the prothrombin time (PT) or activated partial thromboplastin time (aPTT) prior to an invasive procedure is a misuse of this component.

Alternative therapies have been suggested (NIH):

1. Cryoprecipitate should be used when fibrinogen or von Willebrand factor is needed.
2. For treatment of hemophilia A, cryoprecipitate or factor VIII concentrates are available.
3. For the treatment of severe hemophilia B, factor IX complex is preferable. Both of these concentrates are prepared from pooled plasma, and the risk of virus transmission is high in untreated products. Factor IX concentrate carries the additional hazard of thrombogenicity.
4. Crystalloid, colloid solutions containing albumin or plasma protein fraction, hydroxyethyl starch, and dextran are preferred for volume replacement.
5. For nutritional support, amino acid solutions and dextrose are acceptable alternatives.

## PLASMA COMPONENTS

### Cryoprecipitated Antihemophilic Factor

Cryoprecipitated antihemophilic factor (AHF) is the cold insoluble precipitate of plasma remaining after fresh-frozen plasma obtained from whole blood or apheresis has been thawed between 1 and 6° C. Immediately after completion of thawing at 30–37° C and prompt centrifugation at 1–6° C, the plasma must be separated from the cold-insoluble material under sterile conditions. The cryoprecipitated AHF must be refrozen within 1 hour. Quality assurance of this product requires that, in at least 75% of tested units of cryoprecipitated AHF, there must be a minimum of 80 international units of coagulation factor VIII per individual plasma collection. In tests performed on pooled components, at least 75% of the pools tested must have a minimum level of 80 international units times the number of components in the pool. Each bag of cryoprecipitated AHF contains factor VIII von Willebrand factor (VWF) fibrinogen, factor XIII, and fibronectin, between 150 and 250 mg of fibrinogen, and fibronectin in less than 15 mL of plasma. Cryoprecipitate is the only concentrated fibrinogen product available. Fibrinogen preparations that were previously available are no longer prepared because of the high risk of infectious disease transmission.

### Clinical Indications

Because cryoprecipitated AHF is a source of coagulation factor VIII, von Willebrand's factor (vWF), factor XIII, fibrinogen, and fibronectin, it is useful in the control of bleeding in a variety of clinical disorders. These conditions include factor VIII deficiency, von Willebrand's disease, factor XIII deficiency, and hypofibrinogenemia.

The National Hemophilia Foundation recommends that hemophiliacs, particularly children, receive cryoprecipitate. However, in mild or moderate cases, an attempt should be made to use desmopressin, an analog of the naturally occurring antidiuretic hormone, vasopressin, which has been shown to raise factor VIII levels in normal subjects and patients with mild to moderate hemophilia A and von Willebrand's disease.

For the treatment of bleeding in factor VIII-deficient patients, rapid infusion of cryoprecipitate (about 10 mL of diluted component per minute) of a loading dose is generally expected to produce the initial desired level of factor VIII with smaller maintenance doses very 8 to 12 hours. Patients should be monitored periodically by means of factor VIII plasma assays. A regimen of therapy for 10 or more days may be required to maintain hemostasis in afflicted patients after surgery.

The level of factor VIII needed for therapy or prophylaxis is not exactly predictable and varies with each clinical situation. A rule-of-thumb calculation of the number of bags of cryoprecipitate needed by factor VIII-deficient patients has been formulated. If a patient has antibodies to factor VIII, larger doses or more frequent doses may be needed to achieve hemostasis. The degree of factor VIII saturation of the extravascular space, which is equivalent to approximately 1.5 times the size of the intravascular space, can affect a patient's response to therapy. A lower dose response than expected can reflect the degree of extravascular space saturation.

Patients with von Willebrand's disease require smaller amounts of cryoprecipitate. Laboratory assays are helpful in monitoring patients with von Willebrand's disease as well as those suffering from hypofibrinogenemia.

Determination of Cryoprecipitate Quantity (Dosage) in
Factor VIII Deficient Patients
Number of bags of cryoprecipitate required =

$$\frac{\text{Desired level of Factor VIII (\%)} \times \text{Patient's Plasma Volume (mL)*}}{80**}$$

* In lieu of an exact measure of plasma volume, 4% of the patient's body weight (Kg) × 1000 may be substituted.
** 80 represents the average number of units of factor VIII in a single unpooled bag of cryoprecipitate. If several bags of cryoprecipitate are pooled into one unit, the number of original bags should be multiplied by 80 to obtain the number in the denominator.
EXAMPLE:
If the desired level of factor VIII activity is 70% and the patient's plasma volume is 2500 mL, the number of single bags of cryoprecipitate needed would be 22.

$$\text{Number of bags required} = \frac{0.70 \times 2500 \text{ mL}}{80} = 22 \text{ bags}$$

## Methods

Plasma should be separated from erythrocytes within four hours of collection by heavy centrifugation. The plasma should be frozen within 2 hours of separation (or 8 hours of collection) in a freezer at $-30°$ C or less. Frozen plasma should then be thawed at 1 to 6° C. The AHF-poor plasma is then separated from the cryoprecipitate after centrifugation, leaving about 15 mL of plasma with the cryoprecipitate. The precipitate should be refrozen within 1 hour and stored at $-18°$ C or below.

Units of cryoprecipitate can be pooled into groups of two to six units prior to freezing. They should be pooled promptly after preparation, using aseptic technique, and then refrozen immediately to prevent possible bacterial growth and loss of labile coagulation factors. These units must be labeled as pooled units.

## Storage Requirements

The shelf-life of cryoprecipitate when stored at $-18°$ C or below is 12 months. On request, cryoprecipitate is thawed in a 37° C waterbath for up to 15 minutes. The cryoprecipitate should be resuspended in the residual 10 to 15 mL of plasma in the bag of wet cryoprecipitate or by adding 10 to 15 mL of sterile diluent (0.9% sodium chloride injection, USP, is preferred) and gently resuspending.

If several bags of cryoprecipitate are pooled, the precipitate in each concentrate should be mixed with 10 to 15 mL of sterile diluent (0.9% sodium chloride injection, USP) to ensure complete removal of all precipitate from the container. Cryoprecipitate that has been pooled prior to freezing usually requires no extra diluent.

Thawed units should be kept at room temperature and used as soon as possible. Storage in the refrigerator may cause reprecipitation of concentrated factor VIII. Cryoprecipitate must be administered within 6 hours of thawing, if it is being used for factor VIII content, and within 4 hours of pooling. Thawed units may not be refrozen.

## Advantages

Because of the small volume, cryoprecipitate is preferable to fresh-frozen plasma in the correction of bleeding conditions in certain disorders, for example, factor VIII deficiency. This component, however, should not be used unless a specific hemostatic defect for which this product is useful has been identified. Compatibility testing is not necessary unless large volumes are transfused. Although an ABO-compatible product is preferred, it is not essential, nor is Rh status a consideration.

## Disadvantages

If cryoprecipitate is used for bleeding disorders other than those previously identified, it will be ineffective. Other disadvantages can include:

1. Febrile or allergic reactions
2. Bacterial contamination
3. Air embolism during administration
4. Hyperfibrinogenemia in massively transfused patients
5. Development of a positive direct antiglobulin test
6. Transmission of blood-borne diseases

## Special Notes

Crossmatching is not required for this component.

The transmission of blood-borne viruses in coagulation factor concentrates and other plasma products remains a serious health concern. Factor VIII and factor IX concentrates that have not been treated have been implicated in the transmission of a number of viral diseases, most notably hepatitis B, hepatitis C, and AIDS.

Approaches to virus inactivation in plasma products include:

1. Heating in the liquid state in the presence of low molecular weight stabilizers
2. Heating in the lyophilized state
3. Ultraviolet (UV) irradiation

The major problem with heat inactivation is achieving a balance between optimum viral destruction and retention of biologic activity of the heat-labile coagulation factors. To inactivate viruses with heat without a substantial loss of protein biologic activity in the liquid state requires the inclusion of high concentrations of stabilizers such as amino acids, sugars, and salts, or mixtures such as 2.75 M glycine and 50% sucrose. However, the inclusion of additives decreases the rate of virus inactivation at 60° C. An alternate approach is to remove excess water through lyophilization before heating. Heating at 60° C for 10 hours inactivates 104 infectious units of HBV virus, but increasing the temperature from 60 to 70 or 80° C causes a 90% or greater loss in AHF activity. An even greater decline in the rate of virus inactivation has been observed on heating AHF in the lyophilized state at temperatures greater than 60° C, although no loss in AHF activity has been observed after 72 hours of heating at 60° C. Several proteins present in lyophilized AHF concentrates display an altered electrophoretic mobility as a result of exposure to 60° C for 24 hours.

Newer techniques to increase the yield and/or purity of AHF in concentrates include polyethylene glycol precipitation, solid- and liquid-phase chromatography with heparin, and polyelectrolytes. Direct adsorption of factor VIII:C from plasma by polyelectrolytes results in an overall yield of about 50% and a purity of approximately 1000-fold.

***Monoclonal Absorption of Cryoprecipitate.*** The newest method of processing and purifying AHF concentrates is by monoclonal absorption. The purification of plasma proteins is achieved by using immunoaffinity chromatography.

With cryoprecipitate as the starting material, two methods of production are presently being used. These methods have some common characteristics, but differ in the specificity of the monoclonal antibody used for the purification of factor VIII and the method of viral inactivation. One product uses a monoclonal antibody directed toward the vWF portion of the factor VIII/vWF complex; the other product uses a monoclonal antibody specifically directed toward the factor VIII portion of the factor VIII/vWF complex. The other major processing difference is the method of virus inactivation. One method uses heat treatment of the product in a freeze-dried state at 60° C for 30 hours; the other uses a solvent/detergent treatment which is a chemical viral inactivation procedure.

Initial clinical trials have demonstrated no immediate adverse effects or symptoms of blood-borne diseases to date.

### Factor IX Complex

Factor IX complex, Konyne$^R$, is a commercially prepared, heat-treated plasma product that contains coagulation factors II, IX, and X and low levels of factor VII. This product is approximately 50 times more purified over whole plasma, and when reconstituted as directed, contains 25 times as much factor IX as an equal volume of fresh plasma.

#### Clinical Indications

The main indication for using factor IX complex is in the treatment of conditions caused by factor IX (hemophilia B or Christmas disease) deficiency. The use of factor IX complex for patients with factors II or X or mild cases of hemophilia B should be used if treatment with fresh-frozen plasma is not feasible or has proven ineffective. Other clinical indications include reversal of coumarin anticoagulant-induced hemorrhage as a secondary approach, if the risk of transmitting hepatitis is considered justifiable, and in the treatment of bleeding episodes in patients with hemophilia A (factor VIII deficiency) who have inhibitors to factor VIII.

#### Methods

Reconstitute with Sterile Water for Injection, USP, and administer within 3 hours after reconstitution. Do not refrigerate after reconstitution. Administer by the intravenous route.

#### Storage Requirements

Must be stored under refrigeration (2 to 8° C). Freezing should be avoided because breakage of the diluent bottle might occur. The product may be stored for a period of up to 1 month at a temperature not exceeding 25° C during travel.

#### Advantages

Factor IX complex is a rapid method of achieving and maintaining hemostasis in appropriate patients.

#### Disadvantages

Factor IX complex is prepared from paid donors, in whom the risk of blood-borne disease is high. Heat treatment may not completely eliminate the risk of exposure to infectious agents. Cases of postoperative thrombosis have also been reported after the administration of this product.

#### Special Notes

U.S. federal law prohibits dispensing factor IX complex without a prescription. In the treatment of specific coagulation disorders, deficiencies of factors II or X, and even cases of mild hemophilia B, the use of fresh-frozen plasma should be initially considered.

## OTHER BLOOD DERIVATIVES

### Intravenous Immunoglobulin

Intravenous immunoglobulin (IgG) is prepared by modifying Cohn fraction II to render it safe for intravenous injection. This product differs from blood derivates produced for intramuscular injection, which are not suitable for intravenous use. If IgG prepared for intramuscular use is administered intravenously, immunoglobulin aggregates may activate the complement and kinin systems and produce hypotensive and/or anaphylactic reactions. Potential indications and clinical uses for intravenous immunoglobulin preparations include congenital immune deficiencies, acquired antibody deficiency, and prophylaxis or treatment of bacterial and viral diseases. Other indications can include the treatment of disorders such as posttransfusion purpura or Kawasaki syndrome.

The risks associated with administration of IgG include allergic reactions, pulmonary reactions, and volume overload. Some patients with other than group O blood may develop a positive DAT caused by ABO unexpected antibodies.

### Antiprotease Concentrates

A purified, heat-treated concentrate of antithrombin III (AT III) is available in addition to liquid plasma and FFP as sources of treatment in patients deficient in AT III. Other manufactured antiproteases include alpha$_1$-antitrypsin and C1-esterase inhibitor.

Patients who are deficient in AT-III do not effectively inhibit thrombin activity and are prone to thromboembolic diseases (e.g., venous thrombosis).

## Colloid Plasma Substitutes

Human albumin (5% and 25%) and plasma protein fraction (PPF) are colloid plasma substitutes. PPF is similar in composition to 5% albumin, but it has a greater concentration of nonalbumin plasma proteins. These solutions are commonly used for volume expansion and colloid replacement. Pharmacological agents (e.g., dextran) are also used as plasma substitutes for volume expansion.

Albumin is appropriately used to correct acute, massive loss of colloid (e.g., in patients with hypovolemic shock or severe burns). Take care to avoid inappropriate use of albumin therapy. In cases of patients with hypoalbuminemia, the clinical benefit of albumin transfusion is doubtful.

Although the use of colloidal plasma substitutes assists in the efficient utilization of blood products and reduces the risk of transmission of blood-borne pathogens, complications are possible. These include anaphylactic reactions, cardiac overload and/or interstitial dehydration subsequent to the rapid infusion of large quantities of 25% albumin, and possible hypotensive episodes due to rapid infusion of PPF.

## BLOOD SUBSTITUTES

Although saline solutions were used as early as 1833 for the treatment of cholera, the use of crystalloid solutions as substitutes for blood began around 1875. These solutions were developed because of the increasing incidence of complications associated with blood transfusion. The discovery of the ABO blood group system and the many scientific discoveries that followed led to the present era of blood transfusion.

While the use of human whole blood and blood components has many benefits, problems are also associated with it including the following:

1. An increasing demand for blood and blood products and a concomitant shortage of donors
2. The risk of transmitting blood-borne diseases
3. Cultural and religious objections to blood transfusion
4. Difficulty with collecting, storing, and transporting blood or blood components in underdeveloped countries or at disaster sites or in military situations
5. The time and cost factors associated with crossmatching

The traditional blood supply system is expected to continue to function for many years, but in the future the increasing demand may not be met. As an alternative to human-derived blood and blood components, substitutes and alternate sources are being developed. Substitutes must be nontoxic, nonpyrogenic, nonallergic, sterile, and easy to store at normal temperatures. These alternate blood replacement fluids must be equivalent to human blood in viscosity and osmotic pressure, and retained in the vascular system for a sufficient time to exert the required therapeutic effect. In addition, these substances must be eliminated by normal metabolism or excretion and must not affect normal hemostasis. They must also be relatively cheap to produce and easily administered. In the case of red cell substitutes, an additional requirement is that the substitute be able to give up oxygen to the tissues within the normal physiologic range of partial pressures.

Blood substitutes, whether they result from synthesis by organic chemistry procedures or from biologic processes through genetic engineering, are likely to make broad contributions to transfusion medicine. Approximately twenty companies are vying for a share of the $1 billion blood substitute market. Blood substitutes prepared from organic processes, hemoglobin extracted from outdated human red blood cells, or recombinant DNA products are either FDA approved or are being tested. Recombinant DNA is already a reality in the production of products such as erythropoietin.

## Red Cell Substitutes

Recent phase I clinical trials with polymerized, hemoglobin-based oxygen carriers have proven successful on healthy volunteers. A safe dosage level has been established in volunteers; however, its efficacy in patients for whom blood loss is an issue (e.g., hypovolemic shock or trauma) has not been established. Benefits of this product include no necessity to crossmatch before transfusion because of the lack of cellular antigens, less viscosity, and a nonrefrigerated shelf life of more than one year. Recurring blood shortages and potential disease transmission continue to drive the quest for an artificial product. Although the risk of contracting HIV from blood transfusion is estimated at 1:225,000 and the risk of contracting hepatitis is 1:3,000, the perception of danger remains.

Several types of synthetic red blood cell surrogates exist. These include the following:

1. Emulsions of perfluorocarbons
2. Stroma-free hemoglobin
3. Polymerized hemoglobin
4. Liposome-encapsulated hemoglobin

### Perfluorocarbons

Perfluorochemicals (PFCs) are large organic compounds in which all the hydrogen atoms have been replaced by fluorine atoms. They are chemically inert, immiscible in water, and not metabolized. Oxygen transported by a PFC is carried in solution and has approximately 20 times the solubility for oxygen and carbon dioxide as does water, which is almost three times the oxygen-carrying capacity of blood. The PFC solution Fluosol-DA 20% was first administered to volunteers in 1979. American clinical trials were strictly limited to acutely anemic Jehovah's Witness patients who refused blood transfusion on religious grounds.

Experiments with Fluosol-DA have demonstrated a circulation half-life of about 13 hours and a tissue half-life of 9 days. These substances do not preferentially extract oxygen from the air. Because Fluosol-DA 20% does not contain sufficient PFC, only 10% by volume, the concurrent administration of 60 to 100% oxygen is required to dissolve a significant amount of oxygen, which can render the patient vulnerable to oxygen toxicity. The safety of PFCs has not yet been established, but pulmonary hypertension, bronchospasm, cytotoxicity, and retention by the liver and spleen have been reported. In addition, the emulsifying agent Pluronic F-68 may cause a clinical reaction involving the activation of complement. The stability of the current emulsion limits the shelf-life, even though it can be stored frozen for up to 1 year.

When PFC was assessed as a red cell substitute in acutely anemic patients, no adverse reactions were noted, but no significant beneficial effects were obvious because of the small increase in arterial oxygen content, brief half-life, and limited total dose. Further assessment of PFCs concluded that the solution was unnecessary in moderately anemic patients and ineffective in severely anemic patients.

Fluosol, a 20% intravascular perfluorochemical emulsion, was approved by the FDA in 1990 specifically for use on patients with high risk of ischemic complications in percutaneous transluminal coronary angioplasty (PTCA).

Many of the limitations of PFCs will be lessened when a better biologically inert surfactant becomes available. New formulations of perfluorochemicals that correct the observed shortcomings of Fluosol-DA may be more effective.

***Characteristics.*** The advantages of perfluorocarbons are as follows:

1. Contain no antigens; no typing and crossmatching necessary
2. Easily synthesized from readily available materials
3. Free of infectious diseases
4. Do not carry carbon monoxide and could provide oxygen to a carbon monoxide victim until the patient replaces abnormal red cells
5. Small particle size enables the suspension to penetrate occluded vessels in conditions such as cerebral ischemia or myocardial infarction

The disadvantages of perfluorocarbons are as follows:

1. Potentially cause oxygen toxicity
2. Unstable in vitro—need to be frozen
3. Retention by liver and spleen and other adverse reactions
4. Have not been proven beneficial in severely anemic patients

## Hemoglobin Solutions

Hemoglobin solutions, such as stroma-free hemoglobin or polymerized hemoglobin, may be used as free solutions in the circulation, or may be encapsulated in a membrane.

***Stroma-Free Hemoglobin.*** Stroma-free hemoglobin solution is another example of an oxygen-carrying blood substitute. In 1967, a major improvement was made in the preparation of free hemoglobin by removing the membrane fragments (stroma) from hemolyzed erythrocytes. Stroma-free hemoglobin is prepared by slowly lysing washed red cells with a buffered solution of water, followed by high-speed centrifugation and micropore filtration. This procedure separates the fragmented cell membrane into relatively large pieces that can be removed.

Removal of the stroma eliminated the earlier renal, cardiovascular, and coagulation problems, but free native tetrameric hemoglobin has an undesirably high oxygen affinity. To avoid excessively high colloid osmotic pressure, stroma-free hemoglobin is used at half the oxygen-carrying capacity of whole blood.

One of the disadvantages of free hemoglobin solutions as a blood substitute is the low circulation retention time, which is less than 8 hours. It is rapidly filtered by the kidneys, and may cause some nephrotoxicity. This can be improved by coupling the beta-chains of hemoglobin (cross-linked hemoglobin) through an organic phosphate compound.

***Characteristics.*** The advantages of stroma-free hemoglobin are as follows:

1. Excellent volume expanders
2. Potential candidate for an emergency resuscitative fluid

The disadvantages of stroma-free hemoglobin are as follows:

1. Toxicity
2. Can activate the complement system
3. Short half-life in the circulation
4. Significant oncotic effect and unacceptably high affinity for oxygen
5. Must be refrigerated or frozen

***Polymerized Hemoglobin.*** The limitations of stroma-free hemoglobin (SFH) solutions have been partly removed by pyridoxylation (SFH-P) followed by polymerization (poly SFH-P) of hemoglobin. Polymerized pyridoxylated hemoglobin is currently the only modification of hemoglobin solution that approximates the oxygen-carrying capacity of whole blood and can be infused without altering the patient oncotic pressure. It supports life in the absence of red cells while maintaining baseline hemodynamics and oxygen consumption. Poly SFH-P achieves a near-normal patient hemoglobin and has a longer intravascular persistence than any unpolymerized product. These solutions have a normal oxygen-carrying capacity and a circulation half-life of 38 hours. The total hemoglobin concentration is 14 to 16 g/dL compared to the stroma-free hemoglobin concentration of 7 g/dL.

Poly SFH-P is an improved short-term red cell substitute. Because it is an effective oxygen carrier, it persists in the circulation much longer than SFH, and the tissue oxygenation effect is significantly improved. It has, however, a higher affinity for oxygen than erythrocytes and a higher content of nonfunctional methemoglobin. Polymerization also causes a reduction in colloid osmotic pressure (COP) while maintaining a constant hemoglobin concentration.

Although nephrotoxicity is less likely with a polymer than with the hemoglobin tetramer, a major area of concern are toxicity problems associated with the administration of poly SFH-P. Nephrotoxicity is transient and is not believed to be associated with permanent renal damage. The cause of toxicity may be the presence of vasoactive substances in the hemoglobin solution, which affects renal blood flow. This belief is supported by the fact that the majority of recipients have developed transient bradycardia and mild hypertension during infusion. Another possibility is that the changes in renal function are related to the filtration of free hemoglobin through the kidneys because once hemoglobinemia disappears, renal function returns to normal.

An additional problem is that polymerized hemoglobin solutions may be immunogenic. Polymerized hemoglobin survives for a much longer time in the circulation than free hemoglobin, and these solutions retain a significant fraction of the tetramer. The question of the immunogenicity of the polymer is currently being investigated.

*Characteristics.* The advantages of polymerized hemoglobin are as follows:

1. Relative simplicity of preparation
2. Approximates the oxygen carrying capacity of whole blood
3. Can be infused without altering the patient oncotic pressure
4. Near-normal patient hemoglobin
5. Longer intravascular persistence than any unpolymerized product
6. Tissue oxygenation effect is significantly improved in comparison to stroma-free hemoglobin

The disadvantages of polymerized hemoglobin are as follows:

1. A higher affinity for oxygen than erythrocytes
2. A higher content of nonfunctional methemoglobin
3. Nephrotoxicity
4. May be immunogenic

### Encapsulated Hemoglobin

Another general approach for producing surrogate erythrocytes that seems to eliminate many of the problems plaguing SFH and poly SFH-P hemoglobin solutions is based on the concept of encapsulation of hemoglobin in membranes. The use of encapsulated hemoglobin as a red cell substitute has received relatively little attention in comparison to the research on PFCs and hemoglobin solutions.

Encapsulation dates back to 1964, when Chang first encapsulated hemoglobin in nylon membranes. Artificial cell membranes can now be formed using a variety of synthetic or biologic materials to produce desired variations in characteristics such as permeability and surface properties. Almost any substance, such as enzyme systems, cell extracts, or hormones, can be included in artificial cells.

The ideal biophysical criteria for artificial red cells include the following:

1. Adequate oxygen-carrying capacity and appropriate oxygen affinity
2. Rapid gas exchange
3. Satisfactory circulating half-life and thromboresistance
4. Chemical and physical stability
5. Biologic inertness (low pathogenic potential)
6. Satisfactory viscosity
7. Storage stability
8. Low immunogenicity

Encapsulation of hemoglobin in liposomes (hemosomes) is an alternative approach that minimizes many of the problems associated with the other methods of cell preparation. Liposomes can be prepared from a single phospholipid, a mixture of phospholipids, or mixtures of phospholipids and neutral lipids, for example phosphatidylcholine plus cholesterol. Hemosomes composed of polymeric phospholipids may offer specific advantages because of their reduced permeability and rate of aggregation, their increased resistance to hydrodynamic shear and chemical disruption, and their apparent thromboresistance. Because the toxicity, stability, and storage of these preparations still presents problems, recent research has been concerned with improving encapsulation techniques and producing nontoxic biodegradable membranes.

Hemoglobin has been successfully encapsulated in lipid vesicles at concentrations equal to that found in erythrocytes. A 10 g/dL quantity of hemoglobin encapsulated in an artificial cell results in an intracellular environment comparable to that of normal red blood cells. In this way, the enzymes enclosed in the artificial cells are stabilized by the high concentration of protein. Such vesicles can be stabilized by polymerization and have a half-life of several months.

A different approach to the preparation of vesicles is to encapsulate stroma-free hemoglobin in a polymerized hemoglobin membrane. The crosslinked membrane is permeable to oxygen and impermeable to hemoglobin in solution. These vesicles are capable of reversibly binding oxygen, are less than 4 $\mu$m in diameter, and have been reported to be stable under conditions of normal blood flow.

Liposome-embedded heme is also being investigated because oxygen binding is reversible and very rapid. In addition, oxygen volume dissolved in the solution is similar or superior to that of blood and the oxygen-binding affinity is close to that of blood. The particle is small in size and composed of bioacceptable heme and phospholipid. In vivo oxygenation of tissues, however, has not been extensively investigated.

A significant advance has been achieved by the development of neohemocytes, which are microcapsules containing purified human hemoglobin and 2,3-diphosphoglycerate. The microcapsule membrane is composed of phospholipids and cholesterol molecules that are biodegradable and biocompatible. Neohemocytes are substantially smaller than erythrocytes. The size range (0.1–1.0 $\mu$m) is small enough to allow free passage through capillaries.

Neohemocytes rather than hemosomes qualify as prototype artificial red cells because, in addition to having the general characteristics of hemosomes, they meet other essential specifications including lack of degradation of the encapsulated hemoglobin and a physiologically acceptable oxygen affinity. The six essential specifications for prototype cells include the following:

1. The microcapsule membrane must be biodegradable and physiologically compatible.
2. The encapsulation process must avoid significant hemoglobin degradation.
3. The oxygen affinity of hemoglobin must be reduced relative to that of free human hemoglobin.
4. The encapsulated hemoglobin must be sufficiently concentrated (more than 33% of that in erythrocytes).
5. There should be no evidence of overt intravascular coagulopathy.
6. The artificial cells must be small enough to pass unrestricted through normal capillaries.

For typical liposomes, emulsions, and microcapsules, the mononuclear phagocytic clearance process is dominant. Natural and synthetic glycolipids have been inserted into the liposomal membrane and tested for their ability to alter liposome clearance. Incorporation of these glycolipids did decrease uptake by the mononuclear phagocytic system, but many natural glycolipids are antigenic and thus would not be suitable for insertion. Inert carbohydrates attached to lipids may reduce clearance and binding of liposomes to tissues.

The overall clearance of neohemocytes consists of three processes: clearance resulting from irreversible binding to tissues followed by breakdown; clearance caused by rapid or early destruction or breakdown; and clearance from uptake by the mononuclear phagocytic system. The objective of neohemocytes is to have cells that do not result in blockage, that interact minimally with tissues, and that are relatively invisible to the mononuclear phagocytic system.

Encapsulation appears to be the approach most likely to lead to a blood substitute that has all the properties of erythrocytes, but major obstacles remain, including toxicity, stability, storage, and the question as to whether mass production can be cost-effective. Further studies are needed to resolve the problems of selecting an acceptable microencapsulating material, developing a microencapsulation process that yields the desired range but avoids denaturation of hemoglobin and encapsulating a sufficient amount of hemoglobin while maintaining an acceptable final viscosity. Development of a nontoxic product that combines the functions of a plasma expander with the ability to carry and deliver oxygen to tissues could prove useful in the treatment of trauma, as a temporary substitute for red cells, and for the treatment of tissue ischemia.

***Characteristics.*** The advantages of encapsulated hemoglobin are as follows:

1. Reduced permeability and rate of aggregation
2. Increased resistance to hydrodynamic shear and chemical disruption
3. Apparent thromboresistance
4. Substantially smaller than erythrocytes (neohemocytes)

The disadvantages of encapsulated hemoglobin are as follows:

1. Toxicity
2. Stability
3. Storage
4. Questionable cost-effectiveness

## Alternate Cellular Technology

### In Vitro Stem Cell Culturing

It is conceivable that pluripotent stem cells could be maintained in culture to replicate and differentiate into mature blood cells. Although it has been shown that cultures of human bone marrow cells may survive for several months, more basic information is needed about the processes that regulate the balance between self-renewal and differentiation of cells. Major problems associated with this technology include the production and harvesting of a sufficient number of functional cells ($10^{10}$ to $10^{12}$) for transfusion and the harvesting of mature functional cells free from microbial contamination.

Compatibility testing between donor and recipient will probably be necessary, thus negating the advantage of a universally compatible product. Questions remain as to whether in vitro stem cell culturing can be expanded to produce sufficient numbers of functional cells in a cost-effective way.

### Artificial Platelets

Platelet substitute approaches have been similar to those of red cells. Although attempts to use phospholipids and the reconstitution of platelet membrane glycoproteins into lipid vesicles have been made, these experiments have failed to construct an artificial platelet that will mimic platelet function. Recent studies with liposomes as artificial red cells provide some encouragement, but researchers have been faced with the same problems. Another approach, the use of freeze-dried or fragmented platelets, has been unsuccessful in controlling bleeding.

## Alternate Sources of Blood Products

### Recombinant DNA Technology

Recombinant DNA technology is believed to hold much promise as an alternate source of plasma proteins. Within the next decade, recombinant DNA products will probably replace at least several plasma derivatives, but each plasma protein will present its own collection of specific problems to the industry.

The major proteins currently recovered from human plasma fractionation are albumin, factor VIII, prothrombin complex, and immunoglobulins. Human plasma fractionation supplies the need for these products in the United States, but the world need is not being met. In addition, other plasma proteins cannot be recovered in high yield from plasma, or can be recovered only at the expense of another product. In 1982, 3.5 million liters of plasma were fractionated to meet American demands for plasma products. Large-scale production and purification capabilities must be available before genetic engineering can meet even the demand for plasma products in the United States.

Genetic engineering is a method by which proteins from sources such as human blood are produced. Bacteria, yeast, and, for very large molecules, mammalian cells are used because they replicate proteins more accurately. Because nonpathogenic microorganisms are used, the supply of protein becomes unlimited, is less expensive, and has a high degree of purity.

Recombinant DNA (rDNA) is a combination of gene identification and cloning techniques. A strand of DNA (gene) which codes for a specific product can be isolated, characterized, sequenced, and subjected to a series of chemical and enzymatic reactions. Genetic engineers identify the section of human DNA that governs the manufacture of a specific protein, enzymatically snip out that single gene, and then insert it into the DNA of a microorganism. The selected microorganism than reproduces it in sufficient quantities for collection and purification. A major challenge facing gene-cloning technology is expansion of production to meet the demand. In addition, although products produced by DNA technology would substantially eliminate the risk of blood-borne disease, care must be taken to avoid introducing new diseases from cell cultures.

### Substitutes for Plasma Products

Plasma proteins can potentially be produced by microorganisms carrying the genetic code for these proteins. The

first attempts at recombinant DNA technology have been successful in the cloning and expression of albumin, antithrombin III, urokinase, tissue plasminogen activator, alpha-1-antitrypsin, and factor IX; and recently factor VIII and von Willebrand factor.

The largest recombinant protein expressed to date is albumin. This required the ligation of separate DNA fragments to obtain the complete, circulating form of the molecule. Cloning, however, is not the most difficult aspect of producing factor IX and factor VIII. For example, factor VIII is believed to be large (molecular weight 100,000 and 300,000).

The number of DNA fragments required for a complete factor VII molecule could be a major complication, compounded by the fact that the messenger RNA for the protein is probably an extremely small trace. In fact, it is still not known in which organ the protein is synthesized. Factor VIII is extremely sensitive to proteases, and thus it is essential to ensure that organisms synthesizing the molecules have low endogenous levels of proteases. Because disrupting virtually any cell results in the release of proteases, it is desirable that a recombinant organism synthesizing factor VIII secrete the molecule into the medium. This puts severe limitations on purification procedures. In addition, factor IX is posttranslationally modified by the action of liver enzymes dependent on vitamin K. Bacteria and yeast are not known to possess the vitamin K-dependent carboxylase system before it can deliver the functional factor IX zymogen. Therefore, a chemical modification procedure and/or expression in mammalian cells (resulting in the proper modification) is required to obtain a functioning protein.

The plasma fractionation industry currently isolates immunoglobulin fractions from plasma of donors hyperimmunized against known antigens. Production of immunoglobulins by methods other than plasma fractionation will be by cell fusion technique. Most companies are producing mouse-derived monoclonal antibodies. This experience should prove valuable for increased human antibody production. One major problem in the use of monoclonal antibodies as therapeutic agents is the proof that a product derived from a cancerous cell line is free of carcinogenic agents. This is particularly important because it has recently been shown that some types of human leukemia are caused by viral infections.

Albumin might be the first DNA recombinant transfusion product to be available in the field of transfusion. In 1985, several manufacturers announced that recombinant factor VIII would be available. These firms claim that the functional portion of the molecules has been cloned and synthesized by a recombinant mammalian cell line. The predicted expression and actual commercial use and performance of DNA recombinant products have exceeded the projections:

| Product | Expression | | Commercialization | |
|---|---|---|---|---|
| | Predicted | Actual | Predicted | Actual |
| HB Vaccine | 1982 | 1981 | 1990 | 1987 |
| Factor VIII | 1991 | 1984 | 1997 | ? |
| Albumin | 1982 | 1981 | 1991 | ? |

The ultimate success of recombinant DNA in producing plasma proteins will depend on the cost of these products compared to the cost of using human plasma fractions. The costs of these procedures differ for various products. It is crucial to take into account the interrelationships among demands for various plasma derivatives, some of which drive the plasma market. If albumin needs could be met by recombinant DNA but no hemophilia factors were produced, the cost of producing coagulation factors would be prohibitive. When large-scale production becomes a reality, the simultaneous manufacturing of a variety of derivatives must be guaranteed to have an adequate and continuous supply of products for patients who depend on these derivatives for survival. The biotechnology industry must be prepared to deal with changing economic patterns as recombinant DNA products affect traditional markets.

### Erythropoietin

Erythropoietin (EPO) is a glycoprotein hormone synthesized mostly by the kidneys in response to renal hypoxia. This hormone acts upon erythroid progenitor cells in the bone marrow, causing them to differentiate and produce red blood cells. Once the red blood cells are produced, an increase in oxygen is detected by the renal oxygen sensor cells and EPO is no longer secreted by the kidneys.

Recombinant human EPO is used today for treatment of patients (e.g., hemodialysis patients who suffer from severe chronic anemia because of inadequate EPO). This product is 98% pure and stable. It produces an increase in reticulocytes in 2.7–3.5 days and an increase in hematocrit in 7 days. Another possible use for recombinant EPO is to stimulate hematopoiesis in autologous blood donors. It also could be used to treat anemia in premature infants, or in patients with anemia associated with chronic diseases.

### Pharmacologic Alternatives

DDAVP is a synthetic analog of vasopressin. Because of its effect on factor VIII or vWF, DDAVP was originally used to treat patients suffering from mild to moderate hemophilia A or von Willebrand syndrome. Today, it is used to treat bleeding, or prophylactically in patients with a wide variety of disorders including uremia, drug-induced platelet dysfunction, and primary platelet disorders. The reported side effects are infrequent and usually mild. However, DDAVP is contraindicated in the rare Type IIb form of von Willebrand syndrome.

Vitamin K and fibrinolytic inhibitors may be appropriate forms of alternative therapy. Vitamin K is required for normal hemostasis. A deficiency will produce abnormal, liver-related blood coagulation tests (prothrombin time, for example). Epsilon aminocaproic acid and tranexamic acid are inhibitors of the fibrinolytic system. These drugs offer specific correction of the hemostatic defect in specialized circumstances of generalized fibrinolysis.

## HEMAPHERESIS

Platelets, granulocytes, plasma, and plasma components such as factor VIII are frequently collected by the technique of hemapheresis. Using hemapheresis, the harvesting of blood components is efficient and the remaining constituents of whole blood can be immediately returned to the donor. This technique may also be used for the therapeutic withdrawal of unwanted or harmful components from a patient's blood.

### Initial Development of Equipment

Early in the twentieth century, attempts were made to separate leukocytes from whole blood, but in the 1950s, the need to use blood and its derivatives efficiently produced the first actual equipment for separating blood continuously in a closed system. Prototype models of the present continuous flow blood cell separators were developed in the 1960s. The objective of the first equipment was to improve the efficiency of separating plasma and formed elements, but the modern continuous-flow blood cell separators were initially designed to harvest leukocytes.

Development of biomechanical equipment to fractionate whole blood was largely due to the influence of Dr. Edwin J. Cohn. During World War II, the need for plasma led Cohn to adapt De Laval's cream separator for separation of plasma from whole blood. The decade following the advent of the Cohn Fractionator was filled with experiments designed to separate leukocytes from whole blood by fractionation.

In 1961, Bierman reported the hematologic changes observed in donors after leukapheresis. Further studies of leukocyte depletion and replenishment led to improved designs of the separation bowls and equipment. Allen Latham, Jr. and the Arthur D. Little Company developed a discontinuous-flow set of bowls based on the basic principles of the Cohn Fractionator without its inherent cost and complexity. After the granting of the initial patent for this equipment, Latham supervised the first clinical trials of the equipment at the Boston Red Cross in 1973.

Later research was directed at refining the basic system and developing disposable equipment for the separation of blood into components. The results of these studies led to development of three separate pieces of equipment: one that automatically fractionated banked blood into plasma and packed red cells, a density-gradient centrifuge used to separate fractions of blood, a separator designed for use with healthy donors. The collaborative efforts of many scientists resulted in a reasonably effective, closed, continuous-flow centrifuge primarily designed to separate whole blood into individual cellular and plasma portions.

## Continuous-flow Cell Separation

In response to the need for processing large volumes of blood from healthy donors to obtain an adequate collection, NCI and IBM announced the development of a continuous-flow blood cell separator. This was the first closed-centrifuge system in which it was possible to subject whole blood to an uninterrupted flow and a constant force field while collecting all of its components. Field testing of this equipment began in 1966, and it was manufactured to order through 1975.

In the early 1970s, a new automated continuous-flow system for granulocyte-only collection was developed and marketed. Rather than using a force field to separate individual components by densities, this system was based on the principle of filtration leukapheresis. This method had been used for 50 years to selectively remove granulocytes from whole blood. The principle of filtration leukapheresis relies on selective and reversible adherence of granulocytes to nylon wool fibers. The remaining components pass through the filter and are returned to the donor. This method produces the highest granulocyte yields per unit of donor time and minimizes unwanted cellular elements such as lymphocytes, platelets, and erythrocytes.

In 1978, another model that maintained the basic ideas of continuous flow centrifugation, selective separation by means of collection ports and concentric channels, and a rotating seal was introduced. The flexibility of this equipment was enhanced in 1980 by the addition of a variation to the separation channel. The dual-stage separation channel was introduced as a means of obtaining platelet concentrates with minimal leukocyte contamination.

Computer technology was applied to hemapheresis equipment in 1979. A microprocessor was introduced to control machine operation with a sealless system. Whole blood separation and component collection are performed in the centrifuge by means of specifically designed chambers that interconnect. This permits blood flow from the donor vein into the separation bag of the centrifuge, transfer of component-rich plasma within the centrifuge to the collection bag, and subsequent return of recombined fractions to the donor's vein. With this system, whole blood enters the chamber, the packed red cells are forced to the outside wall and extracted for return to the donor, and the plasma, rich in the desired cell fraction, is transferred to the collection bag, where the transferred component is concentrated along the periphery and cell-poor plasma is removed for reinfusion with the red cells. This entire sterile procedure is monitored continuously by the microprocessor.

## Plasmapheresis

If plasmapheresis donors undergo the procedure no more often than once in every 8 weeks, the standards that apply to whole-blood donation apply to the selection and care of the donor. If *serial plasmapheresis* is performed (donation of plasma more frequently than once every 8 weeks), the FDA requirements and recommendations must be followed. Deviation from the requirements necessitates the approval of a physician.

The system used in performing phlebotomy and processing the blood must be designed to ensure safe reinfusion of autologous red blood cells. Plasmapheresis must be performed under conditions that prevent the possibility of an air embolism. If a manual system of separation is used, the donor's blood must bear two separate and independent means of identification that enable the donor and phlebotomist to determine with certainty that the contents of the bag are the donor's own autologous red blood cells. All of the available red blood cells should be returned to the donor before collecting a second unit of blood, or within 2 hours of the phlebotomy.

The current AABB *Standards* require that the amount of whole blood, not including anticoagulant, withdrawn for processing from a donor during plasmapheresis using a manual method must not exceed 500 mL at one time or 1000 mL during the entire session or within a 48 hour period. If the donor's weight is or exceeds 176 lb (80 kg), the amount of whole blood withdrawn at one time shall not exceed 600 mL, or 1200 mL during the entire plasmapheresis session or within a 48-hour period.

Automated devices for plasma procurement are available. This equipment makes possible the on-line collection of plasma from each donor without separating the donor from his/her own red cells. The amount of plasma shall not exceed the amount approved by the FDA for that instrument. Automation of plasmapheresis improves on the time-consuming process of manual collection and eliminates the risk of returning the wrong red cells to a donor.

The use of automated equipment will alleviate some of the problems associated with obtaining a sufficient supply of normal human plasma and donor identification. Plasmapheresis has been proposed and in some countries is actually used to supplement the plasma collected in other ways. Plasma and plasma components, such as cryoprecipitate for the initial isolation of factor VIII complex, can be obtained in greater quantity and more cost-effectively by automated plasmapheresis.

## Therapeutic Hemapheresis

Therapeutic hemapheresis is the process of separating and removing a harmful constituent from a patient through the use of a blood cell separator. Plasma exchange is the most common form of therapeutic hemapheresis. In this procedure, aliquots of the patient's plasma are removed and replaced with either 5% albumin or normal plasma. The patient's red blood cells are returned with the replacement solution.

Removal of harmful substances in the plasma, such as antibodies or immune complexes and concurrent administration of immunosuppressive or cytotoxic therapy are combined in most diseases treated by plasma exchange. The procedure can only be done at the written request of the patient's physician and with the consent of the blood bank physician.

Plasma exchange is believed generally to be effective in the treatment of the following diseases:

1. Hyperviscosity syndrome
2. Cryoglobulinemia
3. Myasthenia gravis
4. Goodpasture's syndrome
5. Thrombotic thrombocytopenia purpura
6. Guillain-Barré syndrome

The level of high-titer factor VIII inhibitor can be temporarily reduced by plasma exchange and may bring about some remission in post-transfusion purpura. Plasma exchange may be a useful adjunct to dietary treatment in reducing the circulating blood levels of phytanic acid in *Refsum's disease*. The efficacy of plasma exchange is less certain in conditions such as *systemic lupus erythematosus* and *rheumatoid arthritis*.

## CHAPTER SUMMARY

### Whole Blood

The use of anticoagulated whole blood has been drastically reduced over the past two decades in favor of component therapy. Whole blood is appropriate for use if enhanced oxygen-carrying capacity and blood volume replacement are needed.

### Red Blood Cell Products

Patients in need of the oxygen-carrying capabilities of hemoglobin are candidates for red blood cells. Because of extended in vivo survival time, infusion of these red cells can theoretically reduce blood requirements in transfusion-dependent patients. Leukocyte-poor blood is most frequently indicated for use in patients who have suffered from febrile transfusion reactions due to leukocytes. Frozen deglycerolized red cells allow preservation and extended storage of erythrocytes. This is particularly advan-

tageous for patients with rare blood types or multiple antibody problems.

### Platelets

The introduction of blood platelets as a blood component became possible when plastic whole blood donor collection bags with multiple satellite containers became readily available. This technology permitted the separation, storage, and transport of platelet concentrates to produce readily available blood bank components.

### Granulocytes

Leukocyte concentrates, primarily neutrophils, may be of value to patients with severe neutropenia who have a life-threatening systemic infection uncontrolled by antibiotics.

### Irradiated Blood and Blood Components

Graft-versus-host disease can occur after transfusion of blood or various blood products. The risk of graft-versus-host disease can be minimized, if not eliminated, by irradiating whole and various other components immediately before infusion.

### Plasma

Plasma can be separated from units of whole blood and stored as either single-donor plasma or fresh frozen plasma. Either form of plasma can be used for temporary volume replacement in patients who are depleted of whole blood or protein. Plasma may also be appropriate for coagulation factor replacement. Components such as cryoprecipitate are prepared from human plasma. Fractionation of human plasma can be into albumin or immune globulins.

### Plasma Components

Cryoprecipitated antihemophilic factor (AHF) is the cold insoluble precipitate of plasma remaining after fresh-frozen plasma obtained from whole blood or apheresis has been thawed between 1 and 6° C. Because cryoprecipitated AHF is a source of coagulation factor VIII, von Willebrand's factor (AHF-VWF), factor XIII, fibrinogen, and fibronectin, it is useful in the control of bleeding in various clinical disorders including factor VIII deficiency, von Willebrand's disease, factor XIII deficiency, and hypofibrinogenemia.

Factor IX complex, Konyne[R], is a commercially prepared, heat-treated plasma product that contains coagulation factors II, IX, X, and low levels of factor VII. The main indication for factor IX complex is in the treatment of conditions caused by factor IX (hemophilia B or Christmas disease) deficiency. The use of factor IX complex for patients with factors II or X or mild cases of hemophilia B should be considered if treatment with fresh-frozen plasma is not feasible or has proven ineffective.

## Blood Substitutes and Alternate Sources of Blood Components

While the use of human whole blood and blood components has many benefits, problems are associated with the use of these products. It is expected that the traditional blood supply system will continue to function for many years, but in the future the increasing demand may not be met. Substitutes and alternate sources are being developed as an alternative to human-derived blood or blood components.

Several types of synthetic red blood cell surrogates exist, including emulsions of perfluorocarbons, stroma-free hemoglobin, polymerized hemoglobin, and liposome-encapsulated hemoglobin.

It is conceivable that pluripotent stem cells could be maintained in culture to replicate and differentiate into mature blood cells. Major problems associated with this technology include the production and harvesting of a sufficient number of functional cells for transfusion and the harvesting of mature functional cells free from microbial contamination.

Although attempts to use phospholipids and the reconstitution of platelet membrane glycoproteins into lipid vesicles have been made, these experiments have failed to construct an artificial platelet that mimics platelet function.

Recombinant DNA technology is believed to hold much promise as an alternate source of plasma proteins. Within the next decade recombinant DNA products will probably replace at least several plasma derivatives. The major proteins currently recovered from human plasma fractionation are albumin, factor VIII, prothrombin complex, and immunoglobulins.

## Hemapheresis

Platelets, granulocytes, plasma and plasma components such as factor VIII are frequently collected by the technique of hemapheresis.

Therapeutic hemapheresis is the process of separating and removing a harmful constituent from a patient through the use of a blood cell separator. Plasma exchange is the most common form of therapeutic hemapheresis and is believed to be generally effective in the treatment of hyperviscosity syndrome, cryoglobulinemia, myasthenia gravis, Goodpasture's syndrome, thrombotic thrombocytopenia purpura, and Guillain-Barré syndrome.

---

## REVIEW QUESTIONS

1–4. Match the following blood products with the most appropriate clinical application:
  1. Whole blood (less than 4 or 5 days old)
  2. Packed red blood cells
  3. Washed red cells
  4. Neocyte-enriched packed cells
  A. Exchange transfusion in newborn infants
  B. Patients with *paroxysmal nocturnal hemoglobinuria*
  C. If oxygen-carrying capacity and volume replacement are needed
  D. Patients with thalassemia
  E. If the oxygen-carrying capabilities of hemoglobin are needed

5. The currently approved FDA approved shelf-life of whole blood drawn into CPDA-1 is _____ days.
  A. 21
  B. 28
  C. 32
  D. 35

6. Whole blood has the advantage of:
  A. Increasing the availability of components.
  B. Being less expensive than combined component therapy.
  C. Reducing the risks of combined component therapy.
  D. Both B and C.

7. Packed red blood cells prepared in an open system have an expiration time of:
  A. 24 hours
  B. 48 hours
  C. 72 hours
  D. 21 days

8 and 9. Packed red blood cells have the advantage of
  8. _____ but the disadvantage of
  9. _____ .
  8.
  A. Decreased exposure to infectious diseases
  B. Volume reduction
  C. Increased concentration of anticoagulant
  D. Increased $K^+$
  E. Increased viscosity
  9.
  A. Increased cost
  B. Increased $K^+$
  C. Increased concentration of anticoagulant
  D. Increased viscosity
  E. No known disadvantages

10. The purpose of rejuvenation of packed red cells is:
  A. Depletion of 2,3 DPG
  B. Depletion of ATP
  C. Restoration of normal oxygen transport
  D. Reduction of the risk of hepatitis transmission

11. A characteristic of neocytes is:
  A. A lower level of pyruvate kinase activity
  B. Longer transfusion survival time
  C. Greater density than mature erythrocytes
  D. Shorter transfusion survival time

12. Hemochromatosis may be reduced by transfusing:
    A. Packed red blood cells
    B. Whole blood
    C. Washed red cells
    D. Neocytes

**13 and 14**

13. For blood to be considered to be leukocyte-poor by current standards and to be suitable for transfusion, the unit of blood must remove
    13. _____% of leukocytes and retain
    14. _____% of erythrocytes.

13.
    A. 30
    B. 50
    C. 70
    D. 90
    E. 100

14.
    A. 30
    B. 50
    C. 70
    D. 90
    E. 100

15. The standards require that units having leukocytes removed by washing should contain *no more* than _____ leukocytes.
    A. $0.2 \times 10^9$/L
    B. $0.5 \times 10^9$/L
    C. $1.0 \times 10^9$/L
    D. $2.0 \times 10^9$/L

16. Leukocyte-poor blood is most frequently indicated clinically in patients who have:
    A. A high titer of antibodies to erythrocytes
    B. A high titer of antibodies to leukocytes
    C. Congestive heart failure
    D. Previously experienced febrile transfusion reactions

17. Of the available techniques used to prepare leukocyte-poor blood, the technique that has the greatest number of advantages for most alloimmunized patients is:
    A. Spin-cool-filter
    B. Upright spin
    C. Inverted spin
    D. Spin-filter

18. The most commonly used methods for depleting red cells of leukocytes are:
    A. Washing and buffy-coated removal
    B. Inverted spin and washing
    C. Upright spin and inverted spin
    D. Spin-filter and washing

19. The percentage of red cells recovered after thawing and deglycerolization of frozen blood is:
    A. 35%
    B. 50%

C. 75%
D. 85%

20. Which of the following is *not* a clinical indication for frozen/deglycerolized red cells?
    A. An alloimmunized patient who has previously experienced nonhemolytic febrile transfusion reactions
    B. A patient with an IgA deficiency
    C. A patient who is allergic to plasma proteins
    D. None of the above

21. Which of the following is a cryoprotective additive?
    A. Glycerol
    B. Dimethyl sulfoxide
    C. Polyvinylpyrrolidone (PVP)
    D. All of the above

**22 and 23**

22. Under current regulations, frozen blood can be stored for up to **22.** _____ at **23.** _____

22.
    A. 35 days
    B. 90 days
    C. 1 year
    D. 10 years

23.
    A. 4° C
    B. 0° C
    C. −20° C
    D. −65° C or colder

24. The *most common* application of deglycerolized red cells is:
    A. Autologous transfusion
    B. Prevention of febrile reactions caused by leukoagglutinins
    C. Prevention of febrile reactions caused by platelet antibodies
    D. Decreased sensitization to platelet antigens

25. The average total leukocyte count in a unit of deglycerolized red cells is:
    A. $0.1 \times 10^9$/L
    B. $0.3 \times 10^9$/L
    C. $0.5 \times 10^9$/L
    D. $5.0 \times 10^9$/L

26. Which of the following is *not* an advantage of deglycerolized red cells?
    A. Reduction of leukocytes
    B. Reduction of platelets
    C. Plasma protein removal
    D. Lower cost

27. The proper storage temperature for platelet concentrates for a 3-day period of time is _____° C.
    A. −1 to 0
    B. 1 to 6
    C. 10 to 15
    D. 20 to 24

28. The pH of stored platelet concentrates must *not* fall below:
    A. 4.5
    B. 5.5

**C.** 6.0

**D.** 7.0

29. According to Federal regulations, _____ of random donor platelet concentrates must contain _____ platelets.

    **A.** 30% − 5.5 × $10^{10}$

    **B.** 50% − 1.5 × $10^{10}$

    **C.** 50% − 5.5 × $10^{10}$

    **D.** 75% − 5.5 × $10^{10}$

30. The pH of platelet concentrates at maximum storage depends on:

    **A.** Type of plastic bag

    **B.** Concentration of platelets

    **C.** Method of preparation

    **D.** Type of anticoagulant that the initial blood was drawn in

31. The best storage condition for platelet concentrates is:

    **A.** On a 6 rpm elliptical rotator

    **B.** On a 1 rpm elliptical rotator

    **C.** On a 2 rpm circular rotator

    **D.** All of the above, except A

32. Which of the following is *not* a possible consequence of the transfusion of platelet concentrates?

    **A.** Bacterial contamination

    **B.** Hemolytic transfusion reaction

    **C.** Pulmonary edema

    **D.** Febrile reactions to plasma proteins

33. Granulocyte transfusions are clinically appropriate for:

    **A.** Patients with severe neutropenia

    **B.** Patients who have infections

    **C.** Patients who have life-threatening systemic infections that are uncontrolled by antibiotics

    **D.** Patients needing granulocytes from a single unit of blood

34. Graft-versus-host disease is caused by:

    **A.** Granulocytes

    **B.** Platelets

    **C.** Lymphocytes

    **D.** Erythrocytes

35. Which of the following blood components has *not* been documented to cause GVHD?

    **A.** Single units of fresh plasma

    **B.** Fresh frozen plasma

    **C.** Stored whole blood

    **D.** Washed red cells

36. The types of patients at highest risk of developing GVHD are:

    **A.** Infants receiving intra-uterine transfusions

    **B.** Children with severe congenital AIDS

    **C.** Patients with acute leukemia receiving total body radiation

    **D.** Patients with solid tumors

37. The radiation source for irradiation of blood products is:

    **A.** $^{131}$I

    **B.** $^{137}$Ce

    **C.** $^{14}$C

    **D.** $^{131}$Te

38. The effect of radiation on lymphocytes is that it:

    **A.** Inhibits lymphocyte mitotic activity

    **B.** Inhibits lymphocyte blast transformation

    **C.** Affects locomotion

    **D.** Both A and B

39. Single-donor plasma can appropriately be used for patients with:

    **A.** Dehydration

    **B.** Severe burns

    **C.** Hypovolemic shock

    **D.** Both B and C

40. An appropriate use of fresh-frozen plasma is:

    **A.** Volume replacement

    **B.** Protein replacement

    **C.** Coagulation factors replacement

    **D.** Carbohydrate and mineral supplementation

41. If a unit of fresh frozen plasma is stored at 1 to 6° C, it *must* be used within _____ hours after thawing to correct a labile coagulation deficiency.

    **A.** 2

    **B.** 4

    **C.** 6

    **D.** 12

42. Which of the following is a characteristic of cryoprecipitated antihemophiliac factor?

    **A.** Contains platelets

    **B.** Contains factor VIII

    **C.** Contains fibrinogen

    **D.** All of the above except A

43. How many bags of cryoprecipitate are required if the desired level of factor VIII is 60% and the patient's plasma volume is 2500 mL?

    **A.** 13

    **B.** 15

    **C.** 17

    **D.** 19

44. Once defrosted, cryoprecipitate must be administered within _____ hours of thawing.

    **A.** 2

    **B.** 4

    **C.** 6

    **D.** 12

45. Transmission of viruses in cryoprecipitate may be eliminated by:

    **A.** Heating in the liquid form

    **B.** Heating in a lyopholized form

    **C.** Irradiating with ultraviolet light

    **D.** All of the above

46. A major disadvantage of factor IX complex is the:
    A. High risk of hepatitis
    B. Lack of other coagulation factors
    C. Lack of platelets
    D. Need to administer one hour after reconstitution
47. Perfluorocarbons have been investigated as:
    A. Platelet substitutes
    B. Granulocyte substitutes
    C. Red blood cell substitutes
    D. Plasma substitutes
48. One of the major disadvantages of stroma-free and polymerized hemoglobin is:
    A. Poor volume expansion
    B. Toxicity
    C. Decreased tissue oxygenation effects
    D. Difficulty of preparation
49. Neohemocytes are closer to being prototype artificial red cells because of the following characteristic(s):
    A. Lack of degradation of encapsulated hemoglobin
    B. Physiologically acceptable oxygen affinity
    C. Resistance to biodegradation
50. Recombinant DNA technology has been successful in the cloning and expression of all of the following except:
    A. Albumin
    B. Factor VIII
    C. Factor IX
    D. Factor X

## Bibliography

Bacterial contamination of platelet pools—Ohio, 1991. MMWR, 41(3), Jan. 24, 1992.
Banzhaf, J.: Technical Quarterly (Am. Red Cross Blood Services, Rochester Region). Summer, 1988, pp. 1–2.
Beissinger, R.L., Farmer, M.C., and Gossage, J.L.: Liposome-encapsulated hemoglobin as a red cell surrogate. Am. Soc. for Artificial Internal Organs, 32(1):58–63, 1986.
Biotechnology. Parenterals, 4(5):1–5, 1986.
Blomback, M.J., Chmielewska, et al.: Activation of blood coagulation, fibrinolytic and kallikrein systems during storage of plasma. Vox Sang., 47(5):335–342, 1984.
Blumberg, N., et al.: A critical survey of fresh-frozen plasma use. Transfusion, 26(6):551–553, 1986.
Boral, L.I.: Platelet transfusion therapy. Lab. Med., 16(4):221–226, 1985.
Buccino, L.A.: Blood substitute potential thrusts research into high gear. Advance for medical laboratory professionals. October 19, 1992 (12–13).
Button, L., et al.: Rejuvenation of red cells drawn in Adsol to extend autologous red cell storage. Transfusion, 26(6):558, 1986.
Campbell, J. (Ed.): AABB News Briefs, 11(6):3, 1988.
Castro, O.L.: Long-term cryopreservation of red cells from patients with sickle cell disease. Transfusion, 25(1):70–72, 1985.
Chang, T.M.: Artificial cells in medicine and biotechnology. Appl. Biochem. Biotechnol., 10:5–24, 1984.

Dwyer, J.M.: Manipulating the immune system with immune globulin. New Engl. J. Med., 326(2):107, 1992.
Eisenstaedt, R.S.: Concurrent audit of fresh frozen plasma use. Abstract of a paper presented at the Annual American Association of Blood Banks Meeting. Transfusion, 25(5):466, 1985.
Factor IX Complex Product Brochure. Berkeley, CA, Cutter Biological, May, 1986.
Fratantoni, J.C.: Comment on standardized procedures the regulatory process. Transfusion, 26:(1):36–37, 1986.
Gottschall, J.L., et al.: Studies of the minimum temperature at which human platelets can be stored with full maintenance of viability. Transfusion, 26(5):460–462, 1986.
Gould, S.A., et al.: The development of polymerized pyridoxylated hemoglobin solution as a red cell substitute. Ann. Emerg. Med., 15(12):1416–1419.
Gould, S.A.: Fluosol-DA as a red-cell substitute in acute anemia. N. Engl. J. Med., 314(26):1653–1656, 1986.
Harley, K.M., et al.: Platelet temperature in transport under warm and cold conditions. Abstract of a paper to be presented at the Annual American Asociation of Blood Banks Meeting. Transfusion, 26(6):558, 1986.
Hayward, J.A., et al.: Polymerized liposomes as stable oxygen-carriers. Fed. Eur. Biochem. Soc., 187(2):261–266, 1985.
Head, D.R.: Whole blood versus packed red cells. Transfusion, 25(6):591, 1985.
Hedlund, B.E., et al. Polymerized Hemoglobins. In Transfusion Medicine: Recent Technological Advances. New York, Alan R. Liss, Inc., pp. 39–48, 1986.
Heldenbrant, C.M., et al.: Evaluation of two viral inactivation methods for the preparation of safer factor VIII and factor IX concentrates. Transfusion, 25(6):510–515, 1985.
Henry, J.B. (Ed.): Clinical Diagnosis and Management by Laboratory Methods, 17th ed. Philadelphia, W.B. Saunders Co., 1982, pp. 1020–1022.
Hogan, V.A., et al.: A simple method for preparing neocyte-enriched Leukocyte-Poor Blood for Transfusion-Dependent Patients. Transfusion, 26(3):253–257, 1986.
Hogge, D.E., et al.: Platelet Storage for 7 Days in Second-Generation Blood Bags. Transfusion, 26(2):131–135, 1986.
Horowitz, B., et al.: Inactivation of viruses in labile blood derivatives. Transfusion, 25(6):523–527, 1985.
Huestis, D.W., Boue, J.R., and Case, J.: Practical Blood Transfusion, 4th ed. Boston, Little, Brown and Co., 1988, pp. 328–336.
Huggins, C.: Preparation and usefulness of frozen blood. Annual Review of Medicine, 36:499–503, 1985.
Hunt, C.A., et al.: Synthesis and evaluation of a prototypal artificial red cell. Science, 230:1165B, 1985.
Hunt, C.A., and Burnette, R.R.: Lipid microencapsulation of hemoglobin. Appl. Biochem. Biotechnol, 10:147–149, 1984.
International Forum: What is the Prospective Impact of the Recombinant DNA Technique on the Production of Human Plasma Derivatives? Which are the Derivates Where Donor Plasma Could be Replaced? Vox Sang., 44:390–395, 1983.
Iwasaki, K., et al.: Efficacy and safety of hemoglobin-polyethylene glycol conjugate (pyridoxylated polyethylene glycol hemoglobin) as an oxygen-carrying resuscitation fluid. Artif. Organs, 10(6):470–474, 1986.
Janco, R.L., et al.: Perfluorochemical blood substitutes differentially alter human monocyte procoagulant generation and oxidative metabolism. Transfusion, 25(6):578–582, 1985.
Kahn, R.A., Allen, R.W., and Baldassare, J.: Alternate sources and substitutes for therapeutic blood components. Blood, 66(1):1–12, 1985.
Kevy, S.V., et al.: A seven year evaluation of extended storage of deglycerolized red cells. Abstract of Paper Presented at the Annual Meeting of the American Association of Blood Banks. Transfusion, 25(5):476, 1985.

Kim, H.C., et al.: The role of frozen-thawed-washed red blood cells (FTW-RBC) in preventing transfusion acquired CMV infection (TA-CMVI) in the neonate. Abstract of paper to be presented at the American Association of Blood Banks Annual Meeting. Transfusion, 25(5):472, 1985.

Lane, T.A., et al.: Leukocyte reduction in blood component therapy. Annals Int. Med, 117(2):151–162, July 15, 1992.

Lane, T.A., and Lamkin, G.E.: Glycogen metabolism in stored granulocytes. Transfusion, 25(3):246–250, 1985.

Lane, T.A., and Lamkin, G.E.: The effect of storage on degranulation by human neutrophils. Transfusion, 25(2):155–161, 1985.

Leitman, S.F., and Holland, P.V.: Irradiation of blood products: Indications and guidelines. Transfusion, 25(4):293–300, 1985.

Lowe, K.C.: Blood transfusion or blood substitution? Vox Sang., 51(4):257–263, 1986.

Luff, R.D., et al.: Microwave technology for the rapid thawing of frozen blood components. Am. J. Clin. Pathol., Vol. 83, No. 1:59–64, 1985.

McGill, M.: Blood product irradiation recommendations. Transfusion, 26(6):542, 1986.

McLoud, B.C., Sassetto, R.J., Cole, E.R., and Pierce, M.I.: Factor VIII collection by pheresis. Lancet, Sept. 27:671–673, 1980.

McMican, A., Luban, N.L.C., and Sacher, R.A.: Practical aspects of blood irradiation. Lab. Med., 18(5):299–303, 1987.

Menache, D.: Mesures to Inactivate Viral Contaminants of Pooled Plasma Products. Infection, Immunity and Blood Transfusion. New York, Alan R. Liss, Inc., 1985. pp. 407–423.

Menitove, et al.: Stability of protein C and protein S in blood components. Abstract of a paper presented at the Annual American Association of Blood Banks Meeting. Transfusion, 25:466, 1985.

Meryman, H.T., and Hornblower, M.: The preparation of red cells depleted of leukocytes. Transfusion, 26(1):101–106, 1986.

Millward, B.L., and Hoeltge, G.A.: The historical development of automated hemapheresis. J. Clin. Apheresis, 1:25–32, 1982.

Mitra, G., et al.: Elimination of infectious retroviruses during preparation of immunoglobulins. Transfusion, 26(4):94, 1986.

Moore, G.L., and Ledford, M.E.: Effects of 4000 Rad irradiation on the in vitro storage properties of packed red cells. Transfusion, 25(6):583–585, 1985.

Moss, G.S., et al.: Hemoglobin solution—from tetramer to polymer. Surgery, 95(3):249–255, 1984.

Murphy, S.: Guidelines for platelet transfusion. JAMA, 259(16):2453–2454, 1988.

National Institutes of Health. Fresh-Frozen Plasma: Indications and Risks. Connecticut Medicine, 49(5):295–297, 1985.

Oberman, H.A.: Transfusion Classics. Transfusion, 25:359, 1985.

Overby, L.R.: Challenges and Opportunities in Biotechnology. In Infection, Immunity, and Blood Transfusion. New York: Alan R. Liss, Inc., 1985, pp. 425–443.

Peetoom, F.: Closing: Transfusion Medicine, Recent Technological Advances. In Transfusion Medicine, Recent Technological Advances. New York, Alan R. Liss, Inc., pp. 343–346.

Read, E.J., and Klein, H.G.: Fresh frozen plasma transfusion: A perspective surgery. Abstract of AABB Meeting. Transfusion, 25(5):465, 1985.

Rock, G., et al.: Plasma Collection using an automated membrane device. Transfusion, 26(3):269–271, 1986.

Rodgers, G.P., et al.: Augmentation by erythropoietin of the fetal-hemoglobin response to hydroxyuria in sickle cell disease. New Engl. J. Med., 328(21):73–80, 1993.

Schwartz, G.J., and Diller, K.R.: Intracellular freezing of human granulocytes. Cryobiology, 21:654–660, 1984.

Sehgal, L.R., et al.: Polymerized pyridoxylated hemoglobin: Evolution of a new blood substitute. Am. Clin. Prod. Rev., 6(7):10–13, 1987.

Sehgal, L.R., et al.: Polymerized pyridoxylated hemoglobin: A red cell substitute with normal oxygen capacity. Surgery, 95(4):433–438, 1984.

Siber, G.R.: Immune globulin to prevent nosocomial infections. N Engl. J. Med., 327(4):269–270, 1992.

Sirchia, G., et al.: Leukocyte depletion of red cell units at the bedside by transfusion through a new filter. Transfusion, 27(3):402–405, 1987.

Snyder, E.L., et al.: The effect of mode of agitation and type of plastic bag on storage characteristics and in vivo kinetics of platelet concentrates. Transfusion, 26(2):125–130, 1986.

Snyder, A.J., et al.: Why is fresh-frozen plasma transfused? Transfusion, 26:107–112, 1986.

*Standards for Blood Banks and Transfusion Services,* American Association of Blood Banks: 15th ed. Bethesda, MD. 1993.

Towell, B.L., et al.: A comparison of frozen and fresh platelet concentrates in the support of thrombocytopenic patients. Transfusion, 26(6):525–530, 1986.

Tremper, K.K., and Anderson, S.T.: Perfluorochemical emulsion oxygen transport fluids: A clinical review. Ann. Rev. Med., 36:309–313, 1985.

Tsuchida, E.: Liposome-embedded iron-porphyrins as an artificial oxygen carrier. Ann. N. Y. Acad. Sci., 446:429–442, 1985.

Turgeon, M.L.: Should a community hospital establish a frozen blood program? Med Lab., September:20–23, 1972.

Van Aken, W.G.: Future trends in blood component preparation. Vox Sang., 51(Suppl.1):67–71, 1986.

Widmann, F.K.: Technical Manual. (9th Ed.) Arlington, Va., American Association of Blood Banks, 1985. pp. 41–42, 44, 45, 46, 50, 52, 55, 269.

Yomtovian, R.: From ABO to HTLV: changing trends in blood transfusion safety. Minn. Med., 68:587–589, 1985.

Zeiner, D.E.: Many transfusion substitutes on the horizon but few used so far. Adv. Med. Lab. Professionals, 38:20–21, 1991.

# Clinical Conditions Associated
# with Immunohematology

# 11

# Hemolytic Disease of the Newborn

At the conclusion of this chapter, the reader should be able to:

- Briefly define the cause (etiology) and consequences of hemolytic disease of the newborn (HDN).
- Describe the consequences of the coating of fetal erythrocytes with maternal antibody.
- Define the term "extramedullary hematopoiesis."
- Name the antibodies most frequently responsible for HDN in descending order of severity and describe the mechanism of HDN.
- Describe the in utero consequences of extensive hemolysis and explain how the fetus attempts to compensate for hemolysis.
- Compare the consequences of hemolysis to the fetus versus those to the newborn baby.
- Name the major immunoglobulin class responsible for HDN.
- Explain the basic antigen-antibody reaction that produces HDN.
- List and briefly explain the factors that affect the production of antibodies in the maternal circulation.
- Name at least three causes of transplacental hemorrhage and the volume of fetal blood that is considered significant in fetal-maternal hemorrhage.
- Name procedures generally used in prenatal testing and describe the procedure of amniocentesis and the significance of the results.
- Name procedures used in postnatal assessment of potential HDN. Describe the significance of each procedure to the diagnosis.
- Describe the etiology, genetic frequency, symptoms, physiology, laboratory diagnosis, and treatment of HDN caused by ABO incompatibility.
- Describe the etiology, genetic frequency, symptoms, physiology, laboratory assessment, and treatment of HDN caused by Rh and other blood group incompatibilities.
- Compare the relationship of HDN caused by ABO incompatibility to HDN caused by Rh incompatibility.
- Name and describe the prenatal tests and treatments that are significant in HDN caused by anti-D.
- Calculate the appropriate number of vials of Rh IG when given the Kleihauer-Betke value.
- List and describe the general and laboratory criteria for the administration of Rh IG.

## Chapter Outline

Hemolytic disease of the newborn (HDN) or erythroblastosis fetalis results from excessive destruction of fetal red cells by maternal antibodies. This condition in the fetus or newborn infant is clinically characterized by anemia and jaundice. If the hemoglobin breakdown product, bilirubin, which visibly produces jaundice, reaches excessive levels in the newborn infant's circulation, it accumulates in lipid-rich nervous tissue. This deposition of bilirubin (kernicterus) can cause mental retardation or death.

## THE GENERAL CHARACTERISTICS OF HDN

### Basic Physiology of HDN

In hemolytic disease of the newborn (Fig. 11-1), the erythrocytes of the fetus become coated with maternal antibod-

ies that correspond to specific fetal antigens. This hemolytic process reduces the normal 45- to 70-day life span of fetal erythrocytes.

The fetal hematopoietic tissues (the liver, spleen and bone marrow) respond to hemolysis by increasing production of erythrocytes. Increased erythrocyte production outside the bone marrow, *extramedullary hematopoiesis,* can result in enlargement of the liver and spleen. There is also premature release from the bone marrow, predominantly of many nucleated erythrocytes into the fetal circulation. If increased erythropoiesis cannot compensate for erythrocyte destruction, a progressively severe anemia develops. This severe anemia may cause the fetus to develop cardiac failure with generalized edema (hydrops fetalis), resulting in death in utero. In newborn infants, severe anemia can produce heart failure shortly after birth.

Less severely affected infants continue after birth to experience erythrocyte destruction, which generates large quantities of unconjugated bilirubin. Before birth, unconjugated bilirubin is normally bound to albumin and forms conjugated bilirubin in the mother's liver through the action of the enzyme glucuronidase. The newborn infant's immature liver does not efficiently synthesize glucuronidase during the first few days of life. This results in low amounts of the enzyme in the newborn infant's circulation. Additionally, the albumin, which is necessary to form conjugated bilirubin, is limited. This combination of factors in the newborn, who must excrete large quantities of bilirubin resulting from excessive hemolysis, can produce the threat of accumulation of free bilirubin in lipid-rich tissue of the central nervous system. Total plasma bilirubin levels approaching 20 mg/dL can cause mental retardation or death.

### The Mechanism of Antibody Transfer from Mother to Fetus

The transfer of antibodies from the maternal circulation to the fetal circulation occurs through the placenta. The only immunoglobulin that is selectively transported to the fetus is IgG. Although the fetus produces some IgG, IgG in cord serum is derived almost entirely from the maternal circulation. Among the five classes of immunoglobulins in humans, only IgG is found in cord blood in a concentration equivalent to the concentration found in maternal blood. The other immunoglobulin classes, such as IgM, are either present in much lower concentrations in the newborn than in the mother or entirely absent.

In the first 12 weeks of gestation, only small amounts of IgG are synthesized. This concentration of IgG continues to rise until birth. Evidence suggests that the levels of the IgG subclass, IgG1, rise at an earlier stage of gestation than IgG3 subclass levels. At birth, IgG1 levels are higher than those of IgG3 compared to maternal concentrations. The fetal concentrations of IgG2 are distinctly lower than those of the other IgG subclasses.

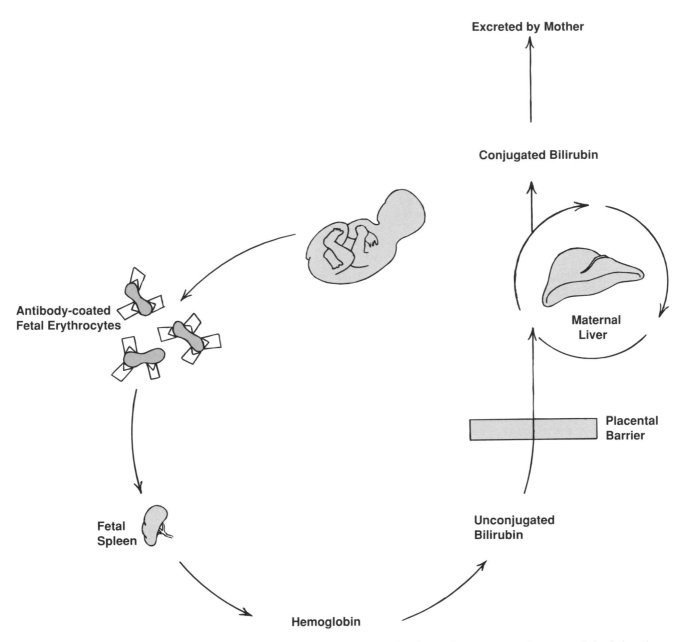

**Figure 11-1.** Basic physiology of hemolytic disease of the newborn. If D antigen-bearing erythrocytes enter the maternal circulation, these antigens are recognized as foreign by the D negative mother. If antigenic stimulation or an anamnestic response caused by anti-D occurs in subsequent pregnancies, high titers of anti-D are produced in the maternal circulation. These anti-D antibodies can cross the placental barrier and attach to the D positive erythrocytes of the fetus in the current pregnancy. These antibody-coated erythrocytes have a shortened survival and the fetus suffers from anemia. The bilirubin resulting from erythrocyte (hemoglobin) breakdown is excreted through the maternal circulation and does not injure the fetus.

The mechanism by which IgG passes through the placenta is accomplished by an active transport mechanism determined by the Fc portion of the Ig molecule. Each immunoglobulin class is characterized by its heavy polypeptide chain. Therefore, the structure of IgG responsible for transplacental passage should reside in the ($\gamma$) chain. Most research on the subject of transplacental passage supports the hypothesis that all IgG subclasses are capable of crossing the placental barrier between mother and fetus.

## Blood Systems Involved in Causing HDN

The categories of HDN include virtually every blood group antibody that can occur as IgG (Table 11-1). In a survey of antibodies that have caused HDN, over 70 different antibodies were identified. Based on specific IgG antibody type, the causes of HDN in descending order of severity are:

1. Anti-D, either alone or in combination with anti-C or anti-E.

**Table 11-1. Antibodies Causing HDN***

| Blood Group System | Related Antigens | Severity of HDN |
|---|---|---|
| ABO | A and B | Mild |
| Rh | D | Mild to severe |
| | C | Mild to moderate |
| | c | Mild to severe |
| | E | Mild to severe |
| | e | Mild to moderate |
| Kell | K | Mild to severe |
| | k | Mild to severe |
| Duffy | Fy$^a$ | Mild to severe |
| | Fy$^b$ | Not implicated in HDN |
| Kidd | Jk$^a$ | Mild to severe |
| | Jk$^b$ | Mild to severe |
| Lutheran | Lu$^a$ | Mild |
| | Lu$^b$ | Mild |
| Lewis | Le$^a$ | Rare |
| MNSs | M | Mild to severe |
| | N | Mild |
| | S | Mild to severe |
| | s | Mild to severe |
| P | PP$_1$P$^k$ (Tj$^a$) | Mild to severe |
| I | | Not a proven cause of HDN |
| Xg | Xg$^a$ | Mild |
| Colton | Co$^a$ | Severe |
| | Co$^{a-b}$ | Mild |
| Cartwright | Yt$^a$ | Moderate to severe |
| | Yt$^b$ | Mild |
| Diego | Di$^a$ | Mild to severe |
| | Di$^b$ | Mild to severe |
| Wright | Wr$^a$ | Severe |
| Other antigens | At$_a$ | Mild |
| | Batty | Mild |
| | Becker | Mild |
| | Berrens | Mild |
| | Biles | Moderate |
| | En$^a$ | Moderate |
| | Evans | Mild |
| | Ge | Mild |
| | Gonzales | Mild |
| | Good | Severe |
| | Heibel | Moderate |
| | Hunt | Mild |
| | Jobbins | Mild |
| | Jr$^a$ | Mild |
| | Lan | Mild |
| | Radin | Moderate |
| | Rm | Mild |
| | Ven | Mild |
| | Zd | Moderate |

* Modified from Weinstein, L.: Irregular Antibodies Causing Hemolytic Disease of the Newborn Clin. Obstet. Gynecol. *25*(2):321–332, 1982.

2. Other Rh antibodies, such as anti-c.
3. Other blood group system antibodies, such as anti-Kell, anti-Duffy, and anti-Kidd.
4. ABO antibodies.

High titers of anti-A, B of the IgG type in group O mothers commonly cause a mild hemolytic disease of the newborn in approximately 1 in 150 births. Rarely is this form of HDN severe. This is chiefly because the A and B antigens are not fully expressed in the erythrocytes of the fetus and newborn.

Until the early 1970s, anti-D was the most frequent cause of moderate or severe forms of HDN. Before modern treatment for Rh$_o$ (D)-induced HDN prevention, anti-D, either alone or in combination with anti-C, accounted for approximately 93% of the cases of non-ABO HDN. Other forms of HDN related to the Rh blood group system, such as anti-c and anti-E, or anti-C and anti-e, accounted for about 6% of the cases. Only a small fraction, approximately 1%, of the cases of HDN was caused by antibodies outside the Rh system, such as anti-Kell or anti-Duffy. Since the development of modern treatment, however, against immunization to the D antigen, the frequency of HDN caused by anti-D has significantly decreased.

**Mechanism of HDN**

HDN results from the production of antibodies in the mother that have been stimulated by foreign antigens. These immune antibodies subsequently react with fetal antigens if the latter are present. Erythrocytic antigens and leukocyte and platelet antigens can all induce maternal immunization by the formation of IgG antibodies.

Manifestations of fetal-maternal incompatibility are not usually apparent in a firstborn infant. The first exposure to a foreign antigen "sensitizes" an immunocompetent mother and a low titer of IgM antibody is produced. IgM cannot cross the fetal-maternal placental barrier. In a second or subsequent pregnancy, repeated exposure can lead to the production of IgG antibody that can cross the fetal-maternal barrier.

The actual production of antibodies depends on a variety of factors: the genetic makeup of an individual, the antigenicity of a specific antigen, and the actual amount of antigen introduced into the maternal circulation.

### Genetic Makeup

For antibody formation to take place, the mother must genetically lack the trait and the fetus must genetically possess the trait, which has been inherited from the father. This genetic inheritance expresses itself in the mother as her being negative for an antigen, whereas the fetus possesses the antigen.

### Immunogenicity

Antigens vary in terms of the number of receptor sites on the erythrocyte membrane and their immunogenic strength. Certain antigens, such as D, c, and Kell, are known to be very potent in stimulating the immune system.

### Transplacental Hemorrhage

Transplacental hemorrhage (TPH) can occur at any stage of pregnancy. Immunization resulting from TPH can result from negligible doses during the first 6 months in utero; however, significant immunizing hemorrhage usually occurs during the third trimester or at delivery. Fetal erythrocytes can also enter the maternal circulation as the result of physical trauma due to an injury, abortion, ectopic pregnancy, amniocentesis or normal delivery. Abruptio placentae, cesarean section, and manual removal of the placenta are often associated with a considerable increase in TPH. A significant fetal-maternal hemorrhage is considered to be 30 mL or greater; evidence exists to support the theory that a minimal dose for inducing a primary immunization is probably less than 0.1 mL for some of the more immunogenic antigens.

## ASSESSMENT OF HDN

### Prenatal Testing

The following procedures are generally used in prenatal testing under various conditions:

1. ABO grouping.
2. Rh testing for D and weak D ($D^u$).
3. Alloantibody screening; if negative, it should be repeated again at 34 weeks of gestation.
4. Alloantibody identification, if the antibody screening test is positive.
5. Antibody titer, if an alloantibody is present.
6. Amniocentesis.

### Amniocentesis

Amniocentesis is an analysis of fluid from the amniotic cavity obtained by the transabdominal insertion of a needle. This analysis provides the physician with an assessment of fetal development and well-being. Using a prediction table, an estimate of cord hemoglobin concentration can be determined based on the optical density of the amniotic fluid during gestation. Other factors, such as genetic disorders and chromosomal abnormalities, can be determined through amniotic fluid.

Some of the clinical criteria used in deciding to perform an amniocentesis include the following:

1. If a previous infant had HDN, amniocentesis may be performed as early as 28 weeks of gestation, even if the antibody titer remains constant. If a previous child was severely afflicted, an amniocentesis may be performed as early as the 22nd week of gestation.
2. When the maternal antibody level accelerates before the 34th week of gestation.

The severity of hemolysis is related to the amount of bilirubin in the amniotic fluid as measured by spectrophotometry. The optical density (OD) of normal amniotic fluid forms a smooth curve at different wavelengths over the range of 400 to 600 nm. According to Liley, the OD

of amniotic fluid at 450 to 460 nm in normal pregnancy is about 0.05 at 30 weeks and falls to about 0.02 at term. Fluid from an infant with severe HDN has a greatly increased optical density with a peak at 450 to 460, the so-called bilirubin bulge. There is a tendency for the bilirubin to decrease in mild cases of HDN as the pregnancy advances.

At 450 nm, the difference between the infant's OD and a baseline value is determined. This value is plotted on a Liley graph. On this graph, three zones are associated with the status of the severity of HDN. Zone 1 represents an unaffected state in which the fetus is considered not to be in danger. Zone 2 indicates that the fetus needs monitoring and the amniotic fluid should be retested. Zone 3 indicates that the fetus is in danger.

Amniotic fluid can also be analyzed to aid in making a decision regarding early delivery of the infant. Absorbance at 650 nm may be useful as a screen or as part of a battery of lung maturity estimates. If a fetus is under 34 weeks of gestation or immature for its gestational age, an intrauterine transfusion may be indicated rather than premature delivery.

### Percutaneous Umbilical Blood Sampling

Percutaneous umbilical blood sampling (PUBS), also referred to as *cordocentesis,* is becoming an important tool in fetal-maternal medicine. This technique allows for diagnosis, through fetal blood aspiration and therapy, because of direct access to the fetal circulation. Using an ultrasound-guided needle, the umbilical cord is punctured close to its placental insertion. Most physicians prefer the umbilical vein over the artery because the vein is larger, straighter, and has a thinner wall. A small blood sample can be aspirated and sent for study, which can include the Kleihauer-Betke test and mean corpuscular volume (MCV). The MCV is much higher in the fetus than the mother. Therefore, the MCV offers a confirmation that the blood is fetal in origin.

PUBS can be performed after the 17th week of gestation. Indications for the procedure include prenatal diagnosis of:

1. Inherited and acquired blood disorders.
2. Infections (e.g., rubella, cytomegalovirus, and toxoplasmosis).
3. Inherited metabolic disorders.
4. Hypoxia and/or acid-base imbalance associated with fetal distress.

In addition, PUBS allows for direct intravascular transfusions in the fetus. This replaces injection of red blood cells into the fetus intraperitoneally. This allows therapy to begin earlier and provides for a better and more rapid therapeutic response.

Major procedural complications are blood extravasation from the puncture site, fetal bradycardia, and chorioamnionitis. Antibiotics can be administered as prophylaxis against chorioamnionitis.

Rh negative women should receive Rh immune globulin (RhIG), preferably within 72 hours following amniocentesis or any other procedure that could cause fetal-maternal hemorrhage or the end of a pregnancy. Exceptions are: the fetus is Rh negative, or there is evidence of immunization to D antigen not related to antepartum RhIG therapy.

### Postpartum Testing

In addition to the clinical signs of anemia and jaundice in the newborn (Fig. 11-2), various laboratory procedures are helpful in addition to procedures 1 through 5 listed previously under Prenatal Testing. These postpartum procedures may be useful in determining the presence and assessing the severity of HDN:

1. Hemoglobin and hematocrit determination of cord or infant blood.
2. Serum bilirubin of cord or infant blood.
3. ABO grouping and Rh typing of cord or infant blood.
4. Direct antiglobulin test of cord or infant blood.
5. Antibody elution and identification, if the DAT is positive.
6. Peripheral blood smear.

### Tests for Assessing Fetal Maternal Hemorrhage

Tests for quantitating the extent of fetal-maternal hemorrhage include:

1. The weak D ($D^u$) rosette test.
2. The Kleihauer-Betke test.

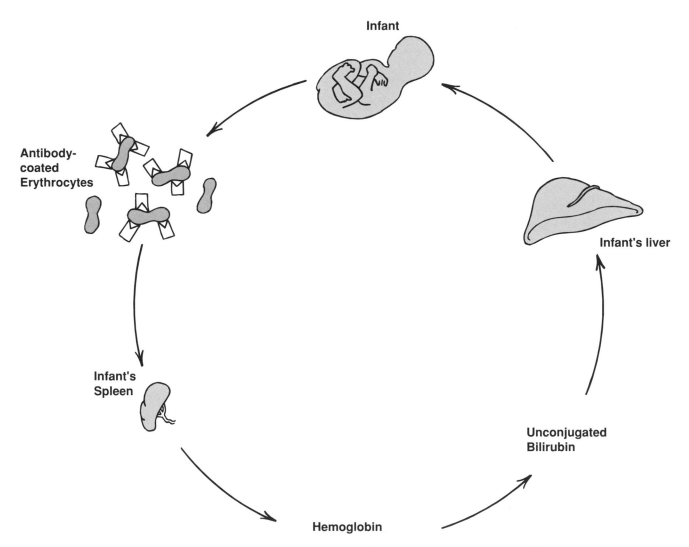

**Figure 11-2.** Postpartum effects of hemolytic disease of the newborn. After delivery, the accumulation of bilirubin can severely harm an infant. The liver of the newborn does not produce glucuronyl transferase, which is necessary for converting bilirubin to an excretable form. Consequently, bilirubin accumulates, and if not removed, will be deposited in lipid-rich tissues such as the brain. Excessive bilirubin in the circulation also produces jaundice.

## Hemoglobin Determination

Most neonatologists refer to the cord hemoglobin as the reference criterion of the severity of the hemolytic process. The normal range for cord hemoglobin during the first day of life is 14.5 to 22.5 g/dL. Moderately afflicted infants suffering from HDN may have cord hemoglobins ranging from 10.5 g/dL to 14.5 g/dL. The cord hemoglobin levels in severely afflicted infants can range from 3.4 g/dL to 10.4 g/dL. Most infants with levels of cord hemoglobin concentration within the normal range do not require exchange transfusion.

## Bilirubin Assay

Serum bilirubin is one of the most frequently used indices in decision-making related to exchange transfusion.

An analysis of bilirubin is valuable in determining the severity of HDN because a relationship exists between cord bilirubin concentration and the severity of HDN. This relationship is less closely correlated than the relationship between cord hemoglobin levels and severity.

The normal infant's cord bilirubin level ranges from 0.7 to 3.5 mg/dL. A cord bilirubin of 4 mg/dL or more may be an indication for exchange transfusion. Severe cases of HDN frequently have cord bilirubin values in excess of 6.0 mg/dL.

## Direct Antiglobulin Testing (DAT)

About 40% of infants born with a positive DAT require no treatment; others need exchange transfusions to prevent kernicterus. The presence of a positive DAT is associated with hemolytic anemias, including HDN.

## ABO Grouping and Rh Testing

All women admitted for delivery, abortion, or invasive obstetric procedures should have their Rh type determined. When the test for either D or weak D (D$^u$) is positive, the woman should be designated Rh positive. When the tests for both D and weak D (D$^u$) are negative, the woman should be designated Rh negative. Mistyping of an Rh negative mother as Rh positive must be avoided in cases of a large fetal-maternal hemorrhage of Rh positive blood.

The relationship among specific ABO groups and Rh types and HDN is explained in the appropriate section of each discussion on HDN of various etiologies in this chapter. Problems in blood typing specific to the neonate or in the presence of a positive DAT are discussed in the procedures section for each test.

## Antibody Elution and Identification

The coating of erythrocytes with antibodies can frequently be demonstrated through the use of an elution technique (see Chapter 15 for a full discussion) that removes the antibodies from the erythrocytic membrane. The quantity of antibody on fetal erythrocytes is not highly correlated with either the infant's cord hemoglobin concentration or the cord serum bilirubin concentration.

## Peripheral Blood Smear

Hypochromic erythrocytes and spherocytes are commonly seen in HDN. The number of immature nucleated erythrocytes is helpful in assessing the erythropoietic response to hemolysis.

## Determination of Fetal-Maternal Bleed

A postpartum maternal blood sample from all Rh negative women at risk should be tested to detect a fetal-maternal hemorrhage in an amount sufficient to require more than one dose of RhIG for effective prophylaxis.

## D$^u$ Rosette Test

The D$^u$ rosette test (see Chapter 15) was developed and reported by Sebring and Polesky in 1982. This test will detect fetal-maternal hemorrhage of approximately 10 mL in the maternal circulation.

The principle of the test is to identify D$^+$ fetal cells that may be in maternal circulation of a D negative mother. Because this is a qualitative test, positive results must be followed by a quantitative procedure such as the Kleihauer-Betke test. This is particularly important in cases where weak D (D$^u$) positive infant erythrocytes react as strongly as D$^+$ erythrocytes, or, if the mother is weak D (D$^u$) positive, the rosette test is also positive.

The weak D (D$^u$) rosette procedure has advantages over the conventional weak D (D$^u$) test. The risk of false negatives is too great for the weak D (D$^u$) test to be the only method used to detect significant fetal-maternal hemorrhage. The incidence of false negative results with an approximately 30 mL hemorrhage is 12%. Additionally, it is difficult to recognize Rh positive cells by the weak D (D$^u$) procedure unless they constitute at least 2% of the total number of erythrocytes present.

## Kleihauer-Betke Test

The Kleihauer-Betke test can detect a fetal-maternal hemorrhage as small as 7.5 mL of packed erythrocytes or 15 mL of whole blood. This procedure tests for fetal hemoglobin rather than the presence of erythrocytes. Fetal erythrocytes contain 53 to 95% hemoglobin F.

The principle of this procedure is that adult hemoglobin (hemoglobin A) is soluble in acid, while fetal hemoglobin (hemoglobin F) is insoluble at this low pH and not eluted. The disadvantages of this procedure include false positive results in cases of Rh negative mothers with high levels of fetal hemoglobin due to sickle trait or the hereditary persistence of fetal hemoglobin and the subjective nature of test interpretation.

## HDN CAUSED BY ABO INCOMPATIBILITY

### Etiology

In the white population, in 15% of all pregnancies, the mother has blood group O and the baby either blood group A or B. Although ABO incompatibilities between mother and baby occur frequently and represent a common form of HDN, the symptoms are usually mild and may not be clinically obvious. In cases where jaundice develops within 24 hours of birth, the incidence of HDN due to ABO incompatibility ranges from 1 in 70 to 1 in 180 with an estimated average of 1 in 150 births. The most frequent form of ABO incompatibility occurs when the mother is group O and the baby is group A or group B, usually group A. Although anti-A and anti-B are present in the absence of their corresponding antigens as environmentally stimulated (IgM) antibodies, infrequent IgG forms may be responsible for HDN caused by ABO incompatibility. Anti A,B can also be found in group O persons. This IgG antibody reacts with both A and B antigens. Consequently, anti A, B found in group O individuals is primarily the antibody responsible for this type of HDN.

### Genetic Frequency

The actual frequency of incompatible antigens can be determined by multiplying the maternal phenotype O with a frequency in the White population of 0.44 by the fetal gene frequency for A (0.27). This results in a chance combination of 0.12 or 12%. If the mother is group O, frequency 0.44 times the gene frequency for group B (0.07) produces a chance combination of 0.03 or 3%.

### Signs, Symptoms, and Physiology

If a mother's first baby is mildly affected, subsequent ABO incompatible babies may be clinically unaffected; however, if the first child is severely affected, it is likely that subsequent ABO incompatible infants will also be severely affected. In the Black population, HDN caused by anti-B seems to be more severe than HDN caused by anti-A.

Anti-A and anti-B antibodies are usually 19S (IgM) in character and are unable to pass through the placental barrier. If antibodies of the IgG class are present, they are able to pass through the placental barrier.

The generally mild nature of this form of HDN may be due to several factors: fewer A and B antigen sites on the fetal/newborn erythrocytes, weaker antigen strength of fetal/newborn A and B antigens, and competition for anti-A and anti-B between tissues as well as erythrocytes. The number and strength of A and B antigen sites on fetal erythrocytes are less than on adult erythrocytic membranes. Newborn erythrocytes of blood group $A_1$ have an average of 300,000 A antigen sites compared to adult erythrocytes of blood group $A_1$, which have an average of 900,000 A antigen sites. Although A and B antigens are detectable before birth, the strength of the A and B antigens does not increase during fetal life; however, these antigens do gain in strength shortly after birth. Additionally, A and B substances are not confined to the red cells, so that only a small fraction of IgG anti-A and anti-B which crosses the placenta combines with the infant's erythrocytes.

### Laboratory Diagnosis

Hemolytic disease caused by ABO incompatibility is clinically mild, with jaundice most frequently developing within 24 hours after birth. The laboratory profile of this form of HDN consists of:

1. ABO grouping of mother and baby.
2. Direct antiglobulin test.
3. Antibody elution testing.
4. Hemoglobin assay.
5. Bilirubin assay.
6. Peripheral blood smear.

### ABO Grouping of Mother and Baby

ABO grouping most commonly reveals the mother to be group O and the baby to be group A or possibly group B.

### Direct Antiglobulin Testing

A DAT performed on cord or infant blood may be either negative or weakly positive. The lack of consistency in this test may be due to a weak antigen-antibody interaction which causes antibody to be removed during the washing phase of the DAT, an antibody titer that may be too low to be detectable, extensive intravascular hemolysis of coated erythrocytes, or variation in fetal erythrocyte antigen development.

### Antibody Elution

Antibody elution of cord blood may reveal the presence of immune anti-A or anti-B. An eluate is often more useful than the direct antiglobulin test in assessing HDN caused by ABO incompatibility. The demonstration of antibodies using an elution technique is positive in about one third of cases.

### Hemoglobin Determination

Hemoglobin may be slightly lower than in ABO compatible infants. Normal hemoglobin concentrations of cord and venous blood samples from newborn infants range from 15 to 20 g/dL.

## Bilirubin Assay

The bilirubin assay may exceed the normal values of cord total serum bilirubin of 1 to 3 mg/mL. Hyperbilirubinemia may also be seen in conditions such as premature birth or maternal diabetes. HDN is judged to be clinically significant if the peak bilirubin level reaches 12 mg/dL or more.

## Peripheral Blood Smear Morphology

This may reveal an anemia with erythrocyte abnormalities such as hypochromia, microspherocytosis, and reticulocytosis. Immature nucleated erythrocytes may be seen in small numbers.

## Treatment

Except in the extremely rare cases of severe HDN produced by ABO incompatibility, phototherapy is the usual treatment. Phototherapy uses ultraviolet light that reacts with bilirubin near the surface of the skin. This process slowly decomposes/converts bilirubin into a nontoxic isomer, photobilirubin, which is transported in the plasma to the liver. There the molecules are rapidly excreted in the form of bile without being conjugated.

The need for exchange transfusion is rare in cases of ABO incompatibility because of the generally mild nature of this type of HDN. One of the risks of exchange transfusion in these cases is the triggering of yet more hemolysis. These hemolytic transfusion reactions may result from transfusing a baby with adult A or B cells that will interact with circulating maternal IgG anti-A,B in the baby's circulation.

## HDN CAUSED BY Rh INCOMPATIBILITY

## Etiology

In the early 1930s, Diamond, Blackfan and Baty made the classic observations that icterus gravis, hydrops fetalis, and anemia in the newborn represented different grades of clinical severity of the same unknown process. Unfortunately, they did not suspect that this syndrome was a manifestation of hemolytic anemia affecting the fetus. This process was originally referred to as erythroblastosis fetalis.

In 1938, Darrow suggested that this process was a hemolytic anemia caused by the transfer of immune bodies from the mother to the fetus. Because she had no data to support her hypothesis, she incorrectly selected fetal hemoglobin as the causative agent.

The development work on the Rh factor conducted by the major investigators, Landsteiner and Wiener, led Levine to establish that the Rh antigen was the immunizing agent in the blood and/or tissues of the fetus. He speculated that the Rh factor was not present in the mother but inherited by the fetus from the father. In 1941, Levine

concluded, based on experimental and case study data, that the majority of cases of hemolysis in the fetus/newborn resulted from isoimmunization of an Rh negative mother by the Rh positive erythrocytes of the fetus.

## Types of Responses to Rh Immunization

The immunization of Rh [D and weak D (D$^u$)] mothers depends on both the dosage of Rh D positive erythrocytes and the mother's ability to respond to these foreign D antigens. About one third of all Rh (D) negative persons are classified as nonresponders. Nonresponders fail to form anti-D despite intentional repeated injections of Rh (D) positive erythrocytes.

In addition to the nonresponder status, two other categories of individuals exist: responders and hyperresponders. Responders and hyperresponders differ in terms of the type and quantity of anti-D antibody that they produce. Responders form anti-G, a component of anti-D. Hyperresponders produce extremely high titers of both IgM and IgG types of anti-D. Some hyperresponders may additionally produce antibodies to antigens to which they were never exposed. This hyperresponsive condition is referred to as augmentation. The Rh-augmented immune response is responsible for very rare cases of primary Rh immunization.

The normal pattern of immunization in an Rh negative mother involves primary immunization due to a previously incompatible Rh positive pregnancy or blood transfusion which stimulates the production of low titered anti-D, predominantly of the IgM class. Subsequent antigenic stimulation such as fetal-maternal hemorrhage in a woman pregnant with an Rh positive fetus elicits a secondary (anamnestic) response, characterized by the predominance of increasing titers of anti-D of the IgG class.

Levine observed as early as 1943 that a condition of HDN due to ABO incompatibility between the mother and fetus reduced the chance of maternal immunization to the D antigen. Rh negative women with group O blood were more strongly protected than Rh women of other blood types to immunization by the D antigen. In the most representative cases, a group O Rh negative mother pregnant with a group A Rh positive fetus is less likely to develop HDN due to anti-D. This situation exists presumably because the fetal erythrocytes that enter the maternal circulation contain both the A antigen and the D antigen. These cells react with the anti A,B in the maternal circulation and are destroyed before they can immunize the mother to the D antigen.

This observation led to the pioneering experiments which demonstrated that D negative individuals failed to produce anti-D antibodies after repeated injections of D positive cells that had been coated with anti-D antibodies in vitro. As a result of this work, the development and clinical use of Rh IgG in the prevention of HDN due to anti-D became a reality.

## Genetic Frequency

Before the advent of modern prophylaxis to D, anti-D was the most frequent cause of severe HDN. Based on gene frequency, it is fairly easy to see why this situation existed.

When the homozygous Rh negative mother's genotype dd is crossed with a father's genotype of DD, the offspring will all have the genotype Dd, phenotype Rh positive. In cases where the father has a heterozygous genotype (Dd), a 50% probability exists for the offspring to be phenotypically Rh$_0$ positive with half of the offspring having the genotype Dd and the other half having the genotype dd.

If the frequency of antigens in the general White population is taken into consideration, the theoretic probability that a D− woman (0.16) with a D+ husband (0.84) will produce a D+ fetus is 0.134, or 13%. In reality, factors such as the ABO status of the mother and baby and the volume of transplacental hemorrhage will affect the rate of immunization in pregnant women without a history of prior pregnancies or blood transfusions. With the established rate of immunization, D negative women who did not receive immunosuppressive therapy after their first D positive infant and who are pregnant for the second time may demonstrate anti-D and have an affected infant.

## Signs, Symptoms, and Physiology

Except in rare instances, the firstborn Rh positive infant of an Rh negative mother seldom shows clinical signs of HDN and may simply have a positive direct antiglobulin test. If severe HDN is observed in a firstborn D positive infant, it must always be suspected that the mother was previously immunized before the pregnancy by means of a previous blood transfusion, abortion, etc. Although the second D can be severely affected, subsequent incompatible infants have no tendency for the disorder to become progressively more severe.

When the mother has been previously immunized and subsequently produces anti-D of the IgG type in response to a D positive fetus, the following activities occur: the passage of IgG Rh antibodies into the fetal circulation induces erythrocyte hemolysis and anemia of varying degrees of severity. This anemia may produce heart failure and hypoxia in the unborn child, causing stillbirth or rapid accumulation of bilirubin in the newborn.

## The Effect of Antibody Titer

Once an unexpected antibody such as anti-D has been identified in maternal serum, a rising antibody titer is evidence of a presently active immune response. The severity of HDN, however, does not correlate well with maternal anti-D antibody titer.

The discrepancy observed between the severity of HDN and the antibody titer may be due to differences in the nature of IgG antibodies. Fetal hemolysis is essentially due to antibodies of the IgG1 and IgG3 subclasses.

## The Role of Antibody Subclasses

Antibodies of the IgG1, IgG2, IgG3, and IgG4 subclasses are all generally believed to be able to pass through the placental barrier. Because IgG subclasses have different properties such as their rate of transfer across the placenta and complement fixation, their hemolytic capacity varies.

Fetal hemolysis is primarily due to antibodies of the IgG1 and IgG3 subclasses. When IgG1 antibodies are absent, a lower frequency of severe forms of HDN is observed. The frequency of severe forms of HDN also decreases if IgG1 is found in association with IgG3. The molecular characteristics of IgG1 and IgG3 are undoubtedly responsible for their role in the hemolytic process.

The IgG1 antibodies transfer through the placenta earlier, have less difficulty in transfer, and have a longer half-life than IgG3 antibodies. Because IgG1 antibodies cross the placenta with greater ease and earlier (approximately 2 months before IgG3 antibodies), they are exposed to erythrocyte antigens for a longer period. This makes IgG1 antibodies more competitive in binding to erythrocytic antigens than IgG3 antibodies. Although both IgG1 and IgG3 antibodies bind to macrophages, IgG3 antibodies have a better binding and are more hemolytic when linked to erythrocytes.

## Gm Allotypes of Anti-D Antibodies

A greater understanding of HDN due to anti-D has resulted from the accidental discovery of the Gm allotypic markers on the heavy chain of the IgG molecule. The structural differences among the immunoglobulin classes themselves and among the allotypes of IgG are situated at the level of the Fc fragment. Because of its placental transfer site and its macrophage binding site, the Fc fragment is responsible for the hemolytic properties of the anti-D antibodies.

In an analysis of the correlation between the severity of HDN and the type of anti-D antibodies, greater hemolytic action occurs when the IgG1 subclass is present. The greatest proportion of clinically severe cases had not only the IgG1 anti-D antibody, but within this class the antibody population marked by the G1m(4) allotype.

In cases of anemia (cord blood hemoglobin of less than 10 g/dL), the presence of G1m(1) and G1m(4) allotypes has been observed; however, when cord bilirubin and other criteria are used, severe forms of HDN are significantly higher when the G1m(4) allotype is present than when it is absent. The severity of hemolysis is not affected by the presence or absence of other allotypes. The prognostic value of anti-D antibody titers during pregnancy could be enhanced by a study of the IgG subclasses and their allotypes.

## Laboratory Diagnosis

### Prenatal Assessment

Prenatal testing in the case of D negative mothers has some special considerations in addition to the procedures already discussed in the section on assessment of HDN.

A detectable antibody titer (see Chapter 14, Special Procedures) is rarely demonstrated before 28 weeks of gestation in the first immunizing pregnancy. When anti-D develops during the first pregnancy, it is most commonly detected at about the 35th week of gestation or later. The titer is usually low. Rarely is there a significant rise in the anti-D titer if a subsequent D fetus is present. If anti-D is detected and identified, attention should be paid to the presence of other antibodies of the Rh system or other antibodies such as anti-Duffy, anti-Kidd, and anti-S, which are common secondary antibodies in Rh immunization.

Amniocentesis may be performed in cases where the serum titer of anti-D is 1:16 or higher with a history of a previous stillbirth due to anti-D, a serum titer of 32 or higher in a pregnant woman with a history of a previous child who needed an exchange transfusion, or a progressive rise of anti-D to 1:64 without a history of an affected fetus or child. In such cases, an initial amniocentesis would be done at 24 to 28 weeks of gestation or 6 to 8 weeks before the gestational age of previous fetal loss due to D antigen. Two sequential amniotic specimens are required to assess change in the status of the fetus. The noninvasive monocyte monolayer assay is also believed to be efficient in predicting which infants are at risk of severe HDN, thus reducing the number of amniocenteses required.

### Postpartum Assessment

The identification of HDN due to anti-D is characterized by the following test results:

1. *Rh blood typing* with D or weak D (D^u) positive results of the cord or infant's blood show the mother as D and weak D (D^u) negative.
2. *Direct antiglobulin* test is positive and the mother demonstrates a positive indirect antiglobulin test with anti-D the identified antibody.
3. *Antibody elution* of cord blood cells reveals the presence of anti-D.
4. *Hemoglobin* levels of cord blood may be moderately to severely decreased. Levels ranging from 10.5 to 14.5/dL are seen in moderately afflicted infants, while levels ranging from 3.4 to 10.4 g/dL are seen in severe cases.
5. *Bilirubin* levels on cord serum range from 3.5 mg/dL to more than 6.0 mg/dL in the most severely afflicted infants.
6. *Peripheral blood smears* demonstrate the presence of immature erythrocytes with a range of over 5 or 6 per 100 leukocytes.

## Treatment

### Prenatal Treatment

***Plasma Exchange.*** Plasma exchange is a therapeutic tool in the treatment of immune-mediated disease. An application of this can be in the treatment of pregnant women in whom a high antibody titer, coupled with a past history of delivering a stillborn infant due to HDN, indicates a significant possibility of another fetal loss due to HDN. Although results of this technique indicate that plasma exchange is a useful therapeutic tool in the treatment of high-risk HDN pregnancies, plasma exchange is not accepted by many clinicians for routine use. Some of the disadvantages include high cost, discomfort and inconvenience to the patient, and the non-selective removal of all plasma proteins.

***Intraperitoneal and Intrauterine Transfusion.*** Severe intrauterine hemolysis in the fetus can be treated by intraperitoneal fetal transfusion (IPT) or intrauterine transfusion. In this procedure, blood is usually selected on the basis of compatibility with maternal serum and the matching of donor and maternal erythrocytes with respect to the antigen causing the hemolysis. Because of the high mortality in infants with severe HDN born before the thirtieth week of gestation, premature delivery may not be an option. Therefore, blood transfusion may be the only choice if the infant is to be saved.

One of the risks of transfusion is the introduction of other antigens into the circulation. Enhanced antibody production has been observed after intrauterine transfusion of common nonrhesus antigens which may also cause HDN, for example, Kidd (Jk) and Duffy (Fy). The risk may be greater for intravascular fetal transfusions in which a larger dose of antigen enters directly and more rapidly into the fetal vascular system, in contrast with the gradual absorption of antigen in IPT. Destruction of fetal erythrocytes could depend on whether the corresponding antigen had been inherited from the father. It has been suggested that the donor blood lack the Rh_o, Kell, Kidd, Duffy, and S antigens whenever any of these are absent from the maternal cells, even if the father also lacks them.

***Prenatal Prevention of HDN.*** In 1900, Von Dungern initiated the first step in the prevention of HDN, when he discovered that active immunization is suppressed by a passive antibody. Forty years later, based on the pioneering work on the Rh_o factor by Landsteiner and Weiner, Levine demonstrated that a form of HDN was the direct result of a D incompatibility between a D negative mother and a D positive fetus. Later, three independent research teams demonstrated that a passive antibody, Rh IG, could protect most D negative mothers from becoming immunized after the delivery of a D positive infant or similar obstetric conditions.

In 1968, Rh IG was licensed for administration in the United States. Since that time, a dramatic decrease in the incidence of anti-D HDN has taken place. Although complete elimination may never occur because of the cases in which anti-D is formed prior to delivery, all pregnant Rh negative women should receive Rh IG even if the Rh status of the fetus is unknown because fetal D antigen is present in fetal erythrocytes as early as 38 days from conception.

Administration of Rh immune globulin (Rh IG) at 28 weeks gestation (antenatal) has decreased the incidence of primary immunization in D negative women to 0.07%. In addition to this, the use of Rh IG after conditions such as abortion, ectopic pregnancy, or antepartum hemorrhage has contributed to the decreased incidence of D antigen immunization. Antenatal treatment is most effective if initiated by the 28th week of gestation.

In the United States in 1980, more than 203,000 Rh negative primiparous women gave birth. In the absence of an antepartum program, among the future second births of these women, an estimated 300 infants will have Rh HDN attributable to antepartum sensitization. In about 2% of cases, an Rh negative mother is immunized by the time her first Rh positive infant is delivered.

Questions continue to remain concerning the cost-effectiveness of antepartum administration of Rh IG. The major objection to this mode of treatment is the cost associated with the treatment of all pregnant Rh negative women who may be pregnant with an Rh positive fetus. Opponents to antenatal administration of Rh IG cite that the value would be evident only if the mother conceived another Rh positive fetus or received an Rh positive transfusion. Other clinicians feel that the timing of administration and size of the dose need more research. Women who have received antepartum Rh IG must be considered for additional treatment with this product postpartum.

### Postpartum Treatment

***Exchange Transfusion.*** Infants who are severely afflicted with HDN may require an exchange transfusion shortly after birth. An exchange transfusion removes bilirubin and circulating maternal antibodies from an infant's plasma and replaces antibody-coated erythrocytes with compatible donor cells.

Several criteria may be applied in determining whether or not an exchange transfusion is warranted. If the cord bilirubin is 5 mg/dL at birth, with the plasma bilirubin rising to above 11.5 mg/dL at 12 hours after birth and above 16 mg/dL after 24 hours, the need for an exchange transfusion is indicated. If the rate of increase in plasma bilirubin is more than 0.5 mg/dL/hour or anemia (hemoglobin below 14 g/dL) exists, exchange transfusion may be necessary. Prematurity is also a consideration. In premature infants, the threshold for bilirubin toxicity occurs at lower levels, along with decreased albumin binding capacity as well as a higher risk of acidosis, hypoglycemia, hypothermia, hypoxia, and sepsis.

The selection of blood, appropriate anticoagulants, and crossmatch procedures for exchange transfusions are discussed in the previous procedures section. The actual procedure of transfusion takes place by way of umbilical vessels.

The immediate effectiveness of a two-volume exchange transfusion is 45 to 50%; however, re-equilibration between bilirubin in plasma and extravascular bilirubin takes place. The plasma bilirubin tends to rise or rebound after an exchange transfusion, partly because of the entry of bilirubin from the extravascular spaces and partly because of continued production of bilirubin from residual maternal antibody coating newly released erythrocytes. If, following the first exchange transfusion, bilirubin threatens to exceed 20 mg/dL in a full-term infant, subsequent exchanges may be necessary. Additional exchanges are less effective in controlling the bilirubin level than are initial transfusions because they mainly remove bilirubin in the infant's plasma rather than removing the infant's D positive erythrocytes. Phototherapy is used as an adjunct therapy in this situation.

In a newborn infant needing exchange transfusion because of Rh hemolytic disease, the production of bilirubin can be modulated, with concurrent reduction in the number of exchange transfusions. This can be accomplished through the use of high-dose intravenous immune globulin therapy. The mechanism responsible for reduction of bilirubin is unknown at this time, but it is hypothesized that high-dose intravenous immune globulin blocks the Fc receptors and resultant inhibition of hemolysis. The optimal dose, number of infusions, and best preparation remain to be determined.

***Postpartum Prevention of HDN Caused by Anti-D.*** The frequency of HDN caused by anti-D has declined dramatically in the United States since the introduction of widespread postpartum administration of Rh immune globulin (Rh IG) (Fig. 11-3). In 1968, Rh IG began to become available to postpartum Rh negative women who had delivered an Rh positive infant. In a relatively short time, the incidence of immunization with the demonstration of anti-D dramatically dropped from 8% after the first pregnancy, with an additional 8% developing anti-D during their second pregnancy, to 1 or 2%. Although postpartum administration of Rh IG averts sensitization in most D negative women with D positive incompatible pregnancies, it cannot help the 1 or 2% of mothers who are immunized due to significant prenatal fetal-maternal hemorrhage.

RELATED LABORATORY PROCEDURES. Up to 50% of $Rh_o$ negative mothers with an incompatible fetus may demonstrate varying quantities of fetal erythrocytes after delivery (postpartum). One to 2% of women who received Rh IG at the termination of their previous pregnancy have detectable Rh antibodies on delivery of a subsequent Rh positive infant. A major cause of these failures is the administration of inadequate amounts of Rh IG. Various

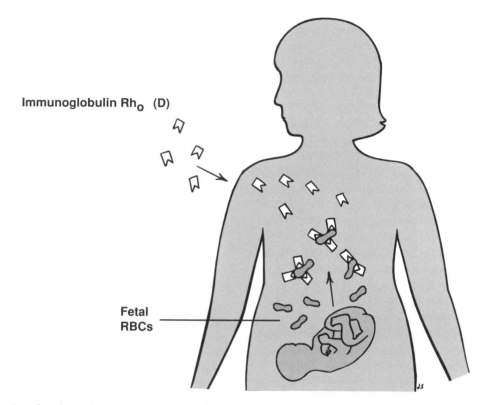

**Immunoglobulin Rh$_o$ (D)**

**Fetal RBCs**

**Figure 11-3.** Prevention of a primary immune response to an Rh$_o$ (D) incompatible fetus. Prevention of sensitization of an Rh$_o$ (D) negative mother to an Rh$_o$ (D) positive can be accomplished by the antenatal or postnatal administration of immune globulin-D. The passively administered anti-D binds with the D antigen of the fetal erythrocytes. These cells are subsequently phagocytized and removed from the maternal circulation without foreign antigen recognition by the mother's immune system.

laboratory techniques (see Chapter 15 for a full discussion) can be used to detect the extent of fetal-maternal hemorrhage, such as the weak D (D$^u$) rosette test, the Kleihauer-Betke acid elution test, an enzyme-linked antiglobulin test, or flow cytometry. A single vial of Rh IG is sufficient to compensate for up to 15 mL of D antigen-bearing fetal erythrocytes or 30 mL of fetal whole blood.

With an assay such as the Kleihauer-Betke test, the number of vials of Rh IG can be determined. In this procedure, the volume of fetal-maternal hemorrhage can be calculated by multiplying the percentage (%) of fetal cells by a factor of 50. The volume of fetal blood is divided by 30 to determine the number of vials of Rh IG needed (Table 11-2).

Example:

1. Kleihauer-Betke reported as 3%
2. 3% × 50* = 150 mL of fetal blood
3. $\frac{150 \text{ mL}}{30}$ = 5.0 = 6** doses of Rh IG

* Factor of 50 = 5000 mL (estimated maternal blood volume) × 1/100 (%).

** If the number to the right of the decimal point is less than 5, round down and add one vial. If the number to the right of the decimal point is 5 or greater, round up to the next number and then add one vial. Example: an answer of 2.4 will yield 3 doses and an answer of 2.9 will yield 4 doses.

CRITERIA FOR THE ADMINISTRATION OF RH IG. For prophylactic treatment using Rh IG to be effective, appropriate amounts must be administered under the following general conditions to previously unsensitized D negative women within 72 hours of delivery or obstetric intervention:

1. After delivery of a D positive infant.
2. After amniocentesis, abortion, miscarriage, or ectopic pregnancy.
3. Before delivery in selected cases (antenatal).

**Table 11-2. Typical Rh Ig Dosage for Massive Fetomaternal Hemorrhage***

| % | Volume (mL whole blood) | | Vials (Rh IG) |
|---|---|---|---|
| Fetal Cells | Average | Range | to Inject |
| 0.3–0.5 | 20 | <50 | 2 |
| 0.6–0.8 | 35 | 15–80 | 3 |
| 0.9–1.1 | 50 | 22–110 | 4 |
| 1.2–1.4 | 65 | 30–140 | 5 |
| 1.5–2.0 | 88 | 37–200 | 6 |
| 2.1–2.5 | 115 | 52–250 | 6 |

* Recommendations based on the use of 1 vial for each 15 mL of red blood cells or 30 mL of whole blood of fetal origin estimated to be in the maternal circulation.

The laboratory criteria for Rh IG administration are:

1. The mother is D and weak D (D^u) negative.
2. The screening test for alloantibodies is negative for anti-D antibody.
3. The infant is D or weak D (D^u) positive. In obstetric cases where the Rh cannot be determined, it must be assumed that this criteria has been met.
4. The direct antiglobulin test on cord cells or infant's cells, if available, is negative. If a positive DAT test result is obtained, an elution technique should be used to establish that anti-D is not the coating antibody.

Administration of Rh IG is indicated, but sometimes inadvertently omitted, after several common events: abortion, ectopic pregnancy, amniocentesis, chorionic villi sampling, antepartum hemorrhage, or fetal death. Treatment with Rh IG for the prevention of immunization to D may be appropriate for a D negative patient who has received D positive red blood cells, including those transfused with platelets or granulocytes.

If pregnancy in an Rh negative woman terminates before 13 weeks of gestation, a low-dose vial of 50 $\mu$g is adequate to cover the small fetal blood volume during the first trimester. From 13 weeks until term, the standard full-dose vial (300 $\mu$g) should be given.

## OTHER BLOOD GROUP ANTIGENS

### Etiology

Although the occurrence of HDN due to the D antigen has significantly decreased, the frequency of HDN due to other antigens has not and, in fact, is equally important to detect. Any fetal antigen that is recognized by the maternal immune system as foreign may prompt antigen-specific IgG production that can potentially result in fetal erythrocyte destruction. More than 40 antigens have been identified in cases of HDN. Sensitization to antigens of blood group systems other than ABO and Rh is reported to account for as high as 5% of all neonatal immune hemolytic disease. Although many of the cases of HDN caused by antibodies other than anti-D have been generally reported as clinically mild, some severe forms have been noted.

### Signs, Symptoms, and Physiology

The frequency of various types of HDN due to antibodies reflects the antigen incidence in the general population. The developmental time of an antigen on fetal erythrocytes is another major determinant of its ability to stimulate immunization or react with corresponding maternal antibody.

#### Rh Antigens Other than D

Anti-c is less severe than anti-D. In severe cases, the cord hemoglobin average is 7.5 g/dL (rare). Most cases are in the range of 13 gm/dL. A history of previous blood transfusion is present in a substantial proportion of cases.

#### Kell Antigens

Kell (K) antigen can be found to react as strongly on fetal erythrocytes of 10 weeks gestation and later as on adult erythrocytes. Cellano (k) is clearly detectable as early as 6 to 7 weeks of gestation. Kp^a can be detected as early as 16 weeks of gestation and as strongly as on adult erythrocytes.

Sensitization to subgroups (antithetical antigens of the Kell system (Kp^a, Kp^b, Js^a, and Js^b)) has been reported to occur only occasionally and to result in mild HDN. Although anti-Kp^b is generally reported to produce only mild hemolysis, cases of severe hemolysis have been reported.

#### Duffy Antigens

Both Fy^a and Fy^b have been found to be well developed during intrauterine life. At the earliest, Fy^a has been reported in a fetus of 6 weeks of gestation and Fy^b in one of 6½ weeks. In these few cases, fetal erythrocytes have a weaker reaction than adult erythrocytes. At the twelfth week of gestation, Fy^a and Fy^b antigens were found on fetal erythrocytes in the same frequency and strength as on adult erythrocytes.

#### Kidd Antigens

Kidd blood group antigens have been found to be well developed during intrauterine life. The Jk^b antigen has been found in fetuses as early as 6 to 7 weeks of gestation and Jk^a has been detected beginning at the tenth week of gestation. Both the Jk^a and Jk^b antigens occur in the same frequency and strength on fetal erythrocytes as on adult erythrocytes.

#### Lewis Antigens

Lewis antibodies are almost invariably IgM. It is rare to find an IgG Lewis antibody by indirect antiglobin test. Cases of HDN due to Lewis antigens are rare. One case of mild HDN and another case of a potent IgG anti-Le^a in cord serum have been reported. In the latter case, the cord bilirubin was 4.6 mg/dL and a positive direct antiglobulin test was obtained; however, the case was diagnosed as an ABO incompatibility. The anti-Le^a was not identified as contributing to the HDN caused by the ABO incompatibility.

#### Lutheran Antigens

Antigens Lu^a and Lu^b have been reported as being more poorly developed on fetal erythrocytes than on adult erythrocytes, both in frequency and in strength. The Lu^a antigen was found at the earliest in a fetus of 14 weeks gestation and Lu^b was found in two cases at 10 weeks of gestation. The failure of these antigens to cause severe HDN is attributed to their weak expression during fetal development. Although the Lu$^b$ antigen is of high frequency (99.8% in Whites), the antibody is IgM, IgA, or occasionally IgG.

In 1961, the first example of HDN due to Lu$^a$ was identified. An example of mild HDN caused by anti-Lu$^a$ in a primiparous woman has been reported. In this case, the bilirubin was 15.8 mg/dL when the infant was 4 days old and was treated with phototherapy.

## Other Antigens

Rare examples of other antigens, such as Lan, have been identified as the cause of mild HDN.

Antigen Lan belongs to the Langereis blood group system, a high incidence antigen. Anti-Lan is usually IgG and is stimulated by red cells. This antibody has been implicated in transfusion reactions and HDN.

Other examples of HDN have been attributed to the MNSs system. This system is normally a cold-reacting system; however, examples of anti-M and anti-U have been noted in rare cases of severe HDN which required exchange transfusion. Some of the cases, caused by anti-U, have been mild.

## Laboratory Assessment

Laboratory assessment of HDN due to other blood group systems should follow the protocol outlined in the preceding sections on prenatal and postnatal testing. Evidence of an alloantibody in maternal serum, a positive direct anti-globulin test on cord cells, and the clinical symptoms of HDN are all important parameters in the assessment of this type of HDN.

## Treatment

The prenatal treatment is in the manner described for Rh$_o$ (D), including serial amniocentesis when previous obstetric history and antibody titers are significant. Postnatal treatment of the infant may require exchange transfusion or phototherapy.

## CASE STUDIES OF MATERNAL AND RELATED CASE STUDIES OF HEMOLYTIC DISEASE OF THE NEWBORN

### Case 1

#### History and Laboratory Data

A well-hydrated White baby boy was 1 day old when the neonatalogist observed that he was beginning to appear jaundiced. This baby was the first child of a 28-year-old computer analyst who had no previous obstetric history or history of prior blood transfusion. The pregnancy had been normal.

Stat total bilirubin, hemoglobin and hematocrit, blood type and Rh, and direct antiglobulin tests were ordered on the baby. A cord blood sample had not been collected at delivery. A blood grouping and Rh testing and a screening test for unexpected antibodies were requested on the mother.

***Laboratory Data.*** The baby's laboratory results:

| | |
|---|---|
| Total bilirubin | 10.8 mg/dL |
| Hemoglobin | 16.9 g/dL |
| Hematocrit | 0.52 |
| Blood group and Rh | A$_1$, Rh Positive |
| Direct antiglobulin test | Negative |

The mother's laboratory results:

| | |
|---|---|
| Blood group and Rh | O, Rh Negative |
| Unexpected antibody screen | Negative |

#### Treatment

The baby was immediately started on phototherapy. Subsequent total bilirubin tests were no higher than the 24-hour value and continued to decrease over the next 48 hours. At the time of discharge, the total bilirubin was 6.9 mg/dL.

#### Questions

1. What was the most probable cause of this infant's jaundice?
2. What additional laboratory tests could have been of value?
3. Why was phototherapy the treatment of choice?

#### Discussion

1. Although the mother was Rh negative and the baby was Rh positive, the absence of prior exposure to red cell antigens through pregnancy, miscarriage, abortion, or blood transfusion makes the presence of anti-D antibody highly unlikely even if fetal maternal hemorrhage had occurred during the pregnancy. The fact that the mother is Group O and the baby Group A, suggests an ABO incompatibility, which is particularly common between Group O mothers and Group A babies.

Clinical signs and symptoms are usually mild if the HDN is associated with ABO incompatibility. The laboratory data further suggest that the baby's jaundice was the result of anti-A antibodies. The laboratory results of normal hemoglobin and hematocrit, moderately elevated total bilirubin, and a negative direct antiglobulin test are typical in cases such as this.

2. An elution procedure on the infant's erythrocytes may have demonstrated the presence of anti-A.

3. Phototherapy is a commonly used noninvasive method of treatment in cases of jaundice. The ultraviolet light increases the breakdown of bilirubin pigment that has accumulated in the skin. This treatment is effective in mild cases of jaundice.

## Conclusion

Hemolytic disease of the newborn caused by ABO incompatibility.

## Case 2

### History and Laboratory Data

A 34-year-old geologist was initially seen by her obstetrician at 10 weeks gestation. This was her first pregnancy. She had no previous history of miscarriage, abortion, or prior blood transfusion. A routine prenatal laboratory workup included blood group and Rh type, and unexpected antibody screening.

***Laboratory Data.***

| | |
|---|---|
| Blood group A, D | negative, weak |
| D (D$^u$) | negative |
| Unexpected antibody screen | negative |

***Supplementary Clinical Data.*** At 22 weeks gestation, the patient fell down a steep embankment while on a geologic field survey for her company. She was taken to the emergency room of a nearby hospital because she sustained some minor cuts. No vaginal bleeding, uterine tenderness, or abdominal pain were noted by the emergency room physician. A subsequent visit to her obstetrician a week later also revealed no abnormalities.

The remainder of this woman's pregnancy proceeded normally. She went into spontaneous labor at 40 weeks (full term) of gestation. A normally developed baby girl was subsequently delivered. The baby had no signs of pallor or jaundice.

The following routine laboratory tests were ordered on the cord blood: blood grouping, total bilirubin, hemoglobin, hematocrit, and direct antiglobulin test. Immune globulin (Rh IG) was ordered for the mother.

***Supplementary Laboratory Data.*** The baby's cord blood test results are:

| | |
|---|---|
| Blood group and Rh | A, Rh(D) Positive |
| Total bilirubin | 2.4 mg/dL |
| Hemoglobin | 19.8 g/dL |
| Hematocrit | 0.58 |
| Direct antiglobulin test (DAT) | Positive (3+) |

A postpartum blood specimen from the mother revealed that she was Group A, Rh(D) negative and weak D (D$^u$) negative with a positive unexpected antibody screen. The antibody was identified as anti-D, present in a titer of 1:64. A subsequent elution of the baby's red blood cells also revealed the presence of anti-D.

***Follow-Up Data.*** At 24 hours of age, the baby began to develop jaundice. A blood sample from the baby's heel for total bilirubin was 4.3 mg/dL. Phototherapy was begun immediately. On day 2, the baby's bilirubin rose to its maximum value of 9.8 mg/dL. Both the mother and baby were discharged on the third day postpartum.

### Questions

1. Is this patient a candidate for Rh IG?
2. What is the possible cause of the anti-D antibody in this case?
3. Could this situation have been averted or anticipated?

### Discussion

1. The three *exclusionary* criteria for Rh immune globulin (Rh IG) are:

A. If the mother is Rh(D) positive or weak D (D$^u$) positive. In mothers with the weak D (D$^u$) phenotype, however, the situation is controversial. If these women are also C+, the weak D (D$^u$) phenotype is the result of gene suppression caused by the presence of the C gene in a "trans" position. Mothers with this type of weak D (D$^u$) *cannot* be immunized to D or produce anti-D antibodies. Other weak D (D$^u$) phenotypes, which are rare, can produce anti-D but are not usually given Rh immune globulin prophylactically.

B. If both mother and baby are Rh(D) negative.

C. Rh(D) negative mothers who demonstrate anti-D antibody due to active immunization are not candidates for Rh Ig prophylaxis. However, the sole presence of anti-D, is *not* definitive proof that active immunization has occurred. Administration of antenatal Rh IG could contribute to a positive test for unexpected antibodies and must be ruled out through either documentation of the patient's obstetric history or laboratory testing. Anti-D antibody that has been passively acquired is usually weakly reactive. However, anti-D that results from active antibody production is generally high-titered and can be inactivated by treating the serum with substances such as 2-mercaptoethanol. Mothers who received antenatal Rh immune globulin should also receive postpartum Rh Ig. In this case, the mother is *not* a candidate for Rh Ig.

2. Because this patient had no prior history of miscarriage, abortion, or previous pregnancies, it must be assumed that feto-maternal hemorrhage occurred after the trauma of falling.

3. Rh immune globulin is a concentrated solution of IgG anti-D antibody. A normal dose contains 300 $\mu$g, which is sufficient to counteract the immunizing effects of 15 mL of Rh positive fetal erythrocytes or 30 mL of fetal whole blood.

The Kleihauer-Betke or weak D (D$^u$) rosette procedures are helpful in identifying and determining a semiquantitative estimate of the amount of fetal erythrocytes in the maternal circulation. This allows calculation of the total dose of Rh Ig required.

## Case 3

### Laboratory Data

**Reagent Red Blood Cell Screening Cells Partial Listing of Antigens Present**

| Cell No. | Rh-hr | | | | | Kell | | Duffy | | Kidd | | Lewis | | MNS | | | | P |
|---|---|---|---|---|---|---|---|---|---|---|---|---|---|---|---|---|---|---|
| | D | C | E | c | e | K | k | Fy$^a$ | Fy$^b$ | Jk$^a$ | Jk$^b$ | Le$^a$ | Le$^b$ | S | s | M | N | P$_1$ |
| I | + | 0 | + | + | + | 0 | + | + | 0 | + | + | 0 | + | + | + | + | 0 | + |
| II | 0 | + | 0 | + | 0 | 0 | + | 0 | + | + | 0 | 0 | + | 0 | + | + | 0 | + |

**Patient Results**

| Cell No. | Immediate Spin | 37° C | AHG | Coombs Control |
|---|---|---|---|---|
| I | Neg | Neg | 2+ | |
| II | Neg | Neg | Neg | 2+ |

**Reagent Red Blood Cell Panel Antigen Profile Partial Listing of Antigens Present**

| Cell No. | Rh-hr | | | | | Kell | | Duffy | | Kidd | | Lewis | | MNS | | | | P |
|---|---|---|---|---|---|---|---|---|---|---|---|---|---|---|---|---|---|---|
| | D | C | E | c | e | K | k | Fy$^a$ | Fy$^b$ | Jk$^a$ | Jk$^b$ | Le$^a$ | Le$^b$ | S | s | M | N | P$_1$ |
| 1 | 0 | 0 | 0 | + | + | 0 | + | + | + | + | 0 | 0 | 0 | + | 0 | + | + | + |
| 2 | 0 | 0 | 0 | + | + | 0 | + | 0 | + | + | + | 0 | + | + | + | + | 0 | 0 |
| 3 | 0 | + | 0 | + | + | 0 | + | 0 | + | + | + | 0 | + | + | + | + | 0 | + |
| 4 | + | 0 | + | + | 0 | 0 | + | + | 0 | + | 0 | 0 | + | 0 | + | + | 0 | + |
| 5 | + | 0 | + | + | 0 | 0 | + | + | + | 0 | + | 0 | + | 0 | + | + | + | + |
| 6 | + | + | 0 | 0 | + | + | + | + | + | + | 0 | 0 | + | + | + | + | + | + |
| 7 | + | + | 0 | 0 | + | 0 | + | 0 | + | + | + | 0 | + | 0 | + | + | + | + |
| 8 | + | + | + | 0 | + | 0 | + | + | 0 | 0 | + | + | 0 | 0 | + | + | 0 | 0 |
| 9 | + | + | 0 | + | + | 0 | + | + | + | + | + | + | 0 | + | 0 | 0 | + | + |
| 10 | + | + | 0 | 0 | + | + | 0 | 0 | + | + | + | 0 | + | 0 | + | + | + | + |
| 11 | + | 0 | 0 | + | + | 0 | + | 0 | + | + | + | + | 0 | 0 | 0 | 0 | + | + |

**Patient Results**

| Cell No. | Immediate Spin | 37° C | AHG | Coombs Control |
|---|---|---|---|---|
| 1 | Neg | Neg | Neg | 2+ |
| 2 | Neg | Neg | Neg | 2+ |
| 3 | Neg | Neg | Neg | 2+ |
| 4 | Neg | 1+ | 2+ | |
| 5 | Neg | Neg | 2+ | |
| 6 | Neg | Neg | 2+ | |
| 7 | Neg | 1+ | 3+ | |
| 8 | Neg | ± | 2+ | |
| 9 | Neg | ± | 1+ | |
| 10 | Neg | Neg | 1+ | |
| 11 | Neg | Neg | 2+ | |

### Questions

1. What is the identity of the unexpected antibody in the patient's serum and the eluate of the baby's erythrocytes?
2. What is the most probable explanation for the presence of this antibody?
3. What further tests should be considered?
4. Is this situation common?
5. Is antenatal Rh immune globulin administration an effective method of prevention of HDN due to anti-D?

### Discussion

1. Although both anti-D and anti-E are the most probable unexpected antibodies in this case, the unexpected antibody was anti-D.

2. Occasionally strong reactions (2 to 3 +), including reactions in the albumin 37° C phase, may be seen 3 months after administration of Rh IG. A positive cord blood DAT with anti-D demonstrated by elution may also be expected.

3. It is suggested that the patient be rechecked in 6 months to totally exclude the possibility of an additional actively acquired unexpected antibody.

4. According to Bowman,* 28% of ABO-compatible babies born to mothers who have received antenatal Rh IG will have a positive DAT (weak). One-fourth of women receiving Rh IG at 28 weeks, 34 weeks, and delivery will have residual passively acquired anti-D at 6 to 9 months postpartum. Another poorly referenced "rule of thumb" is that the anti-D titer at 8 to 12 weeks after the administration of Rh IG should be 1 : 4 or less if caused by passively acquired antibody and greater than 1 : 4 if caused by immunization.

5. Rh immunization may be prevented in at least 94% of instances by antenatal prophylaxis at 28 weeks' gestation.

### Conclusion

Anti-D (probably passively acquired antenatal immune globulin).

* Bowman, John M.: *Eradication of Rh Hemolytic Disease of the Fetus and Newborn,* presented at the Harvard Medical School Course in Eradication of Rh Hemolytic Disease of the Fetus and Newborn, May 21–22, 1981.

## Case 4

### History and Laboratory Data

A 38 year-old woman was 4 months pregnant (gravida 3, para 2). Her husband is homozygous for the D antigen. She was being followed for anti-D sensitization and possible HDN because she is group O Rh negative with a positive indirect antiglobulin test at room temperature, 37° C, and AHG phases. The unexpected antibody had been previously identified as anti-D. Anti-D was again the only unexpected antibody recognized in the patient's serum. Her anti-D titers follow.

### One Month Ago

| Dilution | IS | 37° C | AHG |
|----------|-----|-------|-----|
| 1:1 | 3+ | 4+ | 3+ |
| 1:2 | 3+ | 3+ | 3+ |
| 1:4 | 3+ | 3+ | 3+ |
| 1:8 | ± | 3+ | 3+ |
| 1:16 | Neg | 2+ | 3+ |
| 1:32 | ± | 2+ | 2+ |
| 1:64 | Neg | 1+ | 1+ |
| 1:128 | Neg | Neg | 1+ |
| 1:256 | Neg | Neg | Neg |
| 1:512 | Neg | Neg | Neg |
| 1:1024 | Neg | Neg | Neg |

### Present

| Dilution | IS | 37° C | AHG |
|----------|-----|-------|-----|
| 1:1 | 4+ | 3+ | 3+ |
| 1:2 | 3+ | 3+ | 3+ |
| 1:4 | 3+ | 3+ | 3+ |
| 1:8 | 2+ | 3+ | 3+ |
| 1:16 | 1+ | 2+ | 2+ |
| 1:32 | ± | 2+ | 2+ |
| 1:64 | Neg | 1+ | 2+ |
| 1:128 | Neg | 1+ | 1+ |
| 1:256 | Neg | 1+ | 1+ |
| 1:512 | Neg | ± | ± |
| 1:1024 | Neg | Neg | Neg |

### Questions

1. Based on the previous and current agglutination results, what are the patient's anti-D titers?
2. Comment on the observations in question 1.
3. What is the significance of the results of the present titer?
4. What is the probable Rh phenotype of the fetus?
5. Will interventions be necessary before delivery of this infant?

### Discussion

1. The patient's previous anti-D titer was 1:64 (albumin) and 1:128 (AHG). The present titer is 1:512 (albumin and AHG).
2. There was a fourfold increase in strength of the anti-

D in the mother's serum since the previous study one month before.
3. A rising titer indicates antigenic stimulation that is encouraging antibody production. Another method of assessing antibody avidity is to score the titer. The scoring of this titer follows:

### One Month Previously

| Dilution | AHG | Score |
|----------|-----|-------|
| 1:1 | 3+ | 10 |
| 1:2 | 3+ | 10 |
| 1:4 | 3+ | 10 |
| 1:8 | 3+ | 10 |
| 1:16 | 3+ | 10 |
| 1:32 | 2+ | 8 |
| 1:64 | 1+ | 5 |
| 1:128 | 1+ | 5 |
| 1:256 | Neg | 0 |
| 1:512 | Neg | 0 |
| 1:1024 | Neg | 0 |
|         |     | 68 Total |

### Present

| Dilution | AHG | Score |
|----------|-----|-------|
| 1:1 | 3+ | 10 |
| 1:2 | 3+ | 10 |
| 1:4 | 3+ | 10 |
| 1:8 | 3+ | 10 |
| 1:16 | 2+ | 8 |
| 1:32 | 2+ | 8 |
| 1:64 | 2+ | 8 |
| 1:128 | 1+ | 5 |
| 1:256 | 1+ | 5 |
| 1:512 | ± | 2 |
| 1:1024 | Neg | 0 |
|         |     | 76 Total |

4. The fetus is probably Rh(D) positive.
5. An assortment of diagnostic and therapeutic interventions may be necessary in this case. Various procedures are discussed in Chapter 10; intrauterine transfusion may be necessary.

### Conclusion

Hemolytic disease of the newborn caused by anti-D.

## Case 5

### History and Laboratory Data

A 40-year-old black lawyer was referred to a medical center obstetrician by her family physician after she was diagnosed as pregnant (approximately 8 weeks gestation). Her medical history indicated that she had received 2 units of Group O, Rh negative packed red cells during the delivery of her first child. Rh immune globulin was administered postnatally because she was a suitable candidate. Routine prenatal laboratory testing was ordered.

### Laboratory Data

| Blood group and Rh | O, D and weak D (D$^u$) negative |
|---|---|
| Unexpected antibody screen | Positive |
| Antibody identification | Anti-Kell antibody, titer 1:32 |

***Supplementary Testing.*** A *repeat* titer of anti-Kell was performed at 28 weeks gestation; this titer was 1:128.

### Questions

1. What tests should be performed routinely at delivery?
2. Would prophylactic treatment with immune globulin D have protected the mother against development of this antibody?
3. What is the significance of a rising titer?

### Discussion

1. Current standards do not require that Rh negative mothers be tested at delivery for unexpected antibodies or have a repeat Rh testing. If, however, the Rh status has not been previously determined in prenatal cases or in patients admitted for abortion or amniocentesis, they must be performed on delivery or hospital admission.

The cord blood from newborn infants of Rh(D) and weak D (D$^u$) negative mothers should be tested for D antigen. The presence of unexpected antibodies in the mother's serum and the infant's clinical condition determine whether or not a DAT should be done. Routine protocols differ from one hospital to another.

2. No. Immune globulin Rh IG is effective *only* against the D antigen. It would not protect the mother against immunization to any other foreign antigen.

3. A fourfold or greater increase in unexpected antibody titer suggests an active immunologic response. In this case, the increase of the anti-Kell titer suggests that fetal erythrocytes bearing the Kell antigen have entered the maternal circulation and are stimulating antibody production. The performance of antibody titers is presented in Chapter 14. Although the numeric value of an unexpected antibody titer is not positively correlated to the severity of HDN, the patient should be closely monitored. Tests such as paternal Kell antigen typing or amniocentesis would be of value.

### Conclusion

Hemolytic disease of the newborn caused by anti-Kell.

### CHAPTER SUMMARY

Hemolytic disease of the newborn (HDN) or erythroblastosis fetalis is caused by excessive destruction of fetal erythrocytes by maternal antibodies. This process produces jaundice and can cause mental retardation or death in severe cases.

### The General Characteristics of HDN

In HDN, the erythrocytes of the fetus or newborn are coated with maternal antibodies that correspond to specific fetal antigens. This action results in hemolysis with subsequent increased erythropoiesis both within the bone marrow and in the liver and spleen (extramedullary hematopoiesis). When the rate of erythrocytic hemolysis exceeds the ability to replace lost cells, anemia develops. The accumulated erythrocytic byproducts, specifically hemoglobin, are removed by way of the maternal circulation before birth; however, accumulation of these products can produce serious problems in the newborn infant.

The antibodies capable of causing HDN include blood antibodies that can occur as IgG. Based on severity, the most common causes of HDN are anti-D alone or in combination with anti-C or anti-E; other Rh antibodies; other blood group system antibodies, such as anti-Kell, anti-Duffy, and anti-Kidd; and anti-A and anti-B. Most cases of HDN due to anti-A or anti-B are clinically mild.

For HDN to occur, the mother must lack the antigen that is expressed on the fetal erythrocyte. This antigen must be introduced into the maternal circulation as either the primary immunizing event or the result of transplacental hemorrhage (TPH).

### Assessment of HDN

Prenatal assessment of potential cases of HDN include the following tests: ABO grouping D and weak D (D$^u$) testing, a screening test for unexpected antibodies with the identification and titering of any antibodies, and amniocentesis. Amniocentesis is performed only when certain clinical criteria exist.

Postpartum testing should include the tests suggested for prenatal testing, if not previously performed, as well as several other tests. A hemoglobin, hematocrit, serum bilirubin, and direct antiglobulin test (DAT) should be performed on cord blood if indicated on the basis of the prenatal testing results and clinical status of the infant. If the DAT is positive, an antibody elution and identification should be performed. A peripheral blood smear from the infant is an additional assessment tool. The mother's blood can also be tested by the weak D (D$^u$) rosette test or Kleihauer-Betke test.

### HDN Caused by ABO Incompatibility

ABO blood group incompatibility between mother and fetus occurs frequently and represents a common form of HDN; however, the symptoms are usually mild. The occurrence of this cause of HDN is most frequent if the mother is group O and the baby group A.

## HDN Caused by Rh Incompatibility

Immunization to Rh [D and weak D (D^u)] mothers depends on both the dosage of Rh (D) positive erythrocytes and the mother's ability to respond to these foreign D antigens. The normal pattern of immunization involves primary immunization due to a previously incompatible Rh positive pregnancy or blood transfusion which stimulates the production of low titered anti-D, predominantly of the IgM class. Subsequent antigenic stimulation, such as fetal-maternal hemorrhage during pregnancy with an Rh positive fetus, elicits a secondary (anamnestic) response. This response is characterized by the predominance of increasing titers of anti-D of the IgG class.

The incidence of HDN due to anti-D was the second most common cause of HDN before modern prophylaxis.

HDN due to anti-D may be treated prenatally by prenatal plasma exchange, prenatal intraperitoneal and intrauterine transfusion, or antenatal prophylaxis. Postpartum treatment includes exchange transfusion of the infant in severe cases. Prevention of HDN due to anti-D has significantly decreased the incidence of this form of HDN. In previously nonimmunized women, the administration of immune globulin D is advised. The Kleihauer-Betke test is frequently used to assess the extent of fetal-maternal hemorrhage. The dosage can be determined on the basis of this assessment.

## Other Blood Group Systems

The frequency of HDN due to other blood group antigens continues to exist. More than 40 antigens have been identified as causing HDN. Depending on the antigen strength and other variables, the severity of the disorder can range from mild to severe. Kell, Duffy, Kidd, Lewis, and Lutheran are major categories of antigens in this category.

## REVIEW QUESTIONS

1. In hemolytic disease of the newborn, the mother's _____ is directed against fetal _____.
   A. Antigen—antibody
   B. Antibody—antigen
   C. Antigen—antigen
   D. Antibody—antibody
2. The normal life span of fetal erythrocytes is _____ days.
   A. 30–45
   B. 45–70
   C. 70–95
   D. 95–120
3. Extramedullary hematopoiesis results in increased:
   A. Leukocyte production
   B. Bilirubin production
   C. Erythrocyte destruction
   D. Liver and spleen size

4. Which of the following is not true of unconjugated bilirubin?
   A. Results from erythrocyte destruction
   B. Is bound to albumin by the action of glucuronidase
   C. Becomes conjugated with albumin
   D. Is attracted to tissue proteins
5. The antibody class implicated in hemolytic disease of the newborn is:
   A. IgM
   B. IgG
   C. IgD
   D. IgE
6. The most severe form of hemolytic disease of the newborn is associated with:
   A. Anti-A
   B. Anti-B
   C. Anti-D
   D. Anti-K
7. Production of maternal antibodies depends on all of the following factors except:
   A. Lack of a specific antigen in the mother
   B. Presence of a specific antigen in the fetus
   C. Presence of a specific antibody in the fetus
   D. Immunogenic strength of an antigen
8. Prenatal testing routinely includes all of the following, except:
   A. ABO grouping
   B. D typing
   C. Weak D (D^u) testing if D is negative
   D. Amniocentesis
9. The normal cord hemoglobin (at birth) is:
   A. 0.7–3.4 mg/dL
   B. 3.4–10.4 g/dL
   C. 10.5–14.5 g/dL
   D. 14.5–22.5 g/dL
10. A cord bilirubin of _____ may be an indication for exchange transfusion.
   A. 0.1–0.5 mg/dL
   B. 0.5–1.0 mg/dL
   C. 1.0–2.5 mg/dL
   D. 4.0 mg/dL or greater
11. Both the D^u rosette test and the Kleihauer-Betke test are performed on a:
   A. Baby's cord blood specimen
   B. Baby's circulating blood specimen
   C. Mother's circulating blood specimen
   D. Both A and B
12. The purpose of both the D^u rosette test and the Kleihauer-Betke test is to detect:
   A. Maternal D antigen
   B. Maternal D antibody
   C. Fetal D antigen
   D. Fetal-maternal hemorrhage
13. The most frequent cause of ABO hemolytic disease of the newborn is:

A. Mother group O, baby group A
B. Mother group O, baby group B
C. Mother group A, baby group O
D. Mother group A, baby group B

14. Hemolytic disease of the newborn due to ABO incompatibility is usually milder than other types of HDN due to all of the following factors *except:*
    A. There are fewer A and B antigen sites on fetal erythrocytes
    B. Fetal A and B antigens have weaker antigenic strength
    C. The presence of the D antigen has a protective effect
    D. Competition for anti-A and anti-B exists between the tissues and erythrocytes

15. Rh sensitization is *least* likely to occur in an Rh negative woman if her ABO type is _____:
    A. A
    B. B
    C. O

16. The typical laboratory profile of hemolytic disease of the newborn caused by ABO incompatibility is:
    A. Mother group O, baby group A, DAT negative, cord bilirubin 3.0 mg/dL
    B. Mother group A, baby group O, antibody elution from cord blood positive, cord bilirubin 1.0 mg/dL
    C. Mother group O, baby group A, DAT strongly positive, cord bilirubin 10.0 g/dL.
    D. Mother group O, baby group B, DAT strongly positive, cord hemoglobin 10.0 g/dL

17. All of the following characteristics are typical of hemolytic disease of the newborn caused by the D antigen *except:*
    A. Depends on the dosage of D antigen on fetal erythrocytes
    B. Depends on the mother's ability to respond to foreign D antigens
    C. Usually does not occur in the first pregnancy
    D. May require an exchange transfusion

18. Antenatal Rh immune globulin should be administered at:
    A. 12 weeks gestation
    B. 24 weeks gestation
    C. 28 weeks gestation
    D. 32 weeks gestation

19. Rh immune globulin provides _____ protection against fetal D antigen.
    A. Active
    B. Passive
    C. Antigen-stimulated
    D. Antibody-stimulated

20. An exchange transfusion is warranted if the:
    A. Cord bilirubin is 2.5 mg/dL, plasma bilirubin 10.0 mg/dL at 12 hours, and 10.0 mg/dL at 24 hours

B. Cord bilirubin is 5.0 mg/dL or higher, plasma bilirubin over 11.5 mg/dL at 12 hours, and over 16.0 mg/dL at 24 hours
    C. Increase in plasma bilirubin is more than 0.2 mg/dL/hour
    D. Infant is full-term

21. If an $Rh_o$ (D) negative woman recently delivered an $Rh_o$ (D) positive baby and the Kleihauer-Betke test result is 5%, how many vials of immunoglobulin D should be administered?
    A. 6
    B. 7
    C. 8
    D. 9

22. Which of the following does *not* partially meet the criteria for postpartum administration of immune globulin D?
    A. Mother D negative, infant D positive, cord cell elution revealed anti-Kell
    B. Mother D negative, unexpected antibody screen anti-c, infant D positive, DAT negative
    C. Mother D negative, unexpected antibody screen negative, infant D negative, DAT negative.
    D. Mother D negative, infant's type unknown, unexpected antibody screen positive (anti-K)

23. In addition to the A, B, and D antigens, hemolytic disease of the newborn can be caused by:
    A. Only c antigen
    B. c and Kell antigens
    C. More than 20 different antigens
    D. More than 40 different antigens

24–25. Match the following (an answer may be used more than once):
    24. Anti-Lu$^a$
    25. Anti-M
    A. Has been reported to produce *severe* forms of HDN
    B. Has been reported to produce mild forms of HDN
    C. Has not been identified as a cause of HDN

## Bibliography

Adams, M.M., et al.: Cost implications of routine antenatal administration of Rh immune globulin. Am. J. Obstet. Gynecol., *149*(6): 633–638, 1984.

Barrie, J.U., and Quinn, M.A.: Selection of donor red cells for fetal intravenous transfusion in severe haemolytic disease of the newborn. The Lancet, *i*(8441):1327–1328, 1985.

Bergstrom, H., et al.: Demonstration of Rh antigens in a 38-day-old fetus. Am. J. Obstet. Gynecol., *99*:130–133, 1967.

Boral, L.I., and Henry, J.B.: Transfusion Medicine. *In* Clinical diagnosis and management by laboratory methods, 18th ed. John B. Henry (Ed). Philadelphia, PA: Saunders, 1991, pp. 957–958.

Bowman, J.M.: Prevention of rhesus isoimmunization. Am. J. Obstet. Gynecol., *148*(8):1151–1153, 1984.

Bowman, M. (Ed): $Rh_o$ (D) Immune Globulin. Berkeley, CA, Cutter Biological, 1984.

Bradshaw, D.A.: Red blood cell antibody testing of obstetric patients. Lab. Med., 18(2):77–81, 1987.

Branch, D.R.: Fetal death due to extreme maternal Rh immune augmentation. Transfusion, 21(3):281–284, 1981.

Buck, S.A.: Hemolytic Disease of the Newborn. In Modern Blood Banking and Transfusion Practices, D. H. Pittiglio (Ed.). Philadelphia, F. A. Davis, pp. 399–421.

Caswell, A.K., and Caswell, M.: Antenatal treatment to prevent Rh immunization. Lab. Med., 14(10):655–658, 1983.

Characteristics of Blood Group Antibodies (Product Brochure). Miami, FL, Baxter Healthcare Corp., 1987.

Cheng, M.S., and Lukomskyj, L.: Postpartum D^u-positive women and Rh immune globulin. Lab. Med., 17(12):748–749, 1986.

Chibber, G., et al.: Rh Isoimmunization following abdominal trauma: A case report. Am. J. Obstet. Gynecol., 149(6):692, 1984.

Culver, P.L., Brubaker, D.B., Sheldon, R.E., Martin, M., and Richter, C.A.: Anti-At^a causing mild hemolytic disease of the newborn. Transfusion, 27(5):468–470, 1987.

Dacus, J.V., and Spinnato, J.A.: Severe erythroblastosis fetalis secondary to Anti-Kp^b sensitization. Am. J. Obstet. Gynecol., 150(7):888–890, 1984.

Davey, M.G.: Nonresponders and hyperresponders to Rh antigens. Proceedings of a symposium on Rh antibody mediated immunosuppression. Ortho Diagnostics, 1976.

Dopp, S.L., and Isham, B.E.: Anti-U and hemolytic disease of the newborn. Transfusion, 23(3):273, 1983.

Drozda, E.A., and Ciotola, R.: Unexpected hemolytic disease of the newborn. Lab. Med., 15(7):486–487, 1984.

Dube, V.E., and Zoes, C.S.: Subclinical hemolytic disease of the newborn associated with IgG anti-Lu^b. Transfusion, 22(3): 251–253, 1982.

Fudenberg, H.H., et al.: Basic and Clinical Immunology. 2nd Ed. Los Altos, CA; Lange Medical Publications, 1978, p. 63.

Greenwalt, T.J.: Rh Isoimmunization. JAMA, 251(10):1318–1320, 1984.

Henry, John B. (Ed.): Clinical Diagnosis and Management by Laboratory Methods, 17th Ed. Philadelphia, W. B. Saunders Co., 1982, pp. 503–506, 694, 1055–1059.

Inderbitzen, P.E., and Windle, B.: An example of HDN probably due to anti-Lu^a. Transfusion, 22(6):542, 1982.

Kolins, J.: D^u and rosetting tests for FMH. Diagn. Med., 23, May, 1984.

Krauss, J.S., et al.: Detection of fetomaternal hemorrhage in a mother with sickle trait and hereditary persistence of fetal hemoglobin. Transfusion, 23(6):530–531, 1983.

LaFerla, J.J., and Butch, S.: Fetal Rh blood group determination in pregnancy termination by dilatation and evacuation. Transfusion, 23(1):67–68, 1983.

Mellbye, N.: Presence and origin of human IgG subclass proteins in newborns. Vox Sang., 24:206–215, 1973.

Mollison, P.L.: Blood Transfusion in Clinical Medicine. 5th Ed. Oxford, Blackwell Scientific Publications, 1983.

Nance, S.J., Nelson, J., Horenstein, J., O'Neill, P., and Garratty, G.: Predictive value of amniocentesis versus monocyte monolayer assays in pregnant women with Rh antibodies (Abstract of paper presented at the 39th Annual Meeting of the American Association of Blood Banks). Transfusion, 26(6):570, 1986.

Nance, S.J., Nelson, J., O'Neill, P., Lam, H., and Garratty, G.: Quantitation of fetal-maternal hemorrhage by flow cytometry. Transfusion, 26(6):571, 1986.

Nance, S.J., Nelson, J., O'Neill, P., and Garratty, G.: Correlation of monocyte monolayer assays, maternal antibody titers, and clinical course in hemolytic disease of the newborn (Abstract of paper presented at the 37th Annual Meeting of the American Association of Blood Banks). Transfusion, 24:415, 1984.

Page, P.L.: Hemolytic disease of the newborn due to anti-Lan. Transfusion, 23(3):256–257, 1983.

Parinaud, J., et al.: IgG subclasses and Gm allotypes of anti-D antibodies during pregnancy: Correlation with the gravity of the fetal disease. Am. J. Obstet. Gynecol., 151(8):1111–1115, 1985.

Pittiglio, D.H. (Ed.): Modern Blood Banking and Transfusion Practices. Philadelphia, F. A. Davis, 1983. pp. 399–421.

Riley, J.Z., et al.: Detection and quantitation of fetal maternal hemorrhage utilizing an enzyme-linked antiglobulin test. Transfusion, 22(6):472–474, 1982.

Roitt, I.: Essential Immunology. 4th Ed. Oxford, Blackwell Scientific Publications, 1983. p. 41.

Rubo, J., et al.: High-dose intravenous immune globulin therapy for hyperbilirubinemia caused by Rh hemolytic disease. J Peds., 121(1):93–97, 1992.

Sbarra, A.J.: Amniotic fluid optical density, lecithin-sphingomyelin ratio, and phosphatidylglycerol comparisons. Am. J. Obstet. Gynecol., 148(8):1151–1153, 1984.

Sebring, E.S., and Polesky, H.F.: Detection of fetal maternal hemorrhage in Rh immune globulin candidates. Transfusion, 22(6): 468–471, 1982.

Shah, V.P., and Gilja, B.K.: Hemolytic disease of newborn due to anti-Duffy (Fy^a). N.Y. State J. Med., 244–245, Feb. 1983.

Shirey, R.S., et al.: The association of anti-P and early abortion. Transfusion, 27(2):189–191, 1987.

Toivanen, P., and Hirvonen, T.: Antigens: Duffy, Kell, Kidd, Lutheran and Xg^a on fetal red cells. Vox Sang., 24:372–376, 1973.

Tovey, L.A., and Taverner, J.M.: A case for the antenatal administration of anti-D immunoglobulin to primigravidae. Lancet, i: 878–881, 1981.

Walker, R.H.: Standards for Blood Banks and Transfusion Services, 15th Ed. Bethesda, MD. 1993.

White, P., Hendrick, E., and Mark D. Kolins, M.D.: Fetomaternal hemorrhage revisited. Lab. Med., 16(7):428–430, 1985.

Widmann, F.K. (Ed.).: Standards for blood banks and transfusion services. 15th ed. Bethesda, Md.: American Association of Blood Banks, 1993, pp. 31–32.

Yesus, Y.W.: Hemolytic disease of the newborn due to anti-C and anti-G masquerading as anti-D. Am. J. Clin. Pathol., 84(6): 769–772, 1985.

# 12

# Transfusion Reactions

At the conclusion of this chapter, the reader should be able to:

- Define the term "transfusion reaction."
- State the most frequent cause of fatal transfusion reactions.
- Cite at least one example for each of the following types of transfusion reactions: immediate hemolytic, immediate nonhemolytic, delayed hemolytic, and delayed nonhemolytic.
- State the most severe form of a transfusion reaction.
- Name the factors that determine whether a transfusion reaction will be acute or delayed and intravascular or extravascular.
- State the most frequent cause of an acute hemolytic transfusion and name the nonantibody cause or causes of acute hemolytic reactions.
- Explain the clinical manifestations of an acute hemolytic transfusion reaction.
- Describe the most common initial symptoms of an acute hemolytic reaction in an unanesthetized patient.
- Explain the in vivo consequences of the interaction between antigens and their corresponding antibodies.
- List the characteristics of a delayed hemolytic transfusion reaction, including the usual consequence of such a reaction.

- Cite one of the ways in which this type of reaction can be prevented.
- Name the most frequent cause of febrile transfusion reaction and describe the clinical manifestations of febrile (nonhemolytic) transfusion reactions.
- State the immediate reactions to plasma constituents.
- Cite the most common cause of transfusion-related sepsis and describe the consequences of contaminated blood in transfusion.
- Discuss the features of graft-versus-host disease including etiology and prevention.
- Explain cardiopulmonary and embolic reactions to blood transfusion.
- List and briefly describe some of the other adverse reactions to the infusion of blood or blood components.
- Describe the protocol for the investigation of a transfusion reaction.
- Arrange the steps in a post-transfusion workup in the appropriate sequence and list the supplementary tests that can be performed in a transfusion reaction workup.

## Chapter Outline

## DEFINITION AND CAUSES

The term *transfusion reaction* generally refers to the adverse symptoms produced by an erythrocyte incompatibility between a patient and a unit of donor blood. Typically, visible symptoms occur during or shortly after a transfusion; however, conditions such as shortened posttransfusion survival of erythrocytes, an allergic response, and disease transmission also constitute transfusion reactions. Each blood bank or transfusion service must have a system for detection, reporting, and evaluation of suspected complications of transfusion.

When a physician makes the clinical judgment to transfuse a patient, the expected benefits of the product must be weighed against the known risks. In the event of a suspected transfusion reaction, the personnel responsible for the patient must notify the ordering physician and the transfusion service immediately.

The risk of a transfusion reaction is minimal, but it is not unimportant! Although one estimate of the fatality rate due to blood transfusion is approximately one per million units transfused, the rate of all types of adverse reactions to transfused blood or blood components is assessed to be about 1 in every 200 transfusions.

All suspected transfusion reactions should be evaluated promptly and, to the extent considered appropriate by the medical director. This evaluation should not delay proper clinical management of the patient.

The vast majority of fatal transfusion reactions result from misidentification or clerical errors rather than technical limitations. Causes of fatal reactions in order of frequency are:

1. Misidentification of patients
2. Mislabelling of blood samples
3. Errors in laboratory records
4. Mistakes in blood typing
5. Inaccurate antibody screening or crossmatching

Transfusion reactions can be divided into hemolytic and nonhemolytic types. Hemolytic reactions are associated with the transfusion of incompatible erythrocytes. Transfusion reactions can be further classified into acute (immediate) or delayed in their manifestations (Table 12-1).

Acute hemolytic reactions occur during or immediately after blood has been transfused; delayed reactions may not express themselves until 7 to 10 days post-transfusion. Many reactions demonstrate both extravascular and intravascular hemolysis.

**Table 12-1. Types of Transfusion Reactions**

| Type of Reaction | Manifestations |
|---|---|
| Immediate hemolytic | Intravascular hemolysis of erythrocytes |
| Delayed hemolytic | Extravascular hemolysis of erythrocytes |
| Immediate nonhemolytic | Febrile reactions |
| | Anaphylaxis |
| | Urticaria |
| | Noncardiac pulmonary edema |
| | Fever and shock |
| | Congestive heart failure |
| | Myocardial failure |
| Delayed nonhemolytic | Graft-versus-Host disease |
| | Post-transfusion purpura |
| | Iron overload |
| | Alloimmunization to erythrocytes, leukocytes, and/or platelet antigens or plasma proteins |
| | Infectious diseases |

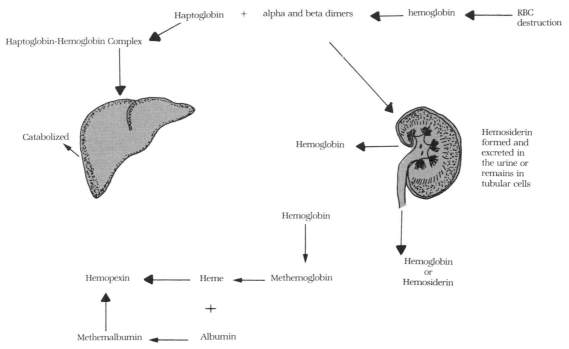

**Figure 12-1.** Intravascular metabolism of erythrocytes.

chapter) but, in some cases, complement-coated erythrocytes survive normally. Renal damage resulting from nonfatal hemolysis is believed to be caused by the presence of antibody-coated cell membrane (stroma).

Intravascular destruction of erythrocytes (Fig. 12-1) accounts for less than 10% of normal erythrocytic destruction. If antigen-antibody complexes activate complement and produce rapid lysis of erythrocytes, hemoglobin is released directly into the blood stream and undergoes dissociation into alpha-beta dimers, which are quickly bound to the plasma globulin, haptoglobin. The formation of the large molecular haptoglobin-hemoglobin complex prevents urinary excretion of plasma hemoglobin. This stable complex is removed from the circulation by the hepatocytes, in which it is processed by the cells in a manner similar to normal intact (extravascular) erythrocytic breakdown. Because haptoglobin is removed from the circulation as part of the haptoglobin-hemoglobin complex, the level of plasma haptoglobin decreases with hemolysis. Once plasma haptoglobin is depleted in the blood circulation, unbound hemoglobin alpha and beta dimers are rapidly filtered by the kidney's glomeruli, reabsorbed by the renal tubular cells, and converted to hemosiderin. Renal tubular uptake can process up to 5 g of filtered hemoglobin per day. Once the capacity for renal tubular uptake has been exceeded, however, free hemoglobin and methemoglobin begin to appear in the urine. Hemoglobin appears in the urine when plasma-free hemoglobin (unbound to haptoglobin) reaches 25 mg/dL or more. The renal processing of filtered hemoglobin can produce excretion of the following:

1. Hemoglobin alone, if hemolysis is severe,
2. Hemosiderin by itself.
3. Both hemosiderin and hemoglobin. If desquamated tubular cells contain hemosiderin granules, this is evidence of a previous condition of hemoglobinemia.

Hemoglobin which is neither bound by haptoglobin nor directly excreted in the urine is oxidized to the methemoglobin. The heme groups in methemoglobin are released and taken up by another transport protein, hemopexin. This complex is removed from the circulation by hepatocytes and catabolized. Heme groups in excess of the hemopexin-binding capacity combine with albumin to form methemalbumin until more hemopexin is available. Once this needed hemopexin becomes available, the complex is subsequently phagocytized by hepatocytes.

The combined depletion of haptoglobin and hemopexin and the presence of methemalbuminemia and hemosiderinuria can be seen in conditions such as intravascular hemolysis. The presence of methemalbumin accompanied by hemopexin depletion *without* hemosiderinuria is associated with bleeding into the tissues, such as intraabdominal bleeding in ectopic pregnancy.

### Hemostasis and Disseminated Intravascular Coagulation

Antigen-antibody complexes can activate the intrinsic coagulation mechanism by way of factor XIIa or directly by the presence of erythrocyte stroma. Plasma activators of plasminogen include plasma kallikrein, activated plasma thromboplastin antecedents (factor XI), and activated Hageman factor (factor XIIa).

Through its lysis of fibrin, plasmin is responsible for forming degradation or fibrin split products consisting of intermediate fragments that exert an antithrombin effect, inhibit the hemostasis system through interference with fibrin monomer polymerization, and interfere with platelet function.

***Pathologic Activation of Coagulation Factors.*** Primary and secondary fibrinolysis are recognized as extreme complications of various intravascular and extravascular disorders and may lead to life-threatening consequences. Primary fibrinolysis is associated with conditions in which gross activation of the fibrinolytic mechanism with subsequent fibrinogen and coagulation factor consumption occurs. The important characteristic of primary fibrinolysis is that no evidence of fibrin deposition appears. Primary fibrinolysis occurs when large amounts of plasminogen activator enter the circulatory system.

Although the same clinical conditions may also induce secondary fibrinolysis or disseminated intravascular coagulation (DIC), the distinction between the two is essentially in the demonstration of fibrin formation. In secondary fibrinolysis, excessive clotting and fibrinolytic activity occur. Increased amounts of fibrin-split (degradation) products (FSPs) and fibrin monomers are detectable because of the action of thrombin on the fibrinogen molecule. This fibrinolytic process is due only to excessive clotting; therefore, it is a secondary condition.

DISSEMINATED INTRAVASCULAR COAGULATION (DIC). Initiation of DIC can be caused by several factors, most commonly tissue thromboplastin introduced into the circulation. This introduction of tissue thromboplastin activates the extrinsic coagulation pathway and platelets, which may result in intravascular consumption of factors V, VIII, fibrinogen, and platelets in the formation of intravascular thrombi. Antithrombin III also appears to be consumed during this process and a deficiency of antithrombin III may contribute to further thrombosis.

DIC may initially occur with varying degrees of thrombosis and hemorrhage, but bleeding is usually the major symptom, particularly in acute cases. The process involves coagulation factors, platelets, vascular endothelial cells, fibrinolysis, and plasma inhibitors. This major breakdown of the hemostatic mechanism occurs when the procoagulant factors outweigh the anticoagulant mechanisms. The generation of microthrombi can cause small blood vessel obstruction and tissue necrosis. Abnormal secondary bleeding is produced by the FSPs, which are produced in time by the increased destruction of fibrinogen. The FSPs disrupt fibrin monomer polymerization by exerting an antithrombin effect and preventing normal platelet function.

The stimuli that can induce DIC may ultimately result in abnormal levels of protein C. Monitoring of patients reveals that protein C antigen and activity decrease progressively during the initial stages of DIC and remain at a low level for 24 to 48 hours before gradually returning toward normal in nonfatal cases.

THROMBIN. Mechanisms involved in DIC result in the formation of thrombin in the circulating blood. Among its many feedback reactions, thrombin indirectly participates in the activation of the fibrinolytic system secondary to DIC and activates protein C. The latter reaction is accelerated by the presence of the endothelial cell cofactor, protein S. Once the generation of excess thrombin is decreased by the action of activated protein C and other regulatory mechanisms, the coagulation process can return to normal. This negative feedback mechanism has the potential to slow down the formation of excess thrombin and stop DIC.

## Prevention

Acute hemolytic transfusion reactions can be prevented by the proper identification of patients and patient samples, and error-free laboratory record-keeping, blood grouping, and crossmatching. The autologous-donor patient must also be carefully identified. Multiple cross-checks should be a routine procedure to prevent inadvertent misidentification of the patient and/or donor unit.

## DELAYED HEMOLYTIC REACTIONS

### Etiology

Delayed hemolytic transfusion reactions can occur from two days to several months post-transfusion. This type of hemolytic reaction is underdiagnosed, under-reported, and under-rated in terms of complications, and is far more frequent than the acute hemolytic reaction.

Delayed hemolytic transfusion reactions may be of two types. They may represent an anamnestic antibody response in a previously immunized recipient on secondary exposure to transfused erythrocyte antigens or result from primary alloimmunization. In an anamnestic response, the antibodies are to antigens to which recipients have been previously immunized by transfusion or pregnancy.

The incidence of primary alloimmunization, excluding D antigen, is 1 to 6% for each unit of blood transfused. Antibodies implicated in delayed hemolytic reactions are anti-E, anti-C, anti-M, anti-Lu$^a$, anti-K, anti-Ce, anti-Jk$^a$, anti-Jk$^b$, anti-k, anti-Fy$^a$, anti-U, and anti-Co$^b$.

### Signs and Symptoms

The most common clinical sign is fever. The triad of anemia, fever, and recent transfusion suggests a delayed hemolytic reaction. Symptoms can range from an asymptomatic state to oliguria or renal shutdown in less than 10% of cases to DIC in very rare cases. Commonly, the accidental discovery of a positive DAT in a subsequent crossmatch reveals that a patient has antibody-coated erythrocytes in the circulation.

In a patient demonstrating an anamnestic response, fever, post-transfusion jaundice, and a sudden drop in the hemoglobin and packed cell volume (hematocrit) with no evidence of hemorrhage or hemodilution may occur within as few as 2 days post-transfusion. A patient exhibiting primary alloimmunization may suffer from a sudden drop in hemoglobin and packed cell volume (hematocrit) several weeks post-transfusion.

## Physiology

An anamnestic antibody response usually begins to occur from 2 or 3 to 7 days post-transfusion. Despite a visibly compatible crossmatch, transfused erythrocytes are removed from the circulating blood and the products of the *extravascular hemolysis* of erythrocytes, such as bilirubin, increase.

In primary alloimmunization, antibody production begins no earlier than 7 to 10 days post-transfusion, but it is several weeks or months before antibodies can be detected clinically. In vivo erythrocyte survival, however, is shortened, with the degree of the decrease depending on the quantity of antibody produced and the quantity of transfused erythrocytes remaining.

Because the antibody produced in a delayed transfusion reaction is largely of the IgG class, it rarely causes *intravascular* hemolysis as seen in an acute hemolytic reaction. The pathologic destruction of erythrocytes is by *extravascular* hemolysis.

When an erythrocyte is phagocytized and digested by the macrophages of the reticuloendothelial system, the hemoglobin molecule is disassembled (Fig. 12-2). The resulting components are iron, protoporphyrin, and globin. Iron is transported in the plasma by transferrin to be recycled by the red bone marrow in the manufacture of new hemoglobin. Globin is catabolized in the liver into its constituent amino acids and enters the circulating amino acid pool. The porphyrin ring is broken at the alpha methene bridge by the heme oxidase enzyme. The alpha carbon leaves as carbon monoxide. The tetrapyrrole (bilirubin) resulting from the opened porphyrin ring is carried by plasma albumin to the liver, where it is conjugated to form glucuronide and excreted in the bile. Both unconjugated (prehepatic) and conjugated (posthepatic) bilirubin are present in the plasma. Bilirubin glucuronide is excreted into the gut, converted by bacterial action, and excreted in the feces as stercobilinogen. A small amount of urobilinogen is reabsorbed into the blood circulation and excreted in the urine.

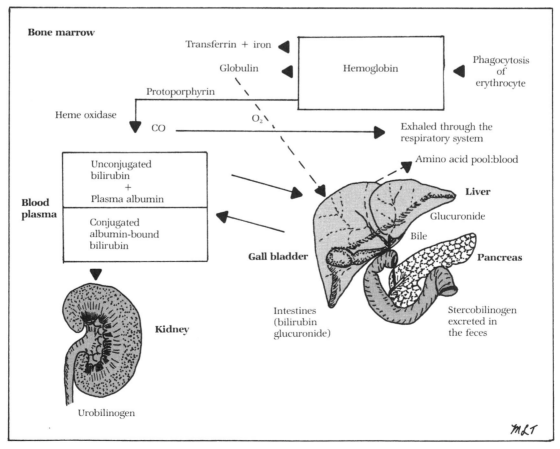

**Figure 12-2.** Extravascular catabolism of erythrocytes.

If a delayed hemolytic transfusion reaction is detected or suspected, tests should be done to determine and confirm the cause of the reaction. This evaluation should be recorded in the patient's chart.

In the case of a suspected delayed hemolytic transfusion reaction, demonstrating the existence of hemolysis by measuring haptoglobin, hemoglobin or bilirubin in serum, and hemoglobin, hemosiderin or urobilinogen in urine may be confirmatory. Often these tests are ordered later than the time at which maximally abnormal findings exist. Increased extravascular catabolism can produce a decreased haptoglobin level, increased indirect bilirubin, and the presence of hemosiderin in urinary epithelial cells.

## Prevention

The blood specimens used for compatibility testing should be *no more* than 3 days old at the time of transfusion if a patient has been previously transfused or pregnant within the preceding 3 months. Although a patient's serum may not demonstrate alloantibodies when antibody attachment and hemolysis first occur, circulating antibody concentrations usually reach detectable levels within several days; however, this may not be the case if the alloantibody produced has been completely absorbed onto the erythrocytes. A low-titered primary immune response may fail to demonstrate detectable levels of the antibody in the patient's serum compared to the level of antibody produced from an anamnestic response.

Elution and identification of antibody are necessary if a positive DAT has been newly discovered. If the patient's serum is negative for alloantibodies or questionable, and the DAT is positive, crossmatching should be done using an eluate. When a positive DAT is present, performing an elution is necessary to identify the specificity of the immunoglobulin absorbed on the cells. A stronger reaction may be achieved by using enhancement media such as LISS. Stronger serum reactions may also be observed by using selected cells that are homozygous for antigens in systems such as Rh, Duffy, and Kidd. Antibodies in these systems sometimes react more strongly with red cells that are homozygous for the corresponding antigen.

After the accelerated destruction and removal of incompatible donor erythrocytes, a delayed hemolytic transfusion reaction is no longer characterized by either a positive DAT or positive eluates. The persistence of a positive DAT with autologous antibodies characterizes a warm acquired hemolytic anemia (discussed in Chapter 6).

## IMMEDIATE NONHEMOLYTIC REACTIONS

In this section, reactions that are not usually associated with erythrocyte hemolysis are discussed. Nonhemolytic reactions, like hemolytic reactions, may be of an immediate or delayed nature.

## Febrile Reactions

### Etiology

Febrile reactions are the most commonly reported transfusion reactions. The most common type of febrile transfusion reaction is due to cytotoxic antibodies or leukoagglutinins (leukocyte antibodies). If these antibodies are present in the recipient's plasma, a reaction occurs between the antibodies and the antigens present on the cell membrane of transfused leukocytes or platelets. In one study, granulocytes were found to be responsible for 91% of leukocyte reactions. Patients who have received multiple platelet transfusions have a high incidence of febrile reactions. Nonspecific leukoagglutinins, as well as those of HLA origin, have been implicated in febrile reactions. Although cytotoxic antibodies and leukoagglutinins can often be demonstrated in patients with febrile reactions, the cause of many of these reactions is obscure and cannot be readily documented by laboratory testing. Frequently the diagnosis is by exclusion of other causes. Leukoagglutinins have also been implicated in a specific type of delayed reaction referred to as the *noncardiac pulmonary edema syndrome.*

### Signs and Symptoms

The most common symptom is fever, often accompanied by chills, which begins during or soon after transfusion. Although a nonhemolytic febrile reaction is rarely harmful, fever may be one of the clinical symptoms of a hemolytic transfusion reaction. Evidence of chills and fever should be investigated as a *potential* hemolytic transfusion reaction.

The fever associated with a febrile nonhemolytic reaction is defined as a rise in body temperature of 1° C or more, occurring in association with the transfusion of blood or components and with no other explanation. Febrile reactions may be mild to severe and may begin early in the transfusion to an hour or two after the reaction has been completed. Fever is more common in patients receiving granulocytes than in those receiving other blood products and tends to occur more often in repeatedly transfused patients and in women who have had multiple pregnancies.

### Prevention

Documenting the existence of leukoagglutinins may be helpful in patients who are expected to need additional transfusions. Tests such as leukoagglutinin and microlymphocytotoxicity assays can be performed. With or without documentation of the existence of specific antibodies, the use of leukocyte-poor preparations (see Chapter 9) is recommended *only* after a patient has had two or more febrile nonhemolytic reactions.

## Platelet Reactions

Two types of immediate reactions to transfused platelets have been documented. These are febrile reactions and hemolytic reactions.

### Febrile Etiology

Febrile reactions to platelet transfusions are probably related to the presence of large numbers of leukocytes in the platelet concentrate component.

### Febrile Signs, Symptoms, and Prevention

Refer to previous discussion of febrile reactions.

### Hemolytic Etiology

The hemolytic reaction to platelet components is related to the common practice of transfusing ABO-incompatible platelets when group-specific platelets are not available.

Transfusions which are not group-specific are generally considered safe and are accepted as clinically effective. Transfusions of incompatible platelets are not, however, without risks related to passively transfused antibodies. In a typical platelet concentrate, a relatively small volume of plasma (commonly 50 to 70 mL) and few erythrocytes (less than 0.1 mL) may be present. Two hemolytic reactions, one fatal, have been reported. Both were related to isoagglutinins present in group O platelet concentrates. One pediatric patient was a group A who received 200 mL of plasma in two aliquots containing a hemolytic anti-A (1:16) and an IgG anti-A (1:32,000). The second patient, who was group B, received between 50 and 70 mL of O plasma with a titer (1:16,000) of anti-B.

### Hemolytic Signs

In the group A patient, in addition to the patient's pre-existing sepsis, a classic case of DIC resulted and the patient expired. In the group B patient, the platelet concentrate produced hemolysis of 40% of the patient's erythrocytes.

### Hemolytic Prevention

The use of group-specific or group-compatible platelets is preferred. In cases of ABO-incompatible platelet preparations, however, it is recommended that as much plasma as possible be removed. Observation of patients during transfusion of any blood product is important in the identification of *immediate* transfusion reactions.

## Reactions to Plasma Constituents

Immediate reactions to plasma constituents may be classified as *allergic, anaphylactoid,* or *anaphylactic* in nature.

### Allergic and Anaphylactoid Reactions

*Etiology.* Although the mechanism of this type of reaction is unclear, most authorities agree that it is a reaction to soluble constituents in donor plasma. There is more discomfort than danger. Allergic reactions are the second most common type of transfusion reaction. When the reaction is extensive or produces edema, it is referred to as anaphylactoid. Anaphylactoid reactions are not uncommon following intramuscular injection of serum immune globulins that have detectable amounts of IgA.

*Signs and Symptoms.* This type of reaction develops during or shortly after transfusion. Allergic reactions are manifested by urticaria (hives), itching, and local erythema, but usually no fever. If the cutaneous reaction is extensive or produces oral, pharyngeal, or laryngeal edema, it is known as an anaphylactoid reaction.

*Prevention.* Laboratory investigation usually yields little information; however, reactions can be well controlled with antihistamines. In repeated or severe reactions, washed or deglycerolized frozen erythrocytes are recommended.

### Anaphylactic Reactions

*Etiology.* Anaphylactic reactions occur in IgA-deficient patients who have developed anti-IgA antibodies. Patients lacking IgA have an increased risk of forming anti-IgA antibodies. Anti-IgA antibody formation can result from immunization due to previous transfusions or pregnancy; however, patients often have anti-IgA without a known source of stimulation.

IgA deficiency is the most frequent of all of the selective deficiencies of serum immunoglobulins, occurring in about 1 in 700 persons. In these patients, 10% develop antibodies to IgA protein and can suffer acute anaphylactic reactions when infused with blood products containing the protein. Anti-IgA antibodies exist in 86% of patients with anaphylactic or anaphylactoid reactions.

Fortunately, anaphylactic reactions due to anti-IgA are very rare. Other potential causes of anaphylactic reaction are the presence of antibodies to soluble plasma antigens or to drugs contained in transfused blood, such as penicillin.

*Signs and Symptoms.* Anaphylactic reactions are dramatic and rapid in their onset. Clinical signs are seen suddenly after exposure to the IgA protein, often before 10 mL of plasma have been infused. Symptoms include nausea, abdominal cramps, emesis, and diarrhea. Transient hypertension is followed by hypotension. Shock and loss of consciousness follow. Medical assistance must be sought immediately if anaphylaxis is suspected.

It is important to distinguish an anaphylactic reaction from other immediate reactions. In an anaphylactic reaction, symptoms become obvious after the transfusion of only a few milliliters of blood or plasma, and fever is absent.

***Prevention.*** Demonstration of antibody to IgA remains a research procedure, but evidence can be obtained by documenting the absence of serum IgA in the patient through immunodiffusion or immunoelectrophoresis techniques.

Avoiding exposure to IgA is mandatory in previously immunized IgA-deficient patients. These patients *must* be transfused with blood components that lack IgA. In some cases, it may be possible to collect and store frozen autologous components for known IgA-deficient patients. When that is not possible, files of such donors are maintained by the AABB Rare Donor File, the Irwin Memorial Blood Bank (San Francisco), the American National Red Cross (Washington), and the Canadian Red Cross (Toronto, Ontario, Canada).

## Bacterial Endotoxemia and Sepsis

### Etiology

Although transfusion reactions are rarely due to bacterial contamination of whole blood and other selected components, an increased number of deaths caused by bacterial contamination of platelet concentrates have been reported to the FDA since 1980. In contrast to a report in 1980, when two fatalities were attributed to contaminated blood or blood components in the previous 2½ years, six deaths due to bacterial contamination of platelet concentrates were reported between January 1980 and December 1983. A report in 1986 stated that, in a three-month period, four episodes of bacterial sepsis related to contaminated random donor platelet concentrates were observed at one medical center. Platelet concentrates that, by contemporary standard practice, are stored at room temperature are now the most common cause of transfusion-related sepsis.

Bacterial endotoxemia in whole blood or blood components stored under refrigeration is usually due to the endotoxins produced by psychrophilic (cold-growing) gram-negative bacteria, such as the *Pseudomonas* species. In products such as platelet concentrates stored at room temperature, bacterial isolates have included *Salmonella heidelberg,* the *Corynebacterium JK* group, *Staphylococcus epidermidis, Staphylococcus aureus, Yersinia,* and *listeria.*

### Signs and Symptoms

The appearance of signs and symptoms caused by bacterial endotoxemia begins within 30 minutes and may follow the infusion of as little as 50 mL of blood. Initial symptoms may include characteristic shaking chills, severe hypotension, pain in the abdomen, generalized muscle pain, vomiting, and bloody diarrhea. The manifestation of shock syndrome is unusual because it appears as dry flushed skin and fever. Renal failure and possibly DIC may follow. If this type of transfusion reaction is not immediately recognized and treated, it can be fatal. Treatment usually consists of the administration of broad-spectrum antibiotics, fluid replacement, respiratory support, corticosteroids, and vasopressors to maintain blood pressure and urinary output.

Reactions caused by recent bacterial contamination are usually manifested within minutes of completing a transfusion. Fever, chills and hypotension are common symptoms. If a transfusion reaction is suggestive of bacterial contamination, it must be reported immediately to the attending physician. Antibiotic treatment of the patient must be initiated immediately. Other forms of treatment should be consistent with the patient's clinical condition.

### Prevention

Maintenance of sterility is essential to the prevention of bacterial contamination. Caution must be exercised before and during blood collection and component preparation. Unit dose dispensing of small quantities of blood to neonatal patients has not led to bacterial contamination. Storage temperature and length of storage are critical considerations. The length of storage time currently approved for platelet concentrates is being questioned.

It is important to inspect blood and blood components visually before issue. If a unit has a brownish or purple discoloration, bacterial contamination should be strongly suspected. Units should also *not* be issued if clots are apparent or if the interface between plasma and erythrocytes has a fuzzy or blurred appearance. Plasma should be inspected for an opaque or muddy look at evidence of bacterial contamination.

Current regulations impose only limited sterility constraints on perishable products such as packed erythrocytes and fresh-frozen plasma. It is essential to monitor the sterility of blood products resulting from aseptic donations. The effectiveness of available methods has been questioned because the integrity of a closed system may be destroyed. Accidental contamination during sterility testing can never be totally excluded; however, a safer technique using a simple, permanently closed system has been recently described.

## Circulatory Overload

### Etiology

Circulatory overload can result from rapid transfusion of large volumes of blood without equivalent blood loss. It can also occur after transfusion of small amounts of blood to patients with abnormal cardiac function and reserve.

## Signs and Symptoms

Typical symptoms include severe headache, dyspnea, cyanosis, and congestive heart failure. Pulmonary edema can subsequently develop as a result of congestive heart failure. In infants with high cardiac reserve function, the prodromal symptoms may be hidden, with complications emerging rapidly and proving fatal.

## Prevention

The use of packed erythrocytes rather than whole blood substantially reduces the risk of circulatory overload. In patients who are not actively bleeding or who are susceptible to circulatory overload, such as those with chronic heart disease, blood should be administered slowly. The usual rate of blood administration, 200 mL/hour, should be reduced to 100 mL/hour, although prolonging the time does increase the risk of bacterial growth. In addition, it is preferable to have the patient in a sitting rather than a reclining position. Some clinicians prefer to divide full units of packed red cells in half. One divided unit can be transfused while the other remains refrigerated. The attending physician may also order the administration of a diuretic medication to reduce fluid retention. In patients with low hematocrits (15 to 20%), phlebotomy of whole blood followed by the transfusion of packed red cells may be useful in increasing oxygen-carrying capacity without expanding blood volume. The protocol for this technique must be approved by the blood bank director and medical staff.

## Other Immediate Adverse Effects

Rapid transfusion of 10 or more units of citrated blood can elevate plasma citrate levels. Clinical and experimental studies have demonstrated that rapid transfusion with citrated bank blood components can cause hypocalcemic myocardial depression.

Hypocalcemia is usually self-compensated, with no need for calcium therapy. Acute cardiac failure and cardiac arrest are rare and have been observed primarily in association with exchange transfusion in infants.

Two additional complications that can precipitate arrhythmias are hyperkalemia (an increase in plasma potassium) and transfusion of a large volume of cold blood, which lowers body temperature.

## DELAYED NONHEMOLYTIC REACTIONS

### Graft-versus-Host Disease

Cases of transfusion-related GVHD have increased significantly in the past several decades. Graft-versus-host disease (GVHD) can be an unintentional consequence of blood transfusion or transplantation in severely immunocom-

promised or immunosuppressed patients. The degree of immunodeficiency in the host, rather than the number of transfused immunocompetent lymphocytes, determines whether or not GVHD will occur.

## Etiology

When immunocompetent T lymphocytes are transfused from a donor to an immunodeficient or immunosuppressed recipient, the transfused, or *grafted*, lymphocytes recognize the antigens of the host as foreign and react immunologically against them (Table 12-2). Instead of the usual transplantation reaction of host against graft, the reverse graft versus host reaction occurs and produces an inflammatory response.

In a normal lymphocyte transfer reaction, the recipient is capable of destroying the foreign lymphocytes; therefore, GVHD is not expected to develop. Engraftment and multiplication of donor lymphocytes in an immunosuppressed recipient is a real possibility, because lymphocytes capable of mitosis can be found in stored blood products. If the recipient cannot reject the transfused lymphocytes, the grafted lymphocytes may cause uncontrolled destruction of the host's tissues and, eventually, death. A patient can develop acute or chronic GVHD. Where the donor and recipient differ at HLA loci, the reaction can be fatal. The stronger the antigen difference, the more severe the reaction.

## Epidemiology

It is now accepted that GVHD can occur whenever immunologically competent allogeneic lymphocytes are transferred into a severely immunocompromised host. Patients at risk include those who are immunodeficient or immunosuppressed with severe lymphocytopenia and bone marrow suppression. In addition, GVHD can occur in healthy recipients receiving blood products from a first-degree relative.

Graft-versus-host disease has been reported subsequent to blood transfusion in bone marrow transplant recipients following total-body irradiation, adults receiving intensive chemotherapy for hematological malignancies, and infants

**Table 12-2. Requirements for Potential Graft-versus-Host Disease**

| Factor | Comments |
| --- | --- |
| 1. A source of immunocompetent lymphocytes | Blood products, bone marrow transplant, organ transport |
| 2. HLA differences between patient and recipient | Differences at HLA locus can be fatal. The stronger the antigen difference, the more severe the reaction |
| 3. Inability to reject donor cells | Patients are severely immunocompromised or immunosuppressed |

with severe congenital immunodeficiency. Despite chemotherapy at the time of bone marrow transplantation, 20–50% of patients will develop acute GVHD, and 20–40% of these patients will die of GVHD or associated infections. GVHD has also occurred in infants who received intrauterine transfusions followed by exchange transfusion. Nearly 90% of patients with post-transfusion GVHD will die of acute complications of the disease. The usual cause of death is generalized infection.

Chronic GVHD affects 20–40% of patients within more than 6 months after transplantation. Two factors closely associated with the development of chronic GVHD are increasing age and a preceding episode of acute GVHD.

### Signs and Symptoms

GVHD cause an inflammatory response. Post-transfusion symptoms begin within 3 to 30 days after transfusion. Because of lymphocytic infiltration of the intestine, skin, and liver, mucosal destruction including ulcerative skin and mouth lesions, diarrhea, and liver destruction result. Other clinical symptoms include jaundice, fever, anemia, weight loss, skin rash and splenomegaly.

In bone marrow transplant patients, acute GVHD develops within the first 3 months of transplantation. The initial manifestations are lesions of the skin, liver, and gastrointestinal tract. An erythematous, maculopapular, skin rash, particularly on the palms and soles, is usually the first sign of GVHD. Disease progression is characterized by diarrhea. Other signs and symptoms of complications related to therapy in potential GVHD patients include fever, granulocytopenia, and bacteremia. Interstitial pneumonia, frequently associated with cytomegalovirus (CMV), can also occur.

Chronic GVHD resembles a collagen vascular disease with skin changes, such as erythema and cutaneous ulcers, and liver dysfunction, characterized by bile duct degeneration and cholestasis. Patients with chronic GVHD are susceptible to bacterial infections. For example, advancing age and preexisting lung disease increase the incidence of interstitial pneumonia.

### Prevention

The risk of graft-versus-host disease can be minimized, if not eliminated, by irradiating whole blood and various other components immediately before infusion (see Chapter 12, Blood and Blood Components). Administration of intravenous immunoglobulin to patients undergoing bone marrow transplantation has been reported as having beneficial effects with regard to the progression of graft-versus-host disease, interstitial pneumonia, and infections such as gram-negative sepsis. However, the cost of this immunomodulatory therapy may be prohibitive.

The efficacy of irradiating blood and components prior to storage is being evaluated. Prophylactic irradiation of whole blood products and components prior to transfusion is presently the most efficient way to prevent post-transfusion GVHD.

There are several clinical indications for blood that reduces the risk of potential GVHD as the result of infused lymphocytes. Patients most at risk who are in absolute need of irradiated blood products include recipients of autologous or allogeneic bone marrow grafts and children with severe congenital immune deficiency syndromes involving T lymphocytes. Patients considered to be at less of a risk of developing GVHD include infants receiving intrauterine transfusions followed by exchange transfusions—and possibly infants receiving only exchange transfusions. The immune mechanism of the fetus and newborn infant may not be sufficiently mature to reject foreign lymphocytes, and prior transfusions may induce a state of immune tolerance in the newborn. Patients receiving total body radiation or immunosuppressive therapy for disorders such as lymphoma and acute leukemia are usually unable to mount an immune response that produces GVHD.

## Noncardiac Pulmonary Edema Syndrome

### Etiology

This disorder is characteristically a complication of granulocyte transfusion. It has occurred, however, after the transfusion of whole blood or plasma, and there are isolated reports of its occurring after cryoprecipitate infusion. The precise cause is not known, but leukoagglutinins have been implicated. The incidence of noncardiac pulmonary edema increases with parity in women.

Two mechanisms have been postulated. In one mechanism, the reaction between donor leukoagglutinins and recipient leukocytes produces leukocyte aggregates that are trapped in the pulmonary microcirculation and produce changes in vascular permeability. If granulocyte concentrates are administered, the reaction involves recipient leukoagglutinins that aggregate the transfused granulocytes. An alternate proposed mechanism is the activation of complement to generate the anaphylatoxins C3a and C5a. These complement components stimulate the release of histamine and serotonin from tissue basophils and platelets in addition to directly aggregating granulocytes. Directly aggregated granulocytes produce leukocytic emboli that lodge in the microvascular circulation of the lungs.

### Signs and Symptoms

The reaction may be mild and respond to supportive therapy but it is characteristically severe and delayed, occurring 1 to 6 hours after transfusion. Respiratory distress can begin after the infusion of amounts of blood too small to produce hypervolemia. Clinical signs include chills, fever, dyspnea, nonproductive cough, hypotension, and cyanosis. Blood eosinophilia is common.

Prevention

Washed or frozen-deglycerolized units of blood may be used to avoid some of these reactions because leukocytes and leukoagglutinins are almost completely eliminated.

**Post-Transfusion Purpura**

Etiology

Post-transfusion purpura is a rare event that may develop after the administration of blood or platelet-containing components. Most patients have been women, most of whom appear to have been immunized by previous pregnancies or, less frequently, by previous transfusions. The severe thrombocytopenia that develops in the disorder is associated with platelet alloantibodies. Almost all affected patients have been shown to be P1$^{A1}$ negative with anti-P1$^{A1}$ antibodies in their plasma at the time of thrombocytopenia. This antibody was directed against platelet membrane glycoprotein III. P1$^{A1}$ antigen is present in 98.3% of the U.S. population. The P1$^{A1}$ antibody destroys not only the transfused platelets but the patient's own P1$^{A1}$ negative platelets. The mechanism of destruction of the patient's own platelets or of P1$^{A1}$ negative platelets from normal donors during the acute phase of post-transfusion purpura is unknown. In three cases, the patients were P1$^{A1}$ positive with an antibody specificity that may have been anti-P1$^{A2}$.

Signs and Symptoms

Clinical signs generally manifest themselves about a week after transfusion due to a sudden decrease in the patient's platelet count. This severe thrombocytopenia produces generalized purpura. In addition to purpura and petechiae, occult or obvious hemorrhage may be present.

Prevention

In patients with severe thrombocytopenia who need treatment, exchange plasmapheresis is a possible mode of therapy. The thrombocytopenia in this disorder is usually self-limiting. Platelet transfusions are usually not beneficial.

**Iron Overload**

Etiology

A delayed effect of multiple transfusions of erythrocytes in nonbleeding, chronically anemic patients is iron overload from transfusion hypersiderosis or hemosiderosis. Patients at risk of iron overload include those with hemoglobinopathies, such as the thalassemias, and aplastic or sideroblastic anemias. Every unit of erythrocytes contains approximately 250 mg of iron. When patients have received more than 100 transfusions, significant iron deposition may occur.

Signs and Symptoms

Deposits of iron in parenchymal cells cause damage to many organs, most significantly the liver, heart, and endocrine glands. Dysfunctions of specific body systems, such as jaundice or cardiac dysfunction, represent manifestations of this condition.

Prevention

Iron-chelating agents may be useful in reducing body storage iron; however, it has not been proven that such treatment can reverse the tissue damage that has already occurred, nor has it been demonstrated that consistent long-term iron balance can be achieved with this therapy. A recent approach to reducing the risk of transfusion-induced iron overload is transfusion with erythrocytes that have been enriched with younger erythrocytes, *neocytes.* Neocytes survive longer in the circulation and result in a greater interval between transfusions, with subsequent reduction in the total iron infused over an extended period of time.

**Other Delayed Adverse Effects**

Two significant consequences of blood transfusion are immunization to foreign antigens and the transmission of disease. Immunization to antigens is described in detail in Chapter 3. Because the transmission of disease through transfusion is critical, it is discussed separately in Chapter 12.

## LABORATORY INVESTIGATION OF TRANSFUSION REACTIONS

Any adverse reaction experienced by a patient in association with a transfusion is to be regarded as a suspected transfusion reaction. All suspected transfusion reactions must be reported to the blood bank or transfusion service and should be evaluated on a timely basis. Circulatory overload or allergic reactions need not be evaluated as possible hemolytic transfusion reactions.

Records must be kept of all reports of transfusion complications. These complications should be reviewed periodically by the hospital transfusion committee. In addition, fatalities resulting directly from transfusion complications, such as hemolytic reactions or viral hepatitis, must be reported to the Food and Drug Administration, Office of Compliance, Center for Biologics Evaluation and Research. This notification must be by phone (301-295-8191) within 24 hours and by written report within 7 days.

Investigation of possible transfusion reactions is important to the immediate and long-term safety of patients. The breadth of the evaluation should be to the degree considered appropriate by the medical director of the blood bank/transfusion service. Further consultation intervention, sometimes with the assistance of computers

**Table 12-3. Conditions and Actions in Cases of Transfusion Reaction**

| Clinical Condition | Preventive Action |
| --- | --- |
| Delayed hemolytic transfusion reaction due to serologic incompatibility | If red blood cell antigen-directed, unexpected antibody is detected, all red blood cell components shall be screened for the specific antigen |
| Anaphylaxis, such as IgA deficiency | Without plasma and multiply wash plasma-containing components with saline prior to issue or administer products from IgA-deficient donors |
| Febrile, nonhemolytic reaction due to presumed sensitization to leukocyte or plasma antigens | Warning label of previous reaction |
| Urticarial reaction due to presumed sensitization to plasma proteins | Warning label of previous reaction |

Adapted from Effect of Transfusion Reaction Consultations on Subsequent Transfusion Practices, *Lab Med 21*(7):444–447, July 1991.

(Table 12-3) may be needed should a subsequent component be ordered in cases such as:

1. Delayed hemolytic transfusion reaction due to serologic incompatibility
2. Febrile, nonhemolytic reaction due to presumed sensitization to leukocyte or plasma antigens
3. Urticarial reaction due to presumed sensitization to plasma proteins
4. Anaphylaxis such as that due to IgA deficiency

Although the protocol may vary depending on the patient's signs and symptoms, the generally accepted procedure for the investigation of a transfusion reaction includes the following:

### Immediate Steps

1. Check the identification of the patient and the transfused unit of blood or component. The label on the blood container(s) and all other records must be examined to determine if there has been an error in identifying the patient or the blood. Notify appropriate persons if any clerical or identification error exists. If a discrepancy is noted, check to see if any other patients are at risk.
2. Obtain a posttransfusion blood specimen from the patient. Label it as the post-transfusion specimen. Obtain the discontinued bag of blood, administration set, and any attached IV solutions.
3. Visually examine the patient's post-transfusion serum or plasma for hemolysis. Prereaction samples should be used for comparison. In a properly drawn specimen, a pink color indicates that intravascular hemolysis may have taken place. If massive hemolysis has taken place, free hemoglobin will be apparent at once. It may be

detectable with the onset of clinical signs and symptoms. Free hemoglobin is cleared from the plasma in 5–12 hours.

4. Perform a direct antiglobulin test on an anticoagulated post-transfusion blood specimen from the patient. In the case of an incompatible transfusion, if the transfused red cells are not immediately destroyed, the direct AHG test will be positive with a mixed-field appearance. If this post-transfusion specimen is positive, the pretransfusion DAT should be also be checked. If only the DAT on the post-transfusion test is positive, the patient's erythrocytes have been coated with antibody or complement. Procedures for investigation of a positive DAT should be followed to determine the cause.
5. Perform an ABO grouping and Rh typing of the patient's pretransfusion and post-transfusion blood specimen, and a specimen from the bag or a segment attached to the transfused unit. If a discrepancy occurs between the ABO group or Rh type of the patient's pretransfusion and post-transfusion specimens or the donor unit, an error in patient identification, specimen labeling, donor unit identification, or other clerical error is responsible. Crosscheck the results against all past records as well as the labeling of the blood product itself. Any other patient specimens drawn at approximately the same time should be rechecked, if the possibility exists of having another patient at risk. Interpretation of the evaluation must be recorded in the patient's chart and, if it is suggestive of a hemolytic reaction or of bacterial contamination, it must be reported immediately to the patient's physician.

### Follow-up Steps. 
Depending on the patient's signs and symptoms (see Case Studies), additional testing may be indicated. There must be a written protocol indicating the circumstances requiring additional testing. This protocol should also outline the needed tests. Followup procedures may include:

1. Repeat the crossmatch with the pretransfusion and post-transfusion specimen. An incompatible crossmatch with the pretransfusion specimen indicates that an error existed in the patient or donor specimen during pretransfusion testing. If the crossmatch is incompatible only with the post-transfusion specimen, an anamnestic reaction is suspect.
2. Repeat the unexpected antibody screening tests on the pretransfusion and donor units as well as on the post-transfusion specimen. If either the pretransfusion or donor unit specimen has a previously unreported unexpected antibody, check for clerical errors in the pretransfusion testing. If the post-transfusion specimen has an antibody not present in the pretransfusion specimen, an anamnestic reaction or passive administration of antibody in a recently infused blood component should be suspected.
3. If any of the unexpected antibody screening tests are positive, identify the antibody. The presence of an un-

expected antibody does not necessarily indicate that it is the cause of the reaction, the corresponding antigen must also be present. Test the patient or donor erythrocytes for the corresponding antigen.

4. Request the collection of a urine sample from the patient as soon as possible. Intact red cells indicate hemorrhage into the urinary tract—not hemolysis. Test the urine specimen for the presence of free hemoglobin. If the urine specimen is not collected for several days, it may be tested for hemosiderin.

## Supplementary Tests

If routine testing fails to provide information and immune hemolysis is suspected, the following tests may be helpful:

1. Antibody screening and compatibility tests with enhancement media or by increasing the ratio of serum to cells.
2. DAT and unexpected antibody screening tests on several post-transfusion specimens collected from the patient at daily or frequent intervals.
3. Monitoring of hemoglobin/hematocrit levels. In a nonbleeding patient, a unit of packed erythrocytes should produce an increase of 1 g/dL or packed cell volume (hematocrit) of 3%.
4. Genotyping of the erythrocytes of the patient's pretransfusion specimen and the donor cells The patient's postreaction specimen must be examined for the presence of cells bearing foreign antigens. If an antigen can be found that is present on the donor cells and absent on the patient's cells, its presence or absence in the post-transfusion sample indicates the degree to which the transfused cells have survived and remain in the circulation.
5. Testing of post-transfusion serum samples for the presence of unconjugated bilirubin. A rising bilirubin may be detectable as early as 1 hour post-transfusion. Peak levels occur at 3 to 6 hours. The degree of hyperbilirubinemia depends on the extent and rapidity of hemolysis and the rate of bilirubin excretion.
6. Measuring of serum haptoglobin in pre- and post-transfusion patient specimens. When haptoglobin is

fully saturated, free hemoglobin appears in the plasma. A decline in haptoglobin is useful in detecting chronic hemolysis. If studies are performed several days after a hemolytic episode, normal levels may be restored because haptoglobin is an acute-phase reactant that may regenerate rapidly after depletion.

### Tests for Fibrinolysis (DIC)

Because the manifestations of fibrinolysis and DIC are extremely variable, diagnosis depends on laboratory testing. The key feature is an elevation of circulating fibrinogen-fibrin split products (FSPs).

Typical results in DIC include prolonged activated partial thromboplastin time (APPT), prothrombin time (PT), and thrombin time. Fibrinogen levels and the total platelet count may vary, although thrombocytopenia and a decrease in fibrinogen are common. Excessive fibrinolysis with the release of FSPs occurs secondary to intravascular fibrin formation. While the presence of FSPs is characteristic, the finding of FSPs is not specific for DIC and cannot be used as the sole criterion for diagnosis.

### Infectious Diseases

According to the Standards of the American Association of Blood Banks, there must be a procedure to encourage reporting suspected cases of transfusion-transmitted diseases. These diseases include but are not limited to hepatitis B, hepatitis C, and transfusion-associated AIDS. Transfusion services must investigate each report. If transmission is confirmed, or at least not ruled out, the blood collecting facility must be notified in writing, and the units of donor blood and components involved in the incident must be identified in the report. The collecting facility shall evaluate each report.

It is also required that appropriate record-keeping procedures exist in order to evaluate the incidence of transfusion-transmitted diseases from blood obtained from each collecting facility. Look-back procedures must exist to identify and notify recipients of the risk of infection from blood or components that came from donors subsequently found to be infected with HIV or HTLV-I/-II.

## CASE STUDIES OF TRANSFUSION REACTIONS

### Case 1

An 18-year-old man was admitted with multiple injuries after he and a passenger, another 18-year-old man, were in a motor vehicle accident. After receiving 50 mL of the first unit of blood, the patient developed shaking chills and became hypotensive. The unit of blood was immediately discontinued and the blood bank was asked to recheck the crossmatch (STAT).

Laboratory Testing

*Clerical Check.* No evidence of blood bank clerical errors.

*Hemoglobinemia.* Slight hemolysis observed.

*Direct Antiglobulin Test.* Patient pretransfusion specimen: Negative Patient post-transfusion specimen: Weakly positive (mixed field)

### *Recheck of Blood Grouping*

| | Anti-A | Anti-B | Anti-A,B | Anti-D | A₁ Cells | B Cells | Int. |
|---|---|---|---|---|---|---|---|
| Patient: | | | | | | | |
| Pretransfusion | 4+ | Neg | 4+ | 3+ | Neg | 4+ | A+ |
| Post-transfusion | Neg | Neg | Neg | 3+ | 4+ | 4+ | O+ |
| Donor segment | 4+ | Neg | 4+ | 2+ | Neg | 3+ | A+ |

***Recheck of Crossmatching.*** Patient pretransfusion specimen and donor segment: Compatible (immediate spin).

Patient post-transfusion specimen and donor segment: Incompatible (immediate spin).

### Interpretation

This is a life-threatening emergency because the patient has the signs of an acute hemolytic transfusion reaction. The emergency room physician and the medical director of the blood bank were immediately notified and treat-

ment was initiated. A rapid check of the passenger's blood status revealed that he was group A and was incorrectly receiving group O blood. The patient was group O and had received group A blood. Further investigation revealed that the original patient blood specimen labels had been reversed when the emergency room personnel handed the already drawn tubes of blood to the phlebotomist.

### Conclusion

Acute hemolytic transfusion reaction.

## Case 2

A 38-year-old woman was admitted for thoracic surgery. She had received 2 units of packed red blood cells following the birth of her third child 10 years ago. During her present hospitalization, she developed a fever 72 hours after receiving 3 units of blood during surgery. On her fifth postoperative day, she began to appear mildly jaundiced and experienced a sudden drop in her hemoglobin and hematocrit, with no evidence of hemorrhage. A transfusion reaction workup was ordered.

### Laboratory Testing

***Clerical Check.*** No evidence of blood bank clerical errors.

***Hemoglobinemia.*** Absent from fifth-day post-transfusion specimen.

***Direct Antiglobulin Test.*** Patient post-transfusion specimen: Positive (polyspecific and IgG antisera).

Patient pretransfusion specimen: Negative.

### *Recheck of Blood Grouping*

| | Anti-A | Anti-B | Anti-A,B | Anti-D | A₁ Cells | B Cells | Int. |
|---|---|---|---|---|---|---|---|
| Patient: | | | | | | | |
| Pretransfusion | Neg | Neg | Neg | 3+ | 4+ | 4+ | O+ |
| Post-transfusion | Neg | Neg | Neg | 3+ | 4+ | 4+ | O+ |
| Donor segment 1 | Neg | Neg | Neg | 2+ | | | O+ |
| Donor segment 2 | Neg | Neg | Neg | 4+ | | | O+ |
| Donor segment 3 | Neg | Neg | Neg | 3+ | | | O+ |

***Recheck of Crossmatching.*** Patient pretransfusion specimen and donor segment: Compatible

Patient post-transfusion specimen and donor segment 1: Compatible

Patient post-transfusion specimen and donor segment 2: Incompatible (microscopically in AHG)

Patient post-transfusion specimen and donor segment 3: Incompatible (microscopically in AHG)

### *Genotyping*

***Unexpected Antibody Screening.***
Patient pretransfusion specimen: Negative
Patient post-transfusion specimen: Weekly positive (AHG)

***Unexpected Antibody Identification.*** Patient post-transfusion specimen: Anti-E (enzyme technique only)

Eluate of patient red blood cells: Anti-E (enzyme technique only)

| Patient | E negative e positive | Genotype: ee |
|---|---|---|
| Donor #1 | E negative e positive | Genotype: ee |
| Donor #2 | E positive e positive | Genotype: Ee |
| Donor #3 | E positive e negative | Genotype: EE |

## Interpretation

This patient exhibits the signs and symptoms of a delayed hemolytic transfusion reaction caused by anti-E. The rapid development of the antibody suggests an anamnestic response. Previous exposure to the E antigen, which the patient lacks, may have occurred during pregnancy or prior transfusion. The patient was transfused with two units of donor blood possessing the E antigen 5 days before development of signs and symptoms of a reaction. If future transfusions are required, the patient should receive blood that lacks the E antigen.

## Conclusion

Delayed hemolytic transfusion reaction.

## Case 3

A 69-year-old woman was being transfused because of a low postoperative hematocrit. She had a history of anemia and had received multiple previous transfusions. She had experienced a febrile transfusion reaction 4 years ago while receiving washed red cells, but had received two units of blood two years ago while in surgery without demonstrating a reaction. During the present episode, she displayed signs and symptoms of a reaction 20 minutes after the initiation of the infusion of a unit of centrifuged red cells. Her temperature rose from 97.5° F to 102.9° F and her blood pressure rose from 130/70 to 150/80. She also experienced chills. The unit of blood was discontinued and ¾ of it was returned to the blood bank.

### Laboratory Testing

*Clerical Check.* No evidence of blood bank clerical errors.
*Hemoglobinemia.* Absent from post-transfusion specimen.
*Direct Antiglobulin Test.* Patient post-transfusion specimen: Negative.

### *Recheck of Blood Grouping*

|  | Anti-A | Anti-B | Anti-A,B | Anti-D | A₁ Cells | B Cells | Int. |
|---|---|---|---|---|---|---|---|
| Patient: |  |  |  |  |  |  |  |
| Pretransfusion | Neg | Neg | Neg | 2+ | 4+ | 4+ | O+ |
| Post-transfusion | Neg | Neg | Neg | 2+ | 4+ | 4+ | O+ |
| Donor segment | Neg | Neg | Neg | 2+ |  |  | O+ |

## Interpretation

There is no evidence of a hemolytic transfusion reaction. This patient exhibits the signs and symptoms of a febrile transfusion reaction. It is recommended that she receive leukocyte-depleted red blood cells if future transfusions are indicated.

## Conclusion

Febrillar transfusion reaction, probably due to leukoagglutinins.

## Case 4

A 58-year-old woman was admitted with the diagnosis of a fractured hip and anemia. She had no prior history of transfusion, but was the mother of three children. Two hours and 45 minutes after initiation of the infusion of a unit of packed red cells, the patient's blood pressure rose from 128/70 to 180/90 and her temperature rose from 98.7° F to 100.6° F. She did not exhibit chills. The transfusion was discontinued and ⅓ of the unit was returned to the blood bank.

### Laboratory testing

*Clerical Check.* No evidence of blood bank clerical error.
*Direct Antiglobulin Test.* Patient post-transfusion specimen: Negative
*Hemoglobinemia.* Absent from post-transfusion specimen.

### *Recheck of Blood Grouping*

|  | Anti-A | Anti-B | Anti-A,B | Anti-D | A₁ Cells | B Cells | Int. |
|---|---|---|---|---|---|---|---|
| Patient: |  |  |  |  |  |  |  |
| Pretransfusion | Neg | Neg | Neg | 3+ | 2+ | 1+ | O+ |
| Post-transfusion | Neg | Neg | Neg | 3+ | 2+ | 1+ | O+ |
| Donor segment | Neg | Neg | Neg | 2+ |  |  | O+ |

## Interpretation

There is no evidence of a hemolytic transfusion reaction. This patient exhibits the signs and symptoms of a mild febrile transfusion reaction. If a subsequent transfusion produces a similar reaction, it is recommended that she receive leukocyte-depleted red blood cells.

## Conclusion

Febrile transfusion reaction, probable leukoagglutinins.

---

## Case 5

An 81-year-old man was admitted with a diagnosis of chronic anemia. He had no history of previous transfusion. One hour after the initiation of the transfusion of a unit of packed red blood cells, he developed hives and his blood pressure increased from 140/70 to 168/76. His temperature remained normal. Approximately 35 mL of blood remained in the donor unit that was returned to the blood bank.

## Laboratory Testing

*Clerical Check.* No evidence of blood bank clerical error.

*Direct Antiglobulin Test.* Patient post-transfusion specimen: Negative.

*Hemoglobinemia.* Absent from post-transfusion specimen.

### *Recheck of Blood Grouping*

|  | Anti-A | Anti-B | Anti-A,B | Anti-D | $A_1$ Cells | B Cells | Int. |
|---|---|---|---|---|---|---|---|
| Patient: |  |  |  |  |  |  |  |
| Pretransfusion | Neg | 3+ | 3+ | Pos | 3+ | Neg | B+ |
| Post-transfusion | Neg | 3+ | 3+ | Pos | 3+ | Neg | B+ |
| Donor segment | Neg | 3+ | 3+ | Pos |  |  | B+ |

## Interpretation

There is no evidence of a hemolytic transfusion reaction. This patient demonstrates the signs and symptoms of an allergic reaction to the foreign proteins in the donor plasma. If additional transfusions are required, the patient should receive a plasma protein-deficient red blood cell product or be premedicated with an antihistamine.

## Conclusion

Allergic reaction to plasma protein.

---

## Case 6

A 25-year-old man, a burn patient, had previously received multiple transfusions and had a clinical diagnosis of burn/wound sepsis. Ten minutes after the initiation of an infusion of whole blood, he demonstrated an increased pulse rate (from 112 to 118) and an increased body temperature (from 100° F to 102.4° C). The unit of blood was discontinued and ¾ of it was returned to the blood bank.

## Laboratory Testing

*Clerical Check.* No evidence of clerical error.

*Direct Antiglobulin Test.* Patient post-transfusion specimen: Negative.

*Hemoglobinemia.* Absent from post-transfusion specimen.

### *Recheck of Blood Grouping*

|  | Anti-A | Anti-B | Anti-A,B | Anti-D | $A_1$ Cells | B Cells | Int. |
|---|---|---|---|---|---|---|---|
| Patient: |  |  |  |  |  |  |  |
| Pretransfusion | Neg | 4+ | 4+ | Neg | 4+ | Neg | B− |
| Post-transfusion | Neg | 4+ | 4+ | Neg | 4+ | Neg | B− |
| Donor segment | Neg | 4+ | 4+ | Neg |  |  | B− |

## Interpretation

There is no evidence of a hemolytic transfusion reaction. Although the possibility of a febrile reaction to donor leukocytes cannot be totally excluded, the patient's signs and symptoms are probably due to an endogenous fever.

## Conclusion

Endogenous fever.

## CHAPTER SUMMARY

### Definition and Causes

The term transfusion reaction generally refers to the adverse signs and symptoms produced by incompatibility between a patient and a unit of donor red blood cells or blood component. The risk of a transfusion reaction is minimal but not unimportant. The vast majority of fatal transfusion reactions result from misidentification or clerical errors rather than technical limitations. Transfusion reactions can be divided into hemolytic and nonhemolytic types and can be acute or delayed in their manifestation. Acute hemolytic reactions occur during or immediately after blood has been infused; delayed reactions may not express themselves until 7 to 10 days post-transfusion. Acute hemolytic reactions are the most serious and potentially lethal.

### Acute Hemolytic Reactions

The most common cause of an acute hemolytic transfusion reaction is transfusion of ABO-incompatible blood. Prevention of acute hemolytic reactions rests in the proper identification of patients and patient samples, along with error-free laboratory record-keeping, blood grouping, and crossmatching.

### Delayed Hemolytic Reactions

Delayed hemolytic transfusion reactions can occur from two days to several months post-transfusion. To prevent a delayed transfusion reaction, patient specimens used for compatibility testing should be no more than 3 days old at the time of transfusion if a patient has been previously transfused, pregnant within the past 3 months, or of unknown transfusion status.

### Immediate Nonhemolytic Reactions

Febrile reactions are the most prevalent type of immediate nonhemolytic reaction. Febrile reactions are most commonly due to cytotoxic antibodies or leukoagglutinins. To prevent a reaction, documenting the existence of antibodies may be helpful in patients who are expected to need additional transfusions.

Two types of immediate reactions to transfused platelets have been documented: febrile reactions and hemolytic reactions. Febrile reactions to platelet transfusions are probably related to the presence of large numbers of leukocytes in the platelet concentrate component. A hemolytic reaction to platelet components is related to the common practice of transfusing ABO-incompatible platelets when group-specific platelets are not available.

Immediate reactions to plasma constituents may be classified as allergic, anaphylactoid, or anaphylactic in nature. Although the mechanism of allergic and anaphylactoid reactions is unclear, most authorities agree that it is a reaction to soluble constituents in donor plasma.

Bacterial sepsis is rarely due to bacterial contamination of whole blood and other selected components, but an increased number of deaths caused by bacterial contamination of platelet concentrates have been reported since 1980. Platelet concentrates stored at room temperature are now the commonest cause of transfusion-related sepsis.

Circulatory overload can result from rapid transfusion of large volumes of blood without equivalent blood loss. It can also occur after transfusion of small amounts of blood to patients with abnormal cardiac function and reserve. Circulatory overload can be prevented through the use of red blood cells rather than whole blood.

The rapid transfusion of 10 or more units of citrated blood can elevate plasma citrate levels. Clinical and experimental studies have demonstrated that rapid transfusion with citrated bank blood components can cause hypocalcemic myocardial depression. Hyperkalemia is another theoretic complication. Additionally, transfusing a large volume of cold blood can lower body temperature.

### Delayed Nonhemolytic Reactions

Graft-versus-host disease can develop when immunocompetent lymphocytes are transfused from a donor to a recipient who is not capable of rejecting the transfused or grafted lymphocytes.

Noncardiac pulmonary edema syndrome is chiefly a complication of transfused granulocytes. Washed or frozen deglycerolized red cells eliminate this complication.

Post-transfusion purpura is a rare event that may develop following the administration of blood or platelet containing blood components. The severe thrombocytopenia that develops in the disorder is associated with platelet antibodies.

Iron overload is a delayed manifestation in patients who have received multiple transfusions over an extended period of time. Deposits of iron in parenchymal cells cause damage to many organs, most significantly the liver, heart, or endocrine glands. Iron-chelating agents may be useful in reducing body iron storage and transfusion with neocytes may be useful.

Two additional significant consequences of blood transfusion can be immunization to foreign antigens and transmission of disease.

### Laboratory Investigation of Transfusion Reactions

The investigation of possible transfusion reactions is important to the immediate and long-term safety of patients. Although specific details of the protocol may vary from one blood bank to another, the general approach to the investigation of a transfusion reaction includes immediate steps such as checking the identification of the patient and the transfused unit of blood or component. Additional testing is needed if routine testing fails to provide information and immune hemolysis is suspected.

## REVIEW QUESTIONS

1. A transfusion reaction can include:
   A. Incompatibility between red cell antigens and corresponding antibodies.
   B. Shortened post-transfusion survival of erythrocytes
   C. An allergic response
   D. All of the above

2. The *most* frequent cause of fatal transfusion reactions is:
   A. Mislabelling of blood samples
   B. Errors in laboratory records
   C. Misidentification of patients
   D. Crossmatching that failed to detect antibodies

3–7. Match the type of transfusion reaction with the appropriate condition:
   A. Immediate hemolytic
   B. Immediate nonhemolytic
   C. Delayed hemolytic
   D. Delayed nonhemolytic

3. Urticaria

4. Hemolysis of erythrocytes during or immediately after blood infusion

5. Graft-versus-host disease

6. Hemolysis of erythrocytes 7 to 10 days post-transfusion

7. Infectious diseases

8. The most severe form of a transfusion reaction is:
   A. Intravascular hemolysis
   B. Extravascular hemolysis
   C. Iron overload
   D. Urticaria

9. The factor/factors that determine(s) whether a transfusion reaction will be acute or delayed and intravascular or extravascular is/are:
   A. The volume of incompatible erythrocytes infused
   B. Antibody class and subclass
   C. Achievement of an optimal temperature for antibody binding
   D. All of the above

10. The antibody *most frequently* cited as a cause of an acute hemolytic transfusion reaction is:
    A. Anti-I
    B. Anti-A, anti-B
    C. Anti-Le$^a$
    D. Anti-K

11. Nonantibody causes of *acute* hemolytic reactions include:

   A. Leukocytes
   B. Bacterial contamination
   C. Infusion of hemolyzed erythrocytes
   D. B and C

12. The *most* common initial symptoms of an *acute* hemolytic reaction in unanesthetized patients are:
    A. Fever with or without chills
    B. Shock and urticaria
    C. Pain in the lower back and hypotension
    D. Pain in the lower back and urticaria

13. In vivo interaction between antigens and antibodies results in:
    A. Activation of factor XIIa
    B. Complement activation
    C. Accelerated intravascular hemolysis
    D. All of the above.

14. Of the reactions listed, the most serious consequence of an *acute* hemolytic transfusion reaction is:
    A. Disseminated intravascular coagulation
    B. Alloimmunization to erythrocytic antigens
    C. Urticaria
    D. Graft-versus-host disease

15. Delayed hemolytic transfusion reactions may represent:
    A. An anamnestic antibody response to leukocyte antigens
    B. An anamnestic antibody response to erythrocyte antigens
    C. Primary alloimmunization to erythrocyte antigens
    D. Both B and C

16. Characteristics of a delayed hemolytic transfusion reaction can include:
    A. Anemia, fever, and transfusion history
    B. Jaundice
    C. Positive direct antiglobulin test (DAT)
    D. All of the above

17. Antibody production in primary immunization to erythrocyte antigens begins _____ following transfusion.
    A. Within 2 days
    B. Within 3 days
    C. About 5 days
    D. About 7–10 days

18. The usual consequence(s) of a delayed hemolytic transfusion reaction is/are:
    A. Shortened erythrocyte survival in vivo
    B. Intravascular destruction of erythrocytes
    C. Extravascular destruction of erythrocytes
    D. Both A and C

19. To prevent delayed transfusion reactions, blood specimens used for compatibility testing should be *no more* than _____ old, if a patient has been recently transfused.
    A. 1 day
    B. 2 days

**C.** 3 days

**D.** 5 days

20. The *most frequent* cause of febrile transfusion reaction is the presence of _____ in the recipient.

**A.** Erythrocyte antigens

**B.** Erythrocyte antibodies

**C.** Leukocyte antigens

**D.** Leukocyte antibodies

21. The type of cell *most frequently* responsible for febrile transfusion reactions is the:

**A.** Erythrocyte

**B.** Lymphocyte

**C.** Granulocyte

**D.** Platelet

22. A febrile transfusion reaction is defined as a rise in body temperature of _____ occurring in association with the transfusion of blood or components and *without* any other explanation.

**A.** 1° C or more

**B.** 1° F or more

**C.** 5° C or more

**D.** 5° F or more

23. With or without documentation of the existence of specific antibodies, the AABB recommends leukocyte-poor preparations only after a patient has had at least _____ febrile nonhemolytic transfusion reactions.

**A.** One

**B.** Two

**C.** Three

**D.** Four

24. Transfusion reactions to platelet concentrates can be:

**A.** Febrile reactions

**B.** Hemolytic reactions

**C.** Immediate

**D.** All of the above

25. Immediate reactions to plasma constituents may be _____ in nature:

**A.** Allergic

**B.** Anaphylactoid

**C.** Anaphylactic

**D.** All of the above

26. The *most common* cause of transfusion-related sepsis is:

**A.** Whole blood

**B.** Platelet concentrates

**C.** Packed red cells

**D.** Leukocyte concentrates

27. Graft-versus-host disease can be a consequence of transfusion if _____ are transfused into a recipient who is not capable of rejecting them.

**A.** Granulocytes

**B.** Platelets

**C.** Lymphocytes

**D.** Erythrocytes

28. The patients susceptible to graft-versus-host disease are:

**A.** Immunodeficient

**B.** Immunosuppressed

**C.** Adolescents

**D.** Both A and B

29. Symptoms of graft-versus-host disease begin within _____ after transfusion.

**A.** 1–2 days

**B.** 2–3 days

**C.** 3–30 days

**D.** 2–3 months

30. Graft-versus-host disease can be prevented by:

**A.** Fresh whole blood

**B.** Blood stored for more than 10 days

**C.** Irradiated blood products

**D.** Fresh-frozen plasma

31. Noncardiac pulmonary edema is characteristically a complication of transfused:

**A.** Erythrocytes

**B.** Platelets

**C.** Lymphocytes

**D.** Granulocytes

32. Post-transfusion purpura typically occurs in patients who are:

**A.** Pl$^{A1}$ positive without Pl$^{A1}$ antibodies in their plasma

**B.** Pl$^{A1}$ negative without Pl$^{A1}$ antibodies in their plasma

**C.** Pl$^{A1}$ positive with Pl$^{A1}$ antibodies in their plasma

**D.** Pl$^{A1}$ negative with Pl$^{A1}$ antibodies in their plasma

33. In the investigation of a transfusion reaction, the first step should be:

**A.** Obtain a post-transfusion specimen

**B.** Repeat the initial crossmatch

**C.** Check the identification of the patient and transfused unit

**D.** Visually examine a fresh blood specimen from the patient

34–38. Arrange the following steps in a post-transfusion workup in the appropriate sequence.

**A.** Check the identification of the patient and transfused unit

**B.** Repeat the pretransfusion crossmatch

**C.** Perform a DAT

**D.** Perform an ABO and Rh grouping

**E.** Obtain a post-transfusion specimen from the patient and visually examine it for hemolysis

34. _____

35. _____

36. _____

37. _____

38. _____

39. Supplementary tests for a transfusion reaction workup can include:
    A. Genotyping of patient and donor erythrocytes
    B. Serum bilirubin assay on post-transfusion specimen
    C. Serial post-transfusion DATs
    D. All of the above

40–43. Match the following conditions with the appropriate action or explanation. (Use an answer only once).

40. An ABO discrepancy is detected.
41. Crossmatch is incompatible only with post-transfusion specimen
42. Antibody detected in post-transfusion specimen only
43. Antibody detected in pretransfusion specimen only
    A. Crosscheck past records and the labeling of blood products
    B. Error in patient or donor during pretransfusion testing
    C. A possible anamnestic response
    D. Prior alloimmunization

## Bibliography

Bailey, J.R.: Intravenous IgG to prevent graft-versus-host disease after bone marrow transplant. New Eng. J. Med., *324*(9):632, 1991.

Barton, J.C.: Nonhemolytic, noninfectious transfusion reactions. Seminars in Hematology, *18*:95–121, 1981.

Bashour, T.T., et al.: Hypocalcemic acute myocardial failure secondary to rapid transfusion of citrated blood. Amer. Heart J., *108*(4):1040–1042, 1984.

Berte, L.M., and DeChristopher, P.J.: A phased approach to transfusion reaction investigation. Med. Lab. Obs., November 1992, 49–52.

Bochner, B.S., and Lichtenstein, L.M.: Anaphylaxis. New Eng. J. Med., *324*(25):1785–1790, 1991.

Braine, H.G., et al.: Bacterial sepsis secondary to platelet transfusion: An adverse effect of extended storage at room temperature. Transfusion, *26*(4):391, 1986.

Dunstan, R.A., and Rosse, W.F.: Post-transfusion purpura. Transfusion, *25*(3):219–222, 1985.

Ferrara, J.L.M., and Deeg, H.J.: Graft-versus-host disease. New Eng. J. Med., *324*(10):667–674, 1991.

Ferraro, M.L.: Irradiation removes threat of transfusion-associated GVHD. Advance for Medical Laboratory Professionals, March 15, 1993, pp. 9, 34.

Gerhan, S.L.: Investigation of an apparent delayed transfusion reaction. Lab. Med., *17*(10):607–609, 1986.

Gueguen, M., et al.: A new method for monitoring the sterility of blood donation. Transfusion, *26*(3):293–295, 1986.

Heal, J.M., et al.: Bacterial proliferation in platelet concentrates. Transfusion, *26*(4):388, 1986.

Hoogan, V.A., et al.: A simple method for preparing neocyte-enriched leukocyte-poor blood for transfusion-dependent patients. Transfusion, *26*(3):253–257, 1986.

Houlihan, P.M., Geier, N.A., and Lofsness, K.G.: Post-transfusion detection of donor red cell abnormalities. Lab. Med., *20*(4):254–257, 1989.

Kaitin, K.I.: Graft-versus-host disease. New Eng. J. Med., *325*(5):357–358, 1991.

Moore, G.L., and Ledford, M.E.: Effects of 4000 rad irradiation on the in vitro storage properties of packed red cells. Transfusion, *25*(6):583–585, 1985.

Leitman, S.F., and Holland, P.V.: Irradiation of blood products. Transfusion, *25*(4):293–300, 1985.

Lowenthal, R.M., Challis, D.R., Griffiths, A.E., Chappell, R.A., and Goulder, P.J.R.: Transfusion-associated graft-versus-host disease: Report of an occurrence following the administration of irradiated blood. Transfusion, *33*(6):524–529, 1993.

Myhre, B.A., and Brubaker, D.: Preparation of consultation reports by computer for transfusion reactions. Lab. Med., *21*(4):232–234, 1990.

Ortiz, A., Caramelo, C., and Plaza, J.J.: Transfusion-associated graft-versus-host disease. New Eng. J. Med., *324*(2):128, 1991.

Pierce, R.N., et al.: Hemolysis following platelet transfusions from ABO-incompatible donors. Tranfusion, *25*(1):60–62, 1985.

Rosen, N.R., Weidner, J.G., Bolt, H.D., and Rosen, D.S.: Prevention of transfusion-associated graft-versus-host disease: Selection of an adequate dose of gamma radiation. Transfusion, *33*(2):125–127, 1993.

Rosenfield, R.E.: Two types of delayed hemolytic transfusion reactions. Transfusion, *25*(2):182, 1985.

Ross, R.E.: Transfusion associated graft-vs.-host disease: A wolf in sheep's clothing. Advance for Medical Laboratory Professionals. January 20, 1992, pp. 6–7.

Schwaegerle, S., Sharp, D.E., and Hoeltge, G.A.: Effect of transfusion reaction consultations on subsequent transfusion practices. Lab Med., *21*(7):444–447, 1990.

Strauss, R.G.: Sterility and quality of blood dispensed in syringes for infants. Transfusion, *26*(2):163–166, 1986.

Szymanski, I.O.: Sterility of single-donor apheresis platelets. Transfusion, *25*(3):290, 1985.

Theobald, M., et al.: Host-specific interleukin-2-secreting donor T-cell precursors as predictors of acute graft-versus-host disease in bone marrow transplantation between HLA-identical siblings. New Eng. J. Med., *327*(23):1613–1617, 1992.

Vogelsang, G.B., et al.: Thalidomide for the treatment of chronic graft-versus-host disease. New Eng. J. Med., *326*(16):1055–1058, 1992.

Walker, R.H.: AABB Technical Manual, 11th edition, Bethesda, MD, 1993, pp. 471–487.

Wingard, J.R., Vogelsang, G., and Piantadosi, S.: Intravenous IgG to prevent graft-versus-host disease after bone marrow transplant. New Eng. J. Med., *324*(9):632, 1991.

# Transfusion-Acquired Infectious Diseases

At the conclusion of this chapter, the reader should be able to:

- List at least three factors that have contributed to a reduction in accidental transmission of infectious agents in blood or blood products.
- Name the diseases that can be transmitted through blood or blood components.
- List the patient-related factors that influence the actual development of a blood-borne disease if a potentially infectious virus is present in transfused blood or a blood component.
- Cite the incidence of transfusion-acquired hepatitis B and hepatitis C.
- Describe the characteristics of each of the forms of hepatitis, including features such as the average incubation time and symptoms.
- Discuss the characteristics, including etiology and symptoms, of cytomegalovirus.
- Explain the characteristics of Epstein-Barr virus infection.

- Name the human T-cell leukemia-lymphoma viruses that are transmitted through blood transfusion.
- Analyze the difference between the immunodeficiency viruses (HIV) and other blood-borne viruses.
- Briefly describe the signs and symptoms of HIV infection.
- Describe the methods that are effective in reducing the incidence of blood-borne HIV-1 infection.
- State the blood product that can be responsible for the transmission of parvovirus.
- Name the parasitic diseases that can be transmitted via blood or blood components.
- Rank the blood-borne parasitic diseases in order of frequency in the United States.
- Name the bacterial disorders that can be acquired through blood transfusion.

## Chapter Outline

## BACKGROUND

Many potentially infectious agents can be acquired through blood transfusion. Careful interviewing of blood donors, serologic screening of donated blood, the use of plastic collection bags, and refrigerated storage methods have all helped to reduce accidental transmission of infectious agents. However, the possibility of initially acquiring or reactivating an infectious agent is a constant danger. Factors that can influence the acquisition of a disease from the blood include:

1. Overall incidence of an agent or organism in the donor population
2. Pathogenicity of the agent
3. Actual presence of a large enough dose of the agent or organism in the transfusion to produce an infection
4. Immune status of the recipient
5. Physical condition of the recipient
6. Age of stored blood
7. Type of blood component received
8. Availability of a sensitive screening assay for the presence of the agent/organism
9. Donor screening (appropriate interview) or serologic screening such as HIV-1

Viral agents, parasitic organisms, and bacteria can be transmitted through blood or blood components (Table 13-1). Viral diseases, such as hepatitis C and acquired immunodeficiency syndrome (AIDS), are presently a serious health hazard and may be acquired through transfusion. Although parasitic and bacterial diseases are less common on the North American continent than elsewhere, their significance should not be underrated. Two major parasitic infections, malaria and American trypanosomiasis, are the predominating transfusion-acquired parasitic diseases among patients in the Americas. However, cases of transfusion-acquired babesiosis have recently been documented in southern New England, and toxoplasmosis is increasingly being recognized as a hazard. In areas of the world where parasitic diseases are endemic, various parasites may

be transmitted through blood transfusion. Transfusion-acquired bacterial infections, primarily syphilis, have become less of a risk than in the past but continue to be a problem in underdeveloped countries.

## TRANSFUSION-ASSOCIATED VIRUSES

### General Characteristics

Since the discovery of the Australian antigen [hepatitis B surface antigen, (HBsAg)] in 1966 and the establishment of its relationship to post-transfusion hepatitis, numerous transfusion-associated viruses have been identified. The transmission and potential disorders caused by some of these viruses have become apparent only recently.

Transmission of viruses through blood transfusion is a challenging problem to control. Apparently healthy donors may be suffering from subclinical infections, may be in a carrier state as seen in hepatitis B, or may harbor a latent infection such as cytomegalovirus. If viral antigens or antibodies are not detected by screening methods in donor blood and the virus is stable in stored blood or blood products, transmission of the virus is likely. Untreated blood products, such as factor VIII concentrate prepared from pools of plasma derived from many donors, have an extremely high incidence of transmitting infectious viruses. Depending on the virus and the particular type of blood product, transmission through transfusion can be associated with the cellular components of blood, usually leukocytes, or the plasma alone.

Not all transfusion-acquired viruses manifest themselves as clinical disorders. For a virus present in blood to infect a patient, the recipient must be susceptible to that virus. The immune status of the patient is influenced by age, nutritional status, and previous viral exposure. Whether or not the patient has been previously exposed or is harboring the virus in a dormant condition are also determining factors in the actual development of disease.

### General Prevention of Virus Transmission

Prevention of viral transmission and diseases associated with blood transfusion requires knowledge of the infectious agent in terms of isolation of the virus, identification of associated antigens and/or antibodies, and the mechanism of transmission. In addition to this knowledge, methods for reducing transmission must be recognized and applied. Present methods to reduce the transmission of transfusion-associated viruses include:

1. Self-exclusion of high-risk blood donors through interviewing
2. Serologic screening of donor blood
3. Chemical or physical treatment of blood and blood components

Careful selection of donors and screening of blood for either viral antigens such as hepatitis B surface antigen, or

**Table 13-1. Examples of Agents and Diseases Acquired Through Transfusion**

| Category | Agent | Disease |
| --- | --- | --- |
| Viruses | Hepatitis A | Hepatitis A |
| | Hepatitis B and delta agent | Hepatitis B |
| | Hepatitis C | Hepatitis C |
| | Parvovirus | |
| | Cytomegalovirus | |
| | Epstein-Barr virus | Infectious mononucleosis |
| | HTLV (Human T-cell leukemia virus) | |
| | Type I | T-cell leukemia |
| | Human immunodeficiency viruses HIV-1, HIV-2 | AIDS |
| Parasites | Malaria species | Malaria |
| | Trypanosoma cruzi | American trypanosomiasis |
| | Babesia microti | Babesiosis |
| | Toxoplasma gondii | Toxoplasmosis |
| Bacteria | Treponema pallidum | Syphilis |

the presence of antibodies, such as cytomegalovirus anti-bodies, represent the major means of providing transfusion products that are free of viruses. In the case of newly recognized transfusion-acquired viral diseases, such as AIDS, the importance of excluding high-risk populations and the efforts to develop a serologic antibody screening test as quickly as possible illustrate how important donor selection and screening are to maintaining a safe blood supply.

By understanding the mode of transmission of an infectious virus, physical or chemical treatments of blood or components may be effective in eliminating or reducing the level of the virus present. Methods of preparation, such as freezing and deglycerolizing red cells, are known to reduce viral contamination. Heat inactivation may be appropriate for plasma components if the virus can be destroyed without compromising the biologic activity of the component.

Several developing methods to reduce the transmission of viral disease include:

1. Vaccination, if suitable vaccines are available. This method has proven effective in the prevention of transmission of hepatitis B in high-risk populations, such as health care professionals. Vaccination, however, is not always possible because of the lack of identification of the virus or because efficacy of vaccination has not been proven.
2. The addition of an antibody, possibly even a monoclonal antibody, to blood in an attempt to reduce the infectivity of blood or blood components.
3. Gene cloning and commercialization of recombinant DNA blood products. Three human gene products of importance to transfusion therapy have been cloned and expressed in microorganisms: albumin (1981), hepatitis B vaccine (1981), and factor VIII (1984). Hepatitis B vaccine is now available, and the commercialization of the other products is expected in the near future.

A major issue in prevention of viral disease is cost. The cost of screening blood and of alternative preparations or safe substitutes must be determined for each viral agent. Significant factors in determining when screening should be used or what alternatives are appropriate are definition of the population "at risk" and assessment of the impact of the resulting clinical disease.

## General Characteristics of Hepatitis

### Etiology

Although the incidence of transfusion-associated hepatitis has declined significantly in the last two decades, transfusion-associated hepatitis can be a major complication of blood transfusion. Posttransfusion hepatitis may be caused by the primary hepatitis viruses: hepatitis A virus (rare),

hepatitis B virus (HBV) with or without the delta agent, and hepatitis C virus (HCV), as well as the secondary hepatitis viruses—e.g., cytomegalovirus (CMV).

### Incidence

In patients who received blood from volunteer donors who have been screened for hepatitis B surface antigen (HBsAg) by third-generation tests, hepatitis B infections probably account for very few cases of transfusion-acquired cases of hepatitis. The majority of cases are attributable to HCV. However, HCV as a cause of hepatitis also has decreased dramatically since the discovery of the virus and development of specific screening tests. A small portion of cases may be caused by CMV.

### Signs and Symptoms

As a clinical disease, hepatitis can occur in acute or chronic forms. The signs and symptoms of hepatitis are extremely variable. It can be mild, transient, and completely asymptomatic, or it can be severe, prolonged, and ultimately fatal. The course of viral hepatitis can take one of four forms (Table 13-2).

### Hepatitis A Virus

### Etiology

The hepatitis A (HA) virus is a small RNA virus that belongs to the picornavirus class. The structure is a simple nonenveloped virus with a nucleocapsid designated the hepatitis A antigen (HA Ag). Inside the capsid is a single molecule of single-stranded RNA (Figure 13-1). It is be-

**Table 13-2. Forms of Hepatitis**

| Form | Characteristics |
| --- | --- |
| Acute hepatitis | Typical form having associated jaundice. It has four phases: *incubation, preicteric, icteric,* and *convalescence.* Incubation period, from time of exposure to first day of symptoms, ranges from a few days to many months–average time is 75 days (range, 40–180 days) in hepatitis B. |
| Fulminant acute hepatitis | Rare form associated with hepatic failure. |
| Subclinical hepatitis without jaundice | This form probably accounts for persons with demonstrable antibodies in their serum but no reported history of hepatitis. |
| Chronic hepatitis | This form is accompanied by hepatic inflammation and necrosis that lasts for at least 6 months. Occurs in about 10% of hepatitis B patients, and 10–60% of patients with hepatitis C. |

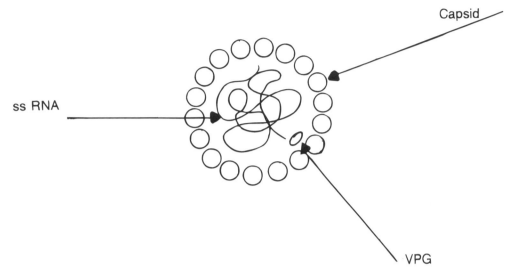

**Figure 13-1.** Hepatitis A virus. The protein capsid is composed of four viral polypeptides. Inside the capsid is a single-strand molecule of RNA, which has a genomic viral protein (VPG) on the 5′ end.

lieved that the RNA has a positive polarity and that proteins are translated directly from the RNA.

## Epidemiology

HA, formerly called *infectious hepatitis* or *short-incubation hepatitis,* is the most common form of hepatitis. Seroepidemiologic studies indicate that the prevalence of antibody in a given population increases with age, reaching approximately 40% of the United States population by age 50. Although hepatitis A occurs worldwide, its incidence in the United States is declining, and areas that have predictable recurrent epidemics are few. In other parts of the world, more than 90% of adults have hepatitis A antibody.

Susceptibility to infection is independent of sex and race. Crowded, unsanitary conditions are a definite risk factor. The hepatitis A virus is transmitted by a fecal-oral route during the early phase of acute illness. Large outbreaks are usually traceable to a common source such as an infected food handler or contaminated water supply. It is noted for occurring in isolated outbreaks or as an epidemic, but it may also occur sporadically.

The incidence of HA is not increased among health care workers or in dialysis patients. HA is very rarely a transfusion-acquired hepatitis, and only rarely causes fulminant acute hepatitis.

## Signs and Symptoms

Nonimmune adult patients infected with HA virus will develop clinical symptoms within 2 to 6 weeks after exposure. Initially elevated serum enzymes are exhibited, with jaundice developing several days later. Many patients will be anicteric. Viremia and fecal shedding of virus disappear at the onset of jaundice. Although protracted illness lasting from 3 to 6 months can occur, protracted cholestasis has been described. A chronic carrier state and chronic hepatitis do not occur.

## Immunologic Manifestation

Shortly after the onset of fecal shedding, an IgM antibody is detectable in serum followed within a few days by the appearance of an IgG antibody. IgM anti-HA is almost always detectable in patients when acute HA reaches undetectable levels within, and disappears within 3 to 6 months after exposure. IgG anti-HA peaks after the acute illness and remains detectable indefinitely, perhaps lifelong.

The finding of IgM anti-HA in a patient with acute viral hepatitis is highly diagnostic of acute HA. Demonstration of IgG anti-HA indicates previous infection. The presence of IgG anti-HA protects against subsequent infection with HA virus, but it is not protective against HBV or other viruses.

## Diagnostic Evaluation

Testing methods for HA include:

1. Total antibody by enzyme immunoassay (EIA)
2. IgM antibody by radioimmunoassay (RIA)
3. HA antigen by radioimmunoassay (RIA)

The short period of viremia makes detection difficult. Specific IgM antibody (measured for total antibodies to HAV) persist for an indefinite time, although the antibody level decreases to undetectable levels in those who are infected when they are very young. Specific IgG antibody apparently protects an individual from symptomatic infection, but an increase in specific IgM may increase with reinfection.

## Prevention

The first effective control measures for the prevention of enterically transmitted viral hepatitis resulted from research conducted during World War II. In 1945, it was demonstrated that infectious virus could be transmitted by contaminated drinking water, that treatment of the water by filtration and chlorination made it safe to drink, and that gamma globulin derived from convalescent-phase serum from patients with hepatitis could protect adults from clinical hepatitis. Except for refinements in the preparation of food and water and the establishment of standards for the preparation and use of immune globulin, no basic changes have been made in the prevention of hepatitis A in almost 50 years.

After close personal contact with a person having hepatitis A, or if traveling to an endemic area, individuals should receive immune globulin intramuscularly. If people remain in an endemic area for more than 3 months, they should receive immune globulin injections every 5 months.

Recent research on the prevention of hepatitis A suggests that a single dose of inactivated, purified hepatitis A virus vaccine derived from cell culture can protect children 2 to 16 years old from acute hepatitis A. Antibodies against hepatitis A (seroconversion) occurs in 99% of vaccine recipients. Universal childhood vaccination may prove to be the most cost-effective method of protecting large populations both nationally and globally.

When vaccines against the hepatitis A virus are licensed, immunization against hepatitis A will benefit many groups. These groups include employees of child-care centers and health care workers. Other groups include international travelers, military personnel, food handlers, prisoners, and consumers of raw shellfish.

## Hepatitis B

Hepatitis B virus (HBV) is the classic example of a virus acquired through blood transfusion. In part, this observation led to the name of "serum hepatitis," by which HBV was previously known. Hepatitis B serves as a model when considering transfusion-transmitted viral infections.

## Etiology

The Australia antigen, now called hepatitis B surface antigen (HBsAg), was discovered in 1966. This discovery and its subsequent association with hepatitis B virus (HBV) permitted characterization of the biochemical and epidemiologic characterization of HBC infection.

HBV is a complex DNA virus that belongs to a new class called the hepadna viruses. The intact virus is a double-shelled particle referred to as the *Dane particle* (Figure 13-2). It has an outer surface structure, hepatitis B surface antigen (HBsAg), and an inner core component, the hepatitis B core antigen (HBcAg). Inside of this core is the

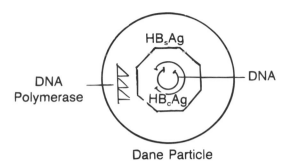

**Figure 13-2.** Hepatitis B virus. The intact hepatitis B virus (HBV) consists of a double-shelled particle referred to as the Dane particle. It has an outer surface component of hepatitis B surface antigen (HBsAg) and an inner core component of hepatitis B core antigen (HBcAg). Inside the core is the genome, a single molecule of partially double-stranded DNA, which contains the genetic information. One of the DNA strands is incomplete, leaving a single-strand or gap region which comprises 10 to 50% of the total length of the molecule.

viral genome, a single molecule of partly double-stranded deoxyribonucleic acid (DNA).

The unique structure of the DNA of HBV is one of the distinguishing characteristics of the hepadna class of viruses. The DNA is circular and double-stranded, but one of the strands is incomplete, leaving a single-stranded or gap region that comprises 10–50% of the total length of the molecule. The other DNA strand is nicked (the 3 and 5 ends are not joined). The entire DNA molecule is small, and all of the genetic information for producing both the surface and core antigens is on the complete strand. In addition to the DNA configuration, the core of virus also contains an enzyme that is a DNA-dependent DNA polymerase. This polymerase acts to complete the single-stranded region of the DNA.

## Epidemiology

Soon after discovery of HBV, the relationship between the presence of the antigen in donor blood and posttransfusion hepatitis B was documented. In the past, HBV infection was one of the most frequent clinical infections transmitted by blood transfusion.

Today, the incidence of HBV infection is increasingly rare posttransfusion (estimated 0.3–0.9%). The incidence of transfusion-acquired HBV has been severely reduced since high-risk donor groups—such as paid donors, prison inmates, and military recruits—have been eliminated as a major source of donated blood and specific serologic screening procedures have been instituted. This shift to an all-voluntary donor supply probably accounts for a 50–60% reduction of transfusion-related hepatitis. The overall incidence of HBV, however, is high among patients who have received multiple transfusions or blood components prepared from multiple donor plasma pools, hemodialysis patients, drug addicts, and medical personnel.

Persons at risk of exposure to HBV, including those mentioned above, comprise members of the following groups: heterosexual men and women and homosexual men with multiple partners, household contacts and sexual partners of HBV carriers, infants born to HBV-infected mothers, patients and staff in custodial institutions for the developmentally disabled, recipients of certain plasma-derived products (including patients with congenital coagulation defects, health and public-safety workers who have contact with blood, and persons born in areas of high HBV endemicity and their children).

HBV does not seem capable of penetrating through the skin or mucous membranes; some break in these barriers is required for disease transmission. Transmission of HBV occurs via percutaneous or permucosal routes, and infective blood or body fluids can be introduced at birth, through sexual contact, or by contaminated needles. Infection can also occur in settings of continuous close personal contact.

HBV is largely a disease spread by the parenteral route through blood transfusion, needlestick accidents, and contaminated needles, although the virus can be transmitted in the absence of obvious parenteral exposure. About half of the patients with acute type B hepatitis have a history of parenteral exposure. Inapparent parenteral exposure involves close intimate or sexual contact with an infectious individual.

HBV has been found in saliva, semen and other biological fluids of HBV carriers. Urine and stool are not believed to be infectious.

## Signs and Symptoms

A number of factors (e.g., the dose of the agent), as well as an individual's immunologic host-response ability, influence the clinical course of the infection.

*Asymptomatic Infection.* The most frequent clinical response to HBV is an asymptomatic or subclinical infection. In patients developing clinical symptoms of transfusion-associated hepatitis B, jaundice and abnormal serum enzymes, transaminase (ALT/SGPT), levels can be manifested from a few weeks to up to 6 months after a single transfusion episode. There is, however, rarely any doubt about the diagnosis in patients with a classic serologic response associated with HBV, even in the absence of significant symptoms. Diagnosis is more difficult to make in asymptomatic patients with negative HBV serology, who a few weeks after a transfusion have a mild elevation of serum enzyme, transaminase, levels that persist for a week or two.

*Chronic Infection.* HBV leads to chronic infection and these patients have been shown to have the viral DNA actually incorporated into their liver cells' DNA. This integration may be an important factor in the eventual development of liver cell cancer, hepatocellular carcinoma, a well-known long-term outcome of chronic HBV infection.

*Carrier State.* Carriers (estimated at 750,000 to 1,000,000 in the United States) can be divided into two categories based upon differing infectivity, depending upon the presence in their serum of another antigen, hepatitis B e antigen (HBeAg) or its antibody, (anti-HBe). The types of carrier states include:

1. The more commonly identified carriers have anti-HBe in their serum and are at a later stage of infection. Anti-HBe carriers are less infectious but may transmit infection through blood transfusion. HBsAg positive carriers will become anti-HBe positive carriers at a rate of about 5 to 10% per year. All HBsAg positive individuals must be excluded from giving blood for transfusion.
2. About one in four carriers have HBeAg in their serum. It is likely that they have recently become carriers and their blood is highly infectious.

## Laboratory Testing—Serologic Markers

Several serologic markers for HBV infection have been defined. These markers are:

1. Hepatitis B surface antigen (HBsAg)
2. Hepatitis B e antigen (HBeAg)
3. Antibody to the hepatitis B core antigen (anti-HBc)
4. Antibody to hepatitis B e antigen (anti-HBe)
5. Antibody to hepatitis B surface antigen (anti-HBs)

*Hepatitis B Surface Antigen (HBsAg).* The initial laboratory screening procedure for hepatitis was for the detection of HBsAg. This procedure screens for the presence of the major coat-protein of the virus (HBsAg) in serum and is considered to be the most reliable method of choice for preventing the transmission of HBV via blood. The presence of HBsAg indicates active HBV infection, either acute or chronic.

The initial detectable marker found in serum during the incubation period of HBV infection is HBsAg. The titer of HBsAg rises and generally peaks at, or shortly after, the onset of elevated serum enzymes (e.g., ALT/SGPT). Clinical improvement of the patient's condition and a decrease in serum enzyme concentrations are paralleled by a fall in the titer of HBsAg, which subsequently disappears. There is, however, variability in the duration of HBsAg positivity and in the relationship between clinical recovery and the disappearance of HBsAG (Figure 13-3).

Among persons infected with HBV with detectable HBsAg in their serum, not all of the HBsAg represents complete Dane particles. HBsAg positive serum also contains two other virus-like structures. These virus-like structures are incomplete spherical and tubular forms, consisting entirely of HBsAg and devoid of any HBcAg, DNA, or DNA polymerase. The incomplete HBsAg particles can be present in serum in extremely high concentrations and form the bulk of the circulating HBsAg.

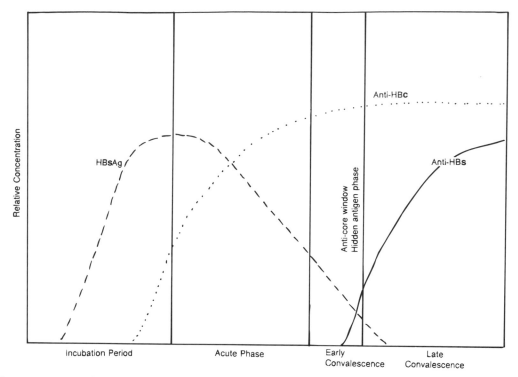

**Figure 13-3.** Representative profile of hepatitis B serum markers. HbSAg = hepatitis B surface antigen, anti-HBc = hepatitis B core antibody; anti-HBs = anti-core window or hidden antigen phase.

***Hepatitis B e Antigen (HBeAg).*** A hepatitis B–related antigen, the hepatitis B e antigen (HBeAg), is found in the serum of some patients who are HBsAg positive. It is rarely found in the absence of HBsAg. HBeAg appears to be associated with the HBV core; however, the relationship between HBeAg and the structure of HBV is unclear. HBeAg appears to be a reliable marker for the presence of high levels of virus and a high degree of infectivity.

***Hepatitis B Core Antibody (anti-HBc).*** During the course of most HBV infections, HBsAg forms immune complexes, with the antibodies produced as part of the recovery process. Because the HBsAg contained in these complexes is usually undetectable, HBsAg disappears from the serum of up to 50% of symptomatic patients. During this phase, an indicator of a recent hepatitis B infection is anti-HBc, the antibody to the core antigen. The period of time between the disappearance of detectable HBsAg and the appearance of detectable antibody to HBsAg (anti-HBs) is called the *anti-core window,* or hidden antigen phase, of hepatitis B virus infection. This window phase may last for a few weeks, several months, or a year, during which anti-HBc may be the only serologic marker. Anti-HBc occurs in 3–5% of persons. Of 100 anti-HBc positive persons, 97 will have anti-HBs, 2 will have HBsAg and 1 may have only anti-HBc.

### Antibodies to HBeAg and HBsAg

Antibodies to HBeAg (anti-HBe) and HBsAg (anti-HBs) develop during convalescence and recovery from HBV in-

fection. The development of anti-HBe in a case of acute hepatitis is the first serologic evidence of the convalescent phase. Antibody to HBsAg (anti-HBs), unlike anti-HBc and anti-HBe, does not arise during the acute disease; it is manifested during convalescence. Anti-HBs is a serologic marker (Table 13-3) of recovery and immunity. Anti-HBs is probably the major protective antibody in this disease. Thus, hepatitis B immune globulin is so named because it contains high levels of anti-HBs.

### Prevention

The most important factors in the prevention of transfusion-acquired hepatitis B are donor interviewing (refer to Chapter 2), screening of donor blood, use of hepatitis-free products, and appropriate use of blood and blood components (refer to Chapter 10). Elimination of high-risk donors has accounted for a substantial reduction in the incidence of hepatitis. Routine testing of donated blood for HBsAg has further reduced the incidence. In addition, testing for anti-HBc detects almost 100% of HBsAg positive persons, the rare asymptomatic donor who is in the core window phase, and the large number of donors who have had subclinical hepatitis B infections and are now immune.

The use of a vaccine against hepatitis, licensed since 1982, is warranted for high-risk persons, among whom are technologists and technicians who handle patient blood specimens. Vaccination offers a new approach to preventing transfusion-acquired hepatitis in patients who are

**Table 13-3. Serologic Markers for Hepatitis B virus (HBV) Infection**

|  | Early (Asymptomatic) | Acute or Chronic | Low-Level Carrier | Immediate Recovery | Long after Infection | Immunized with HBsAg |
|---|---|---|---|---|---|---|
| HBsAg | + | + | − | − | − | − |
| anti-HBs | − | −/+ | − | − | −/+ | + |
| anti-HBc | − | + | + | + | −/+ | − |
| anti-HBc (IgM) | − | + | − | + | − | − |

Adapted from Hoofnagle, Jay H. "Type A and Type B Hepatitis," *Laboratory Medicine*, Vol. 14, No. 11, November, 1983, p. 713.

likely to need ongoing transfusion therapy. Additionally, avoidance of untreated products prepared from multiple donor pools reduces the incidence of HBV infection. Hepatitis B vaccine is also a vaccine against cancer (hepatitic cancer). It is probably the first such vaccine and is very important to Third World countries.

In cases of accidental needlestick exposure or exposure of mucous membranes or open cuts to HBsAg positive blood, hepatitis B immune globulin (HBIG) should be administered within 24 hours of exposure and again 25–30 days later. Infants born to mothers with acute hepatitis B in the third trimester, or with HBsAg at the time of delivery, should be given HBIG as soon as possible and no later than 24 hours after birth, and given the hepatitis B vaccinations series. Persons who are either HBsAg positive or who have anti-HBc need not be given HBIG.

## Delta Hepatitis

### Etiology

The *delta agent* was first described in 1977 as a pathogen that "superinfects" some patients who are already infected with HBV. HBV is required as a "helper" to initiate delta infection. The majority of persons with acute or chronic HBV infection as demonstrated by serum HBsAg can be infected with delta agent, hepatitis D.

The delta agent is a defective, or incomplete, RNA virus that is unable by itself to cause infection. Delta agent consists of viral RNA coated in HBsAg produced by HBV, its "helper" virus. This agent is unique because it can replicate only in HBV-infected hosts. Therefore, the delta virus only infects patients who are HBsAg positive.

### Epidemiology

In Italy and the Middle East, delta infection is common and found in HBsAg carriers. In the United States, northern Europe and Asia, infection is uncommon and occurs only in individuals with multiple parenteral exposures, such as hemophiliacs and intravenous drug addicts.

### Signs and Symptoms

Delta infection can be benign and brief, but fulminate hepatitis and chronic hepatitis are being attributed with increasing frequency to the delta agent. Chronic delta infection is associated with increased hepatic damage and a more severe clinical course than is expected from chronic HBV infection alone. The occurrence of sequential attacks of HBV in the same patient is probably attributable in most cases to delta infection superimposed on a previous acute HBV infection.

Infection with delta agent can occur in several conditions and the symptoms would be typical of either acute or chronic hepatitis. These situations are:

1. Acute delta hepatitis with a concurrent acute type B hepatitis.
2. Acute delta hepatitis in a chronic HBsAg carrier.
3. Chronic delta hepatitis in a chronic HBsAg carrier.

### Immunologic Manifestation

The delta agent probably partially suppresses HBV replication. Delta infection is diagnosed by the appearance of delta antigen in serum or development of IgM or IgG anti-delta antibodies that appear sequentially in a time frame similar to that described for hepatitis A or B antibodies.

### Diagnostic Evaluation

The delta agent appears in the circulating blood as a particle with a core of delta antigen and a surface component of HBsAg. A person with delta hepatitis will have detectable delta antigen in the liver and antibody to the delta agent in the serum. Test methodologies for delta agent include:

1. Total antibody by enzyme immunoassay (EIA).
2. IgM assay by radioimmunoassay (RIA).
3. Antigen detection by double immunodiffusion (DIF).

In addition, delta agent antigen can be demonstrated in liver biopsies by direct immunofluorescence (DIF) and immunoperoxidase (IP) and in serum by cloned DNA (cDNA). The importance of detection of antibodies to delta agent is largely prognostic. Detection of IgG anti-delta in the presence of IgM anti-HBc antibody strongly suggests simultaneous infection (coinfection). Detection of IgM anti-delta in a patient with chronic HBV infection is evidence of HDV superinfection.

Screening for total anti-delta antibodies in serum is important in the identification of a subpopulation of apparently healthy HBsAg carriers whose risk of serious liver damage is fourfold higher than that in anti-delta negative carriers. The combined presence of total anti-delta antibody plus abnormal liver function tests in a symptom-free carrier suggests parenchymal damage and is considered an indication for liver biopsy. Hepatic lesions in anti-delta positive carriers often consist of chronic active hepatitis or advanced cirrhosis. A positive test result for IgM anti-delta increases the likelihood of occult, active HDV infection.

## Hepatitis C

### Etiology

Until recently hepatitis C—previously referred to as non-A, non-B (NANB) hepatitis—was regarded as a diagnosis of exclusion because of the absence of specific serologic markers and unknown viral origin. Recently, the hepatitis C virus (HCV) was identified and immunologic assays developed for its detection. No homology exists between type A or B hepatitis viruses, or the delta agent, and HCV.

### Viral Characteristics

In May 1988, it was announced that the genome of a lipid-encapsulated, single-stranded, positive-sense RNA virus, designated hepatitis C virus (HCV), had been identified and cloned from the liver and plasma of an experimentally infected chimpanzee. This large RNA virus is similar to the Toga and Flavi viruses. HCV contains 10,000 nucleotides of a single-stranded RNA molecule in one common, open reading frame. Expression of a portion of the HCV genome in a recombinant system yields a viral antigen that detects a specific antibody in the serum of many patients with parenterally and community-acquired hepatitis C. Although cases of hepatitis C without seroconversion (demonstrable anti-HCV) may be explained otherwise, they may be caused by another, presently unidentified virus.

### Epidemiology

In the past, hepatitis C was considered to be a disease limited to transfusion recipients. Hepatitis C, however, is now recognized in many other epidemiologic settings. To date, two epidemiologically distinct types of non-A, non-B hepatitis have now been identified worldwide. One type, hepatitis C, is mainly transmitted parenterally and is associated with the form of hepatitis that develops posttransfusion or as sporadic (community-acquired) hepatitis occurring primarily in developed countries. Hepatitis C is prevalent in the United States and western Europe and resembles type B hepatitis (HBV) in terms of transmission characteristics. In contrast, the other form of non-A, non-B hepatitis, hepatitis E, is caused by an entirely different virus, is transmitted by the fecal-oral route, and is primarily associated with epidemic cases of hepatitis in developing countries.

The recently developed ability to detect antibodies to HCV, generally only several months after acute infection, is an important advance that provides a screening procedure for donated blood as well as a potential clinical diagnostic test. A high overall prevalence of HCV antibodies has been noted in various types of patients. Sixty to eighty percent of hemophiliacs receiving clotting factors, 60–70% of patients with chronic active hepatitis or cirrhosis with a history of blood transfusion, and 50–70% of intravenous drug abusers were found to exhibit antibodies in one survey. Other groups with a high incidence of HCV antibodies are homosexual men infected with HIV, some women having sexual contacts with drug abusers, patients with primary hepatocellular carcinoma, and a substantial percentage of patients with primary biliary cirrhosis, alcoholic cirrhosis, or cryptogenic cirrhosis—none of whom had a history of a blood transfusion.

Hepatitis C accounts for a substantial proportion of cases of acute and chronic liver disease in the United States. It is estimated that at least 170,000 new cases of hepatitis C occur in the United States each year. In the United States, parenterally transmitted HCV accounts for 20–40% of cases of acute viral hepatitis. At least half of the patients with acute hepatitis C produce biochemical evidence of chronic liver disease, and some of these cases lead to chronic, active hepatitis or cirrhosis. In addition, the virus may be causally associated with hepatocellular carcinoma.

### Posttransfusion Hepatitis

The most common serious complication of blood transfusion is posttransfusion hepatitis from the hepatitis C virus (HCV). Hepatitis C as a consequence of blood transfusion was first recognized in 1974, after the recognition of the hepatitis B virus (HBV) and the development of a serologic test specifically to identify hepatitis B surface antigen (HBsAg). After the introduction of this serologic test in the screening of blood donors, the rate of posttransfusion hepatitis decreased from 33% to approximately 15%. Cases of posttransfusion hepatitis that were not directly attributable to HBV or other causes remained classified as non-A, non-B hepatitis. Recently, a retrospective study based on the demonstration of antibody to HCV has identified HCV as the etiologic basis for approximately half of the cases of posttransfusion hepatitis, particularly those that developed chronicity.

Prior to laboratory screening, the transfusion of infected blood or blood components, such as Factors VIII or IX, comprised a clearly documented route of transmission of HCV. The annual incidence in the United States of hepatitis C among hemophiliacs receiving coagulation factor replacement therapy was 2–6%. Three to six percent of transfused hemodialysis patients previously developed hepatitis C, and it was also responsible for much of the hepatitis in renal transplant patients.

Although the incidence of posttransfusion hepatitis C declined in the 1980s because of efforts to replace the pool of high risk, paid donors and the surrogate testing of donor blood for antibody to hepatitis B core antigen (HBcAg) and elevations of alanine aminotransferase (ALT) levels, infection with HCV is a serious consequence of blood transfusion. The current risk of posttransfusion hepatitis C is about 3 per 10,000 units transfused. Prospective studies of the risk of posttransfusion hepatitis C in unscreened blood suggest that 1–6% of volunteer blood donors in the United States may be chronic carriers of HCV. These cases, however, account for only 5–10% of all of hepatitis C in the United States each year.

## Parenteral and Occupational Sources of Exposure

Although hepatitis C is traditionally associated with a history of blood transfusion, transmission of HCV is more likely to occur from types of parenteral exposure other than transfusions. The most prevalent type of parenteral exposure has been observed in i.v. drug abusers. Forty-two percent of patients identified with hepatitis C had a history of i.v. drug abuse.

Accidental needlesticks also comprise a clearly documented route of hepatitis transmission, but less than 5% of the patients in one study had a history of medical or dental employment involving frequent blood contact. In addition, hemodialysis staff have been reported to have a rate of 1% for HCV infection.

## Sexual Transmission

The role of sexual transmission of HCV is unclear. The dilemma stems from contradictory research findings. In an unpublished case-control study, the Centers for Disease Control and Prevention (CDC) concluded that sexual activity was significantly associated with acquiring this form of hepatitis. Another study also concluded that sexual transmission is a strong candidate as a route of transmission—or when the source of infection cannot be identified in many patients with hepatitis C. However, other studies of sexual transmission conclude that sexual transmission of HCV appears to occur, but at a lower rate of frequency than with HBV, probably because of lower circulating concentrations of virus.

## Other Sources of Transmission

Mother to infant transmission has been documented. Personal contact is thought to be a route of infection, but it has not been conclusively demonstrated and the actual risk for such transmission is unknown.

Between 25% and 50% of sporadic community-acquired cases of hepatitis cases in the United States are of the HCV type and are unrelated to parenteral exposure.

Some of these cases are believed to result from heterosexual transmission, but in approximately 40 percent of cases the route of infection cannot be identified. Therefore, transmission can occur by inapparent as well as apparent parenteral routes, and this form of hepatitis cannot be distinguished from other types of viral hepatitis solely by epidemiologic characteristics.

In addition, liver disease can occur among the recipients of organs from donors with antibodies to HCV. Nearly all the recipients of organs from anti-HCV positive donors become infected with HCV. The current tests for anti-HCV antibodies may underestimate the incidence of transmission and the prevalence of HCV infection among immunosuppressed organ recipients. However, if the medical condition of the potential recipient is so serious that other options no longer exist, the use of an organ from an anti-HCV seropositive donor should be considered.

## Signs and Symptoms

Although the clinical characteristics of the acute disease of both types of hepatitis C are virtually indistinguishable, the chronic consequences are markedly different. The signs and symptoms of hepatitis C are extremely variable. It can be mild, transient, and completely asymptomatic, or it can be severe, prolonged, and ultimately fatal.

The diagnosis of hepatitis C was previously a diagnosis of exclusion. If viral hepatitis was suspected, the other primary causes—e.g., hepatitis A (HA) and hepatitis B (HBV)—secondary causes—e.g., Epstein-Barr virus (EBV)—and other causes of liver inflammation were excluded before hepatitis C was considered.

Hepatitis C more closely resembles HBV than HA in regard to transmission and clinical features. Hepatitis C, like HBV, can be acute, ranging from mild anicteric illness to fulminant disease. A fulminant course with a rapidly fatal outcome is rare. Most frequently the patient is only mildly symptomatic and nonicteric; less than 25% of patients develop jaundice. Transfusion-associated hepatitis C can be divided into short and long incubation types. Incubation periods for the short-duration type range from 1 or 2 to 5 weeks; the longer duration type ranges from 7 to 12 weeks to 6 months or longer.

Hepatitis C is characterized by alanine aminotransferase (ALT) levels in the 200–800 range and marked fluctuations with rapid rises and falls and intervening periods of normalcy. Mean ALT and bilirubin levels of patients with hepatitis C, however, are significantly lower than those of patients with HBV, and the extensive overlap of the ranges of elevation precludes identification of the type of viral hepatitis by the use of these assays.

The diagnosis of hepatitis C has a guarded prognosis. Although hepatitis C was initially thought to be a relatively benign disease, there is increasing evidence of progression to cirrhosis (in about 20% of patients), liver failure, and even hepatoma. Up to 60% of patients with posttransfusion hepatitis C develop chronic liver disease based on biopsy analysis, and up to 20% of these patients develop cirrhosis.

Posttransfusion hepatitis C affects men and women equally, but it has been demonstrated that 75% of patients developing chronic hepatitis were men. Parenterally acquired (nontransfusion) patients with hepatitis C, including those who have no identifiable source, have the same clinical characteristics and develop chronic liver disease with the same frequency. In addition, an extremely high prevalence of anti-HCV in serum and cryoprecipitate exists along with the frequently associated serum HCV RNA. This suggests a close relationship between essential mixed cryoglobulinemia (type II) and chronic HCV infection. HCV may in fact play a role in the pathogenesis of mixed cryoglobulinemia.

It is important to note that a risk exists for possible clinical misinterpretation because of the absence of surrogate markers or anti-HCV in patients clinically diagnosed as suffering from either acute or chronic hepatitis C.

## Laboratory Testing

Following the development of serologic tests for hepatitis A and hepatitis B, it rapidly became apparent that many cases of posttransfusion hepatitis, as well as many sporadic cases of hepatitis, were not caused by type A or type B viruses or the delta agent (Table 13-4), or by secondary viruses such as EBV or CMV. Because these viruses had been previously isolated and identified, and evidence of viral infection could be documented in the laboratory, hepatitis C was a diagnosis of exclusion. The diagnosis of hepatitis C has been based on the absence of appropriate changes in serologic tests for acute HAV, HBV infection, other hepatotropic disorders, or dysfunctional hepatic disorders such as hepatoma, or the consequences of alcohol abuse.

## Surrogate Testing

In the absence of specific serologic markers, surrogate testing of blood donors was instituted to eliminate donors who might transmit hepatitis C. Although these procedures are nonspecific, high-risk donors could be screened out of the donor pool by these means. These surrogate procedures consist of the transaminase enzyme, alanine aminotransferase (ALT or SGPT), and antibody to hepatitis B core antigen (anti-HBc) tests. It should be noted that the presence of anti-HBc in a donor's serum does not represent any virologic association but implies that a correlational relationship can occur in donors at risk for parenterally transmitted hepatitis C.

In one study of blood donors, it was demonstrated that the chance of hepatitis C occurring in a recipient was eight times greater if the donor's serum ALT was greater than 45 IU/L above normal. In this same study, however, 62% of transfusion-acquired hepatitis C cases occurred in recipients of blood whose values were below the cutoff value. Thus, the predictive effectiveness of ALT screening was difficult to assess. In addition, the test is not specific and is influenced by a large number of physiologic variables. Elevation of ALT can be due to a variety of causes such as medications, alcohol intake, and obesity.

The relationship between the presence of anti-HBc in donor blood and the development of hepatitis in recipients of that blood has been studied. Approximately 12% of recipients of at least 1 unit of blood positive for anti-HBc developed hepatitis C compared with 4% of recipients of only anti-HBc negative blood.

Although surrogate assays for ALT would have detected at least half of the anti-HCV-positive donors involved in the transmission of hepatitis C in transfusion recipients with acute and chronic hepatitis C, surrogate testing fails to catch between one-third and one-half of all (now generally referred to as) HCV-infected blood.

## HCV Testing

With the advent of a testing procedure for antibody to hepatitis C virus (anti-HCV), the significance of using ALT and anti-HBc assays as surrogate markers for hepatitis C in donors can be assessed. Retrospective studies have revealed a high correlation between anti-HCV and both ALT levels and the presence or absence of anti-HBc.

One problem with the new assays for anti-HCV is the variability and length of the window period before seroconversion. Approximately one-third of those infected with HCV manifest anti-HCV antibodies within several weeks, others may take months or, less commonly, some individuals may take as long as a year to express antibodies. The current test antigen represents only 12% of the encod-

**Table 13-4. Characteristics of Viral Hepatitis**

|  | Type A<br>Travelers | Type B<br>Hospital Personnel | Delta | Type C<br>Posttransfusion |
|---|---|---|---|---|
| Agent | Hepatitis A RNA | Hepatitis B DNA | Delta agent RNA | Hepatitis C RNA |
| Antigens | HA Ag | HBsAg, HBcAg, HBcAg, HBeAg | Delta | HCV |
| Antibodies | Anti-HAV | Anti-HBs, Anti-HBc, Anti-HBe | anti-Delta | anti-HCV |
| Epidemiology | Fecal-oral | Parenteral | Parenteral | Parenteral |
| Incubation period (in days) | 15–45 | 40–180 | 30–50 | 15–150 |

Adapted from Hoofnagle, Jay H. "Type A and Type B Hepatitis," *Laboratory Medicine*, Vol. 14, No. 11, November 1983, p. 715.

ing capacity of the virus. Although it is a good marker for chronic viremia, present assays are not comprehensive enough to detect all stages of infection. Therefore, a reactive test implies exposure to HCV, but not infectivity or immunity.

Anti-HCV negative cases may actually be due to HCV, but some patients may not mount an immune response (antibody titer) that is detectable by the current first-generation assays. An undetectable antibody response may be more likely in acute, self-limited disease, in which HCV-related antigen may be only transiently present. Therefore, the presence of detectable HCV antibody may reflect the persistence of a sufficient quantity of HCV antigen to stimulate the immune response repeatedly.

In addition, technical problems with testing for antibody to HCV include the absence of confirmatory tests. Additional specific and sensitive assays are urgently needed for different antibody subclasses and low titers of anti-HCV antibody, for neutralizing antibodies, and for directly detecting HCV antigen and other viral products.

### Prevention

Preventive practices among health care workers (such as the avoidance of needlestick injuries) should be followed. Recent investigations have shown that removing from the blood supply blood from donors with anti-HBcAg may reduce the incidence of posttransfusion HCV.

## Cytomegalovirus

In 1966, it was first reported that cytomegalovirus infection was associated with what is now referred to as posttransfusion mononucleosis. Infants infected with cytomegalovirus can become severely ill, with symptoms including pneumonia and hepatitis. Cytomegalovirus may be associated with transfusion-associated hepatitis and is one of the most important causes of the congenital viral infections in the United States that may cause death in premature infants.

### Etiology

The first descriptive report of histologic changes characteristic of the changes now associated with cytomegalovirus infection was published in 1904, when protozoan-like cells in the lungs, kidneys and liver of a syphilitic fetus were seen. In the 1920s, it was suggested that the large protozoan-like cells with intranuclear inclusions seen in some histologic preparations were not protozoal in origin, but it was not until 1956 that the cytomegalovirus was isolated in the laboratory. In 1966, the actual isolation of the virus after transfusion and the observation of elevated antibody titers were noted.

### Viral Characteristics

Human cytomegalovirus is classified as a member of the herpes family of viruses. There are presently five recog-

nized human herpesviruses: herpes simplex I, herpes simplex II, varicella-zoster virus, Epstein-Barr virus, and cytomegalovirus. All of the herpesviruses are relatively large, enveloped DNA viruses which undergo a replicative cycle involving DNA expression and nucleocapsid assembly within the nucleus. The viral structure gains an envelope, when the virus buds through the nuclear membrane that is altered to contain specific viral proteins.

These viruses are susceptible to lipid solvents, freezing, and heat, and viral isolates are not well preserved at 4° C, 20° C, or higher temperatures. Variables such as the location of the virus (intracellular versus extracellular), the presence of host cells, and soluble substances such as antibodies or complement have been made studying the stability of the virus in biologic situations difficult. If the virus is present in blood, urine, and breast milk, it may be more stable than laboratory isolates of the virus.

Although the herpes family produces diverse clinical diseases, the viruses share the basic characteristics of being cell-associated. The requirements for cell association vary, but all five viruses may spread from cell to cell, presumably by way of intracellular bridges, and in the presence of antibody in the extracellular phase. This common characteristic may play a role in the ability of the virus to produce subclinical infections which can be reactivated under appropriate stimuli.

### Epidemiology

Cytomegalovirus infection is endemic worldwide. Many cases are congenital infections in newborn infants; however, dissemination of the virus may be by oral, respiratory, and venereal routes or parenterally by organ transplantation or by the transfusion of fresh blood. A complete characterization of the transmission of cytomegalovirus from person to person has not been established, but transmission appears to require close, intimate contact with secretions or excretions (primarily urine, respiratory secretions, tears, feces, and genital secretions of infected persons). The most likely mode of acquisition is venereal, through contact with infectious virus in body secretions.

It has been recognized for more than 15 years that transfusion of blood from healthy asymptomatic blood donors is occasionally followed by active cytomegalovirus infection in the recipient. There is strong evidence to incriminate peripheral blood leukocytes and transplanted tissues as sources of cytomegalovirus.

### Incidence

The incidence of primary infection during childhood is low, but the rate of exposure to the virus may be accelerated during the first years of life in toddlers and children in day care centers. During adolescence the infection rate rises significantly. By adulthood, most persons have experienced asymptomatic contact with cytomegalovirus, as demonstrated by the fact that 40–100% of adults have detectable antibodies to cytomegalovirus by age 35. Serologic evidence further demonstrates that adult women have higher rates of antibody responses than men of the same age. The incidence of viral exposure and subsequent antibody formation (seropositivity) varies greatly depending on the socioeconomic status and living conditions of the population surveyed.

Less than 1% of normal healthy adults excrete the virus in their urine, but persons experiencing acquired infection, reinfection with the same or different strains of cytomegalovirus, or reactivation of a latent infection can excrete the virus in titers as high as $10^6$ infective units/mL in the urine and/or saliva for weeks or months. There is an average infection rate of 13% after transfusion to immunocompetent recipients, with most infections being asymptomatic.

## Latent Infection

Persistent infections characterized by periods of reactivation are frequently termed *latent* infections, although this condition has not been clearly defined for cytomegalovirus. True viral latency is defined by the presence of the genetic information in an unexpressed state in the host cell. An operational definition of latency can include the conditions of a dynamic relationship between the virus and the host, along with evidence of latency and reactivation of a latent infection.

Evidence that cytomegalovirus produces latent infections in humans is circumstantial and indirect. The mechanism of latency and the identity of the host cells which harbor the latent virus remain undocumented. Leukocytes from the peripheral blood of patients with active cytomegalovirus infections have been cultured, with subsequent recovery of cytomegalovirus; however, attempts to recover the virus from the leukocytes of healthy donors have been unsuccessful except in one report. In animal models, the virus is present and recoverable from neutrophilic leukocytes in active infections, but it is also believed that splenic B lymphocytes and possibly monocytes may harbor latent infections. Additionally, salivary gland, heart, and prostate tissue may be sites of latent infection. The types of cells and the mechanism of latency remain to be demonstrated in humans. The estimated cytomegalovirus carrier rate among blood donors, which is defined as the number of seroconversions (patients changing from being negative for antibodies to the virus to demonstrating antibodies) per 100 units of blood transfused ranges from 1 to 12%.

## Patients at Risk

Cytomegalovirus is known to cause transfusion-related infections, especially in premature infants, or infants weighing <1200 g at birth, and can be a frequent cause of morbidity and mortality in recipients of organ transplants and patients receiving immunosuppressive chemotherapy. Because cytomegalovirus can persist latently, active infections may develop under a variety of conditions such as pregnancy and immunosuppression, or after organ transplantation. In practice, the greater the degree of immunosuppression, the more likely the patient is to suffer from a cytomegalovirus infection, primary or reactivated. Children with leukemia and premature infants of less than 1200 g birth-weight fare badly, with fatal infections reported.

Patients with the highest risk of mortality from cytomegalovirus infections are transplant-seronegative patients who receive tissue from a seropositive donor. Cytomegalovirus is the most commonly recognized pathogen in the first 6 months after renal transplantation. Infections in cardiac transplant recipients have been reported to occur in association with increased pulmonary superinfections in addition to the clinical signs and symptoms of primary infection. Active cytomegalovirus infection is a major cause of morbidity and often mortality in AIDS patients.

The risk of developing cytomegalovirus infection is greatest for patients who are exposed to cellular blood components from a large number of donors. In heavily transfused patients, blood transfusion becomes a significant risk factor. The transfusion of granulocytes carries a high risk of viral infection in immunocompromised bone marrow recipients, with interstitial pneumonia occurring in 38 to 44% of cases. The relative importance of blood transfusion as a risk factor in organ transplantation patients varies according to the organ or tissue transplanted. The greatest majority of infections in patients are transmitted by the donor kidney or arise from the reactivation of the recipient's latent virus.

Infections in immunosuppressed patients may result in disseminated multisystem involvement including pneumonitis, hepatitis, gastrointestinal ulceration, arthralgias, meningoencephalitis, and retinitis. Interstitial pneumonitis, frequently associated with cytomegalovirus infection, is a major cause of death following allogeneic bone marrow transplantation. In premature infants, acquired cytomegalovirus infection can result in atypical lymphocytosis, hepatosplenomegaly, pneumonia, or death.

## Signs and Symptoms

The classic congenital cytomegalovirus syndrome is manifested by a high incidence of neurologic symptoms. Psychomotor retardation is seen in 51 to 75% of survivors. Hearing loss is observed in 21 to 50% of cases and visual impairment in 20% of cases. Infants without symptoms at birth may develop hearing impairment and neurologic impairment at a later date.

In most patients, cytomegalovirus infection is asymptomatic, with jaundice being rare. Infections occurring in healthy immunocompetent adults usually result in seroconversion. Occasionally a self-limited, heterophile-negative mononucleosis-like syndrome occurs. The symptoms include sore throat and fever, chills, profound malaise, and myalgia. Lymphadenopathy and splenomegaly may be observed.

Infrequent complications of cytomegalovirus infection in previously healthy adults include interstitial pneumonitis, hepatitis, Guillain-Barré syndrome, meningoencephalitis, myocarditis, thrombocytopenia, and hemolytic anemia. However, transfusion-acquired cytomegalovirus infections may cause not only a mononucleosis-like syndrome but hepatitis and an increase in rejection of transplanted organs.

Three types of cytomegalovirus infections are possible in blood transfusion recipients:

1. Primary infection occurs when a previously unexposed (seronegative) recipient is transfused with blood from an actively or latently infected donor. This type of infection is accompanied by the presence of cytomegalovirus in the blood and urine, a transient virus-specific IgM antibody response, and eventual seroconversion to produce IgG antibodies to the virus. Primary infections may be symptomatic, but the great majority are not.
2. Reactivated infections are produced when a seropositive recipient is transfused. Leukocytes from positive or negative donors are thought to trigger an allograft reaction, which in turn reactivates the recipient's latent infection. Such infections may be accompanied by significant increases in IgG antibodies to the virus but no detectable IgM response. Some reactivated infections exhibit viral shedding as their only manifestation. Reactivated infections are largely asymptomatic.
3. Reinfection may be caused by a strain of cytomegalovirus in the donor's blood that is different than the one originally infecting the recipient. A significant antibody response is observed in this situation and viral shedding occurs. Whether or not an IgM response occurs is unknown. Although it is difficult to differentiate a reactivated infection if both patient and donor are cytomegalovirus antibody positive before transfusion, reinfections can be documented if isolates can be obtained from both donor and recipient.

## Alterations in the Immune System

Cytomegalovirus is known to alter the immune system as well as producing overt manifestations of infection. A cytomegalovirus infection interferes with the host's immune responsiveness in both normal and immunocompromised individuals. This diminished responsiveness results in a decreased proliferative response to the cytomegalovirus antigen which persists for several months. In patients with cytomegalovirus mononucleosis, alterations of T lymphocyte subsets produce an increase in the absolute number of suppressor (T8) lymphocytes and a decrease in helper (T4) lymphocytes. These subset abnormalities persist for several months.

Questions have been raised regarding cytomegalovirus as a potentially oncogenic virus because viral antigens and/or nucleic acid have been found in human malignancies, including adenocarcinoma of the colon, carcinoma of the cervix, cancer of the prostate, and Kaposi sarcoma. Cytomegalovirus does have transforming properties in vitro. However, even though considerable circumstantial evidence exists linking cytomegalovirus to human malignancies (especially Kaposi's sarcoma), a direct cause-and-effect relationship has not been established.

## Laboratory Testing

In cytomegalovirus infection, hematologic examination of the blood usually reveals a characteristic leukocytosis. A slight lymphocytosis with over 20% variant lymphocytes is common. Clinical chemistry assays may demonstrate abnormal liver function tests. Elevated concentrations (titers) of several antibodies may occur. These include antinuclear antibody (ANA), rheumatoid factor (RF) antibodies, and nonspecific cold agglutinins. Another assessment of infection is the demonstration of inclusion bodies in leukocytes in urinary sediment.

A definitive diagnosis can be made only by isolating the cytomegalovirus from urine or blood samples or demonstrating of a rise in antibody titer. Human cytomegalovirus is indistinguishable by negative staining electron microscopy from its close relatives, herpes simplex and varicella, the cause of chickenpox. Viral culture is the method of choice for confirming cytomegalovirus infection.

## Serologic Markers

In cells infected by cytomegalovirus, several antigens appear at varying time intervals postinfection. Before replication of viral DNA takes place, immediate-early antigens and early antigens are present in the nuclei of infected cells. Immediate-early antigens appear within one hour of cellular infection, and early antigens are present within 24 hours. At about 72 hours postinfection or at the end of the viral replication cycle, late antigens are demonstrable in the nucleus and cytoplasm of infected cells.

The immune antibody response to these various antigens differs in incidence and significance. The presence of antibodies against immediate-early and early antigens is associated with active infection of either a primary or reactivated nature.

Antibody to early antigen undergoes a relatively rapid decline after recovery but can persist for up to 250 days and may identify patients with recent infections as well as active infections. The presence of antibody to early antigen is strongly associated with viral shedding. Antibodies to late antigens persist in high titer long after the recovery from an active infection.

## Screening of Blood Donors

The morbidity and mortality due to transfusion-acquired cytomegalovirus infection in high-risk patients have prompted serious efforts to provide convenient screening methods. The prevalence of cytomegalovirus antibody varies with age and geographic location but ranges from 40 to 100%. Donors with recent infection may be more likely to shed virus and be more infectious than chronically infected donors.

The incidence of antibodies against cytomegalovirus-induced immediate-early antigens, early antigens, and late antigens was studied in a population of healthy blood donors. Antibodies to immediate-early antigens were found in 9.6%, antibodies to early antigens in 10.2%, and antibodies to late antigens in 76% of the donors. The incidence of antibodies to cytomegalovirus-induced immediate-early and early antigens increased with age and was higher in women than men.

In another study, 51% of donors were seronegative for cytomegalovirus antibodies. The highest percentage of seronegative findings (60%) was among donors 18 to 35 years old. This age group represented 57% of the donors. If viruric donors are a source of transfusion-acquired cytomegalovirus in high-risk patients, screening blood for early antigen antibodies is warranted. In another study of random donors, 28% had antibodies to cytomegalovirus; however, among the 52 homosexual donors who were eligible on the basis of their medical histories, the following results were obtained:

High risk: Of 39 patients, 35 (90%) were seropositive
Low risk: Of 13 patients, 10 (77%) were seropositive
A study at a San Francisco clinic showed 94% of homosexual men and 43% of random donors to have cytomegalovirus antibodies. Detection of IgM anti-CMV that is associated with recent infection should be useful in screening for infectious units.

## Laboratory Procedures

Procedures for the identification of cytomegalovirus infections include:

1. Viral cultures of urine and/or blood
2. ELISA technique for IgG type antibodies
3. Passive latex agglutination (PLA)
4. Indirect immunofluorescence (IFA)
5. Enzyme-linked antigen assay (ELA)
6. A microtiter complement fixation (CF) test
7. Enzyme immunoassay tests (EIA)
8. Indirect hemagglutination (IHA)
9. Solid-phase fluorescence in immunoassay (SFI)

In one investigation comparing IHA, IFA, EIA, and PLA techniques of blood testing within 1 week of collection, the passive latex agglutination technique (PLA) was rated best overall because it was technically the easiest and required the least hands-on and turnaround times. The short turnaround time (10 minutes) rendered the latex technique a more flexible test for blood bank use because both scheduled and emergency screening of donors could be accommodated. The comparatively high reagent cost of the kit could be offset by time savings. IHA, EIA, ELISA, and PLA were found suitable for donor screening.

***Results of EIA Testing of Random Donors.*** IgG antibody tests have the disadvantage of cross-reacting with Epstein-Barr, varicella, and herpes simplex viruses. IgM screening by IFA and ELA does not always identify the viruric donor.

## Prevention

Most transfusion-acquired infections need not be prevented. Those occurring in immunocompetent patients rarely give rise to serious disease. Of patients who are immunosuppressed, only seronegative patients appear to be at significant risk of developing cytomegalovirus infections. Infant recipients weighing less than 1200 grams at birth, when either the infant or mother is CMV-antibody negative, or if this information is unknown, should be protected from the risk of transfusion-associated CMV disease. The use of cytomegalovirus-seronegative blood has been recommended for transfusion of selected premature babies and for recipients of bone marrow transplants. Transmission of this virus by transfusion of blood or components containing white cells is assuming increasing importance in patients with severely impaired immunity who require supportive therapy.

Transfusion-acquired cytomegalovirus infections can be prevented by using blood from donors unlikely to carry the virus, such as those negative for antibodies. Effective antibody screening, leukocyte-depleted blood products, and immune globulin containing passively acquired cytomegalovirus antibodies are all methods of prevention. Immune globulin was found to prevent infections in seronegative patients who did not receive granulocytes. This treatment is promising for preventing cytomegalovirus infections in high-risk patients. Resolution of the mechanism of latency or inapparent infections is critical to the further prevention of transfusion- and transplantation-associated cytomegalovirus infection.

Health care professionals and day care providers are among the groups that are becoming increasingly concerned about the risks associated with exposure to cytomegalovirus. Nosocomial transmission from patients to health care workers has not been documented, and observance of good personal hygiene and hand-washing offers the best measure for preventing transmission. However, children and providers of day care are at an increased risk of infection.

In 1990, the FDA licensed cytomegalovirus immunoglobulin intravenous (human) (CMV-IGIV). CMV-IGIV is indicated for the attenuation of primary (first-degree) cytomegalovirus disease associated with kidney transplantation. CMV-IGIV was previously available as a designated orphan drug. It is to be used for kidney recipients who are CMV seronegative but received a seropositive kidney.

Prophylactic gancyclovir is also used in some transplant protocols, such as liver transplantation or other solid organs. The aim of this treatment is to prevent CMV disease in those who are at high risk, such as seropositive patients or recipients of a CMV positive organ.

### Epstein-Barr Virus

The Epstein-Barr virus (EBV) can be transfusion-acquired. This virus can produce infectious mononucleosis, with hepatitis as the most frequent complication. EBV infection is an infrequent consequence of blood transfusion and does not cause as much of a problem in blood recipients as does cytomegalovirus.

#### Etiology

The Epstein-Barr virus was first discovered in 1964 as the cause of infectious mononucleosis. This same virus is associated with Burkitt's lymphoma, a malignant tumor of the lymphoid tissue occurring mainly in African children, and with nasopharyngeal carcinoma.

#### Viral Characteristics

EBV is a human herpeoncogenic DNA virus which has been isolated with increasing regularity. This virus is found in association with blood leukocytes. In infectious mononucleosis, the virus infects B lymphocytes; however, the variant lymphocytes produced in response to infection and seen in an examination of the peripheral blood have T cell characteristics. Among the habitats of the persisting virus in the carrier state is the B-lymphocyte in lymph nodes and peripheral blood.

#### Epidemiology

Although the Epstein-Barr virus appears to be transmitted primarily by close contact with infective oral-pharyngeal secretions, the virus has been reported to be transmitted by blood transfusion and transplacental routes.

Patients at risk include those who lack antibodies to the Epstein-Barr virus. The frequency of seronegative recipients is nearly 100% in early infancy and declines with increasing age, more or less rapidly depending on socioeconomic conditions, to less than 10% in young adults. Probably because approximately 90% of adult patients already have protective neutralizing antibodies in their serum, most blood transfusion recipients are immune to the virus. If multiple transfusions are received, antibody to the Epstein-Barr virus will be present in one or more of the donations and may have a protective effect. Thus, there is little chance to transmit the virus under ordinary conditions.

Despite the various factors that reduce the transmission of Epstein-Barr virus, cases of transfusion-associated infectious mononucleosis or infectious mononucleosis-like ill-

nesses have been recorded. The Epstein-Barr virus is only a minor problem for immunocompetent individuals but can become a major problem for immunologically compromised patients. Epstein-Barr virus (EBV) associated posttransplantation lymphoproliferation disease develops in 1% to 10% of transplant recipients. Infectious mononucleosis or infectious mononucleosis-like illness following blood transfusion may often be due to concomitant cytomegalovirus infections rather than the Epstein-Barr virus. Therefore, transmission of Epstein-Barr virus may occur only under rather limited conditions:

1. If a single unit of blood is transfused from a donor who is in the viral incubation period. Although transfusion of additional units of blood should theoretically protect the recipient unless the blood came from seronegative donors, on rare occasions single units of blood or platelet-rich plasma from donors who were incubating the virus produced viremia and infectious mononucleosis-like symptoms in recipients from 2 to 17 days later.
2. When the donor is seropositive, based on a test for antibodies to Epstein-Barr viral capsid antigen, but lacks Epstein-Barr neutralizing antibodies or possesses them at a level too low to protect the recipient. Multiple transfusions of blood would probably reduce or eliminate this possibility.
3. When the recipient has a T lymphocyte deficiency which might permit the donor's B lymphocytes, including EBV genome-carrying B cells, to outlast the period of a blood donor's passive antibody protection (approximately 4 weeks). The lymphomas observed in severely immunosuppressed patients could then arise from the recipient's or donor's B lymphocytes.

#### Incidence

Immunosuppressed patients have a higher prevalence of Epstein-Barr infection. The incidence ranges from 35 to 47%. As occurs with other herpesviruses, there is a carrier state after primary infection. More than 90% of blood donors have antibodies to Epstein-Barr virus and thus are carriers of the virus.

#### Signs and Symptoms

Infectious mononucleosis is usually a self-limiting lymphoproliferative disorder. It is a fairly common acute disorder and is usually benign. Although anyone can suffer from this condition, it typically affects young adults. However, an increasing number of older adult cases is being recognized. A case of fatal mononucleosis was recently reported in a young child in Japan.

The incubation period of infectious mononucleosis is from 10 to 50 days and, once fully developed, it lasts for 1 to 4 weeks. Clinical manifestations include extreme fatigue, sore throat, fever, and cervical lymphadenopathy.

Splenomegaly occurs in about 50% of cases. Jaundice is infrequent, although the most common complication is hepatitis.

## Laboratory Testing

In addition to clinical symptoms, hematologic and serologic laboratory testing is necessary to establish a diagnosis. Leukocyte counts range from 10 to 20 $\times$ $10^9$/L in about two thirds of patients. About 10% of the patients with this disorder demonstrate leukopenia. Differential leukocyte examination may reveal neutrophilia, although mononuclear cells usually predominate as the disorder develops. Typical relative lymphocyte counts range from 60 to 90%. Variant lymphocytes with a variety of morphologic features are characteristic and persist for 1 to 2 months or as long as 4 to 6 months.

A definite diagnosis of infectious mononucleosis is established by serologic antibody testing. The antibodies present are heterophil and Epstein-Barr virus antibodies. Other tests may detect viral capsid and nuclear antigens.

*Heterophil antibodies* may be present in a normal person in low concentrations; however, a titer of 1:56 or greater is clinically significant in suspected cases of infectious mononucleosis. Heterophil antibodies are defined as antibodies that are stimulated by one antigen and react with entirely unrelated antigens. Infectious mononucleosis antibodies are one type of heterophil antibody that has a variety of characteristics, which include:

1. Reaction with horse, ox, and sheep erythrocytes
2. Absorption of beef erythrocytes
3. No absorption by guinea pig kidney cells

Rapid slide tests are now available using the principle of agglutination of horse erythrocytes. The use of horse erythrocytes appears to increase the sensitivity of the test.

An assay for IgM and IgG antibodies to the antigens of the Epstein-Barr virus is available. Antibodies to viral antigen develop within the first 2 weeks of disease onset. Other antibodies appear later. Allo-Anti-i is the most clinically significant antibody because it can cause hemolytic anemia.

The EBER-1 gene is expressed early during latent EBV infection. This gene codes for a small-messenger RNA expressed at up to $10^7$ copies per cell. Detection of EBER-1 RNA in tissues (e.g., liver) is valuable because it precedes the occurrence of clinical and histologic EBV-associated, posttransplantation, lymphoproliferative disease.

## Prevention

Transfusion of blood products which contain few viable lymphocytes should reduce the chance of transfusing Epstein-Barr virus to patients at risk. These blood components may be leukocyte-depleted or irradiated products.

## Investigating Post-Transfusion Hepatitis

The viral agents discussed in the preceding sections can be the direct cause of hepatitis or lead to hepatitis as a complication, but documenting transfusion-acquired hepatitis in transfusion recipients is difficult. Two approaches to documentation are available: prospective follow-ups and retrospective assessments.

In prospective follow-ups, serologic and biochemical evaluation of a transfusion recipient could be conducted at periodic intervals following transfusion. In actual practice, prospective follow-ups are not realistic because of cost. In retrospective studies, the identification of clinical cases of hepatitis could be correlated with the patient's transfusion history of the previous 6 months; however, numerous donors may be implicated.

In attempting to identify the cause of the hepatitis, hepatitis B is typically suspect. The incidence of HBsAg in follow-up donor samples is rare. Because all donors have been tested previously, seroconversion indicates that, at the time of the implicated donation, the level of circulating HBsAg was below the detectability of the test used (most third-generation tests detect about 1 $\times$ $10^{-9}$g HBsAg/mL) or that the original test was done incorrectly. In implicated donors, the presence of anti-HBc alone or in combination with an elevated transaminase (ALT/SGPT) level is used by some centers as a reason to permanently defer a donor. If a donor is the only source of blood or a component given to a patient, that donor must be permanently deferred (refer to Chapter 2).

## Human T-Cell Lymphotropic Virus (HTLV)

The HTLV group of viruses is composed of types I, II, and III.

### HTLV I/II

Human T-cell lymphotropic virus type I (HTLV-I) was first isolated in 1978 in an adult black male residing in the southeastern United States. HTLV-I is associated with acute adult T-cell leukemia and chronic neurologic syndrome. Although HTLV-I is known to produce malignant transformation, the exact mechanism is not known. Two cases of malignant transformation have been described in patients previously well, but known to have HTLV-I antibodies for 5 to 10 years. It has been demonstrated that the helper T lymphocytes of seropositive—but clinically normal, unaffected—individuals can release HTLV-I viral particles in vitro when cocultured with normal lymphocytes.

HTLV-I is usually cell-associated, and transmission through blood transfusion has been documented for whole blood and cellular components. HTLV-I is also known to be transmitted by breast feeding and sexual contact. It has been suggested that seropositive individuals excrete a small number of HTLV-I genome-carrying lymphocytes in their saliva. HTLV-I/-II infection has been identified in female prostitutes in some parts of the United States. HTLV infection is common in Japan and the Caribbean. Intravenous drug abuse is the primary mode of transmission of HTLV in Western countries. It has been suggested that infection is mostly caused by HTLV-II rather than HTLV-I.

The association of a group of human retroviruses (the HTLV group) with overt malignant lymphoma/leukemia raises the concern of possible transmission of neoplasia by blood transfusion. When blood from 41 seropositive but healthy individuals was transfused into seronegative recipients, it induced seroconversion in 63% of the recipients. However, seroconversion did not occur in any of 14 recipients of fresh-frozen plasma derived from seropositive donors, and to date none of these patients has developed clinical disease.

Serologic studies of family members of affected patients have revealed a high intrafamilial incidence of HTLV-I antibodies, often in the total absence of clinical disease. The incidence of HTLV-I infection is variable, but in certain areas of the world as many as 1 in 4 adults shows serologic evidence of infection. However, few adults subsequently develop malignancies.

The spectrum of disease associated with HTLV-I infection ranges from the chronic, asymptomatic carrier form to a smoldering chronic form, to the typical acute forms. It is hypothesized that immunologic status, age, and genetic and environmental conditions are all important factors.

Consideration needs to be given to identifying and excluding infected donors. Because blood transmission of HTLV-I had been recognized in Japan, the Japanese began screening donated blood before it became a requirement in the United States. The FDA licensed tests to screen for antibody to HTLV-I in blood and cellular components donated for transfusions on November 29, 1988. In February 1989, the American Association of Blood Banks (AABB) recommended that blood centers implement routine testing of donated blood for anti-HTLV-I. The AABB *Standards* now require testing of all donated blood for anti-HTLV-I and -II. Donors who are repeatedly reactive in the anti-HTLV-I screening tests should be permanently deferred. Note that in 1992 false-positive serologic tests for HTLV-I, HIV-1, and hepatitis C virus were observed following influenza vaccination.

## Human Immunodeficiency Virus

### Etiology

Over the last several years, one of the most publicized transfusion-acquired viruses has been human immunodeficiency virus (HIV). HIV is probably the most intensively studied virus in the history of biomedical research. HIV-1 and HIV-2 are responsible for the clinical disease, acquired immunodeficiency syndrome (AIDS).

### Viral Characteristics

HIV is a member of the family *Retroviridae,* a type-D retrovirus that belongs to the lentivirus subfamily. Included in this family are oncoviruses such as HTLV-I and -II, which primarily induce proliferation of infected cells and formation of tumors. Since the discovery of this virus, much has been learned about the impact of the virus on human cells. HIV-1 virus is composed of a lipid membrane, structural proteins, and glycoproteins that protrude. The viral genome consists of three important structural components: *pol, gag,* and *env.* These components code for various products (Table 13-5). Long terminal repeat segments (ltr) border these three components. HIV-2 has a different envelope and slightly different core proteins.

Retroviruses carry a single, positive-stranded RNA and use a special enzyme, called *reverse transcriptase,* to convert viral RNA into DNA. This reverses the normal process of transcription, where DNA is converted to RNA—hence the term *retrovirus.*

The life cycle of HIV virus consists of five phases:

1. The virus attaches and penetrates target cells such as lymphocytes that express the CD4+ receptor. After penetration, the virus loses its protein coat, exposing the RNA core.
2. Reverse transcriptase converts viral RNA into proviral DNA.
3. The proviral DNA is integrated into the genome.
4. New virus particles are produced as the result of normal cellular activities of transcription and translation.
5. These new particles bud from the cell membrane. Once the viral genome is integrated into host cell DNA, the potential for viral production always exists and the viral infection of new cells can continue.

HIV has a marked preference for the helper-inducer (CD4) subset of T lymphocytes. It displays an affinity for these cells, because a CD4 surface marker protein on these cells serves as a receptor site for the virus. In addition to lymphocytes, cells such as those found in the central nervous system and upper respiratory tract have a similar receptor. Recent studies have demonstrated that immunologic activation of T helper cells latently infected with HIV induces the production of multiple viral particles leading to cell death. The extensive destruction of T cells leads to

**Table 13-5. Viral Genome Components**

| Component | Product |
| --- | --- |
| *pol* | Produces DNA polymerase |
|  | Produces endonuclease |
| *gag* | Codes for p24, and for proteins including p17, p9, and p7 |
| *env* | Codes for 2 glycoproteins: gp41, gp120 |

the gradual depletion of the helper-inducer type of lymphocytes. Defects in immunity are believed to be partially related to this T-cell depletion. Progressive defects in the immune system include a severe B-cell failure, defects in monocyte function, and defects in granulocyte function.

## Epidemiology

Transmission of HIV is believed to be restricted to intimate contact with body fluids, particularly blood or seminal fluid. Casual contact has not been implicated.

The virus can be transmitted through a parenteral route by transfusion with infected blood (if the blood has not been screened for HIV) or among IV drug abusers who use needles contaminated with the virus. Posttransfusion AIDS is well documented. Although it is rare, blood-borne transmission can also occur during medical procedures involving withdrawal and reinjection of blood or blood products.

Sexual transmission is a well-documented route of transmission. HIV is transmitted by infected cells and not free fluid. Relatively low levels of infective HIV particles are present in body fluids. However, genital secretion can contain substantial numbers of virus-infected cells. Up to 5% of white cells in seminal fluid can be HIV-infected. Seropositive individuals do not necessarily transmit the disease, if their genital fluids do not contain a large number of infected cells.

Children born to women with HIV have a 20–30% risk of infection with HIV. Infected mothers can also spread HIV to their newborn infants by breastfeeding. Most transmission of HIV to organ/tissue recipients occurred before 1985, prior to the implementation of donor screening recommendations. Reports of transmission from screened, HIV-antibody negative organ or tissue donors have been rare. Transmission of HIV from infected health care workers has been noted. However, the risk of transmission is very small.

## Incidence

The first cases of acquired immunodeficiency syndrome (AIDS) were reported in June 1981. From 1981 through December 1987, 50,000 AIDS cases were reported to CDC, and by August 1989, 100,000 cases were reported. From September 1989 through November 1991, state and territorial health departments reported 100,000 additional cases (1991—45,506 cases). A total of almost 207,000 cases were reported up to December 31, 1991, with 133,232 reported deaths associated with AIDS. In 1992, another 42,978 cases of AIDS were reported.

The proportion of AIDS cases related to transfusions as a mode of exposure declined in both adults (2.5% to 1.9%) and children (11% to 5.6%) from the first to the second 100,000 cases. Transfusion-associated AIDS is defined as the occurrence of AIDS in persons with no other known risk factor for AIDS and who were transfused with blood or blood components within 5 years of the onset of illness. Reductions in HIV transmission by blood and blood products as a result of screening and other procedures implemented in 1985 are now reflected by decreases in AIDS cases among persons with hemophilia and transfusion recipients. The residual risk for HIV-1 infection from the transfusion of screened blood is estimated at about 1 in 60,000 units of blood.

Blacks and Hispanics continue to be disproportionately represented in both the first and second 100,000 cases (27% and 15%, and 31% and 17%, respectively). Trends in the occurrence of AIDS reflect earlier trends in HIV infection in various populations and regions. An increasing number of persons with AIDS have been reported to have had heterosexual exposure to persons at risk for HIV infection. AIDS in women also increased in the second 100,000 reported cases. In the United States, 8% of all AIDS cases diagnosed in 1991 resulted from heterosexual contact with an injecting drug user. Reports of other sexually transmitted diseases (STDs) serve as a proxy marker for behaviors associated with sexual HIV transmission. The incidence of STDs has declined among homosexual/bisexual men in some regions, but increased in younger age groups. Declines in the incidence of HIV infection, beginning in the mid-1980s, have contributed to the current slower rate of increase in AIDS cases among homosexual/bisexual men.

An estimated 1 in 250 persons in the United States is infected with HIV. About 225,000 HIV-positive persons were hospitalized in 1990, of whom only one-third were admitted for symptomatic HIV infection or AIDS. Routine, voluntary HIV testing of patients 15 to 54 years old in hospitals with one or more patients with newly diagnosed AIDS per 1000 discharges per year could potentially have identified as many as 110,000 patients with HIV infection that was previously unrecognized.

Pediatric AIDS occurs in children below the age of 13, primarily among infants and toddlers. Of these cases of AIDS, the majority of cases were in children under 3 years of age. Most of these children were born to parents with high-risk behaviors or have a parent with AIDS. The next most common cause of pediatric AIDS is transfusion-associated AIDS.

## Signs and Symptoms

It is not known when an exposed individual becomes infectious or how soon infected individuals develop serologic markers of infection. HIV produces a chronic infection, with symptoms that range from asymptomatic to the end stage complications of AIDS.

Typically, patients in the early stages of HIV infection are either completely asymptomatic, or may show mild, chronic lymphadenopathy. The early phase may last from many months to many years after viral exposure. Although the course of HIV-1 infection may vary somewhat among individual patients, a common pattern of development has been recognized. The newly revised HIV classification system provides uniform and simple criteria for categorizing conditions among adolescents and adults with HIV infection. The criteria for HIV infection for persons age 13 years and older:

1. Repeatedly reactive screening tests for HIV antibody, with specific antibody identified by the use of a supplemental test;
2. Direct identification of virus in host tissues by virus isolation;
3. HIV antigen detection; or
4. A positive result on any other highly specific licensed test for HIV.

During the early period after primary infection, widespread dissemination of virus occurs and a sharp decrease in the number of CD4 T cells in peripheral blood is manifested. The early burst of virus in the blood, *viremia,* is often accompanied by flu-like symptoms that can be so severe that those suffering from them may seek help in hospital emergency rooms. An immune response to HIV develops with a concurrent decrease in detectable viremia. It was previously believed that the human immune system could drive the AIDS virus into a latent period that kept it inactive for years. Recently this view has been replaced with a new vision of a virus that is furiously creating copies of itself throughout the course of the disease, even when the patient appears healthy. Even when HIV cannot be detected in the blood, viremia, it infects (in large quantities) the lymphatic tissues, including the tonsils and lymph nodes, throughout the body. The absence of viremia generally lasts until the end stage of the disease.

This phase is followed by a prolonged period of clinical latency (range = 7 to 11 years; median = 10 years). During the period of clinical latency, the patient is usually asymptomatic. Differences in the infecting virus, the genetic makeup of the host, and environmental factors (including concomitant infection) have been suggested as causes of the variation in the duration of clinical latency in persons not receiving antiretroviral therapy. Treatment, with inhibitors of viral reverse transcriptase such as zidovudine (Retrovir) and administration of prophylaxis for pneumonia due to *Pneumocystis carinii,* has increased AIDS-free time in HIV-1 infected persons.

The quantity of CD4 T lymphocytes continues to diminish as the disease progresses, and when the number of cells reaches a critically low level the risk of opportunistic infection increases. The CDC has revised the classification system for HIV infection to emphasize the clinical importance of the CD4+ T-lymphocyte count in the categorization of HIV-related clinical conditions. The measure of severe immunosuppression, as defined by a CD4+ T-lymphocyte count of <200 cells/uL or a CD4+ percentage of <14, represents patients who are at the greatest risk for the full spectrum of severe HIV-related morbidity (Table 13-6). However, some researchers have concluded

**Table 13-6. Revised HIV Classification and AIDS Surveillance for Case Definition for Adolescents and Adults***

| Category | CD4+ T-Lymphocytes Count | CD4+ T-Lymphocytes Percentage |
| --- | --- | --- |
| 1 | ≥500 | ≥29 |
| 2 | 200–499 | 14–28 |
| 3 | <200 | <14 |

Clinical Categories of HIV Infection

A    One or more of the following conditions with documented HIV infection: asymptomatic HIV infection, persistent generalized lymphadenopathy, and/or acute (primary) HIV infection with accompanying illness or history of acute HIV infection. Conditions listed in categories B and C must not have occurred.

B    Symptomatic conditions, such as candidiasis (oropharyngeal or vulvovaginal), cervical dysplasia, fever, diarrhea lasting more than 1 month, that are not included in category C, and that meet at least one of the following criteria:

(a) The conditions are attributed to HIV infection or are indicative of a defect in cell-mediated immunity; or

(b) The conditions are considered by physicians to have a clinical course or to require management that is complicated by HIV infection.

C    Conditions included in the 1993 AIDS surveillance case definition: candidiasis of the bronchi, trachea, lungs, or esophagus; invasive cervical cancer; coccidiomycosis, disseminate or extrapulmonary; cryptococcosis, extrapulmonary; cryptosporidiosis, chronic intestinal and more than 1 month in duration; cytomegalovirus disease (other than liver, spleen, or nodes); cytomegalovirus retinitis (with loss of vision); encephalopathy, HIV–related; herpes simplex: chronic ulcer(s), for more than 1 month, or bronchitis, pneumonitis, esophagitis; histoplasmosis, disseminate or extrapulmonary; isosporiasis, chronic intestinal and for more than 1 month; Kaposi's sarcoma; lymphoma, Burkitt's or equivalent; lymphoma, immunoblastic or equivalent; lymphoma, primary of the brain; *Mycobacterium avium*–complex or *M. kansasii,* disseminated or extrapulmonary; *Mycobacterium tuberculosis* in any site, pulmonary or extrapulmonary; *mycobacterium,* other species or unidentified species, disseminated or extrapulmonary; *Pneumocystis carinii* pneumonia; recurrent pneumonia; progressive multifocal leukoencephalopathy; recurrent *salmonella* septicemia; toxoplasmosis of the brain; wasting syndrome due to HIV.

For classification purposes, once a person has a category C condition, the person will remain in Category C.

* For persons ages ≥ 13 years
Adapted from "1993 Revised Classification System for HIV Infection and Expanded Surveillance Case Definition for AIDS Among Adolescents and Adults," *MMWR,* Vol. 41, No. RR-17, Dec 18, 1992.

that levels of CD4+ lymphocytes are an incomplete surrogate marker for progression to AIDS, and the association is especially weak during the first 16 weeks of zidovudine therapy. The development of addition markers predictive for rapid CD4+ cell decline and disease progression is of major clinical importance. Differences, independent of virus quantity, in biologic properties among HIV-1 isolates—such as syncytium-inducing (SI) capacity, replication rate, and cytotropism—have been suggested as surrogate markers. Appearance of SI variants, occurring 2 years before progression to AIDS on the average, is predictive for a significantly increased rate of CD4+ lymphocyte decline.

Clinical symptoms of the later phase of the disease include extreme weight loss, fever, and multiple secondary infections. End-stage AIDS is characterized by the occurrence of neoplasms and/or opportunistic infections. Opportunistic infections noted with the greatest frequency are due to the following microorganisms: *Pneumocystis carinii,* cytomegalovirus, mycobacterium avium-intracellular, cryptococcus, toxoplasmosis, *Mycobacterium tuberculosis,* herpes simplex and legionella. Histoplasma capsulatum is being recognized with increasing frequency. The most frequent malignancy observed is an aggressive, invasive variant of Kaposi's sarcoma discovered in many cases upon autopsy. Malignant B-cell lymphomas are being recognized with increasing frequency in patients with AIDS, or at high risk for AIDS. AIDS is presently considered fatal. When clinically apparent disease develops, patients usually die within 2 years with current treatment.

## Laboratory Testing

The common denominator of HIV infection is a deficiency of a specific subset of thymus-derived (T) lymphocytes, designated by the phenotypic marker CD4. In this disorder, both a leukopenia and lymphocytopenia exist. T-lymphocyte subset distribution is altered with a decrease in the helper-inducer T cells and an increase in suppressor-cytotoxic T cells. A decreased lymphocyte proliferative response to soluble antigens and mitogens exists in this disorder. This condition additionally demonstrates defective natural killer (NK) cell activity. Functional testing also reveals a diminished response to pokeweed mitogen (PWM). A variety of other ancillary findings including polyclonal hypergammaglobulinemia, elevated levels of alpha interferon, alpha$_1$ ($\alpha_1$) thymosin, and beta microglobulin, and reduced levels of T-cell growth factor or interleukin-2 have been noted.

## Serological Testing

HIV testing of blood donors is usually done by performing an enzyme immunoassay (EIA) test (Table 13-7). Screening tests are designed to have high sensitivity, because the consequence of missing a true positive unit of blood or tissue specimen is grave. If the EIA screening test is repeat-

**Table 13-7. HIV Testing Methods**

Enzyme immunoassay (EIA)
    Enzyme-labeled antiglobulin
    Sandwich
    Competitive binding
Latex
Western blot
Antigen capture
Immunofluorescence assay (IFA)

edly reactive, a confirmatory test must be performed to determine the donor's status (Table 13-8). Technical and biologic factors can produce a false-positive test. Possible causes can include specimen problems such as lipemia, hemolysis, or contamination; technical problems such as improper washing or incorrect reaction temperature; or biologic factors such as recent vaccine recipients or passively acquired antibodies. Re-entry of a donor into the blood-donor pool must follow the protocol developed by the FDA. Important points in the re-entry protocol include:

1. A required 8-week, or 6-month, interval between samples to consider possible seronegative donors in the incubation phase
2. The use of EIA tests based on whole-virus lysate
3. Testing with a licensed Western blot or immunofluorescence assay (IFA) test, so that the appropriate sensitivity for antibody detection is present in the method

The development of first-generation serologic tests was rapid and has had a significant effect on reducing the transmission of HIV by blood. Serologic tests detect antibodies to HIV and are only capable of determining where an individual has had prior HIV viral exposure. Newer techniques are directed at HIV antigen detection. HIV located inside the CD4+ lymphocytes does not produce a protein in excess like HBsAg. Therefore, the quantities of viral protein in the blood of persons infected with HIV is very low. The antibody to HIV is present in much greater quantity, and with present techniques the antibody is much easier to detect.

## Interpretation of Results

A positive test result means only that the antibody to HIV is present. In AIDS patients, 85–90% do have a positive HIV antibody test, as well as increased antibody titers to viruses such as cytomegalovirus, Epstein-Barr virus, hepatitis A and B, and *Toxoplasma gondii;* and circulating immune (antigen-antibody) complexes can be found.

Several problems are associated with the use of crude viral preparations as antigen targets. Because the AIDS virus represents an enveloped particle, its membrane shares many antigenic similarities with the cell line used as the virus producer. These include T-cell antigens, HLA antigens, and other potential targets of the humoral response

**Table 13-8. Reentry of Donors***

| Not Eligible for Reentry into Donor Pool | |
| --- | --- |
| *Testing of initial specimen* | *Result* |
| Anti-HIV-1 or anti-HIV-1/2 | Licensed Western blot positive or indeterminate or immunofluorescent antibody (IFA) reactive |
| Anti-HIV-2 | Repeatedly reactive with another HIV-2 enzyme immunoassay (EIA) procedure |
| HBsAg | Repeatedly reactive anti-HBc test or confirmed by neutralization test |
| **Evaluate for Possible Reentry into Donor Pool** | |
| *Testing of initial specimen* | *Result* |
| Anti-HIV-1 or anti-HIV-1/2 | Licensed Western blot or immunofluorescent antibody (IFA) nonreactive |
| Anti-HIV-2 | Nonreactive with another HIV-2 enzyme immunoassay procedure and Western blot or IFA |
| HBsAg | Nonreactive anti-HBc test or not confirmed by HBs Ag specific |
| **Not Eligible for Reentry into Donor Pool** | |
| *Testing of specimen 6 months later* | *Result* |
| Anti-HIV-1 or anti-HIV-1/2 | Repeatedly reactive EIA or licensed Western blot positive or indeterminate or immunofluorescent antibody (IFA) reactive |
| Anti-HIV-2 | Repeatedly reactive HIV-1 or -2 with another HIV-2 enzyme immunoassay procedure or a licensed Western blot or IFA reactive or indeterminate |
| *Testing of specimen 8 weeks later* | |
| HBsAg | Repeatedly reactive anti-HBc or HBsAg tests |
| **Eligible for Reentry into Donor Pool** | |
| *Testing of specimen 6 months later* | *Result* |
| Anti-HIV-1 or anti-HIV-1/2 | Original EIA method nonreactive and whole-virus lysate anti-HIV-1 EIA nonreactive and licensed Western Blot or immunofluorescent antibody (IFA) nonreactive |
| Anti-HIV-2 | Screening test and a different HIV-2 enzyme immunoassay procedure and Western blot or IFA nonreactive |
| *Testing of specimen 8 weeks later* | |
| HBsAg | Nonreactive anti-HBc and HBsAg tests |

* These donors have demonstrated repeatedly reactive screening tests.

that can produce false-positive results. The sensitivity of ELISA tests with respect to disease detection is also subject to inherent difficulties. Examples of false-negative results can include:

1. AIDS patients with diminished antibody titer associated with late-stage disease or loss of the virus envelope accompanying purification procedures
2. Patients who lack detectable antibody for approximately 6 weeks following infection. Virus-positive, antibody-negative individuals would go undetected in an initial screening assay

At the present time, blood samples from donors that are initially reactive to HIV antibody testing are rechecked in duplicate in order to rule out technical errors. If, upon repeat testing, one or more of the duplicates is positive, the sample is considered "repeatably reactive," and the unit of blood is not used for transfusion. In order to rule out false-positive results, it is necessary to confirm repeatably reactive test results by an alternative protocol (Table 13-9).

***Western Blot Test.*** Before a blood donor is notified of "anti-HIV reactivity" tests demonstrating positive results, the results should be both reproducible and confirmable by at least one additional test. The most frequently used confirmatory test is the Western blot test. This test is an alternative procedure to establish the presence of antibody to HIV in serum or plasma. When the test is positive for bands p41 and/or p24 in conjunction with a positive ELISA test, it can be regarded as a confirmatory test. The test appears to work best with samples that contain high levels of antibody.

In the Western blot procedure, purified HIV viral antigens are electrophoresed on a gel, and the separated polypeptides are then transferred onto sheets of nitrocellulose paper. The nitrocellulose paper is incubated with the serum specimen. Any antibody that binds to the separated peptides present on the nitrocellulose paper is detected by a secondary anti-human antibody and is conjugated to a suitable enzyme marker and incubated with the appropriate enzyme substrate. Antibody specificities against known viral components (generally the core component p24 and envelope component gp41) are considered true-positive results, while antibody specific against nonviral cellular contaminants are nonspecific, false-positive results.

The Western blot is a time-consuming and expensive methodology that is open to considerable interpretation. To confirm antibody reactivities in a more objective manner than that offered by the Western blot methodology, the development of an immunofluorescent test has been sought that could accurately and rapidly confirm initially reactive serum specimens. The simplicity of the test reflects its format: an HIV-induced cell line and an uninfected control cell line are separately deposited onto a microscope slide. The serum specimen to be tested is incubated on each cell spot, followed by an incubation with a goat anti-

**Table 13-9. Sample Blood-Donor Screening Protocol for HIV**

| Enzyme Immunoassay (EIA) | | | | |
|---|---|---|---|---|
| Result | Next Step | Next Step | Next Step | Results |
| Negative | Blood safe for transfusion | | | |
| Reactive | Repeat (duplicate) | | | |
| | Result: Both negative | Blood safe for transfusion | | |
| | Result: One or both reactive | Discard unit and any indate components from the same donor | | |
| | | Perform HIV-1 confirmatory test, e.g., Western blot, etc. | | |
| | | | Result: Negative Test for anti-HIV-2 | Result: Negative/Place on list for possible reentry |
| | | | | Result: Positive/Notify donor and further test for HIV-2 |
| | | | Result: Positive | Notify donor and Health Dept., if required by law |
| | | | Result: Indeterminate | Test for anti-HIV-2 |
| | | | | Result: Negative/Defer as for HIV-1 |
| | | | | Result: Repeat reactive/Notify and further test for HIV-2 |

human antibody conjugated to fluorescein isothiocyanate (FITC), and the microscope slides are examined under an ultraviolet microscope. It is possible to distinguish true- from false-positive test results. A dipstick version has also been developed for clinical labs, physicians' offices, and field testing conditions.

SECOND AND THIRD GENERATION TESTING METHODS. Second-generation tests are similar to the first-generation tests in format and principle, with the exception that the antigen sources are recombinant DNA–derived products rather than crude or purified viral antigens. Sensitivities of gene-derived assays may not be significantly improved, but the specificity of second-generation tests may be superior, because the problems associated with antibody reactivities against cell-substrate components will be nonexistent. Third-generation tests detect actual infectious viral particles. Cell culture methods do provide information regarding the presence of the virus; however, in order to be specific for HIV, a virus capture assay is needed to detect viral antigens in cell culture specimens.

Some patients with HIV infection fail to demonstrate HIV antibodies (seronegative). Therefore, more sensitive antibody tests, assays for HIV-1 p24 antigen, and the use of the polymerase chain reaction (PCR) appear to hold the most promise for future screening of organ and tissue donors. Serologic detection of HIV in neonates is complicated by the presence of immune complexes, consisting of passively transferred maternal antibodies and HIV antigens. A new immune complex–dissociated HIV p24 antigen assay may be of value in diagnosing HIV infection in neonates born to HIV-infected women.

*Prevention.* The first step in prevention of transfusion-acquired HIV virus is careful screening of blood donors. Blood-donor medical history standards have recently undergone extensive revision (refer to Chapter 2, Blood Donors). Low-risk homosexual behavior, according to the American Association of Physicians for Human Rights, is defined as sexual contact with only one, or no, sexual partners for the last 3 years.

The U.S. Public Health Service has recommended that all donated blood and plasma be tested for HIV antibody, and additionally recommends that the blood or serum from donors of organs, tissues, or semen intended for human use be similarly tested and that the test result be used to evaluate the appropriate use of such materials from these donors.

The National Hemophilia Foundation currently recommends that pediatric hemophiliacs receive cryoprecipitate. Patients who have never previously received factor VIII should receive heat-treated products, if no other alternative exists (Refer to Chapter 10, Blood Components, for a discussion of the future applications of biotechnology in the production of factor VIII). Treatment of blood components can be an additional preventive method, if biologic activity of the needed component is not compromised. HIV virus has been demonstrated to be efficiently inactivated by formalin, beta-propiolactone, ethyl ether, detergent, and ultraviolet light plus psoralen. The results are reassuring regarding the potential safety of various biological products.

Guidelines from the CDC for clinical and laboratory personnel who work with AIDS patients and blood specimens suggest that the same precautions should be used as when the risk of hepatitis B infection is present. Specifically, patient care and laboratory personnel should avoid direct contact of nonintact skin and membranes with blood, blood products, secretions, excretions, and tissues.

The CDC developed recommendations for the voluntary and confidential HIV counseling and testing of patients in acute-care hospitals (Table 13-10) to assist in

**Table 13-10. Guidelines for HIV Counseling and Testing**

- Encourage asking patients about their risks for HIV infection.
- Offer HIV counseling to patients at risk.
- Offer voluntary HIV testing services for patients at risk.
- Develop policies regarding provision of routine HIV counseling and voluntary testing services.
- Consider offering HIV counseling and testing routinely to patients of ages 15–54 years if the HIV seroprevalence rate is at least 1% or there is an AIDS diagnosis rate of ≥1.0 per 1000 discharges in the hospital population.
- Counseling and testing should be structured to facilitate confidential, voluntary, patient participation. This should include: (a) pretest information on the testing policies of the institution or physician, and (b) basic information about the medical implications of the test, the patient's option to receive more information, and the documentation of informed consent.
- Offer counseling and testing in nonemergency settings.
- Provide test results in a confidential manner and forward information in accordance with local law.
- Provide optimal care to persons who decline HIV testing or who consent to testing and are HIV antibody positive.
- Protect confidentiality of test results.
- Do not substitute HIV testing programs for universal precautions and other infection-control techniques.

Adapted from "Recommendations for HIV Testing Services for In-patients and Out-patients in Acute Care Hospital Settings," *MMWR*, 42:1–6, 1993.

the diagnosis of medical conditions, initiate early medical management of HIV infection, and inform infected persons or persons at risk for infection about behaviors that can prevent HIV transmission.

### HIV-2

In 1986, a second virus causing the acquired immunodeficiency syndrome, human immunodeficiency virus type 2 (HIV-2), was discovered and found to be relatively common in parts of West Africa. Epidemiologic data indicate that the prevalence of HIV-2 infections in persons in the United States is extremely low (32 reported cases since 1987).

The primary mode of transmission of HIV-2 is heterosexual contact, although HIV-2 infection has been reported in Europe in homosexual men, injecting drug users, transfusion recipients, and men with hemophilia. Portugal and France have reported the highest number of cases of HIV-2 infection in Europe.

Infection with HIV-2 can cause immunosuppression and the development of AIDS. The period between infection and disease may be longer for persons with HIV-2 than for those with HIV-1. Considerable serologic cross-reaction occurs between HIV-1 and HIV-2, but HIV-2 infection may not be diagnosed when screening is done exclusively with HIV-1 tests. Because HIV-2 infections are not always detected by HIV-1 antibody tests, antibody tests for HIV-2 have been developed. In 1990, the FDA licensed an enzyme immunoassay (EIA) test kit for detection of antibodies to HIV-2 in human serum or plasma. An additional combination procedure for screening for

HIV-1 and HIV-2 was licensed in September 1991. Diagnosis of HIV-2 requires more specific supplementary tests, such as an HIV-2 Western blot.

### Human Herpesvirus-6

Human herpesvirus-6 (HBLV, HHV-6) has been suspected as the cause of hepatitis in some organ transplant recipients, and possibly posttransfusion. HHV-6 has been isolated from peripheral blood mononuclear cells and cells of the liver and kidney of transplant recipients. However, the clinical importance of infection with this virus after organ transplantation is unknown. In addition, HHV-6 reactivation may occur during neutropenia a few weeks after bone marrow transplantation. The virus may cause episodes of fever and skin rash that resemble those of acute graft-versus-host disease in some patients.

HHV-6 is often found in saliva, and antibody has been detected in an EIA method in a majority of blood donors. However, a prospective study of transfusion recipients failed to show seroconversion or a significant increase in anti-HHV-6 titer.

### Parvovirus

The parvovirus-like virus of humans has been shown to be transmitted in factor VIII concentrates. Transmission of the virus has been demonstrated in concentrates prepared from donor pools but not from single-donor cryoprecipitate or whole blood. The significance of transmission is uncertain; however, the fact that this virus is transmitted by blood should be kept in mind when considering the transmission of other agents. It is presently believed that the resulting viremia is transient.

## TRANSFUSION-ACQUIRED PARASITES

Transmission of parasitic infections through blood transfusion is infrequent in developed countries. Although deaths caused by transfusion-acquired malaria are rare, fatal cases have occurred in the United States and elsewhere. In many underdeveloped nations where diseases such as African trypanosomiasis (sleeping sickness) are endemic, transfusion-acquired parasitism is a significant problem of nonimmune recipients.

On the North American continent, four parasitic diseases can be seen with greater frequency than others. These are malaria (*Plasmodium* species), Chagas' disease (*Trypanosoma cruzi*), babesiosis (*Babesia microti*), and toxoplasmosis (*Toxoplasma gondii*). In underdeveloped, primarily tropical countries a variety of transfusion acquired parasitic diseases has been observed. In addition to African sleeping sickness (*Trypanosoma brucei rhodesiense* or *Trypanosoma brucei gambiense*), transfusion-acquired parasites include *Wucheria bancrofti, Loa loa,* and *Mansonella ozzardi*.

## Malaria Species

### Etiology

In 1884, two human subjects demonstrated that malaria could be transmitted through blood. The first case of accidental transmission through blood transfusion was described in 1911. The modern tendency is to refer to the various types of malaria by the names of their causative agents: *Plasmodium vivax (P. vivax), Plasmodium falciparum (P. falciparum), Plasmodium malariae (P. malariae)* and *Plasmodium ovale (P. ovale)*. The life cycle of *Plasmodium* is in both humans and mosquitoes.

### Incidence

Although a program coordinated by the World Health Organization from 1960 to 1970 was partially successful in eradicating malaria, the incidence of this disease has progressively increased. The number of cases of malaria reported worldwide increased 2.5 times between 1972 and 1977. In part, the spread of malaria is associated with increased population shifts and travel between temperate and tropical parts of the world.

The resurgence of malaria over most of the tropics continues to endanger the health of developing countries and represents a serious problem for other countries, such as the United States. The total number of people living in endemic areas of malaria in 1982 was 1600 million. The population distribution in some of the endemic areas is as follows:

1. Southeast Asia             920 million
2. Africa                     282 million
3. Eastern Mediterranean      170 million
4. The Americas               130 million
5. Western Pacific             74 million

Species distribution of *Plasmodium* indicates that *P. vivax* is the predominant species worldwide, *P. falciparum* is almost entirely confined to the tropics and subtropics, and *P. malariae* occurs primarily in subtropical and temperate areas where other species of malaria are found. *P. ovale* is rather widely distributed in tropical Africa and replaces *P. vivax* in frequency on the West African coast. *P. ovale* has also been reported in South America and Asia.

It has been estimated that during the period from 1950 to 1982, the total number of recorded cases of transfusion-acquired malaria exceeded 3500. Transfusion-acquired malaria is particularly high in Bangladesh, Brazil, India, Iran, and Mexico. In the United States, 26 cases of transfusion-acquired malaria were reported from 1972 to 1981. A worldwide survey (1973 to 1980) of transfusion-acquired malaria demonstrated that *P. vivax* (together with a few cases of *P. ovale*) was the most common (42%), followed by *P. malariae* (38%) and *P. falciparum* (20%).

### Transmission

Induced malaria is a term that can be applied to accidental or deliberate inoculation of malarial parasites by either a mosquito bite or injection into a human host. Three types of transmission are possible:

1. Transfusion malaria, which is accidentally related to whole blood, blood components, or organ transplants.
2. Accidental "needle" malaria due to the unintentional introduction of parasites by a contaminated needle.
3. Congenital malaria in the newborn who became infected by the transplacental route from the mother.

***The Disease Phase in the Mosquito.*** The disease cycle of malaria is initiated when a female mosquito of various species of anopheline mosquitoes bites an infected human. The infected blood of the person, which may contain male and female gametocytes, is drawn into the stomach of the mosquito. In the mosquito, the male or microgametocyte undergoes maturation and results in the production of microgametes.

Concurrently, the female or macrogametocyte matures into a macrogamete, which may be fertilized by the microgamete to become a zygote. The active zygote is referred to as an ookinete, and after constricting as an oocyst. The growth and development of the oocyte results in the production of a large number of thread-like sporozoites, which circulate throughout the body of the mosquito. The sporozoites that enter the salivary glands of the mosquito are ready to be inoculated into the next person bitten by the mosquito.

The length of this cycle depends upon factors such as the species of *Plasmodium* and the ambient temperature. It may range from as short as 8 days in *Plasmodium vivax (P. vivax)* to as long as 35 days in *P. malariae*.

***The Disease Phase in Humans.*** Sporozoites injected into the bloodstream of a human by an infected mosquito leave the circulatory system within a period of 40 minutes and invade the liver cells of the human host. In the cells of the liver, all four species undergo an asexual multiplication phase. This asexual multiplication produces thousands of tiny merozoites in each infected cell. Subsequent rupture of the infected liver cells releases the merozoites into the circulation.

In the circulation, an asexual cycle takes place within the erythrocytes. This process, referred to as schizogony, results in the formation of from 4 to 36 new parasites in each infected erythrocyte within 48 to 72 hours. At the end of this schizogonoic cycle, the infected erythrocytes rupture, liberating merozoites, which in turn infect new erythrocytes.

Usually, after a patient has become clinically ill, gametocytes appear in circulating erythrocytes. Gametocytes, derived from merozoites, grow but do not divide and finally form the male and female gametocytes. Gametocytes circulate in the blood for some time and, if ingested by an appropriate species of mosquito, undergo the sexual cycle, gametogony, which develops into sporogony in the mosquito.

## Signs and Symptoms

There are usually no symptoms of malaria until several continuous life cycles have been completed. The simultaneous rupturing of erythrocytes liberates toxic products that characteristically produce chills followed by a fever in a few hours. A patient's temperature may rise to 104° or 105° F. The symptoms last from 4 to 6 hours and recur at regular intervals, depending on the type of malaria.

## Laboratory Testing

Examination of blood smears is inappropriate for the screening of asymptomatic blood donors. Serologic techniques for diagnosis of malaria may also be used.

French investigators assessed their 5-year rule, which refers to the amount of time that should elapse after leaving a malarious area before a person can safely be accepted as a blood donor. In this study, potential blood donors who had visited areas where malaria was present had the following rates of positive reactions using the IFA antibody method.

1. Within the past 5 years          14.0%
2. More than 5 years                 4.5%

Screening for the presence of malarial parasites can be performed using automated flow cytometry. With this technique, erythrocytes are stained with acridine orange. Mature erythrocytes contain no DNA and do not fluoresce with this stain. Malaria-infected erythrocytes contain DNA and fluoresce.

## Prevention

Current donor standards of the AABB require that travelers be excluded for 6 months after returning from endemic areas and that persons who have had malaria be deferred for 3 years after therapy (refer to Chapter 2 for complete details). A general consensus supports the view that a single infection with *P. falciparum* does not survive in a human host for more than 2 years; *P. vivax* and *P. ovale* usually die out within 3 years. The survival times of *P. falciparum* and *P. vivax* may be longer in persons who live in endemic areas most of their lives, and infections may be delayed in their reappearance in immune carriers. *P. malariae* may exist with or without symptoms for up to 40 or 50 years. The CDC have proposed that the country of birth of the donor be included as part of the oral and written information required from blood donors to facilitate the detection of those who lived for long periods in malarious areas of the world. The 3-year time limit is a compromise. To retain as many donors as possible, the risk of some cases of transfusion malaria has to be accepted in the hope that

the 3-year limit will minimize the occurrence of *P. falciparum* and *P. vivax* infection.

Because the incidence of malaria worldwide and that of transfusion-acquired malaria have increased to the highest level in the past 25 years, careful interviewing of donors supplemented by serologic screening may become necessary in the future. The importance of donor screening for malarial antibodies was recognized in the 1984 recommendation of the Committee of Ministers of the Council of Europe and also in the regulations of the UK National Blood Transfusion Service. An advantage of the wider use of serologic screening lies in the fact that blood donors who might have been rejected because of the mere suspicion of a previous infection may now be accepted. Screening suspected asymptomatic carriers, however, increases the cost of processing donor blood and the volume of laboratory work in donor processing.

## Special Notes

The ideal policy of detecting and excluding parasitized donors is often impossible in areas where malaria is endemic. In one report, the population of one town in Nigeria is nearly 100% parasitized with *Plasmodium,* mostly *falciparum.* In this circumstance, it is impossible to exclude a donor because of malaria except for those with an active infection. To prevent transfusion-induced malaria, chloroquine prophylaxis is given routinely to all blood recipients. This prophylaxis is also given to all postoperative patients since surgery often activates latent malaria and little, if any, chloroquine resistance has been observed in this particular area. However, in areas with drug resistance, routine prophylaxis is withheld and treatment is administered only to patients in whom symptoms appear after transfusion.

The geographic extension of *P. falciparum* strains resistant to chloroquine has been quite rapid since 1960. Resistant strains of *P. falciparum* species have appeared in large areas of Southeast Asia and also in several countries of Central and South America. Protection of recipients of whole blood in these situations depends on the use of sulphadoxine-pyrimethamine or mefloquine.

## Chagas' Disease

### Etiology

*Trypanosoma cruzi (T. cruzi)* is a parasitic blood and tissue protozoan. This organism has an intracellular state in cardiac muscle and other tissues as well as a trypanosome form in the circulating blood. *T. cruzi* is the causative agent of *Chagas' disease* or *American trypanosomiasis.*

### Incidence

More than 12 million people live in areas in which *T. cruzi* is endemic. Chagas' disease is a serious medical and health problem within the endemic belt of the disease, between northern Argentina and southern Mexico. Of the 65 million people who live within this endemic area, at least 20 million are infected with *T. cruzi*. The risk of transmitting the disease in endemic areas of Chile is between 1 and 7%. Although rare, cases of Chagas' disease have been reported in the United States.

The disease is most commonly seen and most severe in children under 5 years. Older children and adults have milder, subacute, or chronic forms, which generally follow an acute attack.

## Transmission

From the southern parts of the United States through Mexico and Central America and as far south as Argentina, various wild rodents, opossums, and armadillos may be infected and capable of producing disease in humans. Infected potential vectors have been shown to exist farther north.

*T. cruzi* develops in a large number of insects, but reduviid bugs are considered the only important vectors. Only those species that invade houses and habitually defecate during the process of feeding or immediately thereafter are major vectors of the human disease. Most cases of Chagas' disease occur in rural and periurban areas where poor housing conditions, combined with the vector's adaptation to human dwellings, influence the persistence of the domestic cycle, which includes the vector living in intimate contact with man and domestic animal reservoirs.

The trypanosomes develop in the hindgut of the insect and are carried in the feces. The parasite is spread into the skin by scratching near the bite where deposits of infective feces are. The disease may also be transmitted congenitally. Blood transfusion is apparently the second most important mechanism of *T. cruzi* transmission. If no prophylactic measures are taken, the risk of receiving contaminated blood depends on the prevalence of the infection among blood donors and the number of transfusions received.

## Signs and Symptoms

Studies of Chagas' disease indicate that this infection induces a strong immune response, which reduces the infection to subclinical levels. But the infection is lifelong, with progression to clinical symptoms, especially in the myocardium.

At the site of infection, the organisms proliferate, producing an erythematous area known as a chagoma. This lesion occurs most frequently on one side of the face but may appear elsewhere on the body. Incubation varies from 4 to 116 days after exposure. Organisms appear in the blood (in small numbers in persons over 1 year) at about 10 days or persist during the acute stage. Clinical symptoms of the acute stage include generalized malaise, chills, high fever, muscular aches and pains, and increasing ex-

haustion. An acute attack may terminate in a few weeks or the patient may enter the chronic stage of the infection. Variable periods of remission may occur. Exacerbations marked by fever and the appearance of trypanosomes in the circulating blood may serve to separate the two stages of the disease, or the chronic phase may be initially asymptomatic. Lymphadenopathy and splenomegaly are common findings.

Drugs are effective in the early stages of infection and cure from 50 to 90% of cases. If treatment is not administered, 5 to 40% of infected persons (depending on geographic area) enter a silent, latent period of 10 or more years. These patients may subsequently develop the clinical manifestations of cardiopathy, megaesophagus, and/or megacolon which characterize the chronic stage of the disease.

## Laboratory Testing

Confirmation of a suspected case of Chagas' disease can be made through direct blood smear examination, blood culture, animal inoculation, or serologic testing for specific IgM antibodies. Trypanosomes are seldom seen in the circulating blood.

Chronic infections can be detected by the presence of antibodies against *T. cruzi*. Procedures include complement fixation, direct agglutination, indirect hemagglutination (IHA), indirect immunofluorescence (IFA), or ELISA tests. A radioimmunoassay (RIA) has been developed for immunologic diagnosis of Chagas' disease in humans.

The Machado test for diagnosis of Chagas' disease is a complement fixation reaction, using as antigen an extract of the spleen of puppies severely infected with *T. cruzi*. This test is used extensively in the endemic areas of South America and gives a high percentage of positive reactions in patients in the chronic stage of the disease. Direct agglutination is a very sensitive method for the diagnosis of acute cases. High sensitivity and reproducibility of the indirect hemagglutination procedure have been demonstrated.

## Prevention

To prevent transmission of *T. cruzi* in countries where the organism is prevalent, serologic tests should be mandatory for blood donors. In nonendemic areas, screening of donors from endemic areas should be conducted.

Immunologic studies have shown that a chronic, asymptomatic *T. cruzi* infection is characterized by common antigens shared by the parasite and the human host. Unfortunately, this has an adverse effect on the development of a protective vaccine.

### Other Parasitic Diseases

In addition to malaria and *T. cruzi,* a variety of parasitic diseases can be acquired through blood transfusion. Two of these diseases, toxoplasmosis (*T. gondii*) and babesiosis (*Babesia* species), are of importance to blood bank technologists.

## Toxoplasmosis (Toxoplasma gondii)

The hazard of transfusion-transmitted toxoplasmosis has been recently recognized in connection with the use of leukocyte concentrates given to patients. Patients at risk are those who are receiving immunosuppressive agents or corticosteroids.

***Etiology.*** *Toxoplasma* has been recognized as a tissue coccidium. *Toxoxplasma gondii* was first discovered in a North African rodent and has been observed in numerous birds and mammals around the world, including humans. It is a parasite of cosmopolitan distribution that is able to develop in a wide variety of vertebrate hosts. The definitive hosts are the domestic cat and certain other feline animals.

***Incidence.*** Human infections are common in many parts of the world. The incidence rates vary from place to place for unknown reasons. The highest recorded rate (93%) occurs in Parisian women who prefer undercooked or raw meat, and a 50% rate of occurrence exists in their children.

***Transmission.*** Domestic cats are the source of the disease, producing oocysts which are present in their feces. Accidental ingestion of oocysts by humans and animals, including the cat, produce a proliferative infection in the body tissues. Fecal contamination of food and water; soiled hands; inadequately cooked infected meat; and raw milk can be important sources of human infection.

All mammals, including humans, can transmit the infection transplacentally. Transplacental transmission usually takes place in the course of an acute but inapparent or undiagnosed maternal infection. In addition to transplacental transmission, transmission by means of tachyzoites in blood transfusion has been observed, and transmission by means of other body fluids is a theoretic possibility.

THE DISEASE CYCLE IN CATS. Reproduction of *T. gondii* takes place in the intestinal epithelium of cats by both schizogony and gametogony, with the resulting oocysts passed in the feces. This is referred to as the enteric cycle. The cat, as well as humans and other animals, may also have the extraintestinal or proliferative forms in the body tissues (tachyzoites and bradyzoites).

THE DISEASE CYCLE IN HUMANS. The proliferative stage in humans and animals produces the parasites as tachyzoites, which are rapidly multiplying forms characteristic of an acute infection. In the slowly multiplying encysted forms characteristic of chronic infections, the parasitic forms are referred to as bradyzoites. Tachyzoites and bradyzoites comprise the extraintestinal or tissue phase of the cycle, which is the only phase known to exist in humans.

In adults and children other than newborn babies, the disease is usually asymptomatic. A generalized infection

probably occurs. When symptoms are seen, they are frequently mild. The disease picture may simulate infectious mononucleosis, with chills, fever, headache, lymphadenopathy, and extreme fatigue. A chronic form of toxoplasmic lymphadenopathy has been described.

*T. gondii* presents a special problem in immunosuppressed or otherwise compromised hosts. Some of these patients have developed reactivation of a latent toxoplasmosis. This has been observed in Hodgkin's and non-Hodgkin's types of lymphoma as well as recipients of organ transplants. Reactivation of cerebral toxoplasmosis is not uncommon in patients with AIDS. Primary infection may be promoted by immunosuppression. This was the case in two cardiac transplant patients who were seronegative before surgery but received organs from donors who had serologic evidence of acute toxoplasma infection.

Symptoms of the disease vary with most patients demonstrating subclinical or nonspecific illness. Although spontaneous recovery follows acute febrile disease, the organism can localize and multiply in any organ of the body or the circulatory system.

***Laboratory Testing.*** Serologic screening for *T. gondii* can be by indirect fluorescent antibody (IFA), hemagglutination (IHA), and enzyme-linked immunosorbent assay (ELISA). Antibodies are demonstrable within the first 2 weeks after infection, rise to high levels early in the infection, and fall slightly but persist at an elevated level for many months before declining to low levels after many years. Absolute diagnosis must be established by biopsy, necropsy, or intraperitoneal inoculation into mice.

***Prevention.*** Screening of blood donors or potential organ donors for *T. gondii* would prevent the transmission of this parasite to immunocompromised patients.

## Babesiosis

Human babesiosis was first recognized and reported in Europe in 1957. Since that time, human infections by *Babesia* have been reported from North America and Europe. Accidental transmission of *Babesia* is now known as a possible consequence of blood transfusion.

***Etiology.*** European cases of human babesiosis have been demonstrated to be caused by *B. divergens (bovis),* a parasite of cattle. The patients diagnosed in Europe had been associated with land grazed on by cattle with babesiosis. Human babesiosis in North America is usually caused by *B. microti,* a parasite of rodents.

***Incidence.*** In all the European cases, babesiosis occurred in persons who had been splenectomized prior to infection. It is likely that the splenectomy affected patient susceptibility to infection and the severity of illness. North American infections have most often occurred in persons with intact spleens. The majority of North American infections have been associated with people living in or visiting the Cape Cod islands of Nantucket, Martha's Vineyard, Shelter Island, or Long Island. Three asymptomatic cases have been reported in Mexico and another from the state of Georgia. One case of babesiosis has been reported in a splenectomized patient in California.

***Transmission.*** *Babesia* are transmitted by various species of ixodid ticks, in which a sexual multiplicative cycle occurs. Feral mice are reservoir hosts of *B. microti*. Most cases of *Babesia* infection occur in late summer and early fall. It is believed that ticks must feed for at least 12 hours before they transmit the infective organisms.

A carrier state is difficult to confirm in immunologically competent adults. It is known, however, that *Babesia* remain infective in blood drawn from donors with subclinical disease after 14 days of storage.

Of the two confirmed cases of transfusion-associated babesiosis in the United States, one patient received 2 units of packed red cells from a donor who had camped on Cape Cod a week before donation. In the second case, a patient with idiopathic thrombocytopenia who had been treated with corticosteroids had a splenectomy. This patient received 20 units of platelet concentrates from 17 donors, one of whom was a summer resident of Nantucket.

***Signs and Symptoms.*** Five of seven European patients infected with *B. divergens (bovis)* died after a rapidly progressive illness characterized by fever, anemia, jaundice, and renal failure. Most cases of babesiosis in North America have occurred in non-splenectomized patients, and the infection has been self-limited, with an incubation period of 1 to 4 weeks. In these cases, the disease was characterized by gradual onset of malaise followed by fever, headache, chills, sweating, arthralgias, myalgias, fatigue, and weakness. The incubation period of *B. microti* varies from 1 to 4 weeks. However, severe and fatal cases have occurred in persons who underwent splenectomy or were treated by corticosteroids and immunosuppressive drugs.

Chloroquine, which has anti-inflammatory properties, provides symptomatic relief in most cases but seems to have no effect on the degree of parasitemia or its duration.

***Laboratory Testing.*** Human infection is diagnosed by identifying the intraerythrocytic parasites in Giemsa-stained blood films. However, blood film examination is not sensitive enough, and the duration of the asymptomatic carrier state is uncertain.

Serologic testing with the indirect immunofluorescent antibody test (IIF) is useful in diagnosis. Specific serologic tests require the *B. microti* antigen, which is not always easily available.

***Prevention.*** The only recognized control measure is to avoid tick-infested areas. Exclusion of febrile donors who have visited endemic areas or those who have an anti-*Babesia* IFA titer of 1:16 or higher may reduce the risk of accidentally transmitted babesiosis.

### Leishmaniasis

In late 1991, blood banks in the United States were asked to defer temporarily members of the military who served overseas in Operation Desert Storm. Seven members of the military who participated in the Gulf War contracted visceral leishmaniasis from the parasite *Leishmania tropica*. Transmission of the parasite typically occurs through the bite of a sandfly.

No cases of transfusion-transmitted *L. tropica* have been documented, but a theoretical risk exists. This is particularly true because no commercially available screening test exists. Approximately five cases have been reported in the literature of transfusion-associated *L. donovani* infection, which suggests that the potential exists for transfusion transmission of *L. tropica* from individuals infected with this parasite.

Individuals who traveled to Saudi Arabia, Kuwait, Iraq, Oman, Yemen, Qatar, and Bahrain were deferred as donors of transfusable blood components from August 1990 until January 1993. However, donors of plasma intended for further manufacture were not similarly deferred.

## TRANSFUSION-ASSOCIATED BACTERIA

Transfusion reactions due to contamination of donated blood by bacteria such as *Staphylococcus* and *Pseudomonas* were not uncommon in the past. Proper collection, refrigerated storage, disposable containers, and a 24-hour expiration time for components collected or processed in an open system has almost eliminated bacterial contamination and growth in blood and blood components. The exception to this situation is the increased incidence of bacterial contamination in platelet concentrates stored for up to 7 days at room temperature.

Transfusion-acquired blood-borne diseases, such as syphilis, are also less of a hazard due to testing of donor blood and refrigeration. Very few cases of transfusion-acquired syphilis have been reported in recent years. Refrigerated blood storage decreases accidental transmission of the microorganism, because *Treponema* has a short survival in stored blood.

### Syphilis

#### Etiology

The etiologic agent of syphilis, *Treponema pallidum (T. pallidum)* is a thin, spiral-shaped bacterium. Following World War II, the reported incidence of early syphilis in the U.S. declined each year until 1958, when the rate once again began to rise progressively.

#### Transmission

*Treponema pallidum* is usually acquired by the venereal route. However, during the first half of this century, syphilis was a major blood-borne infectious disease which was easily transmitted through the prevailing method of direct donor-to-patient blood transfusion. The hazard of transmission of syphilis or of yaws *(Treponema pertenue)* has not disappeared in some tropical countries, where the organization of blood banks is deficient and direct blood transfusion prevails in emergency situations.

## Incidence

Very few cases of transfusion-acquired syphilis have been reported in recent years. Refrigerated blood storage decreases accidental transmission of the microorganism because *Treponema pallidum* has a short survival in stored blood. Spirochetes do not appear to survive in citrated blood at 4° C for more than 72 hours.

## Signs and Symptoms

After a variable incubation period of 10 days to several months, the primary lesion or chancre appears. This begins as a small nodule that enlarges, forming a relatively painless ulcer. Pus is usually absent and the primary lesion heals spontaneously.

The systemic nature of the disease becomes apparent 6 to 8 weeks after the appearance of the initial chancre, when a generalized rash involving both skin and mucous membranes occurs. During this secondary phase, there may be involvement of the central nervous system, eyes, bones, and liver. *T. pallidum* is more likely to be present in the blood during the secondary stage of syphilis, with symptoms of fever, skin rash, and lymphadenopathy. After a period of weeks to months, the lesions of secondary syphilis resolve spontaneously and the individual enters a latent syphilitic phase. In latent syphilis, serologic tests are reactive but clinical signs or symptoms are absent. One third of untreated latent syphilis cases subsequently develop tertiary syphilis, including neurosyphilis.

## Laboratory Testing

The serologic diagnosis of syphilis can be demonstrated with reagin tests or specific treponemal antigen tests. The reagin tests use a nonspecific antigen which is lipid in character. These tests detect IgG or IgM antibodies produced by the infected host as a result of the interaction of lipids from either the host or spirochetes, or both, with the immune system of the host. Reagin tests use as antigens defined mixtures of cardiolipin, cholesterol, and lecithin. Two commercially available reagin tests are the VDRL (developed by the Venereal Disease Research Laboratories) and RPR (rapid plasma reagin). Positive reagin tests for syphilis occur in a number of other diseases including leprosy, systemic lupus erythematosus, and malaria.

Reactive (positive) reagin tests can be confirmed with two specific treponemal antigen tests: the fluorescent treponemal antibody absorption test and microhemagglutination techniques. The fluorescent treponemal antibody absorption test (FTA-ABS) uses as the antigen a killed

suspension of *T. pallidum* spirochetes. The microhemagglutination assay for *T. pallidum* test is based on agglutination by specific antibodies in the patient's serum with sheep erythrocytes sensitized to *T. pallidum* antigen.

## Lyme Disease

Lyme disease may be a potential problem related to blood transfusion. Because the disease is associated with chronic subclinical infections, transfusion-related cases may appear. Donors with a history of Lyme disease should be asymptomatic, and a full regimen of antibiotic therapy must have been completed before donating blood.

## Etiology

Lyme disease is an infectious disease caused by the spirochete *Borrelia burgdorferi;* it is transmitted by certain ixodes ticks that are part of the *I. ricinus* complex. These include *I. dammini* in the northeastern and midwestern United States, *I. pacificus* in the western United States, *I. ricinus* in Europe, and *I. persulcatus* in Asia. The vector has not been identified in Australia. Although ixodid ticks are also indigenous to Africa and South America, it is not clear whether Lyme borreliosis occurs on these continents.

In the United States, the preferred host for both the larval and nymphal states of *I. dammini* is the white-footed mouse, *Peromyscus leucopus.* White-tailed deer, which are not involved in the life cycle of the spirochete, are the preferred host for *I. dammini's* adult stage, and they seem to be critical to tick survival. Ixodes ticks have also been found on at least 30 types of wild animals and 49 species of birds. Illness is not known to develop in wild animals, but clinical Lyme disease does occur in domestic animals, including dogs, horses, and cattle.

Spirochetes are transmitted from the gut of the tick to human skin at the site of a bite, and then migrate outwardly into the skin, causing the unique expanding skin lesion, erythema migrans (EM). Subsequent dissemination of spirochetes to secondary sites may cause major organ system involvement in humans. In dogs, the most common symptom is arthritis.

## Epidemiology

Retrospectively, it appears that the first symptom of Lyme disease was recognized as early as 1908 in Sweden. In the decades that followed, the rash produced by the disease (erythema chronicum migrans—ECM) was noted elsewhere in Europe, as were other symptoms that seemed to follow ECM's eruption. Secondary symptoms such as impairment of the nervous system were described in France and Germany, and again in Sweden. In the United States, the European rash was virtually unknown until 1969, when a case of a physician bitten by a tick while hunting in Wisconsin was reported. Although a few ECM cases were seen in Americans who had traveled to Europe, there were no further American cases until 1975, when physicians at the U.S. Navy base in Groton, Connecticut, reported seeing four patients with a rash similar to EM. At the same time, an epidemiologist at the Connecticut State Department of Health and a rhematologist at Yale were notified of an unusual cluster of cases of arthritis occurring in children in Lyme, Connecticut. It was not until 1982 that Burgdorfer and Barbour isolated a previously unrecognized spirochete, now called *Borrelia burgdorferi,* from *I. dammini* ticks, and Lyme disease became a recognized infectious disease. Eight states—New York, New Jersey, Pennsylvania, Connecticut, Massachusetts, Rhode Island, Wisconsin, and Minnesota—reported 92% of the nation's cases.

## Signs and Symptoms

The CDC case definition for Lyme disease acquired in endemic areas includes the presence of erythema migrans (EM), regardless of serologic results or neurologic, cardiac, or arthritic manifestations characteristic of Lyme disease, and a positive serologic test for antibody to *Borrelia burgdorferi.*

Lyme borreliosis is a multisystem illness that primarily involves the skin, nervous system, heart, and joints. Clinically, this borrelial infection is comparable to syphilis because of its multisystem involvement, occurrence in stages, and mimicry of other diseases. Lyme disease usually begins during the summer months with EM and flu-like symptoms, and may be accompanied by right upper-quadrant tenderness and a mild hepatitis (stage 1). This stage is followed weeks to months later by acute cardiac or neurologic disease in a minority of untreated individuals (stage 2), and then followed by arthritis and chronic neurologic disease (stage 3) in many untreated patients weeks to years after disease onset. There is considerable overlap between these stages, however; Lyme disease is best characterized as an illness that evolves from early to late without reference to an arbitrary staging system. Therefore, a patient may have one or all of the stages, and the infection may not become symptomatic until stage 2 or 3. The majority of affected patients have EM, 1 in 4 manifest arthritis, and neurologic manifestations and cardiac involvement are infrequent.

Cutaneous manifestations can be demonstrated as early (EM), secondary (disseminated lesions and lymphocytoma), and late lesions (acrodermatitis chromica atrophicans). With the exception of the late lesions, cutaneous manifestations generally resolve spontaneously over weeks to months. Several days to weeks after the onset of EM, nearly one-half of untreated patients develop secondary skin lesions. A rare, early manifestation of Lyme disease is borrelia lymphocytomas, a tumor-like, violaceous swelling or nodules at the base of the earlobe or the nipple, caused by a dense lymphocytic infiltrate of the dermis. This lesion occurs at the site of a tick bite. Acrodermatitis chronica atrophicans (ACA) is a late skin manifestation

of Lyme disease that is more prevalent in Europe than the United States.

Lyme carditis occurs in approximately 8% of untreated patients within 2 to 6 weeks following initial infection, and may be the initial manifestation of Lyme disease. Neurologic abnormalities occur in approximately 15% of untreated patients. These manifestations are usually seen 2 to 8 weeks after disease onset, and may include aseptic meningitis, cranial nerve palsies, peripheral radiculoneuritis, and peripheral neuropathy. The predominant symptoms of Lyme meningitis are severe headache and mild neck stiffness, which may fluctuate for weeks after a post–erythema migrans latent period.

Arthralgia and myalgia are common features of early Lyme disease, but frank arthritis during EM is unusual. Ocular manifestations may occur in Lyme disease, and include cranial nerve palsies, optic neuritis, panophthalmitis with loss of vision, and choroiditis with retinal detachment. A uniform pattern of congenital malformations has not been identified in maternal-fetal transmission of Lyme disease.

## Immunologic Manifestations

Specific IgM or IgG antibodies against *B. burgdorferi* are usually not detectable in a patient's serum unless symptoms have been present for at least 2 to 4 weeks. In cases of Lyme arthritis, tests for serum antinuclear antibodies, rheumatoid factor, and the VDRL (venereal disease research laboratories test) are generally negative. However, anti–*B. burgdorferi* antibodies of the IgG type should be present in the serum of patients with Lyme arthritis.

Assays for the detection of antibodies to *B. burgdorferi* are the most practical means of confirming infection. Several commercial antibody test kits, including a recently introduced latex agglutination procedure, are available for verifying *B. burgdorferi* infection. The most common procedures include indirect fluorescent antibody (IFA) staining methods and enzyme-linked immunosorbent assays (ELISA) for total immunoglobulins (Ig) or IgM and IgG antibodies. Immunoblotting techniques can be used, along with ELISA, to characterize immune response and for diagnosis. Western blot analysis can verify reactivity of antibody to major surface or flagellar proteins of *B. burgdorferi.*

The sensitivities of IFA and ELISA methods are usually low during the initial 3 weeks of infection; therefore, negative results are common. The most serious disadvantages of current techniques are low sensitivity and lengthy processing time. In addition, false-positive reactions resulting from cross-reactivity can occur in tests for Lyme disease. For example, tick-borne relapsing fever spirochetes, *Borrelia hermsii,* are closely related to *B. burgdorferi.* Antibodies to *B. hermsii,* an agent that coexists with the Lyme disease spirochete in portions of the western United States, strongly cross-react with *B. burgdorferi* in IFA staining and ELISA testing. Common antigens are shared among the

Borrelia and even with the Treponemes. Serum from syphilitic patients react positively in assays for Lyme disease. Therefore, serologic test results for antibodies to *B. burgdorferi* should be considered along with clinical data and epidemiologic information when evaluating a patient for Lyme disease.

## CHAPTER SUMMARY

A variety of blood-borne diseases can be acquired through transfusion. Methods such as the careful interviewing of blood donors, serologic screening of blood, use of plastic collection bags, and refrigeration have all contributed to a reduction in the accidental transmission of infectious agents, but the possibility of acquiring or reactivating an infectious agent remains a constant danger.

Viral agents, parasitic organisms, and bacteria can be transmitted through blood or blood components. A variety of viral diseases can be transmitted by transfusion. Blood-borne viral diseases include hepatitis B, hepatitis C, cytomegalovirus infection, infectious mononucleosis, and human immunodeficiency syndrome (HIV-1, HIV-2). Two major parasitic infections, malaria and American trypanosomiasis, are the predominating transfusion-acquired parasitic diseases among patients in the Americas. Transfusion-acquired babesiosis has recently been documented in southern New England, and toxoplasmosis is increasingly being recognized as a hazard. Transfusion-acquired bacterial infections, primarily syphilis, have become less of a risk than in the past, but continue to be a problem in underdeveloped countries. Lyme disease may be transmitted by blood.

### Transfusion-Associated Viruses

In the past, hepatitis B was one of the most frequent clinical infections transmitted by blood transfusion. Hepatitis B virus is largely a disease spread by the parenteral route through blood transfusion, needlestick accidents, and contaminated needles, although the virus can be transmitted in the absence of obvious parenteral exposure.

The existence of transfusion-associated hepatitis C has also been established. Transmission of the hepatitis C virus (HCV) is predominantly by the parenteral route.

Cytomegalovirus infection was previously associated with what is now referred to as posttransfusion mononucleosis. Cytomegalovirus is known to cause transfusion-related infections, especially in premature infants, and can be a frequent cause of morbidity and mortality in recipients of organ transplants and patients receiving immunosuppressive chemotherapy.

The Epstein-Barr virus can be transfusion-acquired. Although the virus can produce infectious mononucleosis,

with hepatitis as the most frequent complication, it is an infrequent consequence of blood transfusion and does not cause as much of a problem in blood recipients as does cytomegalovirus.

Over the last several years one of the most publicized transfusion-acquired viruses has been the human T cell leukemia-lymphoma virus, which is also referred to as the HTLV-III, LAV virus, or the human immunodeficiency virus (HIV). Both HIV-1 and HIV-2 are responsible for the clinical disease, acquired immune deficiency syndrome (AIDS). Transmission of HIV is believed to be restricted to contact with body fluids such as blood or seminal fluid. This virus can be transmitted through a parenteral route by transfusion with infected blood. Posttransfusion AIDS is now well documented. Transfusion-associated AIDS is defined as the occurrence of AIDS in persons with no other known risk factor for AIDS and who were transfused with blood or blood components within a minimum of 5 years of the onset of illness. This parvovirus-like virus of humans has been shown to be transmitted in factor VIII concentrates. Transmission of the virus has been demonstrated in concentrates prepared from donor pools, but not from single-donor cryoprecipitate or whole blood.

### Transfusion-Acquired Parasites

Transmission of parasitic infections through blood transfusion is an infrequent occurrence in developed countries. On the North American continent, four diseases can be seen with greater frequency than other parasitic diseases: malaria (plasmodium species), Chagas' disease *(Trypanosoma cruzi),* babesiosis *(Babesia microti),* and toxoplasmosis *(Toxoplasma gondii).* In underdeveloped, primarily tropical countries, a variety of transfusion-acquired parasitic diseases—African sleeping sickness *(Trypanosoma brucei rhodesiense* or *Trypanosoma brucei gambiense), Wuchereria bancrofti,* loa loa, and *Mansonella ozzardi*—have been observed.

### Transfusion-Associated Bacteria

Transfusion reactions due to contamination of donated blood by bacteria such as staphylococcus and pseudomonas were not uncommon in the past. Proper collection, refrigerated storage, and a 24-hour expiration time for components collected or processed in an open system have almost eliminated bacterial contamination and growth in blood and blood components. The exception to this is the increased incidence of bacterial contamination in platelet concentrates stored for up to 7 days at room temperature.

Transfusion-acquired blood-borne diseases, such as syphilis and Lyme disease, are also less a hazard due to testing of donor blood and refrigeration. Very few cases of transfusion-acquired syphilis have been reported in recent years.

## REVIEW QUESTIONS

1. Which of the following is *not a factor* in the acquisition of an infectious disease through blood or blood-component transfusion?
   A. Incidence of the organism or agent in the donor population
   B. ABO group and Rh type of the donor
   C. Pathogenicity of the agent/organism
   D. Physical and immune status of the patient

2. Which of the following infections can be potentially transmitted through blood or blood-component transfusion?
   A. Hepatitis C
   B. AIDS
   C. Malaria
   D. All of the above

3. If a potentially infectious virus is present in a transfusion, actual development of a clinical disorder depends upon all of the following patient-related factors *except:*
   A. Overall susceptibility
   B. Previous exposure to bacterial organisms
   C. Nutritional status
   D. Previous exposure to that particular virus

4. The most cost-effective method of preventing transmission of viral agents by transfusion is:
   A. Serologic screening of donor blood
   B. Chemical treatment of blood and blood components
   C. Physical treatment (e.g., filtering) of blood and blood components
   D. Self-exclusion of high-risk donors through interviewing

5. Hepatitis B accounts for less than _____% of cases of transfusion-acquired hepatitis.
   A. 5
   B. 10
   C. 25
   D. 75

6. Hepatitis C previously accounted for approximately _____% of cases of transfusion-acquired hepatitis.
   A. 20
   B. 40
   C. 60
   D. 80

7-9. Match the following average incubation times (in days) with the appropriate form of hepatitis.
   7. Hepatitis A
   8. Hepatitis B
   9. Hepatitis C
   A. 5
   B. 25
   C. 50

D. 75
E. 150

10. Which form of hepatitis does *not* have a chronic form of the disease?
    A. Hepatitis A
    B. Hepatitis B
    C. Hepatitis C

11. Another name for hepatitis B infection is:
    A. Infectious hepatitis
    B. Serum hepatitis
    C. Australia antigen
    D. Dane particle

12. The most frequent clinical response to hepatitis B virus is:
    A. Jaundice within 75 days
    B. Asymptomatic infection
    C. Subclinical infection
    D. Both B and C

13. The first laboratory screening test of donor blood was for the detection of:
    A. HBc
    B. HBsAg
    C. HBe
    D. Anti-HBe

14. Which surface marker is reliable for the presence of high levels of hepatitis B virus (HBV) and a high degree of infectivity?
    A. HBeAg
    B. HBsAg
    C. HBcAg
    D. Anti-HBsAg

15. The serologic marker during the "window period" of type B hepatitis is:
    A. Anti-HBs
    B. Anti-HBc
    C. Anti-HBe
    D. HBsAg

16. Which of the following is a characteristic of the delta agent?
    A. A DNA virus
    B. Usually replicates only in hepatitis B virus–infected hosts
    C. Infects patients who are HBcAg positive
    D. Frequently found in the United States

17. Which of the following viruses is *rarely* implicated in transfusion-associated hepatitis (TAH)?
    A. Hepatitis A
    B. Hepatitis B
    C. Hepatitis C
    D. Cytomegalovirus

18. Posttransfusion hepatitis is most frequently due to:
    A. Delta agent
    B. Hepatitis C
    C. Hepatitis A
    D. Hepatitis B

19. The specific diagnostic test for hepatitis C is:
    A. Absence of anti-HAV and anti-HBsAg
    B. An increase in serum ALT
    C. Detection of non-A, non-B antibodies
    D. Anti-HCV
20. Surrogate testing for hepatitis C consists of:
    A. HBsAg and ALT
    B. Anti-HBc and ALT
    C. HBsAg and anti-HBc
    D. Anti-HBs and anti-HBc
21. Human cytomegalovirus is classified as a (an) _____ virus.
    A. Herpes
    B. Hepadna
    C. Retrovirus
    D. RNA
22. Transfusion-related cytomegalovirus infections can occur in:
    A. Premature infants
    B. Seronegative patients who have received seropositive organ transplants
    C. Seronegative patients receiving immunosuppressive chemotherapy
    D. All of the above
23. Cytomegalovirus can be assessed in the laboratory by:
    A. Demonstrating inclusion bodies in leukocytes in urinary sediment
    B. A positive heterophil antibody test
    C. The presence of Epstein-Barr antibodies
    D. A positive test for toxoplasma antibodies
24. The presence of antibodies against immediate-early and early CMV antigens is associated with _____ infection.
    A. Chronic
    B. Active
    C. Latent
    D. Carrier state
25. Characteristics of Epstein-Barr virus include(s):
    A. Transfusion-associated malignancy
    B. Transfusion-associated infectious mononucleosis
    C. Transplacental transmission
    D. Both B and C
26. Transfusion-associated Epstein-Barr virus infections have a higher prevalence in:
    A. Infants
    B. Adolescents
    C. Healthy adults
    D. Immunosuppressed patients
27. Which of the following viruses is most frequently detected in blood intended for transfusion in the United States?
    A. HTLV-I
    B. HTLV-II
    C. HIV
    D. Both A and B

28. The immunodeficiency virus (HIV) differs from viruses such as hepatitis because:
    A. CD4+ lymphocytes are depleted
    B. Helper-inducer lymphocytes are depleted
    C. It carries a single, positive-stranded RNA genome
    D. All of the above
29. The mean period (in months) between viral transmission and the development of AIDS symptoms is:
    A. 6
    B. 12
    C. 15
    D. 27
30. First generation tests for HIV screening detect the presence of _____ in a donor.
    A. Antigen
    B. Antibody
    C. Viral capsid
    D. Genome
31. Parvovirus has been shown to be transmitted in:
    A. Whole blood
    B. Red blood cells
    C. Leukocyte concentrates
    D. Factor VIII concentrates
32. This disease-causing parasite is seen with the greatest frequency in North America:
    A. *Trypanosoma brucei rhodesiense*
    B. *Trypanosoma cruzi*
    C. *Trypanosoma brucei gambiense*
    D. *Mansonella ozzardi*
33. The occurrence of transfusion-acquired malaria is _____ in the United States.
    A. Nonexistent
    B. Decreasing
    C. Remaining the same
    D. Increasing
34–35. The multiplication of the _____ phase of malarial parasite takes place in the human _____.
    34.
       A. Sexual
       B. Asexual
    35.
       A. Bloodstream
       B. Intestine
       C. Liver
       D. Salivary glands
       E. Erythrocytes
36. Using the IFA method, _____% of potential donors have a positive reaction within 5 years of leaving an endemic area.
    A. 50
    B. 28
    C. 14
    D. 7

37. *Trypanosoma cruzi* produces:
    A. Chagas' disease
    B. American trypanosomiasis
    C. African sleeping sickness
    D. Both A and B
38. Toxoplasmosis infection has been recognized in conjunction with _____ transfusions.
    A. Whole blood
    B. Red blood cells
    C. Leukocytes
    D. Factor VIII
39. Transfusion-acquired babesiosis has been recognized primarily in:
    A. South America
    B. Central America
    C. North America
    D. Cape Cod
40. One of the most significant reasons for the decrease of transfusion-acquired syphilis is:
    A. Decreased incidence in donors
    B. More sensitive testing methods
    C. Refrigerated blood storage
    D. Better donor interviewing methods
41. Lyme disease is endemic in:
    A. Connecticut
    B. Northwestern Wisconsin
    C. Florida
    D. Both A and B

## Bibliography

Agnello, V., Chung, R.T., and Kaplan, L.M.: A role for hepatitis C virus infection in type II cryoglobulinemia. New Engl. J. Med., *327*(21):1490–1495, 1992.

Ahtone, J., and Maynard, J.E.: Laboratory diagnosis of hepatitis B. JAMA, *249*:2067–2069, 1983.

Aledort, L.M., et al.: Low CD4 + counts in a study of transfusion safety. New Engl. J. Med., *328*(6):441–442, 1993.

Alter, M., et al.: The natural history of community-acquired hepatitis C in the United States. New Engl. J. Med., *327*(27):1899–1905, 1992.

Alter, H.J., and Holland, P.V.: Indirect test to detect the non-A, non-B hepatitis carrier state. Ann. Intern. Med., *101*:859–861, 1984.

Alter, M.J.: Medical news and perspectives. Blood bank officials hope donor altruism will pass new (anti-HCV) test. JAMA, *263*(13):1749–1750, 1990.

Alter, M.J.: Non-A, non-B hepatitis: Sorting through a diagnosis of exclusion. Ann. Int. Med., *110*(8):583–585, 1989.

Arico, S., et al.: Clinical significance of antibody to the hepatitis delta virus in symptomless HBsAg carriers. Lancet, *2*:356–358, 1985.

Bader, T.F., Krawczynski, K., Polish, L.B., and Favorov, M.O.: Hepatitis E in a U.S. traveler to Mexico. New Engl. J. Med., *325*(23):1660, 1991.

Bancroft, W.H.: Hepatitis A vaccine. New Engl. J. Med., *327*(7):488–490, 1992.

Bloch, K.J.: Cryoglobulinemia and hepatitis C virus. N. Engl. J. Med., *327*(21):1521–1522, Nov. 1992.

Brady, M.T.: Cytomegalovirus infections: Occupational risk for health professionals. Am. J. Infect. Cont., *14*(5):197–203, 1986.

Bruce-Chwatt, L.J.: Transfusion-associated parasitic infections. *In* Infection, Immunity, and Blood Transfusion. New York: Alan R. Liss, 1985, pp. 101–125.

Bush, J.L., and Radich, P.C.: The Epstein-Barr virus receptor. Lab. Med., *20*(5):318–322, 1989.

Caredda, F., Spinello, A., and Moroni, M.: Type D (delta) hepatitis. JAMA, *262*(21):2995–2996, 1989.

Castro, K.G., et al.: 1993 revised classification system for HIV infection and expanded surveillance case definition for AIDS among adolescents and adults. MMWR, *41*(RR-17), December 18, 1992.

Centocor Product Bulletin. Uncovering the hidden antigen phase of hepatitis B infection. 1986.

Choi, S., Lagakos, S.W., Schooley, R.T., and Volverding, P.A.: CD4 + lymphocytes are an incomplete surrogate marker for clinical progression in persons with asymptomatic HIV infection taking zidovudine. Ann. Int. Med., *118*(9):674–680, 1993.

Chokephaibulkit, K., Painter, P.C., and Patamasucon, P.: Overview of hepatitis C. Lab. Med., *23*(12):798–806, 1992.

Constantine, N.T., et al.: Concordance of tests to detect antibodies to hepatitis C virus. Lab. Med., *23*(12):807–810, 1992.

Cowan, D.N., et al.: HIV infection among members of the U.S. Army Reserve components with medical and health occupations. JAMA, *265*(21):2826–2830, 1991.

Czaja, A.J.: Chronic hepatitis C virus infection—A disease in waiting? New Engl. J. Med., *327*(27):1949–1950, 1991.

Davis, G.L., Balart, L.A., Schiff, E.R., Lindsay, K., et al.: Treatment of chronic hepatitis C with recombinant interferon alpha. New Engl. J. Med., *321*(22):1501–1506, 1989.

Dobbins, J.G., and Steward, J.A.: Surveillance of congenital cytomegalovirus disease. MMWR, *41*(SS-2):35–44, 433–434, 1992.

Donahue, J.G., et al.: The declining risk of posttransfusion hepatitis C virus infection. New Engl. J. Med., *327*(6):369–373, 1992.

Egan, B.M., and Nordbo, S.A.: Transmission of HCV by organ transplantation. New Engl. J. Med., *326*(6):410–411, 1992.

Ellerbrock, T.V., et al.: Heterosexually transmitted human immunodeficiency virus infection among pregnant women in a rural Florida hospital. New Engl. J. Med., *327*(24):1704–1709, 1992.

Espanol, T., Caragol, I., and Bertran, J.M.: Postnatal transmission of HIV infection. New Engl. J. Med., *326*(9):642, 1992.

Farci, P., et al.: Diagnostic and prognostic significance of the IgM antibody to the hepatitis delta virus. JAMA, *255*:1443–1446, 1986.

Feng, C.S., Williams, I.B., et al.: A comparison of four commercial test kits for detection of cytomegalovirus antibodies in blood donors. Transfusion, *26*(2):203–204, 1986.

Fiesthumel, S., Lentz, E., Arnold, C., McMahon, C., Dock, N., and Laberson, H.W.: Cytomegalovirus (CMV) infection in blood donors: Correlation of serologic markers with viral shedding. Abstract of a paper presented to the 39th Annual American Association of Blood Banks Meeting, October 1986. Transfusion, *26*(6):554, 1986.

Fody, E.P., and Johnson, D.F.: The serologic diagnosis of viral hepatitis. J. Med. Tech., *4*(2):54–58, 1987.

Fowler, K.B., et al.: The outcome of congenital cytomegalovirus infection in relation to maternal antibody status. New Engl. J. Med., *326*(10):663–667, 1992.

Gudino, M., et al.: Exclusion of HTLV-III antibody positive donors does not decrease the number of donors with elevated ALT levels. Abstract of a paper presented to the 39th Annual AABB Meeting, October 1986. Transfusion, *26*(6):551, 1986.

Hegarty, J., and Williams, R.: Chronic hepatitis in the 1980s. Brit. Med. J., *290*:887–878, 1985.

Heneine, W., et al.: HTLV-II endemicity among Guaymi Indians in Panama. New Engl. J. Med., *324*(8):565, 1991.

Henle, W., and Henle, G.: Epstein-Barr virus and blood transfusions. *In* Infection, Immunity, and Blood Transfusion. New York: Alan R. Liss, 1985, pp. 201–209.

Hollard, P.V., et al.: Anti-HTLV-III testing of blood donors: Reproducibility and confirmability of commercial test kits. Transfusion, (25):395, 1985.

Hoofnagle, J.H.: Type A and Type B hepatitis. Lab. Med., *14*(11): 705–716, 1983.

Ito, S., et al.: Clinical value of the Guanas screening test in donor blood for prevention of posttransfusion non-A, non-B hepatitis. Hepatology, *8*(2):383–384, 1988.

Janssen, R.S., et al.: HIV infection among patients in U.S. acute care hospitals. New Engl. J. Med., *327*(7):445–452, 1993.

Johnson, B., Brown, J.H., and Yoedino, R.L., et al.: Transfusion malaria: Serologic identification of infected donors. MMWR, *32*:222–229, 1983.

J. of Am. Med. Assoc.: The risk of contracting HIV infection in the course of health care. *265*(14):1872–1873, 1991.

Kelen, G.D., et al.: Hepatitis B and hepatitis C in emergency department patients. New Engl. J. Med., *326*(21):1399–1404, 1992.

Khabbaz, R.F., et al.: Seroprevalence of HTLV-I and HTLV-II among intravenous drug users and persons in clinics for sexually transmitted diseases. New Engl. J. Med., February 6, 1992, pp. 375–380.

Khabbaz, R.F., et al.: Seroprevalence and risk factors for HTLV-I/II infection among female prostitutes in the United States. JAMA, *263*(1):60–64, 1990.

Khan, N.C., and Hollinger, F.B.: Non-A, non-B hepatitis agent. Lancet, *1*:41, 1986.

Killian, C.S.: Prevalence of cytomegalovirus antibodies in blood donors. Lab. Med., *19*(2):103–105, 1989.

Kleinman, S., Busch, M., and Holland, P.: Post-transfusion hepatitis C virus infection. New Engl. J. Med., *327*(22):1601, 1992.

Kline, W.E., Schuller, R., and Bowman, R.J.: Comparison of assays for detecting anti-HBcAg. Abstract of paper presented to the 39th Annual American Association of Blood Banks Meeting, October 1986. Transfusion, *26*(6):552, 1986.

Kline, W.E., Bowman, R.J., Sandler, S.G., et al.: Anti-HBcAg screening in blood donors: Test performance and potential impact on the blood supply. Abstract of paper presented to the 39th Annual American Association of Blood Banks Meeting, October 1986. Transfusion, *26*(6):552, 1986.

Koff, W.C., and Hoth, D.F.: Development and testing of AIDS vaccines. Science, *241*:426–432, 1988.

Koot, M., et al.: Prognostic value of HIV-1 syncytium-inducing phenotype for rate of CD4 + cell depletion and progression to AIDS. Ann. Int. Med., *118*(9):674–680, 1993.

Koziol, D.E., et al.: Antibody to hepatitis B core antigen as a paradoxical marker for non-A, non-B hepatitis agents in donated blood. Ann. Int. Med., *104*:488–495, 1986.

Koziol, D.E., et al.: Antibody to hepatitis B core antigen as a paradoxical marker for non-A, non-B hepatitis agents in donated blood. Ann. Int. Med., *104*:488–495, 1986.

La Brecque, D.R.: Viral hepatitis and chronic hepatitis. *In* Internal Medicine (3rd ed.), Jay Stein (Ed.). Boston: Little, Brown, 1989, pp. 478–487.

Lamberson, H.V.: Cytomegalovirus (CMV): The agent, its pathogenesis, and its epidemiology. *In* Infection, Immunity, and Blood Transfusion. New York: Alan R. Liss, 1985, pp. 149–173.

Lemon, S.M.: Type A viral hepatitis. New developments in an old disease. New Engl. J. Med., *313*:1059–1067, 1985.

Lombardo, J.M.: HIV-1 testing: An overview. Am. Cl. Prod. Rev., November 1987, pp. 10, 12–18.

Lurie, P., et al.: Undiagnosed HIV infection in acute care hospitals. New Engl. J. Med., *327*(25):1815–1816, 1992.

Markell, E.K., et al.: *In* Medical Parasitology (6th ed.). Philadelphia: Saunders, 1986, pp. 112–117, 131–138.

Martinez, S., et al.: Heterosexual transmission of HIV—Puerto Rico, 1981–1991. MMWR, *41*(48):899, 905, 1992.

Marwick, C., and Skolnick, A.: Medical News and Perspectives. Research seems to be gaining upper hand on what's been called non-A, non-B hepatitis. JAMA, *263*(1):14, 1990.

McLeod, G., and Hammer, S.M.: Zidovudine: Five years later. Ann. Int. Med., *117*(6):487–501, 1992.

Miles, S.A., et al.: Rapid serologic testing with immune-complex-dissociated HIV p24 antigen for early detection of HIV infection in neonates. New Engl. J. Med., *328*(5):297–302.

Misiani, R., et al.: Hepatitis C virus infection in patients with essential mixed cryoglobulinemia. Ann. Int. Med., *117*(7):573–577, 1992.

Miyoshi, I., et al.: Excretion of HTLV-I in saliva. JAMA, *267*(2): 236, 1992.

Mori, M., et al.: Monoclonal proliferation of T cells containing Epstein-Barr virus in fatal mononucleosis. New Engl. J. Med., *327*(1):58, 1992.

Mosley, J.W., Aach, R.D., Hollinger, F.B., Stevens, C.E., et al.: Non-A, non-B hepatitis and antibody to hepatitis C virus. JAMA, *263*(1):77–78, 1990.

Murph, J.R., et al.: The occupational risk of cytomegalovirus infection among day-care providers. JAMA, *265*(5):603–608, 1991.

Musianim, M., et al.: Serological screening for the prevention of transfusion-acquired cytomegalovirus infections. J. Infection, *9:* 148–152, 1984.

Nath, N., Wilkinson, S., and Dodd, R.Y.: Use of a control serum containing a low level of HBsAg for monitoring proficiency in screening for HBsAg. Transfusion, *26*(6):519–524, 1986.

Nelson, K., et al.: Transmission of retroviruses from seronegative donors by transfusion during cardiac surgery. Ann. Int. Med., *117*(7):554–559, 1992.

Nicholson, K.G.: Hepatitis delta infections. Brit. Med. J., *290:* 1370–1371, 1985.

Nightingale, S.L.: CMV-IGIV. JAMA, *264*(2):168, 1990.

Noall, R., Williams, A., et al.: Inconsistent anti-HBc assay results in blood donors. Abstract of paper presented to the 39th Annual American Association of Blood Banks Meeting, October 1986. Transfusion, *26*(6):552, 1986.

O'Brien, T.R., George, J.R., Epstein, J.S., Holmberg, S.D., and Schochetman, G.: Testing for antibodies to human immunodeficiency virus type 2 in the United States. MMWR, *41*(RR-12): July 17, 1992.

Osmond, D.H., et al.: Risk factors for hepatitis C virus seropositivity in heterosexual couples. JAMA, *269*(3):361–365, 1993.

Overby, L.R.: Challenges and opportunities in biotechnology. *In* Infection, Immunity, and Blood Transfusion. New York: Alan R. Liss, 1985, pp. 425–443.

Pantaleo, G., Graziosi, C., and Fauci, A.S.: The immunopathogenesis of human immunodeficiency virus infection. New Engl. J. Med., *328*(5):327–335, 1993.

Papsidero, L., et al.: Acquired immune deficiency syndrome: Detection of viral exposure and infection. American Clinical Products Review, Octoer 1986, pp. 17–23.

Pate, E.J., et al.: Lack of viral latency of human T-cell lymphotropic virus type I. New Engl. J. Med., *325*(4):284, 1991.

Peetoom, F., and the Cooperative Study Group: Use of an enzyme immunoassay for detection of antibody to human immunodeficiency virus in low-risk populations. Transfusion, *26*(6):591, 1986.

Pereira, B.J.G., et al.: Prevalence of hepatitis C virus RNA in organ donors positive for hepatitis C antibody and in the recipients of their organs. New Engl. J. Med., *327*(13):910–915, 1992.

Phair, J.P.: Estimating prognosis in HIV-1 infection. Ann. Int. Med., *118*(9):742–743, 1993.

Quinnan, G.V., et al.: Inactivation of human T-cell lymphotropic virus, type III by heat, chemical, and irradiation. Transfusion, *26*(5):481, 1985.

Randhawa, P., et al.: Expression of Epstein-Barr virus-encoded small RNA (by the EBER-1 gene in liver specimens from transplant recipients with post-transplantation lymphoproliferative disease. N. Engl. J. Med., *327*(24):1701–1704, 1992.

Rizzetto, M., and Verme, G.: Delta hepatitis—present status. J. Hepatology, *1*:187–193, 1985.

Roth, D., et al.: Detection of hepatitis C virus infection among cadaver organ donors: Evidence for low transmission of disease. Ann. Int. Med., *117*(6):470–475, 1992.

Ruef, C., et al.: Update: HIV-2 infection—United States. JAMA, *262*(12):1579, 1583, 1989.

Schiff, E. (Ed.): Hepatitis forum. North Chicago: Abbott Laboratories, September 1987.

Schmunis, G.A.: Chagas' disease and blood transfusion. *In* Infection, Immunity, and Blood Transfusion. New York: Alan R. Liss, 1985, pp. 127–145.

Seto, B., et al.: Detection of reverse transcriptase activity in association with the non-A, non-B hepatitis agent(s). Lancet, *2*:941–943, 1982.

Stevens, C.E., Taylor, P.E., Pidyck, J., Choo, Q.-L., et al.: Epidemiology of hepatitis C virus. JAMA, *263*(1):49–53, 1990.

Surveillance Branch, Divison of HIV/AIDS, National Center for Infectious Diseases, Centers for Disease Control and Prevention. The Second 100,000 cases of acquired immunodeficiency syndrome—United States, June 1981–December 1991. MMWR, *41*(2):28–29, 1992.

Tarleton, R.L., et al.: Diagnosis of Chagas's disease in humans using a biotin-$^3$H-avidin radioimmunoassay. Am. J. Trop. Med. Hygiene, *33*:34–40, 1984.

Taswell, H.F., Reisner, R.K., et al.: Comparison of three methods for detecting antibody to cytomegalovirus. Transfusion, *26*(3):285–289, 1986.

Tegtmeier, G.E.: Cytomegalovirus and blood transfusion. *In* Infection, Immunity, and Blood Transfusion. New York: Alan R. Liss, 1985, pp. 175–199.

Testing Donors of Organs, Tissues, and Semen for Antibody to Human T-Lymphotropic Virus Type III/Lymphadenopathy-Associated Virus. MMWR, *34*(20):294, 1985.

Turgeon, M.L.: Immunology and Serology in Laboratory Medicine. St. Louis, C.V. Mosby, 1990, pp. 212–220.

U.S. Public Health Service (draft). Guidelines for prevention of transmission of HIV through transplantation of human tissue and organs. Centers for Disease Control and Prevention, Atlanta, GA, March 8, 1993.

Van Der Poel, C.L., Reesink, H.W., Schaasberg, W., Leentvaar-Kuypers, A., et al.: Infectivity of blood seropositive for hepatitis C virus antibodies. Lancet, *335*:558–560, 1990.

Vermund, S.H., Hoover, D.R., and Chen, K.: CD4+ counts in seronegative homosexual men. New Engl. J. Med., *328*(6):442, 1993.

Ward, J.W., Janssen, R.S., and Jaffe, H.W.: Recommendations for HIV testing services for inpatients and outpatients in acute care hospital settings. MMWR, *42*(RR-2):1–6, 1993.

Weiner, A.J., Juo, G., Bradley, D.W., Bonino, F., et al.: Detection of hepatitis C viral sequences in non-A, non-B hepatitis. Lancet, *335*:1–3, 1990.

Wheeler, D.L.: AIDS virus now believed to copy itself throughout course of disease. Ch. Higher Ed., March 31, 1993, p. A9.

White, J.H., et al.: Prevalence of cytomegalovirus antibody in subjects between the ages of 6 and 22 years. J. Infect. Dis., *159*:1013–1017, 1989.

Whitley, R.J., and Gnann, J.W., Jr.: Acyclovir: A decade later. New Engl. J. Med., *327*(11):782–789, 1992.

Wyler, D.J.: Malaria—resurgence, resistance and research. New Engl. J. Med., *308*:875–878, 1983.

Yomtovian, R.: From ABO to HTLV—changing trends in blood transfusion safety. Minnesota Medicine, *68*:587–589, 1985.

Yow, M.D., and Demmler, G.J.: Congenital cytomegalovirus disease—20 years is long enough. New Engl. J. Med., *326*(10):702–703, 1992.

Zarvan, B.S., Hibbard, A.J., Becker, G., and Davis, J.P.: False-positive serologic tests for human T-cell lymphotropic virus type I among blood donors following influenza vaccination, 1992. JAMA, *269*(16):2076–2078, 1993.

Zijlmans, J.M., et al.: Epstein-Barr virus-associated lymphoma in a patient with rheumatoid arthritis treated with cyclosporine. New Engl. J. Med., *326*(20):1364, 1992.

Zuck, T.F., Sherwood, W.C., and Bove, J.R.: Will the real hepatitis C stand up? Lancet, August 5, 1989, pp. 307–308.

Zuckerman, A.J.: The elusive hepatitis C virus. Brit. Med. J., *299*:871–872, 1989.

Part **V**

# Procedures in Blood Banking

# Routine Blood Banking Procedures

At the conclusion of this chapter, the reader should be able to:

- Cite the most frequent source of pretesting error.
- Describe how systematic errors can be eliminated in blood banking.
- Name at least five possible causes of technical errors that can produce false positive or false negative results.
- Describe the safety techniques that should be adhered to in laboratory practice.
- Describe the proper type of specimen, necessary reagents, quality control steps, calculation of applicable results, reference values, sources of error, and clinical applications for each procedure described in this chapter.
- Prepare the necessary reagents and perform the stated procedure.

## Chapter Outline

## GENERAL CONSIDERATIONS IN BLOOD BANK TESTING

The procedures in Chapters 14 and 15 are presented in a format that is consistent with the guidelines set forth by the National Committee for Clinical Laboratory Standards (NCCLS). This format includes:

1. Procedure title and specific method
2. Test principle, including type of reaction and the clinical reasons for the test
3. Specimen collection and preparation
4. Reagents, supplies, and equipment
5. Quality control
6. Procedure
7. Calculations
8. Reporting results
9. Procedure notes, including sources of error, clinical applications, and limitations
10. References

### Accuracy in Pretesting

To eliminate the *most* frequent source of pretesting error, a patient must be positively identified when a blood specimen is obtained. This specimen must be properly collected and labelled (see Chapter 2 for a complete discussion of patient specimen collection and identification). Hemolyzed specimens should not be used for testing.

Blood and blood components must also be correctly collected, labelled and stored (see Chapters 2 and 10 for a complete discussion of collection and storage of blood and blood products).

### Accuracy in Blood Bank Testing

Inaccuracies in testing can be systematic or sporadic. Systematic errors can be eliminated by a continuing quality assurance program that monitors equipment, reagents, and other factors.

The manufacturer's directions for the use of reagent antisera and cells must be followed precisely. For each new lot, package inserts should be saved and the directions reviewed because changes are occasionally introduced. Reagents should be checked for turbidity or an abnormal appearance at each time of use. Contaminated reagents can produce erroneous results.

Test protocols must be *strictly* followed. Techniques such as the sequence of addition of test cells or serum and the time and temperature of incubation must be exact. Sporadic or isolated errors in technique can produce false-positive and/or false-negative results. Other possible causes of technical errors are listed as follows:

Possible causes of false-positive errors:

1. Addition of the wrong antiserum to a test tube
2. Overcentrifugation of a serum-cell mixture
3. Dirty glassware
4. Hemolyzed patient serum or reagent RBCs
5. Inadequate dispersal of centrifuged serum-cell mixture

Possible causes of false-negative errors:

1. Omitting patient or donor serum from the test mixture
2. Omitting antiserum from the test mixture
3. Failure to identify hemolysis of red blood cells by the patient's serum as a positive reaction
4. Inappropriately warming a cell-serum mixture
5. Undercentrifugation of a serum-cell mixture
6. Vigorous shaking of a centrifuged serum-cell mixture

Possible causes of false-positive *or* false-negative errors:

1. Incorrect labeling of test tubes
2. Addition of the wrong antiserum
3. Erroneous reading or interpretation of results
4. Inaccurate recording of results
5. Contamination of antiserum or reagent red cells
6. An inaccurate serum-cell ratio in a test mixture

### Safety in Blood Bank Testing

All specimens should be treated with caution. During the testing of specimens and the handling of blood specimens or blood products, disposable gloves should be worn. Other precautions such as disinfection of work areas and equipment, consistent with the Universal Blood and Body Fluid Precautions (see Chapter 1) must be followed.

## ANTIBODY SCREENING (INDIRECT ANTIGLOBULIN OR INDIRECT COOMBS TEST)

### Principle

The antibody screening test is a qualitative test for the detection of unexpected antibodies in a recipient or donor serum. Serum from patients (surgical, obstetrical) or from blood donors is tested with group O reagent red blood cells from individual donors that represent a variety of the most common blood group antigens.

Detection of an antibody is dependent on the method, medium, and temperature of reactivity as well as the titer of the antibody. Methods approved for unexpected anti-body testing include saline, albumin, low-ionic strength saline (LISS), polyethylene glycol (PEG) and low-ionic Polybrene (LIP) procedures. Enzyme techniques are more appropriate for antibody identification.

Hemolysis or agglutination of reagent red blood cells in the presence of serum at any stage of the test demonstrates the presence of an antibody (a positive test) with specificity to a corresponding antigen on the reagent red blood cells. The absence of hemolysis and/or agglutination indicates that the serum being tested does not contain detectable antibodies directed at antigens present on the reagent red cells being used. Preliminary specificity of an antibody can be established using two or three screening cells; however, the exact specificity of an antibody or antibodies can only be established by further testing with an additional panel of reagent red cells and by comparing the reaction patterns with the known antigens of the panel.

A positive reaction indicates that an antibody is present in the serum being tested. If the antibody is not an autoantibody, a specific blood group antibody directed toward an antigenic determinant that is absent from the patient's own erythrocytes may have been produced as a result of previous transfusions or pregnancies. Infrequently, an antibody may be present that reacts with all red cells tested, including the patient's own cells. This pattern of reactivity is typical of acquired hemolytic anemia.

### Specimen

No special preparation of the patient is required prior to specimen collection. The patient must be positively identified when the specimen is collected. The specimen shall be labeled at the bedside and shall include the patient's first and last name, the date the specimen is collected, and the patient's hospital identification number. The time of collection and the phlebotomist's initials should be written on the required form.

Blood should be drawn by an aseptic technique and the specimen tested as soon as possible. The required specimens are 5–7 mL of clotted blood (red top) evacuated tube and 7 mL of EDTA blood (lavender top) evacuated tube. The presence of hemolysis in the specimen makes the specimen unsuitable for testing.

Antibodies that depend on the binding of complement for their detection may not be detected if aged serum or plasma from an anticoagulated sample are used for anti-body detection testing. Samples for antibody screening may be used up to 72 hours after collection. The specimen must be stored at 1° C to 6° C and kept for 7 days.

### Reagents, Supplies, and Equipment

10 × 75 mm disposable test tubes
Disposable pipettes, 4⅝ inch plastic or Pasteur
Normal saline (0.9%)
Bovine Albumin[1] (Optional)

LISS Additive[1] (Optional)   Prepare by adding 1.75 g NaCl and 18 g glycine to a 1 L volumetric flask. Add 20 mL of phosphate buffer prepared by combining 11.3 mL of 0.15 M $KH_2PO_4$ and 8.5 mL of 0.15 M Na $H_2PO_4$. Add distilled $H_2O$ to the 1 L mark. Adjust pH to 6.7 with NaOH. Add 0.5 g sodium azide as a preservative.

Antiglobulin reagent antisera[1]

Coombs control or check cells (IgG-sensitized cells)[1]

Reagent red blood cells I[1]

Reagent red blood cells II[1]

Patient requisition and patient cumulative cards

Centrifuge

37° C waterbath or heat block

Test-tube rack

High-intensity lamp/optical magnifying lens

Microscope (optional)

## Quality Control

The test reagents should be monitored daily or at the time of use, as described in Chapter 1, and according to the Quality Control Procedure.

An auto-control, a mixture of patient's erythrocytes and serum, may be tested simultaneously with each antibody screening test.

All negative antiglobulin reactions must be tested with Coombs control/check cells. A positive test result at this point will confirm that active antiglobulin was added to the test system and was present when the original antiglobulin test was interpreted as negative. If a positive result is *not* obtained with the control cells, the test is invalid and must be repeated.

## Procedure:

### *Preliminary*

1. Compare information on specimen to request form: first and last name, full hospital number, and date. If this information is *not identical,* obtain a new specimen.
2. Prepare a 2–4% suspension of patient's red cells (see preparation of red cell suspension).
3. Centrifuge the clotted specimen for 5 minutes at 2500 rpm.
4. Determine if the patient has been previously tested by checking records in cumulative patient file.

### *Antibody Screening*

1. Label three 10 × 75 mm test tubes:
   a. I
   b. II
   c. AUTO (optional)
2. Using a disposable pipette, add 2 drops of the patient's serum to each tube.

[1] Should be refrigerated when not in use.

3. Add 2 drops of bovine albumin to each tube (optional).
4. Add 1 drop of reagent red blood cells I to the tube labeled I and 1 drop of reagent red blood cells II to the tube labeled II.
5. Add 1 drop of the patient red cell suspension to the tube labeled AUTO (optional).
6. Mix all tubes and centrifuge for 15 sec at 3400 RPM.
7. Gently resuspend the cells in all three tubes and examine macroscopically for agglutination or hemolysis. Record the results as immediate spin (IS) reactions. Positive reactions should be graded from 1 to 4 + at each stage of observation (see Grading of Agglutination). Complete hemolysis precludes further testing and must be interpreted as a positive result. If partial hemolysis is observed, record and proceed. All positive and negative tests should be continued through all phases of testing.
8. Incubate all tubes for 30 to 60 min at 37° C.
9. Centrifuge all the tubes for 15 sec at 3400 rpm.
10. Gently resuspend the cells in all tubes and examine macroscopically for agglutination or hemolysis. Record results as 37° C reactions.
11. Wash each tube 3 times. Decant completely after the last wash.
12. Add 2 drops of antiglobulin (AHG) reagent to each tube.
13. Mix each tube and centrifuge for 15 sec at 3400 rpm.
14. Gently resuspend the cells and examine macroscopically with the aid of magnification (microscopic examination is optional. Record results as antiglobulin (AHG) reactions.
15. To each tube that exhibits no agglutination, add 1 drop of Coombs check cells. Mix well and centrifuge for 15 sec at 3400 rpm. Resuspend the cells and examine macroscopically for agglutination. Record these results as control cells (CC).

## (Alternate Method) LISS Modification

1. Label 10 × 75 mm test tubes:
   a. I
   b. II
2. Wash reagent red blood cells three times in normal saline. Completely decant saline after the last wash. Resuspend the reagent red blood cells to a 2% suspension in LISS.
3. Using a disposable pipette, add 2 drops of the patient's serum to each tube.
4. Add 1 drop of the LISS suspended reagent red blood cells I to the tube labeled I and one drop of reagent red blood cells II to the tube labeled II.
5. Mix and incubate all tubes for 10 to 15 min at 37° C.
6. Centrifuge all the tubes for 15 sec at 3400 rpm.
7. Gently resuspend the cells in all tubes and examine macroscopically for agglutination or hemolysis.

Record the results. Positive reactions should be graded from 1 to 4+ at each stage of observation (see Grading of Agglutination). Complete hemolysis precludes further testing and must be interpreted as a positive result. If partial hemolysis is observed, record and proceed. All positive and negative tests should be continued through all phases of testing.

8. Wash each tube three times. Decant completely after the last wash.

9. Add 2 drops of antiglobulin (AHG) reagent to each tube.

10. Mix each tube and centrifuge for 15 sec at 3400 rpm.

11. Gently resuspend the cells and examine macroscopically with the aid of magnification (microscopic examination is optional).

12. To each tube that exhibits no agglutination add 1 drop of Coombs check cells. Mix well and centrifuge for 15 sec at 3400 rpm. Resuspend the cells and examine macroscopically for agglutination. Record these results as control cells (CC).

### Reporting Results

Agglutination or hemolysis of any screening cell suspension in the immediate-spin, 37° C, or antiglobulin (AHG) phase indicates a positive reaction. The absence of hemolysis or agglutination constitutes a negative test and indicates the absence of detectable antibodies to specific antigens present on the reagent erythrocytes.

If a pattern of positive and negative reactions is observed with one of the two reagent erythrocytes, antibody identification can be simplified by eliminating antibodies specific for antigens present on the nonreactive cell (see Chapter 6 for the technique of preliminary antibody identification). If one or both reagent screening cells is/are positive, a panel of reagent red cells should be tested to identify the unexpected antibody.

If the autocontrol demonstrates a positive reaction, the serum contains an autoantibody. The presence of an autoantibody can conceal an underlying alloantibody in the serum. Autoabsorption (see sections on absorption of cold and warm agglutinins in Chapter 14) may be required to test the serum for the presence of unexpected antibodies.

If the patient has been recently transfused, a mixed-field reaction in the autocontrol suggests that an unexpected antibody directed at an antigen present on surviving donor cells is present.

### Procedure Notes

Because some antibodies exhibit dosage, practitioners may prefer to use three reagent screening cells instead of two. The use of three cells allows for a greater variety of antigens, particularly cells having homozygous expression of certain antigens. In other cases, one pooled reagent erythrocyte screening cell is used in place of the two or three individual donor reagent erythrocytes. Pooled screening cells do not provide optimum sensitivity for antibody detection and cannot be used when screening potential blood recipients. However, pooled reagent erythrocytes are acceptable for antibody screening tests on blood donors.

The basic screening cell procedure can be modified with enhancement media, such as albumin, enzymes, polybrene (hexadimethrine bromide), or low ionic strength (LISS). If albumin is used as an enhancer, the reactivity of low-titered antibodies may be increased by washing the reagent erythrocytes once with normal saline, decanting the saline completely, and using the "dry button" of cells for the test. If using a LISS additive procedure, the serum volumes should be added according to the manufacturer's directions.

In the absence of hemolysis in the pretest specimen or due to bacterial or chemical contamination, hemolysis may demonstrate that an antigen-antibody reaction has occurred. With the exception of the ABO antibodies that are not detected using group O screening erythrocytes, antibodies capable of producing hemolysis have specificities for the P, Lewis, Kidd, or Vel blood group systems.

### Limitations

The detection of antibodies in serum can be compromised if the ratio of serum to cells in the test or the length of incubation is incorrect. Failure to detect alloantibodies in a serum can result from:

1. Low-titered antibodies that are too weak to be detected by the test methods and/or media being used.
2. An antibody that may be exhibiting a dosage effect.
3. The lack of an antigen on the screening cells to an antibody in the serum.
4. The lack of complement in the test system, e.g., use of plasma or aged serum, which prevents the detection of complement-dependent antibodies.

In rare cases, the presence of an antibody directed at one of the antibiotics in the reagent red cell suspending medium may cause false-positive reactions. Antibodies to both neomycin and chloramphenicol have been reported. False-negative reactions can result from as little as 1/10,000 of a drop of the original serum remaining after cell washing. This produces some neutralization of antiglobulin reagent.

## BLOOD GROUPING AND TYPING

### ABO Blood Grouping (Forward Typing)

#### Principle

The ABO blood groups (A, B, AB, and O) represent the antigens expressed on the erythrocytes of each group.

When an antibody and its corresponding antigen are combined in vitro, clumping of the erythrocytes expressing the antigen results. An antibody and its corresponding antigen are not normally present in the same blood specimen.

Human erythrocytes expressing either A or B antigens agglutinate in the presence of reagent antisera containing IgM anti-A or anti-B. Thus, anti-A will agglutinate all erythrocytes expressing the A antigen; anti-B will agglutinate all erythrocytes containing the B antigen. Determination of ABO grouping is important in pretransfusion studies of patients and donors as well as in specialized cases such as obstetric patients.

## Specimen

No special preparation of the patient is required before specimen collection. The patient must be positively identified when the specimen is collected. The specimen must be labelled at the bedside and the label must include the patient's first and last name, the date when the specimen is collected, and the patient's hospital identification number. The time of collection and the phlebotomist's initials should be written on the required form.

Blood should be drawn by an aseptic technique and the specimen should be tested as soon as possible. Approximately 5 to 7 mL of blood should be collected in a plain (red top) evacuated tube or the specimen may be collected in an EDTA (lavender top) evacuated tube. Newborn or infant samples may be collected in pediatric blood specimen containers or as red cells in normal saline. Cord blood specimens are also appropriate. In forensic laboratories, other types of specimens may be used.

The blood sample should be tested as soon as possible. If a delay in testing is necessary, the blood should be refrigerated.

## Reagents, Supplies and Equipment

Commercial blood grouping antisera:
Anti-A, Anti-B, and Anti-A,B
10 × 75 mm disposable test tubes
Normal saline (0.9% NaCl)
Disposable pipettes, $4\frac{5}{8}''$ plastic or Pasteur
High intensity lamp/optical magnifying lens
Centrifuge

## Quality Control

Reagent antisera should be tested daily with erythrocytes of known antigenicity (see Daily Reagent Quality Assurance, this chapter).

## Procedure

1. Check the patient's name and identification numbers on the blood specimen and requisition.
2. Prepare a 2 to 4% suspension of the patient's red cells in normal saline (see Preparation of Red Cell Suspensions, this chapter).
3. Label three 10 × 75 mm test tubes—one with the letter A, another with the letter B, and a third with A,B.
4. To the tube labeled A, add 1 drop of anti-A antiserum.
5. To the tube labeled B, add 1 drop of anti-B antiserum.
6. To the tube labeled A,B, add 1 drop of anti-A,B antiserum.
7. Using a disposable pipette, add 1 drop of the cell suspension to each of the test tubes.
8. Mix well and centrifuge the test tubes for 15 seconds at 3400 rpm.
9. Resuspend the cells with gentle agitation and examine macroscopically for agglutination (see Grading Agglutination Reactions, this chapter).

## Reporting Results

Agglutination of erythrocytes with a specific antiserum is interpreted as a positive (+) test result and indicates the presence of the corresponding antigen. No agglutination of the erythrocytes produces a negative (0) test indicating that the corresponding antigen is not present.

The various agglutination patterns and their respective interpretations are presented in Table 14-1.

## Procedure Notes

Each manufacturer provides, with each package of antiserum, detailed instructions for the use of anti-A and anti-B. These directions vary in details; therefore, it is important to follow the directions for the specific antiserum in use.

Procedures that apply to all tests for ABO grouping include the following:

1. Do not rely on the color of dyes to identify reagent antisera. All tubes must be properly labelled.
2. Do not perform tests at temperatures higher than room temperature (20 to 24° C).
3. Perform observations of agglutination with a well-lighted background, not a warm viewbox.
4. Record results immediately after observation.
5. Remember that contaminated blood specimens, reagents, or supplies may interfere with the test results.

**Table 14-1. Reactions of Patient Erythrocytes and Known Antisera**

| Anti-A | Anti-B | Anti-A,B | Interpretation Blood Group |
|---|---|---|---|
| 0 | 0 | 0 | O |
| + | 0 | + | A |
| 0 | + | + | B |
| + | + | + | AB |
| 0 | 0 | + | Weak subgroup of group A |

If a patient has been recently transfused with nongroup-specific blood, mixed-field agglutination may be observed. If large quantities of nongroup-specific blood have been transfused, determination of the correct ABO grouping may be impossible. Discrepancies in forward typing can result from conditions such as weak antigens, altered expression of antigens due to disease, chimerism, or excessive blood group substances. Excess amounts of blood group specific soluble substances present in the plasma in certain disorders, for example carcinoma of the stomach and pancreas, neutralize the reagent anti-A or anti-B, leaving no unbound antibody to react with the patient's erythrocytes. This excess of blood group specific substance produces a false-negative or weak reaction in the forward grouping. If the patient's erythrocytes are washed with saline, the substance should be removed and a correct grouping can be observed.

Incorrect typing can also result from additional antigens due to:

1. Polyagglutinable red cells
2. Acquired B-like antigen; acquired A-like antigen
3. Complexes attached to red cells
4. Agents causing nonspecific erythrocyte agglutination
5. Antibody-sensitized red cells—effect of colloids and anti-antibodies, e.g., hemolytic disease of the newborn, incompatible transfusions, or autoimmune processes.

### Limitations

Antisera prepared from human sources are capable of detecting $A_1$ and $A_2$ groups; however, weak subgroups of A may only be detected with anti-A,B reagent antiserum or monoclonal products. Except in the case of newborn and very young infants, a reverse cell typing should also be performed to verify the results of forward typing.

### Title: ABO Blood Grouping (Reverse Typing)

#### Principle

The reverse (serum) grouping procedure to confirm ABO blood grouping is based on the presence or absence of the antibodies, anti-A and anti-B, in serum. If these antibodies are present in serum, agglutination should be demonstrated when the serum is combined with reagent erythrocytes expressing either A or B antigens.

Reverse typing is a crosscheck for forward typing. Because of the lack of synthesized immunoglobulins in newborn and very young infants, this procedure is not performed on specimens from these patients.

#### Specimen

No special preparation of the patient is required before specimen collection. The patient must be positively identified when the specimen is collected. The specimen must be labelled at the bedside and the label must include the patient's first and last name, the date when the specimen is collected, and the patient's hospital identification number. The time of collection and the phlebotomist's initials should be written on the required form.

Blood should be drawn by an aseptic technique and the specimen should be tested as soon as possible. Approximately 5 to 7 mL of blood should be collected in a red top (no anticoagulant) or lavender top (EDTA) evacuated tube.

The blood sample should be tested as soon as possible. Hemolysis is undesirable. If a delay in testing is necessary, the blood should be refrigerated.

#### Reagents, Supplies, and Equipment

Reagent erythrocytes: $A_1$ and B ($A_2$ optional)
$10 \times 75$ mm disposable test tubes
Disposable pipettes, $4\frac{5}{8}''$ plastic or Pasteur
High intensity lamp/optical magnifying lens
Centrifuge

#### Quality Control

Reagent erythrocytes should be tested daily with known antisera (see Daily Reagent Quality Assurance, this chapter).

#### Procedure

1. Label two $10 \times 75$ mm test tubes—one with the letter A, the other with the letter B. Label each with the last three digits of the laboratory number. Note: the letters A and B should be underlined to denote reverse grouping.
2. To each of the two test tubes add 2 drops of the serum or plasma to be tested, using a disposable pipette.
3. To the tube labeled A, add 1 drop of the thoroughly mixed $A_1$ reagent erythrocytes.
4. To the tube labeled B, add 1 drop of the thoroughly mixed B reagent erythrocytes.
5. Mix well and centrifuge both test tubes for 15 seconds at 3400 rpm.
6. Resuspend the cells by gentle agitation and examine macroscopically for agglutination; record results.

#### Reporting Results

Agglutination indicates that an antibody specific for either the A or B antigen is present in the serum or plasma being tested. The blood group of the individual, based on the presence or absence of agglutination, is presented in Table 14-2.

#### Procedure Notes

A hemolyzed specimen is unsuitable for this test. As in the forward typing, testing must be conducted at room

**Table 14-2. Reactions of Patient Serum and Reagent Erythrocytes**

| $A_1$ Cells | B Cells | Antibody | Blood Group |
|---|---|---|---|
| + | + | Anti-A and Anti-B | O |
| 0 | + | Anti-B | A |
| + | 0 | Anti-A | B |
| 0 | 0 | Neither | AB |

temperature or colder. If the expected results of both forward and reverse typing are not demonstrated, either a variation in the patient or a technical error may exist.

Discrepancies in serum (reverse) grouping (see Chapter 4 for a full discussion) can be due to additional or missing antibodies. A brief summary of these situations follows.

Causes of unexpected antibodies:

1. Passively acquired isoagglutinins
2. Alloantibodies
3. Rouleaux formation
4. Auto anti-I; iso anti-I
5. Anti-$A_1$ in $A_x$, $A_2$, and $A_2B$ bloods
6. Anti-H in $A_1B$, $A_1$, B and Bombay bloods
7. Anti-IA and/or iA

Causes of weak or missing antibodies:

1. Deteriorated reagent erythrocytes
2. Hypogammaglobulinemic or elderly patients
3. Newborn infants
4. Chimerism
5. Rare variants of A or B

***Resolution of Technical Error.*** When results of cell and serum tests for ABO do not agree, the discrepancy must be investigated. If the blood is from a donor unit, the unit must not be released for transfusion until the discrepancy is resolved. When the blood is from a potential recipient, it may be necessary to administer group O erythrocytes of the appropriate Rh group before the investigation is complete. Note: It is important to obtain enough of the patient's blood before transfusion that testing can be continued on a sample free of transfused cells.

If the forward and reverse groups do not agree, several immediate steps can be taken. These include the following:

1. Check the quality control results of the antisera and reagent erythrocytes.
2. Recheck the specimen and requisition for accuracy.
3. Recheck the labeling of the erythrocyte preparation.
4. Repeat both the forward (including anti-A,B antiserum) and reverse grouping tests, if the results are the same as the original:
   A. Incubate all test tubes at room temperature for 15 to 30 minutes. This may enhance weak reactions.
   B. Reverse-group the serum, including an autocontrol. Incubate these tubes at 4° C for 15 minutes.

**Table 14-3. Results in ABO Typing**

| Phenotype | Antisera Anti-A* | Antisera Anti-B | Antisera Anti-A,B | Reagent RBCs $A_1$ | Reagent RBCs B |
|---|---|---|---|---|---|
| $A_{sub}B$ with anti-$A_1$ | Neg | Pos | Pos | 2+ | Neg |
| $A_{sub}B$ with no anti-$A_1$ | Neg | Pos | Pos | Neg | Neg |
| A with acquired B | Pos | Pos | Pos | Neg | Pos |
| $A_{sub}$ no anti-$A_1$ | Neg | Neg | Pos | Neg | Pos |
| $A_x$ with anti-$A_1$ | Neg | Neg | Pos | Pos | Pos |
| $A_3$ | Pos (m.f.) | | | | |
| O with autoagglutinins | Pos | Pos | Pos | Pos | Pos |
| O with In-polyagglutinable | Pos | Neg | Pos | Pos | Pos |
| Cord blood AB with weak A antigen | Neg | Pos | Pos | — | — |
| Cord blood A with weak A antigen | Neg | Neg | Pos | — | — |

\* Human anti-A detects Group $A_1$ and $A_2$; BioClone anti-A detects subgroups of A.

This testing may reveal the reason for the original discrepancy. A summary of possible reactions and their causes is presented in Table 14-3.

If this additional testing fails to reveal the source of the discrepancy, the following steps should be taken:

1. Obtain a new blood specimen. This should identify discrepancies due to contaminated or misidentified samples.
2. Wash the patient's erythrocytes 3 or 4 times.

### Additional Erythrocyte Testing

1. Repeat the forward grouping on a 2 to 5% saline suspension of washed cells. Testing of the red blood cells should include anti-A,B, anti-$A_1$, or anti-H, as appropriate to the problem.
2. Perform a DAT on the washed erythrocytes.

ADDITIONAL SERUM TESTING. Test the serum with three examples of $A_1$, $A_2$, and O screening cells. A group B cell and auto control should also be used. It may be helpful to test group O (or ABO compatible) cord cells if anti-I is suspected. If necessary, incubate cell and serum tests at least 30 minutes at room temperature and at 4° C before concluding that the results are negative. Group O and autologous control cells are especially important for tests incubated at 4° C, to prevent misinterpretation of positive reactions due to autoantibodies or alloantibodies reactive at these temperatures.

***Anti-$A_1$.*** Anti-$A_1$ in the serum of A or $A_2B$ individuals usually agglutinates the $A_1$ cells used for serum grouping tests. An antibody can be considered to be anti-$A_1$ if it agglutinates all the $A_1$ cells and none of the $A_2$ or O cells (Table 14-4). Anti-$A_1$ sometimes causes incompatibility on crossmatches. If, on carefully temperature-controlled tests, the antibody is reactive at 35° C, it should be consid-

**Table 14-4. Reactions of Anti-A₁**

| Reagent Cells | Reactions |
|---|---|
| 1. A₁ cell | 3+ |
| 2. A₁ cell | 3+ |
| 3. A₁ cell | 3+ |
| 4. A₂ cell | Neg |
| 5. A₂ cell | Neg |
| 6. A₂ cell | Neg |
| 7. O cell | Neg |
| 8. O cell | Neg |
| 9. O cell | Neg |

ered clinically significant, and only A₂ or O erythrocytes should be used for transfusion.

*Unexpected Antibodies.* Reverse grouping may demonstrate the presence of an unexpected non-ABO antibody. In these cases, either the A or B reagent cell may express the corresponding antigen. If the group O screening cells as well as additional examples of A₁ and B cells are negative, the antigen is uncommon. If the group O cells are positive, the procedure for unexpected antibody screening and identification should be performed.

*Weak or Missing Antibodies.* In patients with agammaglobulinemia or hypogammaglobulinemia, expected isoantibodies may be weak or absent. In addition, ABO antibodies decrease in strength as individuals grow older; thus, in elderly patients, the agglutinins may be difficult to detect. Testing at 4° C may be necessary to demonstrate their presence. If this is done, a control of the patient's own cells and serum is essential to prove that ABO antibodies and not cold-reacting autoagglutinins are being detected.

## Limitations

Reverse grouping must be conducted with forward grouping. By itself, the test is not definitive for ABO grouping.

Reverse grouping performed on cord blood or the serum of a very young infant may give misleading results until the child is approximately 6 months old. Antibodies found in the infant's circulation before this time are usually of maternal origin.

Weak reactions due to a low titer of A or B antibodies (isoagglutinins) may be observed in elderly patients or patients with immune disorders.

## Title: D Typing

### Principle

Human erythrocytes are classified as Rh positive or Rh negative depending solely on the presence or absence of the D antigen. Agglutination will be observed if reagent antiserum containing anti-D is mixed with erythrocytes expressing the D antigen. Determination of the D antigen status of patients is important in pretransfusion and prena-

tal testing because of the immunogenicity of the D antigen. If a D (Rh) negative person is exposed to the D antigen through transfusion or pregnancy, sensitization is likely to occur. This could subsequently result in incompatible crossmatches or hemolytic disease of the newborn.

### Specimen

Approximately 5 to 7 mL of blood should be collected in a red top (no anticoagulant) evacuated tube or a specimen may be collected in a lavender top (EDTA) evacuated tube. The specimen should be properly labeled with the patient's first and last name. Newborn or infant samples may be collected as red cells in normal saline or from a clotted cord sample.

The blood sample should be tested as soon as possible. If a delay in testing is necessary, the specimen should be refrigerated.

### Reagents, Supplies, and Equipment

Commercial blood typing antisera: Anti-D for slide and/or rapid tube tests
Commercial blood typing antisera: Rh control serum
10 × 75 mm disposable test tubes
Normal saline (0.9% NaCl)
Disposable pipettes, 4⅝" plastic or Pasteur
High intensity lamp/optical magnifying lens
Centrifuge

### Quality Control

Reagent antisera should be tested daily with erythrocytes of known antigenicity (see Daily Reagent Quality Assurance, this chapter).

Every specimen tested for the D antigen should have a control run concurrently. Each manufacturer provides, with each package of antiserum, detailed instructions for use. These directions vary in details; therefore, it is important to follow the directions for the specific antisera in use.

### Procedure

1. Label two tubes:
   1. D
   2. D control
2. Prepare a 4% suspension of the erythrocytes (see Preparation of Red Cell Suspensions, this chapter).
3. Place 1 drop of anti-D slide and/or rapid tube antiserum into the test tube labeled D. To the test tube labeled D control, add 1 drop of Rh control.
4. Add 1 drop of the red cell suspension to be tested to each tube.
5. Mix well and allow both tubes to incubate at room temperature for 2 to 5 minutes.
6. Centrifuge for 15 seconds at 3400 rpm.
7. Resuspend the cells by gentle agitation and examine

macroscopically for agglutination (see Grading Agglutination Reactions, this chapter).
8. Record results.

## Reporting Results

Agglutination of the erythrocytes indicates the presence of the D antigen (i.e., Rh positive). No agglutination indicates that the D antigen is not expressed (i.e., Rh negative). Erythrocytes that appear to be Rh negative must be tested for the weak D (D^u) antigen if the specimen is from a blood donor. Weak D (D^u) testing is no longer required on specimens from potential recipients.

If the D control shows agglutination, the test results are invalid. Unless the problem can be resolved, Rh negative blood must be used for transfusion in such cases.

## Procedure Notes

Testing for D antigen may be performed using the slide instead of the tube technique. The test erythrocyte suspension, however, must be 40 to 50% and several sources of false-positive reactions, such as rouleaux, are associated with the slide method.

False-negative results can be encountered with the tube technique if the red blood cell suspension is too strong. Conversely, a false-negative result with the slide technique can be encountered if the suspension is too weak.

If a positive autocontrol is demonstrated, saline or chemically modified anti-D antisera should be used. These reagents should also be used if the erythrocytes have immunoglobulins attached (a positive direct antiglobulin test).

Monoclonal anti-B reagent has been reported to detect weak D antigens that are not demonstrable with antisera of human origin.

Problems that can be encountered in Rh typing and their respective probable explanations are presented in Table 14-5.

## Limitations

Contaminated blood specimens or the presence of materials such as undissolved salt particles or silica may interfere with the test results. Cases of false positive results with chemically modified anti-D have also been reported.

## Title: Weak D (D^u) Typing

### Principle

The weak D (D^u) antigen is a variant of the D antigen. The presence of weak D (D^u) can be demonstrated by an indirect antiglobulin (Coombs) technique, i.e., incubating a red blood cell suspension at 37° C with anti-D antisera. The erythrocytes of donors or selected patients, for example maternity patients, that appear to be Rh negative by direct methods must be further tested for the presence of the weak D (D^u) antigen.

### Specimen

Approximately 5 to 7 mL of blood should be collected in a red top (no anticoagulant) evacuated tube or a specimen may be collected in a lavender top (EDTA) evacuated tube. Newborn or infant samples may be collected as red cells in normal saline or from a clotted cord sample. The specimen must be properly labeled with the patient's first and last name.

The blood sample should be tested as soon as possible. If a delay in testing is necessary, the sample should be refrigerated.

### Table 14-5. Problems in Rh Typing

| Procedure | Anti-D | Rh Control | Cell Suspension | Probable Explanations |
|---|---|---|---|---|
| Slide | Positive | Positive | Serum or plasma | Abnormal serum protein*, positive DAT* |
| | Weakly positive | Negative | Serum or plasma | D^u† |
| | | | | Mixture of Rh positive and Rh negative cells (post-transfusion) |
| Modified tube | Positive | Positive | Saline | Positive DAT** |
| | Positive | Positive | Serum or plasma | Abnormal serum protein*, positive DAT** |
| | Weakly positive | Negative | Saline, plasma or serum | D^u† |
| | | | | Weakly expressed D (Rh₀) antigen, mixture of Rh positive and Rh negative cells (post-transfusion) |
| Weak D (D^u) (AHG phase) | Positive | Positive | Saline, plasma, or serum | Positive DAT** |
| | Weakly positive | Negative | Saline, plasma, or serum | Low-grade D^u |
| | | | | Weakly expressed D (weak D) antigen, post-partum specimen from a large fetal-maternal hemorrhage, mixture of Rh positive and Rh negative cells (post-transfusion) |

\* If washed cells are used, valid results can be obtained.
\*\* Use anti-(D) for saline tube test to obtain valid results.
† Weak D (D^u)
Modified from Ortho Brochure, Ortho Diagnostics, Inc., Raritan, New Jersey, 1976.

## Reagents, Supplies, and Equipment

Commercial blood typing antisera: Anti-D for slide and/
  or rapid tube tests
Commercial blood typing antisera: Rh control serum
$10 \times 75$ mm disposable test tubes
Test tube racks
Normal saline (0.9% NaCl)
Disposable pipettes, $4\frac{5}{8}''$ plastic or Pasteur
$37°$ C waterbath or heat block
Centrifuge
Cell washer (optional)
High intensity lamp/optical magnifying lens

## Quality Control

A negative control AUTO control should be tested concurrently with every patient specimen tested for the D
antigen.

## Procedure

1. Label two tubes:
    1. D
    2. D control
2. Prepare a 2 to 4% suspension of the erythrocytes to
   be tested (see Preparation of Red Cell Suspension,
   later in this chapter).
3. Place 1 drop of anti-D slide and/or rapid tube antiserum into the test tube labeled D. To the test tube
   labeled D control, add 1 drop of Rh control.
4. Add 1 drop of the red cell suspension to be tested to
   each tube.
5. Mix well and allow both tubes to incubate at $37°$ C
   for 15 minutes.
6. Wash the cells three times with normal saline. Decant
   the final wash.
7. Add 2 drops of antiglobulin broad-spectrum antisera
   to each tube.
8. Centrifuge for 15 seconds at 3400 rpm.
9. Resuspend the cells by gentle agitation and examine
   macroscopically for agglutination (see Grading Agglutination Reactions, later in this chapter). Record results.
10. Add 1 drop of Coombs control cells to all negative
    tubes.
11. Centrifuge and examine for agglutination. If the
    Coombs control cells do not agglutinate, repeat the
    weak D ($D^u$) testing. This step verifies the activity of
    AHG antisera. Coombs control cells must agglutinate
    in all tubes that were initially negative.

## Reporting Results

If the weak D ($D^u$) test and control are negative, the blood
is Rh negative, weak D ($D^u$) negative. If the weak D ($D^u$)
test is positive and the control is negative, the individual
has weak D ($D^u$) (see Chapter 5). For purposes of blood

donation, such persons are considered Rh positive. However, as a blood recipient, an individual is regarded as Rh
negative and only Rh negative blood is used for transfusion.

If the control is positive, the test is invalid. In such
cases, the patient may have a positive direct antiglobulin
test, and the weak D ($D^u$) type cannot be determined.

## Procedure Notes

Mixed-field agglutination in a weak D ($D^u$) test from a
postpartum woman may indicate a mixture of maternal
Rh negative and fetal Rh positive cells.

Some weak D ($D^u$) variant individuals may have anti-
D. Their cells may also stimulate the production of anti-
D in an Rh negative person.

## Limitations

If the erythrocytes are coated with immunoglobulins, that
is, demonstrate a positive direct antiglobulin test (DAT),
the weak D ($D^u$) test cannot be performed.

## Title: Compatibility Testing (Crossmatching)

### Principle

Pretransfusion compatibility testing combines a potential
recipient's blood specimen with a blood specimen from
an intended donor. The major crossmatch consists of combining a sample of the recipient's serum with a sample of
erythrocytes from the intended donor. This mixture is
tested at various temperatures and with enhancement
media. If an antibody is present in the potential recipient
that has specificity for an antigen on the donor red cells,
agglutination or hemolysis should be exhibited.

### Specimen

No special preparation of the patient is required before
specimen collection. The patient must be positively identified when the specimen is collected. The specimen must
be labelled at the bedside and the label must include the
patient's first and last name, the date when the specimen is
collected, and the patient's hospital identification number.
The time of collection and the phlebotomist's initials
should be written on the required form.

Blood should be drawn by an aseptic technique and
the specimen should be tested as soon as possible. Approximately 5 to 7 mL of blood should be collected in a plain
red top or lavender top (EDTA) evacuated tube. Hemolysis renders the specimen unsuitable for testing. If a delay
in testing is necessary, the blood should be refrigerated.

If a patient has been pregnant or transfused within the
preceding 3 months, or if the history is uncertain or unavailable, a blood sample for compatibility testing must be
collected within 3 days (72 hours) of red cell transfusions.

In massively transfused (10 units or more) patients, the general rule of thumb is that a new specimen should be drawn after each 10 units of transfused blood. In cases of transfusion with other than group specific blood, a new specimen must be drawn before switching back to the patient's own blood type.

All specimens must be retained under refrigeration for 7 days after transfusion of a unit of blood.

### Reagents, Supplies, and Equipment

Commercial antiglobulin (AHG) reagent (broad-spectrum or IgG)
Commercial 22% albumin (optional)
10 × 75 mm disposable test tubes
Disposable pipettes, 4⅝″ plastic or Pasteur
Scissors
Test tube rack
Normal (0.9%) saline
37° C waterbath or heat block
High intensity lamp/optical magnifying lens
Centrifuge

### Quality Control

Reagent erythrocytes should be tested daily with known antisera (see Daily Reagent Quality Assurance, this chapter). All negative AHG reactions must be tested with IgG sensitized erythrocytes and produce a positive reaction. If the AHG control cells do not agglutinate, the compatibility test is invalid.

### Procedure

#### *Preliminary*

1. Compare the information on the patient's specimen with the information on the test requisition: name, identification number, date. If this information is not identical, obtain a new specimen.
2. Centrifuge the clotted specimen for 5 minutes at 2000 rpm.
3. Check past blood bank records to determine if the patient has ever been screened for antibodies or previously transfused.
4. Perform an ABO grouping (forward and reverse), Rh typing, and unexpected antibody screen on the recipient's specimen. Record all test results in the blood bank log as well as on the crossmatch requisition.
5. Check data on previous records. If the ABO and Rh are not identical, obtain a new specimen for repeat testing.
6. Procure the whole blood or packed cells to be crossmatched from the blood bank refrigerator. Check all identification on the units, for example, group and Rh, expiration date; and the physical characteristics of the units, for example, absence of hemolysis or abnormal color.
7. Detach a segment from the unit of blood. Cut the ends of the segment and drain the contents into a 10 × 75 mm test tube. Label the tube with the donor unit identification number. Recheck the number.
8. Wash the donor specimen 3 times with normal saline. Decant the last wash completely and prepare a 3% suspension of the erythrocytes.
9. Enter the donor number and expiration date on the test requisition. If the donor unit has not been retyped on entering the blood bank inventory, an ABO grouping and Rh typing should be performed.

#### *Compatibility Procedure.*

The compatibility test can be divided into three phases: room temperature (immediate spin), 37° C, and AHG. In some blood banks, only the immediate spin phase is performed if a patient demonstrates a negative antibody screen in the AHG phase using two or three group O screening cells. The following is an example of a typical crossmatch configuration including all phases.

##### ROOM TEMPERATURE (IMMEDIATE SPIN) PHASE

1. Label two 10 × 75 mm test tubes. One tube should have the patient's last name and donor number; the other should be labeled AUTO (control).
2. To tube 1 add:
   2 drops of patient serum
   1 drop of donor's washed cells
   To the AUTO tube add:
   2 drops of patient serum
   1 drop of patient's washed cells
3. Mix and centrifuge for 15 seconds at 3400 rpm.
4. Gently resuspend the cell button and read macroscopically (see Grading Agglutination Reactions, this chapter). If agglutination is observed, do not proceed with the next phases. Agglutination at this phase is considered to indicate an *incompatible* crossmatch. Additional testing may not strengthen the degree of agglutination.
5. Record results. If compatible, proceed with the next phase.

##### 37° C PHASE

1. Potentiators such as 1 drop of 22% albumin or LISS may be added at this phase.
2. Incubate the 2 tubes from the IS phase for 30 minutes at 37° C.
3. Centrifuge for 15 seconds at 3400 rpm.
4. Gently resuspend the cell button and read macroscopically (see Grading Agglutination Reactions, this chapter)
5. Record results.

##### ANTIGLOBULIN PHASE (AHG)

1. Wash the 2 test tubes from the 37° C phase three times with normal saline.

2. After the last wash, decant all saline and add 2 drops of AHG reagent.
3. Mix and centrifuge for 15 seconds at 3400 rpm.
4. Gently resuspend the cell button and examine macroscopically and microscopically.
5. Record results.
6. If either or both of the tubes demonstrate no agglutination, add one drop of IgG sensitized (Coombs control or check cells) to the tube.
7. Centrifuge the tubes for 15 seconds at 3400 rpm and observe and grade for agglutination. *Agglutination must occur.* The test is invalid if the control cells do not agglutinate, and the test must be repeated.
8. Record results.

### Reporting Results

A compatible crossmatch is indicated by the absence of agglutination and/or hemolysis at any stage of the crossmatch. The absence of agglutination indicates that the patient has no demonstrable antibodies with a specificity for any of antigens on the donor erythrocytes.

### Procedure Notes

If incompatibility is demonstrated by agglutination or hemolysis at any stage of the crossmatch, the donor unit should not be used for transfusion. Exceptions might include "least compatible" units in patients with autoantibodies.

If the patient has a positive antibody screen or demonstrates an incompatibility with a donor unit, the antibody specificity should be determined as soon as possible. After antibody identification, corresponding units that are negative for the antigen to the patient's antibody can be crossmatched.

The crossmatch will detect the following:

1. ABO incompatibility
2. Most unexpected antibodies directed against common antigens

If a patient exhibits strong rouleaux formation, a saline replacement technique may be used.

### Saline Replacement Technique

1. Recentrifuge the serum-cell mixture when rouleau formation is suspected.
2. Remove the serum.
3. Replace the serum with an equal volume of saline (2 drops) and mix.
4. Centrifuge the saline-cell mixture.
5. Resuspend the saline-cell mixture and examine for agglutination. *Rouleaux* will disperse. *True agglutination* will remain.

### Limitations

Low-titered antibodies in the patient's serum may not be detectable in the pretransfusion compatibility test. These antibodies may be demonstrable with enhancement methods such as enzyme treatment. In some cases, a delayed hemolytic transfusion reaction may become apparent in 7 to 10 days, if the transfused unit has the antigen corresponding to the patient's antibody.

A crossmatch will not:

1. Prevent immunization of the patient.
2. Guarantee normal survival of transfused erythrocytes.
3. Detect all unexpected antibodies in a patient's serum.

### Title: Cord Blood Workup

#### Principle

Blood drained from the umbilical cord is tested for ABO group, Rh type, and the presence of IgG antibodies on the erythrocytes (DAT). This protocol is followed if the infant's mother is group O or D negative and in other cases where the possibility of hemolytic disease of the newborn (HDN) exists.

#### Specimen

Approximately 5 to 7 mL of blood should be collected in a red top (no anticoagulant) and 3 to 5 mL in a lavender top (EDTA) evacuated tube. The specimen must be properly labeled with the patient's first and last name.

Routinely collected cord blood specimens may be marked HOLD. In cases of potential HDN, the specimen is usually marked STAT. If the specimen is marked HOLD, it should be stored at 1° to 6° C for a minimum of 4 days in a special container for cord blood specimens.

#### Reagents, Supplies, and Equipment

See ABO, Rh, and DAT procedures, described in this chapter.

#### Quality Control

See ABO, Rh, and DAT procedures, described in this chapter.

#### Procedure

1. When a specimen of cord blood arrives, the requisition and blood samples must be checked to ensure that the information on the specimen matches the information on the requisition.
2. If the specimen is STAT, it should be tested for ABO and Rh antigens and a direct antiglobulin test (DAT) should be performed.
3. If the DAT is positive, bilirubin and CBC tests should be performed immediately. An elution (see Elution Techniques in Chapter 15) should be performed on the DAT-positive cells.

## Reporting Results

See ABO, Rh, and DAT procedures, described in this chapter.

## Procedure Notes

It is important to wash cord blood cells appropriately. Cord blood specimens should be washed at least five times before forward blood typing to remove residual proteins. Reverse typing should be omitted because any detectable antibodies are usually of maternal origin.

Washing the erythrocytes with saline or adding a drop or two of saline to the test tube will free the aggregated erythrocytes in case of rouleau formation.

## Limitations

Failure to remove Wharton's jelly or residual protein from a cord blood specimen may produce a false negative DAT.

## Title: Daily Reagent Quality Assurance

### Principle

A comprehensive quality assurance system requires that blood bank reagents be tested on the day of use to ensure that the antisera and reagent erythrocytes are appropriately reactive. Such a system incorporates both positive and negative controls into the procedures recommended by the manufacturer. Any deviation from the expected results warrants investigation before use of the reagent.

### Reagents, Supplies, and Equipment

Commercial antisera: Anti-A, anti-B, anti-AB, anti-D (modified slide/tube test), Rh control, 22% albumin, and antiglobulin (AHG)
Reagent red blood cells: $A_1$, $A_2$, B, group O antibody screening cells, and IgG-sensitized erythrocytes, e.g., Coombs control/check cells
10 × 75 mm test tubes
Test tube racks
Normal saline (0.9% NaCl)
Disposable pipettes: $4\frac{5}{8}''$ plastic or Pasteur, 1 mL graduated serologic, 5 mL graduate serologic
Safety bulb pipettor
37° C waterbath or heat block
Centrifuge
Cell washer (optional)
High intensity lamp/optical magnifying lens

### Procedure

#### Preliminary

1. Prepare a 1:10 dilution of IgG sensitized red blood cells (Coombs' control/check cells) by adding 0.1 mL of red blood cells to 0.9 mL of saline.

2. Prepare a 1:50 dilution of anti-D by adding 0.1 mL of anti-D to 4.9 mL of saline.

#### Antisera and Reagent Red Blood Cell Controls

1. Label a set of 10 × 75 mm test tubes with the numbers 1 through 15.
2. Add undiluted reagent antisera to the labelled tubes as follows:
   A. To tubes 1, 2, and 3, add 1 drop of anti-A.
   B. To tubes 4, 5, and 6, add 1 drop of anti-B.
   C. To tubes 7, 8, and 9, add 1 drop of anti-AB.
   D. To tubes 10 and 11, add 1 drop of anti-D.
   E. To tube 12, add 1 drop of Rh control.
   F. To tubes 13 and 14, add 1 drop of AHG.
   G. To tube 15, add 1 drop of saline.
3. Add undiluted reagent red blood cells to the labelled tubes as follows:
   A. To tubes 1, 4, 7, 10, 12, and 13, add 1 drop of $A_1$ cells.
   B. To tubes 2, 5, and 8, add 1 drop of $A_2$ cells.
   C. To tubes 3, 6, and 9, add 1 drop of B cells.
   D. To tube 13, add 1 drop of $A_1$ cells.
4. Add 1 drop of diluted IgG sensitized red blood cells to tubes 11, 14, and 15.
5. Centrifuge all of the tubes at 3400 rpm for 15 seconds or 1000 rpm for 1 minute.
6. Gently resuspend the cell button and examine macroscopically for agglutination and grade the strength of agglutination.
7. Record the results (see Fig. 1-1).

#### Screening Cells and AHG Reagent Control

1. Label four test tubes with the numbers 16 through 19.
2. Add the following reagents as follows:
   A. To tubes 16 through 19, add 2 drops of albumin.
   B. To tubes 16 and 17, add 1 drop of screening cells I.
   C. To tubes 18 and 19, add 1 drop of screening cells II.
   D. To tubes 16 and 18, add 1 drop of dilute anti-D.
   E. To tubes 17 and 19, add 2 drops of saline.
3. Centrifuge tubes 16 through 19 at 3400 rpm for 15 seconds.
4. Gently resuspend the cell button and examine macroscopically. Record the results as the (IS) room temperature phase.
5. Incubate all of the tubes (16 through 19) for 30 minutes at 37° C.
6. Centrifuge these tubes. Gently resuspend the cell button and examine macroscopically. Record these results as the 37° C phase.
7. Wash the contents of each tube 3 times.
8. To each tube, add 2 drops of AHG.
9. Centrifuge at 3400 rpm for 15 seconds. Gently resus-

pend the cell button and examine macroscopically. Record the results as the AHG phase.

10. To all negative reactions, add 1 drop of IgG sensitized red blood cells. Centrifuge at 3400 rpm for 15 seconds. Gently resuspend the cell button and examine macroscopically. These reactions must demonstrate agglutination or the test is invalid.

## Title: Direct Antiglobulin (Coombs') Test

### Principle

The direct antiglobulin test is based on the principle that antiglobulin antibodies induce in vitro agglutination of erythrocytes with immunologically bound antibodies. After erythrocytes are washed to remove free plasma protein from the test mixture, they are tested directly with reagents containing anti-IgG and anti-C3d (broad spectrum/polyspecific). Monospecific antisera, for example anti-IgG, anti-C3d, and anti-C4, that are specific for immunoglobulins or complement components, may also be used. The DAT procedure is clinically important in the diagnosis of conditions such as hemolytic anemia or delayed hemolytic transfusion reactions.

### Specimen

No special preparation of the patient is required before specimen collection. The patient must be positively identified when the specimen is collected. The specimen must be labelled at the bedside, and the label must include the patient's first and last name, the date when the specimen is collected, and the patient's hospital identification number. The time of collection and the phlebotomist's initials should be written on the required form.

Blood should be drawn by an aseptic technique and tested as soon as possible. The specimen should consist of 5 to 7 mL of clotted blood (red top) evacuated tube and 7 mL of EDTA blood (lavender top) evacuated tube. Newborn or infant samples may be collected as red cells in normal saline or from a cord blood sample.

If a delay in testing occurs, the specimen must be refrigerated. Antibodies dependent for their detection upon the binding of complement may not be detected if aged serum or plasma from an anticoagulated sample is used. Hemolysis of the specimen is undesirable.

### Reagents, Supplies, and Equipment

Antiglobulin serum (polyspecific or monospecific)
IgG sensitized erythrocytes (Coombs control cells)
10 × 75 mm disposable test tubes
Disposable pipettes, 4⅝" plastic or Pasteur
Normal saline (0.9%)
Test tube rack

Centrifuge
Cell washer (optional)
High Intensity lamp/optical magnifying lens

### Quality Control

In addition to the daily reagent quality assurance check, each test must have a saline control run concurrently to rule out autoagglutination. Coombs control/check cells must be added to each test that does not exhibit agglutination. Agglutination of the Coombs control cells verifies the reactivity of the antiglobulin antiserum.

### Procedure

1. Prepare a 2% saline suspension of the patient's erythrocytes (see Preparation of Red Cell Suspension, later in this chapter).
2. Label one 10 × 75 test tube with the letters DAT. Label a second 10 × 75 test tube as DAT Control.
3. Using a disposable pipette, add 1 drop of the red cell suspension to each tube. Note: Some laboratories prefer to add 2 drops of a 3–5% cell suspension in order to retrieve an adequate cell button after washing with saline three times.
4. Wash the contents of both tubes three times. If they are washed by hand, fill both tubes with saline and resuspend the red cells, centrifuge at 3400 rpm for 30 seconds and decant. Repeat three times. Be sure saline is completely decanted after the final wash. Note: Washing should be rapid to prevent elution of the antibody into the saline.
5. Add 2 drops of antiglobulin serum to the tube labelled DAT.
6. Add 2 drops of saline to the tube labelled DAT Control.
7. Resuspend the red cells completely in both tubes and mix well.
8. Centrifuge at 3400 rpm for 15 seconds.
9. Gently resuspend the red cells and examine macroscopically and microscopically for agglutination. Grade the reaction and record results. The DAT control should demonstrate no agglutination (negative reaction). Note: Following addition, the test should be spun and read immediately.
10. Verify the AHG activity if the DAT tube demonstrated no agglutination:
    A. Add 1 drop of Coombs control cells to the DAT tube.
    B. Centrifuge at 3400 rpm for 15 seconds.
    C. Gently resuspend the red cells and examine macroscopically and microscopically for agglutination.
    D. Agglutination *must* be present. If agglutination is not present, the test is invalid and must be repeated.

## Reporting Results

A negative test is demonstrated by the absence of agglutination in the DAT test tube. A positive test is manifested by the presence of agglutination. If a cord blood specimen is positive, the attending physician and the nursery should be notified immediately.

## Procedure Notes

A positive DAT, typically a mixed-field pattern, may be seen following an incompatible transfusion, for example delayed hemolytic transfusion reaction. Additionally, a positive DAT may be exhibited in various disorders including autoimmune hemolytic anemia, lymphoma, chronic lymphocytic leukemia, collagen disorders such as SLE; other diseases such as carcinoma, hepatic disease, or infectious mononucleosis; and illness caused by drugs, such as penicillin and cephalothin. Heterophile antibodies present in equine anti-human lymphocyte globulin (ALG and ATG) that is used to reduce T-cell populations in organ and bone marrow transplant recipients coats recipient red blood cells and causes a positive DAT within a few days. In addition, free unbound ALG/ATG may be found in the plasma. This causes both the unexpected antibody screen and antiglobulin crossmatch to be positive. The results are positive because rabbit anti-human globulin reagents contain antibodies that react with equine immunoglobulin.

Several assumptions are made when interpreting a positive DAT, including the following:

1. The test results are obtained from a properly collected, uncontaminated blood specimen.
2. The red cells are properly washed.
3. The antiglobulin reagent is potent and uncontaminated.

A positive DAT does not imply overt hemolysis; it may occur in healthy persons. The DAT may be negative in individuals with immune hemolytic anemia. In these cases, additional testing should be performed to determine the possible causes of hemolysis. In some circumstances, an alloantibody in the serum may be unrelated to a positive DAT. Patterns of reactivity with AHG antisera vary, depending on the cause. Table 14-6 summarizes some of the typical patterns of AHG reactivity.

To interpret the cause of a positive DAT, the results of the DAT, unexpected antibody screening test, elution studies, and evidence of hemolysis, such as a decreasing hematocrit, can be combined. Examples of such interpretation are given as follows:

### *Situation 1*

Anti-IgG (negative) and anti-C3d (positive)
Antibody screen (negative)
Eluate (negative)
No evidence of hemolysis

**Table 14-6. Examples of Cases of Positive DATs**

| Disorder | AHG Pattern |
|---|---|
| Hemolytic disease of the newborn (HDN) | Anti-IgG |
| Delayed hemolytic transfusion reaction | Anti-IgG |
| Warm autoimmune hemolytic anemia | Anti-IgG or IgG with anti-C3 |
| Cold autoimmune hemolytic anemia | Anti-C3 |
| Acquired hemolytic anemia | Anti-IgG, Anti-IgG + Anti-C3, Anti-C3 only |
| Collagen vascular disease | Anti-C3, weak reactions |
| Chronic lymphocytic leukemia | Anti-IgG |
| Penicillin antibodies | Anti-IgG |

Interpretation: Normal individual, immune disorders, drug-induced.

### *Situation 2*

Anti-IgG (negative) and anti-C3d (positive)
Antibody screen (negative)
Eluate (negative)
Hemolysis
Interpretation: Drug-induced warm autoimmune hemolytic anemia (rare)

### *Situation 3*

Anti-IgG (negative and anti-C3d (positive)
Antibody screen (positive)
Eluate (negative)
Interpretation: Cold agglutinin syndrome, paroxysmal cold hemoglobinuria

### *Situation 4*

Anti-IgG (positive) and anti-C3d (positive or negative)
Antibody screen (negative)
Eluate (negative)
No evidence of hemolysis
Interpretation: Drug-induced

### *Situation 5*

Anti-IgG (positive) and anti-C3d (positive or negative)
Antibody screen (negative)
Eluate (negative)
No evidence of hemolysis
Interpretation: Drug-induced

### *Situation 6*

Anti-IgG (positive) and anti-C3d (positive or negative)
Antibody screen (negative)
Eluate (positive) or
Anti-IgG (positive) and anti-C3d (positive or negative)
Antibody screen (positive)
Eluate (positive)
Interpretation: Warm autoimmune hemolytic anemia, drug induced (methyldopa or derivatives), transfusion

reaction, hemolytic disease of the newborn, antenatal IgG (D)

### Situation 7

Anti-IgG (positive) and anti-C3d (negative)
Antibody screen (negative)
Eluate (negative) or
Anti-IgG (positive) and anti-C3d (negative)
Eluate (negative)
Screening with $A_1$ and/or B red blood cells (positive or negative)
Eluate with $A_1$ and/or B red blood cells (positive or negative)
Interpretation: Hemolytic disease of the newborn, passively acquired antibody, placental transfer of drug antibody

### Situation 8

Anti-IgG (positive) and anti-C3d (negative)
Antibody screen (positive)
Eluate (positive)
Interpretation: Passively acquired antibody

### Limitations

False-positive results may be observed in the DAT due to:

1. Contamination of the AHG antisera or supplies
2. Overcentrifugation
3. Bacterial contamination of specimen or reagents
4. Fibrin clot in cell suspension
5. Overzealous reading of serum-cell mixture
6. Anti-formaldehyde antibodies
7. Variables in sample procurement such as drawing the specimen from a line containing 5% or 10% dextrose, using a clotted specimen rather than an anticoagulated sample or drawing too small a sample in the anticoagulated tube

False-negative results usually result from technical error. They are infrequently caused by a true failure of the antibody-coated red cells to react with the antiglobulin serum. Common causes of false-negative reactions include:

1. Failure to add antiglobulin reagent
2. Inadequate washing of red blood cells
3. Inactivation of AHG sera by exogenous gamma globulin
4. Weak or inactive AHG
5. Lack of broad-spectrum specificity of the AHG
6. Mixing tubes by inverting uncovered tubes with the finger
7. Decreased reactivity of antiserum due to storage
8. Elution of antibody into the supernatant on standing, with subsequent neutralization of AHG
9. Low pH of saline solution (pH less than 6.0)
10. Saline, autoclaved and stored in plastic containers

**Table 14-7. Grading Agglutination Reactions**

| Grade | Description |
|---|---|
| Negative | No aggregates |
| Mixed-field (MF) | Few isolated aggregates, mostly free-floating cells, supernatant appears red |
| Weak | Tiny aggregates that are barely visible macroscopically, many free erythrocytes, turbid and reddish supernatant |
| 1+ | A few small aggregates just visible macroscopically, many free erythrocytes, turbid and reddish supernatant |
| 2+ | Medium-sized aggregates, some free erythrocytes, clear supernatant |
| 3+ | Several large aggregates, some free erythrocytes, clear supernatant |
| 4+ | All of the erythrocytes are combined into one solid aggregate, clear supernatant |

### Title: Grading Agglutination Reactions

Principle

Uniformity in reading reactions is an important aspect of quality assurance. Table 14-7 represents a consistent method of grading agglutination.

### Title: Inspection of Donor Blood

Principle

Each unit of donor red blood cells must be examined when crossmatched and *immediately* before issue to a patient. This inspection must be recorded.

Quality Control

Blood should be rejected for transfusion if:

1. The color is abnormal. Abnormal conditions include purple discoloration of the red cells, or brown or red plasma.
2. Alterations in the physical appearance are present. Clots or hemolysis render a unit unsuitable for transfusion.
3. Contamination is suspected. Cloudy plasma may indicate bacterial contamination.
4. Blood or plasma is present at the sealing ports or tubing. Improper sealing can produce bacterial contamination of a unit

Questionable units of blood must be quarantined until disposition. Evaluation of a questionable unit should include inverting it gently a few times to mix the cells and plasma. Undetected hemolysis, clotting, or other alterations may exist in the undisturbed red blood cell mass. Abnormal blood that cannot be released for transfusion should be returned to the collection center (if imported) or properly disposed of (if drawn in-house).

Notes: *Inspection of Other Components*

Platelets. Before pooling or issuing platelet concentrates should be inspected for the presence of grossly visible aggregates. If aggregates are present, the component should not be used.

Fresh frozen plasma. Each unit of fresh frozen plasma must be inspected to determine that thawing has not occurred when the unit is removed from the freezer. Thawing may be detected because the unit feels soft. Evidence of recrystallization (ice crystals) may make the unit look lumpy.

## Title: Preparation of Red Cell Suspensions

### Principle

The concentration of erythrocytes in a saline suspension is important to the accuracy of testing in the blood bank. With experience, most technologists are able to visually prepare a suspension of the proper concentration; however, students and technologists who work infrequently in the blood bank should follow the methods for preparing an accurate suspension.

### Specimen

No special preparation of the patient is required before specimen collection. The patient must be positively identified when the specimen is collected. The specimen must be labelled at the bedside and the label must include the patient's first and last name, the date when the specimen is collected, and the patient's hospital identification number. The time of collection and the phlebotomist's initials should be written on the required form.

Blood should be drawn by an aseptic technique and tested as soon as possible. The specimen should consist of 7 mL of EDTA blood (lavender top evacuated tube). Newborn or infant samples may be collected as red cells in normal saline or from a cord blood sample.

### Reagents, Supplies, and Equipment

Large disposable test tubes or 10 × 75 mm test tubes
Disposable pipettes: 1 mL, 5 mL, 10 mL, or $4\frac{5}{8}''$ plastic
   or Pasteur
Normal saline (0.9%)
Rubber stoppers or plastic covering
Test tube rack
Centrifuge

### Procedure

Preparation of an approximate 2% red blood cell suspension is as follows:

1. Place 1 to 2 mL of anticoagulated blood in a large tube.
2. Fill the tube with saline and centrifuge the tube.
3. Aspirate or decant the supernatant saline.

4. Repeat washing (steps 2 and 3) until the supernatant saline is clear.
5. Pipette 10 mL of saline into a clean test tube.
6. Add 0.2 mL of the packed cell button to the 10 mL of diluent.
7. Rinse the pipette containing the red cells in the diluent until it is clear of cells.
8. Cover or stopper the tube until time of use. Immediately before use, invert the tube several times until the cells are in suspension.

Preparation of an approximate 5% red blood cell suspension is as follows:

1. Place 1 to 2 mL of anticoagulated blood in a large tube.
2. Fill the tube with saline and centrifuge the tube.
3. Aspirate or decant the supernatant saline.
4. Repeat washing (steps 2 and 3) until the supernatant saline is clear.
5. Pipette 10 mL of saline into a clean test tube.
6. Add 0.5 mL of the packed cell button to the 10 mL of diluent.
7. Rinse the pipette containing the red cells in the diluent until it is clear of cells.
8. Cover or stopper the tube until use. Immediately before use, invert the tube several times until the cells are in suspension.

An alternate procedure is as follows:

1. Using a disposable pipette, transfer approximately 0.2 mL (2 drops) of the patient's packed red cells to a 10 × 75 mm test tube.
2. Fill the tube with normal saline. Cover and mix by inversion.
3. Centrifuge the tube at 3400 rpm for 30 seconds.
4. Decant the saline.
5. Visually prepare a 3% or 5% suspension of red cells in saline by:
   A. Adding approximately 1 mL of saline to the washed red cells to prepare a 3% suspension.
   B. Adding approximately 0.5 mL of saline to the washed red cells to prepare a 5% suspension.
6. The volume of saline (step 5) added to the packed red cells can be adjusted to prepare other percent concentrations, e.g., 2% or 4%.

### Procedure Notes

The supernatant fluid should be clear after the final washing. If any evidence of hemolysis exists, additional washing should be performed.

## Title: Treatment of an Incompletely Clotted Specimen

### Principle

Blood from patients who have received anticoagulant therapy may have a prolonged clotting time. Blood from those

**Table 14-8. Maximum Surgical Blood Order Schedule**

| Type of Surgery | Maximum Standard Crossmatch Order (Units) | Type of Surgery | Maximum Standard Crossmatch Order (Units) |
|---|---|---|---|
| *Dental Surgery* | | Open reduction | T&S |
| Full mouth extraction | 0 | Osteotomy | 1 PC |
| Extraction, impacted molars | 0 | Removal of hip pin | T&S |
| | | Shoulder reconstruction | T&S |
| *General Surgery* | | Spinal fusion | 2 PC |
| Abdominal–perineal resection | 4 PC | Synovectomy | 0 |
| Amputation | T&S | Total hip replacement | 4 PC |
| Anal fistula excision | T&S | Total knee replacement | T&S |
| Aneurysm resection | 6 PC | | |
| Breast biopsy | T&S | *Plastic Surgery* | |
| Cholecystectomy | T&S | Augmentation mammoplasty | T&S |
| Colon resection | 2 PC | Facelift | 0 |
| Colostomy or closure | T&S | Reduction mammoplasty | T&S |
| Esophageal resection | 4 PC | Rhinoplasty | 0 |
| Excision of anal fissure or fistula/sphincterotomy | 0 | Skin flap | T&S |
| Excision of skin lesions | 0 | Skin graft, minor | T&S |
| Exploratory laparotomy | T&S | Skin graft, major (severe burns) | T&S |
| Gastrectomy | 4 PC | | |
| Gastroscopy | 0 | *Pulmonary and Vascular Surgery* | |
| Hemicolectomy | 2 PC | Abdominal aortic aneurysm resection | 4 WB and 2 PC |
| Hemorrhoidectomy | 0 | | |
| Hernia repair, hiatal | 2 PC | Aortofemoral bypass graft | 4 WB and 2 PC |
| Hernia repair, inguinal or femoral | 0 | | |
| Hernia repair, ventral | T&S | Aortoiliac bypass graft | 4 WB and 2 PC |
| Lymph node biopsy | 0 | | |
| Mastectomy, modified radical | 2 PC | Bronchoscopy | 0 |
| Mastectomy, simple | T&S | Endarterectomy: | |
| Parathyroidectomy | T&S | Femoral or carotid | 2 PC |
| Sigmoidectomy | 2 PC | Femoral bypass graft | 2 PC |
| Splenectomy | T&S | Femoral-popliteal bypass graft | 2 PC |
| Thyroid lobectomy | T&S | Thoracotomy | 4 PC |
| Vagotomy and antrectomy | T&S | | |
| Vein stripping | T&S | *Gynecologic and Obstetric Surgery* | |
| | | Cesarean section | T&S |
| *Ear, Nose, and Throat* | | Dilatation, curettage, and conization | 0 |
| Caldwell-LUC | T&S | Hysterectomy, radical and pelvic lymphadenectomy | 4 PC |
| Excision of submandibular gland | 0 | | |
| Myringotomy | 0 | Hysterectomy, simple (including TAH/BSO) | T&S |
| Insertion of ear tubes | 0 | Hysterectomy and antero-posterior repair | 1 PC |
| Laryngectomy | 1 PC | Laparoscopic tubal ligation | T&S |
| Mastoidectomy | 0 | Marshall-Marchetti procedure | 0 |
| Neck dissection (radical) | 4 PC | Ovarian wedge resection, ovarian cystectomy | T&S |
| Parotidectomy | 0 | Stamey procedure | T&S |
| Septoplasty | 0 | Tuboplasty | T&S |
| Tonsillectomy and adenoidectomy | T&S | Uterine suspension, fulguration of endometrial implants | T&S |
| Transantral ethmoidectomy | T&S | | |
| Tympanoplasty | 0 | Vaginal plastic procedures | T&S |
| | | | |
| *Orthopedic Surgery* | | *Neurosurgery* | |
| Amputation, toe | 0 | Carpal tunnel release | T&S |
| Arthroscopy | 0 | Craniotomy for aneurysm | T&S |
| Arthrotomy—removal of loose body | 0 | Craniotomy for tumor | T&S |
| Carpal tunnel repair | 0 | Craniotomy for traumatic hematoma (acute) | T&S |
| Excision, Morton's neuroma | 0 | Craniotomy for chronic subdural hematoma | T&S |
| Fracture, closed reduction | 0 | Craniotomy for AVM | T&S |
| Fracture, open reduction, internal fixation | 2 PC | Craniotomy for rhizotomy | T&S |
| Hip nailing/hip screw | 3 PC | Craniotomy for EC-IC | T&S |
| Leg amputation | T&S | Depressive laminectomy (cervical, thoracic, or lumbar) | T&S |
| Meniscectomy | 0 | | |
| Minor hand or foot surgery | 0 | Laminectomy for disc removal (lumbar) | T&S |

**Table 14-8. (continued)**

| Type of Surgery | Maximum Standard Crossmatch Order (Units) | Type of Surgery | Maximum Standard Crossmatch Order (Units) |
|---|---|---|---|
| Laminectomy for rhizotomy | 2 WB + 2 PC | Cystectomy, segmental | T&S |
| | | Cystourethropexy | 0 |
| Bilteral T$_{2-3}$ sympathectomy | 0 | Fulguration of bleeding bladder tumor | 1 PC |
| Laminectomy for spinal tumor | 2 WB + 2 PC | Hydrocelectomy | 0 |
| | | Ileal conduit-colon conduit | 1 PC |
| Shunts (VP and VA) (if an alloantibody is detected 2 WB should be available) | T&S | Needle biopsy, prostate | 0 |
| | | Nephrectomy, radical | 4 WB |
| Laminectomy for chordotomy | 2 WB + 2 PC | Nephrectomy, simple | T&S |
| | | Nephrostomy | T&S |
| Percutaneous chordotomy | T&S | Orchiectomy | T&S |
| Craniotomy for excision of abscess | 2 WB | Orchiopexy | T&S |
| Burr hole for tapping of cyst or abscess | T&S | Penile prosthesis | T&S |
| Carotid endarterectomy | T&S | Perineal prostatectomy | 2 PC |
| | | Prostate biopsy | 0 |
| *Opthalmologic Surgery* | | Pyelolithotomy | T&S |
| Cataract removal | 0 | Suprapubic prostatectomy | 2 PC |
| Recession, eye | 0 | Transurethral resection of bladder tumor | T&S |
| Entropion or extropion repair | 0 | Transurethral resection of prostate | T&S |
| | | Ureteral dilatation | 0 |
| *Urologic Surgery* | | Ureteral reimplantation | T&S |
| Cystectomy, radical | 4 WB | | |
| Ureterolithotomy | T&S | | |

Key: T&S = Type and Screen

who have received heparin may not clot at all, and blood from patients with excessive fibrinolytic activity may reliquify. Serum separated from an incompletely clotted blood specimen will continue to produce fibrin, especially after 37° C incubation. The resulting strands of protein entrap erythrocytes as clotting progresses and make it difficult to evaluate agglutination.

## Procedure

To accelerate clotting, one of the following techniques can be used:

1. Thrombin solution (50 units/mL) can be added to whole blood at the rate of one drop per mL of blood. Dried thrombin can also be added by placing a small amount on the tip of an applicator stick.
2. Small glass beads can be added to separated serum and gently agitated at 37° C for several minutes. After centrifugation, the supernatant serum can be used.

To neutralize heparin, one or more drops of a 1% saline solution of protamine sulfate (10 mg/mL) can be added to whole blood. Protamine sulfate should be used sparingly because it can promote rouleaux formation or, if added in great excess, can inhibit clotting.

To inhibit fibrinolytic activity, 0.1 mL of a solution containing 5 g epsilon-amino caproic acid in 20 mL saline can be added to 4 mL of freshly drawn whole blood.

## Title: Type and Screen Protocol

### Principle

On the basis of past experience, the amount of blood generally used in a specific surgical procedure can be established in advance. The amount of blood needed varies depending on the technique used by the surgeon and other factors such as the initial condition of the patient due to age or the existence of chronic disease. If the surgeon's order for blood varies from the established protocol of a blood bank (see Chapter 7, Pretransfusion Testing), the physician should be contacted to verify that the type and screen guideline is being overruled.

General guidelines to blood utilization (Table 14-8) can prevent unnecessary crossmatching of blood for procedures in which blood is rarely used. For surgical procedures rarely requiring transfusion, the type and screen procedure has been established as a safe and cost-effective measure that promotes more effective use of the blood supply. If unusual complications produce a need for hemotherapy on a patient who has had a type and screen only, the patient can receive ABO group and Rh type specific blood with safety even without a crossmatch.

## Specimen

A blood specimen from a patient who has been typed and screened for unexpected antibodies can be held for 72 hours. This specimen can be used for crossmatching, if needed.

## Procedure

1. Perform ABO grouping and Rh typing.
2. Perform an indirect antiglobulin test for unexpected antibodies.
   A. If this test is negative, verify that 2 units of the patient's ABO and Rh type are available for crossmatching in case of an emergency.
   B. If this test is positive, identify the antibody.
   C. Prescreen blood for the absence of the corresponding antigen to the patient's unexpected antibody and crossmatch 2 units of appropriate blood to ensure compatibility.
3. If uncrossmatched blood is issued for a patient who has had a type and screen *only,* the physician does not need to sign a special release form intended for the issuing of blood in an emergency with no previous type and screen.

## References

Baumgarten, R.K.: Elimination of the crossmatch, *Transfusion, 27*(5): 445, 1987.

Beattie, K.M.: Discrepancies in ABO Blood Groupings: A Seminar on Problems Encountered in Pre-Transfusion Tests. Washington, D.C., AABB, 1972.

Beattie, K.M., Ferguson, S.J., Burnie, K.L., et al.: Chloramphenicol antibody causing interference in antibody detection and identification tests, *Transfusion, 16:* 174–177, 1976.

*Blood Group Antigens and Antibodies as Applied to the ABO and Rh Systems,* Ortho Diagnostics, Raritan, NJ, 1969, pp. 15–32.

Boral, L.I., and Henry, J.B.: The type and screen: A safe alternative and supplement in selected surgical procedures. Transfusion, *17:* 163–168, 1977.

Bruce, M., Watt, A.H., Hare, W., Blue, A., and Mitchell, R.: A serious source of error in antiglobulin testing. Transfusion, *26*(2): 177–181, 1986.

Dzik, W.H., and Darling, C.A.: Positive direct antiglobulin test (DAT) due to anti-formaldehyde antibodies. Transfusion, *26*(6): 578, 1986.

Epley, K.M., and Klina, L.M.: One step D$^u$ test. Transfusion, *26*(6): 570, 1986.

Gamma Biologicals, Inc., Houston, Texas: *Reagent Red Blood Cells,* package insert, January, 1986.

Gamma package inserts for anti-A, anti-B, anti-D Gamma Biologicals, Inc., Houston, Texas, January, 1986.

Grindon, A.J., and Wilson, M.J. False-positive DAT caused by variables in sample procurement. Transfusion, *21*(3): 313–314, 1981.

Huestis, D. et al.: *Practical Blood Transfusion,* 3rd Ed. Boston, Little, Brown and Co., 1982.

Huestis, D.W., Bove, J.R., and Case, J.: Practical Blood Transfusion. Boston, Little, Brown and Co., 1988.

Issitt, P.: *Applied Blood Group Serology,* 2nd Ed. Oxnard, CA, Spectra Biologics, 1975.

Jones, E.C., Sinclair, M., Unrau, L., and Grawe, G.: False-positive results with chemically modified anti-D. Transfusion, *27:* 142–144, 1987.

Mollison, P.L.: *Blood Transfusion in Clinical Medicine,* 6th Ed. Oxford, Blackwell Scientific Publications, 1979, p. 556.

*Quality Control in Blood Banking,* Ortho Diagnostics, 1973.

Schmidt, P.J., Klein, R.E., and Sherwood, N.C.: D$^u$ confirmation, Tranfusion, *26*(4): 1986, pp. 364–365.

Schmidt, P.J., Samia, C.T., Gregory, K.R., Leparc, G.F.: Rationale reduction in pretransfusion testing. Lab. Med. *17*(8): 467–479, 1986.

Shulman, Ira A.: The abbreviated crossmatch, College of American Pathologists check sample, *Immunohematology, 30*(2): 2–4, 1987.

Turgeon, M.L., and Bender, J.: Routine Analysis. Corning, NY, Corning College Press, 1982.

Walker, R.H. (Ed): AABB Technical Manual, 11th Ed. American Association of Blood Banks, 1993.

# Special Blood Banking Procedures

## Chapter Outline

## TITLE: A, B, H, Le$^a$ AND Le$^b$: SALIVA TESTING

### Principle

Certain blood group substances, namely A, B, H, and Le$^a$, occur in soluble form in secretions such as saliva in a large proportion of individuals, referred to as *secretors*. These water-soluble substances are readily detected in small quantities because they neutralize or inhibit the capacity of their corresponding antibodies to agglutinate erythrocytes possessing the corresponding antigen. These reactions, termed *hemagglutination inhibition,* provide a means of assaying the relative strength or potency of the water-soluble blood group substances. Identifying the presence of ABH or Le$^a$ substance can be important in blood type problem-solving.

### Specimen

The collection and processing of the patient specimen are as follows:

1. Have the patient chew a piece of paraffin wax (gum or anything else that contains sugar or protein cannot be used) to stimulate salivation.
2. Collect about 2 to 3 mL of saliva in a test tube.
3. Place the stoppered tube of saliva in a boiling waterbath for 10 minutes. Heating the specimen inactivates enzymes that might destroy blood group substances.
4. Centrifuge at 3400 rpm for 10 minutes.
5. Transfer the clear or slightly opalescent supernatant to a clean tube. Discard any opaque or semi-solid material.
6. The supernatant fluid should be refrigerated until the time of testing. If testing will not be done on the day of collection and processing, it should be frozen. Frozen samples retain their activity for several years. *Do not refreeze an aliquot once it has been thawed.*

### Reagents, Supplies, and Equipment

Commercial lectin anti-H
2 to 5% washed erythrocytes, group O
10 × 75 mm or 12 × 75 mm disposable test tubes
Disposable pipettes, 4⅝″ plastic or Pasteur
Normal saline (0.9%)
Centrifuge
High intensity lamp/optical magnifying lens
Microscope (optional)

## Quality Control

Saliva from patients who are known ABH secretors, for example of Se and sese, can be used as positive and negative controls, respectively. Aliquots of saliva or processed supernatant from suitable individuals can be frozen for later use.

A reagent control can be simultaneously assayed by:

1. Adding 1 drop of the highest diluted antiserum with 2+ agglutination to a test tube.
2. Adding 1 drop of a 2 to 5% saline cell suspension of the appropriate blood group, e.g., group O.
3. Incubating 30 to 60 minutes (in parallel with testing).
4. Centrifuging for 15 seconds at 3400 rpm.
5. Reading for agglutination. The agglutination should be 2+.

## Procedure

### Preliminary Antisera Dilution

1. Prepare serial dilutions, e.g., 1:2, 1:4, of lectin anti-H.
2. Label a clean 12 × 75 test tube for each dilution and add 1 drop of the dilution to the appropriately labelled tube.
3. Add 1 drop of the 2 to 5% saline suspension of group O red blood cells to each of the tubes.
4. Centrifuge for 15 seconds at 3400 rpm and observe macroscopically for agglutination.
5. Select the highest dilution of antiserum that produces 2+ macroscopic agglutination as the *working antiserum (antibody dilution)*. Record results.
6. Prepare a sufficient quantity of this dilution to complete the test procedure.

### Detection of Secretion

1. Label four 12 × 75 mm test tubes: Patient, Reagent Control, Se, and sese.
2. Add 1 drop of the patient's supernatant saliva to the Reagent Control tube, and 1 drop of known Se and sese controls to their respective tubes.
3. Add 1 drop of working antibody dilution to all tubes.
4. Incubate all of the tubes at room temperature for 10 minutes.
5. Add 1 drop of the 2 to 5% red blood cell saline suspension of group O cells to each tube.
6. Incubate all the tubes at room temperature for 30 to 60 minutes.
7. Centrifuge for 15 seconds at 3400 rpm.
8. Observe for macroscopic agglutination and record results.

## Reporting Results

The reagent control should demonstrate 2+ agglutination. The Se control should demonstrate no agglutination and the sese control should be negative (agglutination). A *nonsecretor* shows agglutination of red blood cells by antiserum-saliva mixture. A *secretor* shows no agglutination of red blood cells by antiserum-saliva mixture.

## Procedure Notes

The absence of agglutination in saliva is a *positive* test for the presence of ABH soluble antigens and indicates that an individual is a secretor The diluted reagent antiserum has been neutralized by soluble blood group antigens in the saliva. Hence, no antibodies in the antiserum are free to react with the antigens on the reagent red cells introduced into the test.

To detect or measure salivary A or B substance in addition to H substance, the same procedure can be used with diluted anti-A and anti-B reagents. The appropriate dilutions of anti-A or anti-B are obtained by preparing serial dilutions with A or B cells, respectively.

The quantity of H as well as A and B substance varies depending on the ABO type of an individual (Table 15-1). The screening procedure just described can be adapted for semiquantitative estimations of blood group activity by testing serial saline dilutions of processed saliva. Processed saliva should be diluted before incubation with diluted antiserum. The higher the dilution needed to remove inhibitory activity, the more salivary blood group substance is present.

Excessive levels of soluble ABH substances can be observed in rare cases, such as ovarian cysts, carcinoma of the stomach or pancreas, or intestinal obstruction. The level of ABH substance in a person's serum may be so high that it inhibits the anti-A or anti-B reagent sera. This interference with ABO blood grouping is due to neutralization of the reagent anti-A or anti-B by the excess specific soluble substances, which leaves no unbound antibody to react with the person's erythrocytes.

### Procedure for Detection of Lewis Secretions

Controls: Use saliva from a person whose red cells are Le$^a$ positive and from one who is Lewis-negative.

**Table 15-1. ABH Substances in Saliva**

|              | ABO Type        | ABH Substances in Saliva | | |
| ------------ | --------------- | ---- | ---- | ---- |
|              |                 | A    | B    | H    |
| Secretors    | A               | Much | None | Some |
|              | B               | None | Much | Some |
|              | O               | None | None | Much |
|              | AB              | Much | Much | Some |
| Nonsecretors | A, B, O, and AB | None | None | None |

1. Prepare working Le$^a$ antiserum in the same manner as lectin anti-H.
2. Label four 12 × 75 mm test tubes: patient, reagent control, Lewis-positive, and Lewis-negative.
3. Add 1 drop of processed saliva to the appropriate tubes and a drop of saline to the reagent tube.
4. Add 1 drop of working diluted antiserum to all of the tubes.
5. Incubate for 10 minutes at room temperature.
6. Add 1 drop of 2 to 5% saline suspension of washed Le$^a$ red blood cells to each tube.
7. Incubate for 30 to 60 minutes at room temperature.
8. Centrifuge at 3400 rpm for 15 seconds.
9. Observe macroscopically for agglutination.
10. Record results.

*Interpretation:* A nonsecretor of Lewis substance demonstrates agglutination; a secretor has no agglutination of the Le$^a$ positive indicator cells. The reagent control should exhibit 2+ agglutination.

A Lewis-positive person who is a secretor of ABH can be assumed to have Le$^b$ as well as Le$^a$ in the saliva. A Le(a+) person who is sese and does not secrete ABH substance will have only Le$^a$ in saliva.

### Limitations

Detection of soluble blood group substances in saliva should be used in conjunction with blood group testing for erythrocyte antigens.

---

## TITLE: ABSORPTION OF COLD AUTOAGGLUTININS

### Principle

Cold-reacting autoantibodies can interfere with the identification of unexpected antibodies in a patient's serum. Absorption of the patient's serum with autologous red blood cells can remove autoantibody from the serum, permitting detection of underlying unexpected antibodies.

### Specimen

No special preparation of the patient is required before specimen collection. The patient must be positively identified when the specimen is collected. The specimen must be labelled at the bedside and the label must include the patient's first and last name, the date when the specimen is collected, and the patient's hospital identification number. The time of collection and the phlebotomist's initials should be written on the required form.

Blood should be drawn by an aseptic technique and the specimen should be tested as soon as possible. The required specimens are 5 to 7 mL of clotted blood (red top) evacuated tube and 7 mL of EDTA blood (lavender top) evacuated tube. Processing of the specimen is described in the following procedure.

### Reagents, Supplies, and Equipment

10 × 75 mm or 12 × 75 mm disposable test tubes
13 × 100 mm or 16 × 100 mm test tubes
Disposable pipettes, 4⅝″ plastic or Pasteur
Normal saline (0.9%) warmed to 37°
Centrifuge
37° C waterbath or heat block
Ice bath
Test tube rack

### Quality Control

An autologous control ( a mixture of 1 drop of patient's absorbed serum + one drop of patient's red blood cells) should be tested at room temperature and with AHG sera. If this control is negative, most of the cold-reacting autoantibody has been removed and further testing should not be compromised.

### Procedure

1. After properly obtaining the specimens, the red top or nonanticoagulated tube may be allowed to clot in the refrigerator. This step is usually *not sufficient* to remove all of the autoagglutinin, but it does begin the process of removing autoantibodies from the serum. If the patient's blood is already clotted or time is limited, this step may be deleted.
2. Wash the patient's own (autologous) red blood cells from the anticoagulated (lavender top or EDTA) specimen tube with warm 37° C saline at least four times. Care should be taken to remove all the saline after each wash.
3. After the last wash, centrifuge the cells for 5 minutes at 3400 rpm.
4. Remove any remaining saline. This step is very important because residual saline may dilute out an alloantibody in the serum that is being autoabsorbed.
5. Obtain the patient's clotted blood from the refrigerator and centrifuge.
6. Remove all available serum from this clotted specimen. If any red blood cells are unintentionally removed with the serum, centrifuge the serum and transfer it to a clean test tube.
7. Transfer enough serum to perform all necessary post-absorption testing, e.g., compatibility tests, antibody screening, etc., in a large test tube, e.g., 13 × 100 mm or 16 × 100 mm.
8. Add an equal volume of the well-washed, tightly-packed autologous red blood cells prepared in steps 2 through 4.
9. Mix the serum and red cells thoroughly and place in a slush ice bath in a 4° C refrigerator for 15 to 30

minutes. Note: A longer incubation of this aliquot of red cells does not remove additional antibody because all the antigen sites are covered within the first 15 to 20 minutes.

10. Remove the tube from the ice bath and centrifuge for 3 minutes at 3400 rpm. Note: A refrigerated centrifuge or an ice-packed test tube holder is preferred.

11. After centrifugation, *immediately* place the tube in the refrigerator without disturbing the red blood cells. This step increases the amount of antibody removed with each absorption.

12. After 5 minutes, carefully transfer the serum to a clean test tube. The serum must be cell-free. Repeat step 10 if necessary.

13. At this point, the serum has been autoabsorbed *once.*

14. To perform subsequent autoabsorption, add the previously autoabsorbed serum to a fresh aliquot of well-washed, tightly packed autologous red blood cells and repeat steps 8 through 12.

15. After the serum has been removed from the last aliquot of autologous red blood cells, it should be warmed up to room temperature before being used for testing.

## Reporting Results

The use of autoabsorbed serum should be noted on any tests performed with this processed serum.

## Procedure Notes

In most cases, at least 2 autoabsorptions are necessary to remove even low-titered cold autoagglutinins. It is preferable to perform several absorptions with fresh aliquots of autologous red blood cells rather than to extend the cold incubation phase. For example, four 15-minute absorptions on four fresh aliquots of autologous RBCs are preferable to one hour-long incubation.

Exercise care when autoabsorbing the serum of a recently transfused patient because an unexpected antibody may be absorbed from the serum. The prewarmed compatibility test may be substituted.

## Limitations

Cold-reacting antibodies, specific as well as nonspecific, will be removed by this procedure if the erythrocytes have expressed the corresponding antigen.

## TITLE: ABSORPTION OF WARM AUTOAGGLUTININS

### Principle

Absorption of a patient's serum with autologous red blood cells can remove autoantibodies from the serum and per-

mits detection of specific unexpected antibodies. Because circulating autologous red blood cells are already coated with autoantibody, they are pretreated with a proteolytic enzyme. This technique uncovers antigen sites, which are then capable of binding free autoantibody from the serum during incubation and producing an absorbed serum. In some cases, warm-reactive autoagglutinins can mask underlying clinically significant unexpected antibodies.

## Specimen

No special preparation of the patient is required before specimen collection. The patient must be positively identified when the specimen is collected. The specimen must be labelled at the bedside and the label must include the patient's first and last name, the date when the specimen is collected, and the patient's hospital identification number. The time of collection and the phlebotomist's initials should be written on the required form.

Blood should be drawn by an aseptic technique and the specimen should be tested as soon as possible. The required specimens are 5 to 7 mL of clotted blood (red top) evacuated tube and 7 mL of EDTA blood (lavender top) evacuated tube. Processing of the specimen is described in the following procedure.

## Reagents, Supplies and Equipment

6% bovine albumin
1% ficin (available commercially or prepared as follows)

### Phosphate Buffer

*Acidic Stock Solution.* Dissolve 22.16 g of $NaH_2PO_4 \cdot H_2O$ in 1 L of distilled $H_2O$. This 0.16M solution of the monobasic phosphate salt (monohydrate) has a pH of 5.0.

*Alkaline Stock Solution.* Dissolve 17.2 g of $Na_2HPO_4$ in 1 L of distilled $H_2O$. This 0.126M solution of the dibasic phosphate salt (anhydrous) has a pH of 9.0.

*Working Buffer Solution (pH 7.3).* Mix 16 mL of acidic stock solution and 84 mL of alkaline stock solution. Check the pH of the working solution before using it.

*Phosphate-Buffered Saline.* The ratio of one volume of working buffer solution (pH 7.3) to nine volumes of normal (0.9%) saline to prepare the phosphate-buffered saline. To prepare a total of 100 mL, 10 mL of working buffer solution is added to 90 mL of normal saline.

### 1% Ficin Solution

*Caution:* Ficin is harmful if it is inhaled or gets in the eyes. Wear gloves, a mask, and an apron, and work under a hood.

Place 1 g of powdered ficin in a 100 mL volumetric flask. Dissolve in phosphate-buffered saline, pH 7.3, to 100 mL. Agitate vigorously by inversion or on a rotator for 15 minutes, or with a magnetic stirrer for 30 to 90 minutes. The powder will not dissolve completely. Collect clear fluid by filtration or centrifugation. Dispense small aliquots of the solution into clear test tubes and stopper. Store aliquots at −20° C. *Do not refreeze thawed solution.*

10 × 75 mm disposable test tubes
13 × 100 mm or 16 × 100 mm test tubes
Test tube rack
Disposable pipettes, 4⅝″ plastic or Pasteur
Normal saline (0.9%)
Centrifuge
37° C waterbath or heat block

## Quality Control

The patient's red blood cells can function as a negative control. If all of the autoantibody can be eluted from the patient's red blood cells (a nonreactive DAT following step 5 of the procedure), these cells can be used to check the efficacy of the absorption process. When the red blood cells no longer demonstrate autoantibody absorption from the serum (a negative DAT), the serum is ready for unexpected antibody testing.

## Procedure

1. Wash 2 mL of patient red blood cells from an EDTA anticoagulated specimen four times in saline. Discard the supernatant fluid from the final centrifugation.
2. Add an equal volume of 6% albumin to the packed red blood cells and mix thoroughly.
3. Incubate the red blood cells-albumin mixture at 56° C for 3 to 5 minutes. Gently agitate the mixture during incubation.
4. Centrifuge at 3400 rpm for 2 minutes.
5. Transfer the supernatant fluid to a clean test tube. Note: this supernatant fluid may be used as an eluate for testing, if a limited quantity of autologous red cells are available.
6. Wash the red cells three times with normal saline. Discard the final supernatant.
7. Add 1 mL of 1% ficin to the packed red cells. Mix thoroughly.
8. Incubate at 37° C for 15 minutes.
9. Wash the ficin-RBC mixture three times in saline.
10. Centrifuge the final wash for at least 5 minutes at 3400 rpm. Remove as much of the supernatant as possible.
11. Divide the red cells into two equal aliquots.
12. Centrifuge the nonanticoagulated red top specimen. To one aliquot of the washed red cells (step 11), add 2 mL of the patient's serum, mix, and incubate at 37° C for 30 minutes.
13. Centrifuge at 3400 rpm for 2 minutes and transfer the serum to the second aliquot of red cells.

14. Mix and incubate this mixture at 37° C for 30 minutes.
15. Centrifuge at 3400 rpm for 2 minutes. Immediately transfer the absorbed serum to a clean test tube. The serum must be cell-free. Recentrifuge the specimen if any red cells are inadvertently transferred with the serum.
16. At least two autoabsorptions are needed to remove enough autoantibodies to test for unexpected antibody reactivity.

If the patient's red cells can be shown to be nonreactive with DAT following step 5, these cells can be used to check the efficacy of the absorption process. When the red cells no longer demonstrate autoantibody absorption from the serum with the DAT procedure, the serum is now ready for unexpected antibody testing using group O reagent screening cells.

## Reporting Results

If no reactivity with group O reagent red cells is observed (see the procedure for this test in Chapter 14, Routine Procedures), it is unlikely that unexpected antibody is present.

## Procedure Notes

If there is reactivity against both the patient's treated red cells and the group O reagent red cells, further absorption of the serum is necessary.

If the absorbed serum reacts with one or both of the group O reagent screening red cells but not with the autologous red cells, the serum contains one or more unexpected antibodies. Further antibody identification (see Unexpected Antibody Identification, this chapter) should be performed using the absorbed serum.

## Limitations

Autoabsorption should not be performed on cells from a recently transfused patient because the circulating allogeneic RBCs may adsorb the unexpected antibodies that are being sought for identification.

## TITLE: ANTIBODY IDENTIFICATION

### Principle

The antibody panel test is a qualitative test for the identification of unexpected antibodies in patient or donor serum. Serum from patients, for example a surgical or obstetric patient, or from a blood donor, which has exhibited reactivity with group O reagent screening red blood cells is further tested against a panel of 8, 10, or more red blood cells that represent a variety of blood group antigens.

Identification and initial detection of an antibody depend on the method, medium, and temperature of reactivity as well as the titer of the antibody. Hemolysis or agglutination of reagent red blood cells in the presence of serum at any stage of the test demonstrates the presence of an antibody (a positive test) with specificity to a corresponding antigen on the reagent red blood cells. The absence of hemolysis and/or agglutination indicates that the serum being tested does not contain detectable antibodies directed at antigens present on the reagent red cells being used.

## Specimen

No special preparation of the patient is required before specimen collection. The patient must be positively identified when the specimen is collected. The specimen must be labelled at the bedside and the label must include the patient's first and last name, the date when the specimen is collected, and the patient's hospital identification number. The time of collection and the phlebotomist's initials should be written on the required form.

Blood should be drawn by an aseptic technique and the specimen should be tested as soon as possible. The required specimens are 5 to 7 mL of clotted blood (red top) evacuated tube and 7 mL of EDTA blood (lavender top) evacuated tube. The presence of hemolysis in the specimen makes the specimen unsuitable for testing.

Antibodies that depend on the binding of complement for their detection may not be detected if aged serum or plasma from an anticoagulated sample is used for antibody detection testing. Samples for antibody screening may be used up to 72 hours after collection. The specimen must be stored at 1 to 6° C and kept for 7 days.

## Reagents, Supplies, and Equipment

10 × 75 mm disposable test tubes
Disposable pipettes, 4⅝″ plastic or Pasteur
Normal saline (0.9%)
Bovine albumin* (Optional)
Antiglobulin reagent antiserum*
Coombs control or check cells (IgG-sensitized cells)*
Group O reagent panel cells*
Centrifuge
37° C waterbath or heat block
Test tube rack
High intensity lamp/optical magnifying lens
Microscope (optional)

## Quality Control

The test reagents should be monitored daily or at the time of use, as described in Chapter 1 and according to the

Daily Reagent Quality Assurance procedure in Chapter 14.

An autocontrol, a mixture of the patient's erythrocytes and serum, must be tested simultaneously with each antibody panel. This control must be negative for the test results to be valid.

All negative antiglobulin reactions must be tested with Coombs control check cells. A positive test result at this point confirms that active antiglobulin was added to the test system and was present when the original antiglobulin test was interpreted as negative. If a positive result is *not* obtained with the control cells, the test is invalid and must be repeated.

## Procedure

1. Label a tube for each of the reagent panel cells, for example, 1–8 or 1–10, and an autocontrol (AUTO).
2. Using a disposable pipette, add 2 drops of the patient's serum to each tube.
3. Add 2 drops of bovine albumin to each tube (optional).
4. Add 1 drop of reagent red blood cells to each, except the autocontrol.
5. Add 1 drop of the patient's 2 to 5% red blood cell suspension to the tube labeled AUTO.
6. Mix all tubes and centrifuge for 15 seconds at 3400 rpm.
7. Gently resuspend the cells in all tubes and examine macroscopically for agglutination or hemolysis. Record the results as immediate spin (IS) reactions. Positive reactions should be graded from 1 to 4+ at each stage of observation (see Grading Agglutination Reactions, Chapter 14). Complete hemolysis precludes further testing and must be interpreted as a positive result. If partial hemolysis is observed, record and proceed. All positive and negative tests should be continued through all phases of testing.
8. Incubate all tubes for 30 minutes at 37° C.
9. Centrifuge all the tubes for 15 seconds at 3400 rpm.
10. Gently resuspend the cells in all tubes and examine macroscopically for agglutination or hemolysis. Record results as 37° C reactions.
11. Wash each tube 3 times. Decant completely after the last wash.
12. Add 2 drops of antiglobulin (AHG) reagent to each tube.
13. Mix and centrifuge for 15 seconds at 3400 rpm.
14. Gently resuspend the cells and examine macroscopically with the aid of magnification (microscopic examination is optional). Record results as antiglobulin (AHG) reactions.
15. To each tube that exhibits no agglutination, add 1 drop of Coombs check cells. Mix well and centrifuge for 15 seconds at 3400 rpm. Resuspend the cells and

* Should be refrigerated when not in use.

examine macroscopically for agglutination. Record these results as control cells (CC).

## Reporting Results

Agglutination or hemolysis of any screening cell suspension in the immediate-spin, 37° C, or antiglobulin (AHG) phase indicates a positive reaction. The absence of hemolysis or agglutination constitutes a negative test and indicates the absence of detectable antibodies to specific antigens present on the reagent erythrocyte.

If a pattern of positive and negative reactions is observed with different test cells, antibody identification is simplified by eliminating antibodies specific for antigens present on any nonreactive cells. Comparisons of the pattern of positive and negative reactions with the known antigen makeup of the reagent red blood cells enable the specificity of the antibodies or antibodies to be determined (see Chapter 7, Pretransfusion Testing).

## Procedure Notes

If the autocontrol is positive, absorption and/or elution tests need to be performed to separate the autoantibody from any underlying unexpected antibody. In the case of a recently transfused patient, a positive autocontrol may indicate the presence of an alloantibody directed at an antigen present on surviving donor cells. In such cases, a mixed-field agglutination reaction may be observed.

The reagent panel cells can be modified with enhancement media such as albumin, enzymes, polybrene, or LISS. If albumin is used as an enhancer, the reactivity of low-titered antibodies may be increased by washing the reagent erythrocytes once with normal saline, decanting the saline completely, and using the "dry button" of cells for the test. If a low ionic strength test procedure is used, the cell suspensions should be prepared according to the manufacturer's directions.

## Limitations

See Antibody Screening (Indirect Antiglobulin or Indirect Coombs' Test with Autocontrol) in Chapter 14.

---

## TITLE: ANTIBODY TITRATION

### Principle

Titration is a semiquantitative method of measuring the concentration of antibody in serum. Serial dilutions, for example, 1:2 or 1:4, of serum containing an antibody are tested with a constant volume of red blood cells. The test result is expressed as the reciprocal of the highest dilution that exhibits agglutination. Observation of agglutination is usually macroscopic; however, it may be microscopic with antibodies such as high-titer, low-avidity antibodies.

Titration is clinically most useful as a comparison of one specimen with another. Although it may be used for other purposes, for instance, to identify "least incompatible" donor units when crossmatching difficulties exist, the antibody titration procedure is most frequently used to detect changing antibody concentrations in obstetrical patients. When a significant increase in antibody concentration does occur, intrauterine transfusions can be performed between 28 and 32 weeks gestation. After 32 weeks, labor is usually induced.

## Specimen

No special preparation of the patient is required before specimen collection. The patient must be positively identified when the specimen is collected. The specimen must be labelled at the bedside and the label must include the patient's first and last name, the date when the specimen is collected, and the patient's hospital identification number. The time of collection and the phlebotomist's initials should be written on the required form.

Blood should be drawn by an aseptic technique and the specimen should be tested as soon as possible. The required specimens are 5 to 7 mL of clotted blood (red top) evacuated tube and 7 mL of EDTA blood (lavender top) evacuated tube. The presence of hemolysis in a specimen makes it unsuitable for testing.

Antibodies that depend on the binding of complement for their detection may not be detected if aged serum or plasma from an anticoagulated sample is used for antibody detection or titration. The serum from this specimen should be *frozen* for future comparative study.
*Note:* The previously titrated serum should be defrosted in a 37° C waterbath for simultaneous testing with the fresh specimen.

## Reagents, Supplies, and Equipment

10 × 75 mm disposable test tubes
Graduated serologic pipettes or disposable pipette tips and aspirator
Normal saline (0.9%)
Bovine albumin* (Optional)
Antiglobulin reagent antisera*
Coombs control or check cells (IgG-sensitized cells)*
Reagent screening red blood cells I*
Reagent screening red blood cells II*
Patient's cumulative record (if previously tested)
Centrifuge
37° C waterbath or heat block
Test tube rack
High intensity lamp/optical magnifying lens
Microscope (optional)

* Should be refrigerated when not in use.

## Quality Control

An autocontrol, a mixture of patient's erythrocytes and serum, must be tested simultaneously with each antibody screening test.

The test reagents should be monitored daily or at the time of use as described in Chapter 1 and according to the Daily Reagent Quality Assurance procedure in Chapter 14.

All negative antiglobulin reactions must be tested with Coombs Control/Check Cells. A positive test result at this point will confirm that active antiglobulin was added to the test system and was present when the original antiglobulin test was interpreted as negative. If a positive result is *not* obtained with the control cells, the test is invalid and must be repeated.

## Procedure

### Preliminary

1. Compare information on specimen with request form: full name, full hospital number, and date. If this information is *not identical,* obtain a new specimen.
2. Prepare a 2 to 4% suspension of patient's red cells (see Preparation of Red Cell Suspensions in Chapter 14).
3. Centrifuge the clotted specimen for 5 minutes at 2500 rpm.
4. Determine if the patient has been previously tested by checking past records in a cumulative patient file.
5. Perform an antibody screening and panel cell procedure. This step is important even if the patient has had an antibody identified previously. It is important to establish the identity of the antibody or antibodies as well as the optimum phase of reactivity.
6. Prepare separate serial dilutions of both the fresh serum and the previous specimen (if available). The dilution should begin with 1:2 and extend to at least 1:132 according to the previous titer. The diluent may be either saline or albumin depending upon the optimum medium of reactivity observed in the screening procedure. If albumin is used as the diluent, the reagent red blood cells must also be suspended in albumin.

### Antibody Titration

1. Label two sets of 10 × 75 mm test tubes, one set for the present serum and the other for the past serum. Each dilution must be represented by a separate tube.
2. Using a disposable pipette, add 2 drops of the diluted serum to each of the respective tubes.
3. Add 1 drop of reagent red cells to each of the tubes. The reagent red cell suspension should be chosen from the most reactive red cells from the screening or panel cells used in the preliminary testing.
4. Mix all tubes and centrifuge for 15 seconds at 3400 rpm.

5. Gently resuspend the cells in all tubes and examine macroscopically for agglutination or hemolysis. Record the results as immediate-spin (IS) reactions. Positive reactions should be graded from 1 to 4+ at each stage of observation (see Grading Agglutination Reactions in Chapter 13). Complete hemolysis precludes further testing and must be interpreted as a positive result. If partial hemolysis is observed, record and proceed. All positive and negative tests should be continued through all phases of testing.
6. Incubate all tubes for 30 minutes at 37° C.
7. Centrifuge all tubes for 15 seconds at 3400 rpm.
8. Gently resuspend the cells in all tubes and examine macroscopically for agglutination or hemolysis. Record results as 37° C reactions.
9. Wash each tube three times. Decant completely after the last wash.
10. Add 2 drops of antiglobulin (AHG) reagent to each tube.
11. Mix each tube and centrifuge for 15 seconds at 3400 rpm.
12. Gently resuspend the cells and examine macroscopically with the aid of magnification (microscopic examination is optional). Record results as antiglobulin (AHG) reactions.
13. To each tube that exhibits no agglutination add 1 drop of Coombs check cells. Mix well and centrifuge for 15 seconds at 3400 rpm. Resuspend the cells and examine macroscopically for agglutination. Record these results as control cells (CC).

### Grading Agglutination Strength

Grading the strength of agglutination is critical to the accuracy of the procedure. It is not uncommon to find that the end point (titer) may be the same for two successive specimens, but the strength of the reactions from the dilutions is not the same. Therefore, to determine antibody strength, both the *avidity* (the strength of the reaction at each dilution) and the titer should be considered. This is done by giving numeric values to each degree of agglutination and totaling the results of all tubes. Although the numeric score may vary from one blood bank to another, uniformity should be demonstrated within a blood bank. An example of a grading system is presented in Table 15-2. Complete or partial hemolysis cannot be easily quanti-

**Table 15-2. Representative Grading System**

| Qualitative Notation | Score |
| --- | --- |
| 4+ | 12 |
| 3+ | 10 |
| 2+ | 8 |
| 1+ | 5 |
| W+ | 2 |
| 0 | 0 |

tated; however, it usually denotes a highly positive reaction.

An example of an antibody titration follows.

| | | | | | | | | | Total Score |
|---|---|---|---|---|---|---|---|---|---|
| **1st specimen** | | | | | | | | | |
| Dilution strength of reaction score | 1 | 2 | 4 | 8 | 16 | 32 | 64 | 128 | |
| | 4+ | 3+ | 3+ | 2+ | 2+ | 1+ | 1+ | 0 | |
| | 12 | 10 | 10 | 8 | 8 | 5 | 5 | 0 | 58 |

| | | | | | | | | | Total Score |
|---|---|---|---|---|---|---|---|---|---|
| **2nd specimen** | | | | | | | | | |
| Dilution strength of reaction score | 1 | 2 | 4 | 8 | 16 | 32 | 64 | 128 | |
| | 4+ | 4+ | 4+ | 4+ | 3+ | 2+ | 1+ | 0 | |
| | 12 | 12 | 12 | 12 | 10 | 8 | 5 | 0 | 71 |

## Reporting Results

The previous and present antibody titers should be reported. If an antibody is increasing in strength but not titer, it should be noted. Only a titer change of two tubes (fourfold) or more is clinically significant.

## Procedure Notes

If the autocontrol demonstrates a positive reaction, the serum contains an autoantibody. The presence of an autoantibody can conceal an underlying alloantibody in the serum. Autoabsorption (see sections on absorption of cold and warm agglutinins, this chapter) may be required to test the serum for the presence of alloantibodies.

The optimum mode and medium of reactivity as well as the most reactive red blood cells should be determined in preliminary evaluation of the antibody. Once determined, these should be used consistently. It is also important to establish the identity of the antibody at each testing and to detect the presence of any additional antibodies.

A variety of factors can affect an antibody titration:

1. The same cell suspension must be used for both sera. Any variation in the strength of suspension or antigen will introduce a variable into the comparison.
2. Meticulous pipetting technique is needed. Mouth pipetting is prohibited. A semi-automatic pipetter is recommended and a clean pipette tip should be used for each dilution.
3. The prozone phenomenon can produce weaker reactions in the initial tubes than in a higher dilution. It is important to evaluate the dilution series starting with the most dilute and ending with the most concentrated specimen.

Some additional applications of antibody titration include:

1. Selection of blood for patients with autoimmune hemolytic anemia
2. Study of the characteristics of one antibody or a mixture of antibodies in a single serum
3. Determination of the reactivity of the antigenic determinants on various red blood cells
4. Testing of antibodies for reagent use

## Limitations

The detection of antibodies in serum can be compromised if the serum dilutions are incorrectly prepared or the ratio of diluted serum to cells in the test is incorrect.

Other limitations are comparable to the limitations encountered in the antibody screening and panel cell identification procedures.

## TITLE: COMPATIBILITY TESTING (CROSSMATCHING): PREWARMED TECHNIQUE

### Principle

Pretransfusion compatibility testing combines a potential recipient's blood specimen with a blood specimen from an intended donor. This procedure is based on the principle that warming the constituent ingredients to 37° C before mixing bypasses the phase in which the cold-reacting antibodies react by either direct agglutination or binding of complement that demonstrates reactivity in the AHG phase. By avoiding the in vitro interference produced by such antibodies, the prewarming technique ensures that agglutination is not present due to clinically significant antibody-antigen reactions that could have in vivo consequences; that is, antibodies that are reactive at 37° C.

### Specimen

No special preparation of the patient is required before specimen collection. The patient must be positively identified when the specimen is collected. The specimen must be labelled at the bedside and the label must include the patient's first and last name, the date when the specimen is collected, and the patient's hospital identification number.

The time of collection and the phlebotomist's initials should be written on the required form.

Blood should be drawn by an aseptic technique and the specimen should be tested as soon as possible. Approximately 5 to 7 mL of blood should be collected in a red top (no anticoagulant) or lavender top (EDTA) evacuated tube.

It is preferable to place the specimens immediately in a container of warm water en route to the blood bank. If the specimen is rapidly centrifuged, special techniques are not usually needed to keep the specimen at 37° C before testing. All specimens must be retained under refrigeration for 7 days after transfusion of a unit of blood.

## Reagents, Supplies, and Equipment

Commercial antiglobulin (AHG) reagent (broad-spectrum or IgG)
   Note: The AHG should be brought to room temperature for this procedure.
10 × 75 mm disposable test tubes
Disposable pipettes, 4⅝" plastic or Pasteur
Scissors
Test tube rack
Normal (0.9%) saline
   Note: Warm saline to 37° C by placing in a 37° C waterbath for at least 30 minutes before beginning the test. Use prewarmed saline throughout the procedure.
37° C waterbath or heat block
High intensity lamp/optical magnifying lens
Centrifuge

## Quality Control

Reagent erythrocytes should be tested daily with known antisera (see Daily Reagent Quality Assurance testing procedure in Chapter 14). All negative AHG reactions must be tested with IgG-sensitized erythrocytes and produce a positive reaction. If the AHG control cells do not agglutinate, the compatibility test is invalid.

## Procedure

### Preliminary

1. Compare the information on the patient's specimen with the information on the test requisition: name, identification number, date. If this information is not identical, obtain a new specimen.
2. Centrifuge the clotted specimen for 5 minutes at 2000 rpm.
3. Check past blood bank records to determine if the patient has ever been screened for antibodies or previously transfused.

4. Perform an ABO grouping (forward and reverse), Rh typing, and antibody screen on the recipient's specimen. Record all test results in the blood bank log as well as on the crossmatch requisition.
5. Check data on previous records. If the ABO and Rh are not identical, obtain a new specimen for repeat testing.
6. Procure the whole blood or packed cells to be crossmatched from the blood bank refrigerator. Check all identification on the units, e.g., group and Rh, expiration date, and the physical characteristics of the units, including absence of hemolysis or abnormal color.
7. Detach a segment from the unit of blood. Cut the ends of the segment and drain the contents into a 10 × 75 mm test tube. Label the tube with the donor unit identification number. Recheck number.
8. Wash the donor specimen 3 times with normal saline. Decant the last wash completely and prepare a 3 to 5% suspension of the erythrocytes.
9. Enter the donor number and expiration date on the test requisition. If the donor unit has not been retyped on entering the blood bank inventory, an ABO typing and Rh typing should be performed.

### Compatibility Procedure

The following is an example of a typical crossmatch configuration including both phases.

1. Label two 10 × 75 mm test tubes. One tube may be labelled Suspension; the other XM for control.
2. To the Suspension tube add 2 or 3 drops of donor cell suspension. To the XM tube add 2 drops of patient serum.
3. Prewarm both tubes at 37° C for 15 minutes.
4. Without removing the tubes from the incubator, add 1 drop of prewarmed cell suspension to the tube labelled XM containing the patient's serum.
5. Mix the XM tube thoroughly.
6. Discard the Suspension tube.
7. Incubate the tube labelled XM at 37° C for 30 minutes.
8. Following the 30-minute incubation, wash the contents of the tube labelled XM three times using the prewarmed saline.
9. Decant completely after the final wash.
10. Add 2 drops of AHG to the tube labelled XM and mix thoroughly. Note: the AHG should be at room temperature.
11. Centrifuge the tube at 3400 rpm for 15 seconds.
12. Gently resuspend the cell button, read macroscopically (see Grading Agglutination Reactions in Chapter 13) and examine for agglutination. Record the results.
13. Add 1 drop of Coombs control check cells to the tube if no agglutination is present. Centrifuge the tube at 3400 rpm for 15 seconds. Gently resuspend the cell button and read macroscopically. Record results.

14. If the Coombs control check cells do *not* agglutinate, the test is not valid and must be repeated.

## Reporting Results

A compatible crossmatch is indicated by the absence of agglutination and/or hemolysis. The absence of agglutination indicates that the patient has no demonstrable antibodies at 37° C with a specificity for any of the antigens on the donor erythrocytes.

## Procedure Notes

Albumin should *not* be used in this technique because it has a tendency to enhance the reactivity of cold agglutinins.

If incompatibility is demonstrated by agglutination or hemolysis at any stage of the crossmatch, the donor unit should not be used for transfusion. Exceptions might include "least compatible" units in patients with autoantibodies.

The crossmatch should be reported as using *prewarmed technique.* The use of a warming coil is generally recommended for the administration of a unit crossmatched by the prewarming technique.

## Limitations

In addition to the general limitations of the routine compatibility procedure, such as failure to prevent immunization of the patient or guaranteeing normal survival of transfused erythrocytes, the prewarming technique does not detect IgM antibodies such as anti-A or anti-B. Cold-reacting alloantibodies such as anti-M may be missed.

## TITLE: DONATH-LANDSTEINER SCREENING TEST

## Principle

The Donath-Landsteiner antibody test is used to demonstrate the presence of this extremely potent hemolysin. This antibody requires cold incubation to exhibit hemolysis in the patient's serum. A positive test is diagnostic of paroxysmal cold hemoglobinuria (PCH), the rarest form of auto-immune hemolytic anemia. See preceding procedure for full details of specimen collection.

## Specimen

Fresh venous blood should be used. Care must be taken to avoid hemolyzing the specimen during venipuncture.

## Reagents, Supplies, and Equipment

1. 16 × 100 mm test tubes
2. Crushed ice water bath (4° C)
3. 37° C water bath or heat block

## Quality Control

A normal patient control specimen is run concurrently with the patient's test specimen.

## Procedure

1. Place two test tubes in a 37° C water bath or heat block. Warm a 10 mL syringe by holding it in the palm of the hand for a few minutes.
2. Draw 10 mL of blood and transfer 5 mL to each test tube. Label one tube "Control" and immediately place at 37° C. Label the other tube "Test" and place in an ice water bath at 4° C. Incubate both tubes for 1 hour. At the end of 1 hour, move the "Test" sample to the 37° C water bath for an additional 30 minutes.
3. At the end of 90 minutes, carefully remove the tubes and examine for hemolysis.

## Reporting Results

If the serum in both tubes is free of hemolysis, the test is negative. If a pink or red color is present in the serum of the "Test" and the "Control" is free of hemolysis, the test is positive. Normal blood will exhibit no hemolysis in either tube.

## Procedure Notes

A positive test is diagnostic of paroxysmal cold hemoglobinuria (PCH). This disease is caused by a cold autoantibody with several unique characteristics. It is a complement-dependent, 7S IgG cold antibody; hemolysis occurs only after warming, even though complement activation may initially occur in the cold. The causative antibody, the Donath-Landsteiner antibody, is extremely lytic and is one of the most potent hemolysins known.

## TITLE: ELUTION TECHNIQUES

## Principle

The purpose of all elution techniques is to interfere with the noncovalent binding forces that hold antigen-antibody complexes together on the red blood cell membrane surface. A number of elution methods that physically disrupt the red blood cell membrane or chemically interfere with the binding forces of these antigen-antibody complexes can be used to detach and retrieve red blood cell antibodies for study. These methods include:

1. Chloroform elution
2. Citric acid elution
3. Cold acid elution
4. Glycine-HCl/EDTA elution
5. Lui easy freeze elution
6. Heat elution
7. Xylene elution

The preparation of an antibody-containing eluate will only be successful if the red blood cells processed are adequately coated with antibody. Before actually performing an elution, free (unbound) antibody is removed from the red blood cell suspension by washing the cells thoroughly with saline. One of the preceding methods is then used to free the antibody bound to the red blood cells. An eluate can be tested for specificity with reagent red blood cells in the same manner as serum.

Elutions are clinically useful in any situation where antibody is attached to red blood cells, e.g., hemolytic disease of the newborn (HDN). Even in cases of very weakly positive (or even negative) direct antiglobulin tests, cell-bound antibody may be present, e.g., hemolytic disease of the newborn caused by ABO incompatibility.

Some elution methods are more satisfactory for certain types of antibodies. The *chloroform elution method* is suitable for the investigation of a positive direct antiglobulin test (DAT) associated with warm-reactive (IgG) auto or unexpected antibodies and, in conjunction with adsorption techniques, the separation of mixtures of IgG red blood cell antibodies. The *heat elution technique* is best suited for the investigation of ABO hemolytic disease of the newborn, and the elution of IgM antibodies from red blood cells. It should not be routinely used for the investigation of immune red blood cell destruction by IgG auto or unexpected antibodies.

An eluate is not stable. If not tested on the day of preparation, an eluate should be promptly frozen and stored at $-20°$ C. Most eluates contain hemoglobin, which does not interfere with their usefulness. Cellular debris, if present, should be completely removed by centrifugation. Eluated antibodies do not always react the same as they did in the serum from which prepared. Serologic behavior of the eluate itself should be determined before extensive tests are started.

## Specimen

An anticoagulated specimen of whole blood in EDTA is taken from an adult, or as a cord specimen from a newborn. Blood should be tested while it is still fresh. If a delay in testing is necessary, the specimen must be stored at $2°$ C to $8°$ C for no longer than 7 days. *Note:* The yield of antibody eluted from stored cells may be less than that from fresh cells.

## Reagents, Supplies, and Equipment

$10 \times 75$ mm disposable test tubes
Disposable pipettes and safety bulb
Normal saline (0.9%)
Antihuman globulin sera
Coombs control check cells
7 mL test tubes
Large centrifuge
$56°$ C water bath
Test-tube rack

## Quality Control

A small volume of thoroughly washed patient red blood cells is tested with AHG to ensure that the cells are coated. Add 2 drops of antiglobulin sera to 2 drops of the final saline wash. Mix well and let stand at room temperature for 5 minutes. Add 1 drop Coombs control cells. Mix and centrifuge at 3400 rpm for 15 seconds. Agglutination indicates the cells have been washed free of any unbound antibody. No agglutination indicates more washing is necessary.

### Chloroform Elution

#### *Reagents*

1. Spectrophometric grade chloroform (very high grade). *Caution:* Store and handle with care.
2. 6% bovine albumin (6% albumin—prepare by adding 4 mL of normal saline to 1.5 mL of 22% bovine albumin).
3. Red blood cells, washed six times in saline.
4. Supernatant saline from final wash.

#### *Procedure*

1. Prepare a 50% suspension of well-washed red blood cells in saline or low ionic strength saline (LISS) in a $13 \times 100$ mm test tube. Use 6% bovine albumin as diluent for increased stability of eluted antibody if it is to be frozen.
2. Add an equal volume of chloroform.
3. Stopper the tube with a cork, and shake the tube vigorously for 10 to 15 seconds. Mix further by inversion for approximately 1 minute.
4. Carefully remove the cork, and place the tube in a $56°$ C waterbath for exactly 5 minutes. *(Do not exceed 5 minutes at $56°$ C).* Vigorously stir the contents of the tube with an applicator stick periodically during this time.
5. Centrifuge the tube at 900–1000 $\times$ g for 4 to 5 minutes.
6. Transfer the supernatant eluate into a clean test tube, and test in parallel with the supernatant saline from the final wash. Note: The use of LISS as the elution diluent and LISS-suspended reagent red blood cells in the detection system can greatly facilitate the detection of eluted antibody.

### Citric Acid Elution

#### *Reagents*

1. Eluting solution: citric acid (monohydrate), 1.3 g; $KH_2PO_4$, 0.65 g; add to volumetric flask and dilute to 100 mL with saline; store at $4°$ C

2. Neutralizing solution: $Na_3PO_4$, 13.0 g; add to volumetric flask and dilute to 100 mL with distilled water; store at 4° C.
3. Red blood cells, washed six times in saline.
4. Supernatant saline from final wash.

## Procedure

1. Chill all reagents to 4° C before use (use an ice bath).
2. Place 1 mL of packed red blood cells in a 13 × 100 mm test tube.
3. Add 1 mL of eluting solution and note the time.
4. Stopper the tube and mix by inversion for exactly 90 seconds.
5. Remove stopper and promptly centrifuge the tube at 900–1000 × g for exactly 45 seconds.
6. Transfer supernatant fluid to a clean test tube and add 5–6 drops of neutralizing solution; save red blood cells for adsorption studies if needed.
7. Check pH; adjust, if necessary, to pH 7.0 by adding more neutralizing solution.
8. Centrifuge at 900–1000 × g for 2 to 3 minutes to remove precipitate that forms after neutralization; harvest the supernatant eluate and test in parallel with the supernatant saline from the final wash.

   *Limitations.* Kell system antigen expression is markedly weakened after citric-acid treatment.

Notes:

1. Citric acid–modified red blood cells may also be protease-treated and used in autologous adsorption studies.
2. Except for Kell-system antigens, red blood cells obtained in step 6 above may be used in tests to determine phenotype if the DAT is negative.

### Lui Easy Freeze Elution Technique

1. To 6–8 drops of washed, red blood cells add 1–2 drops 0.9% NaCl, mix, and stopper.
2. Coat sides of tube by rotation. Place tube at a slant at −6° C to −30° C for 10 minutes.
3. Thaw rapidly (under running tap water).
4. Centrifuge the hemolyzed cells.
5. Test clear hemolysate against A, B, and O cells by routine technique.

### Landstein and Miller Heat Elution Technique

1. Antibody-coated red blood cells are washed four times with normal saline.
2. To one volume of packed red blood cells, add one-half the volume of normal saline.
3. This suspension is agitated *continuously* in a water bath kept at 56° C for 10 minutes.
4. Centrifuge for 3 minutes at 3000 rpm. Preheated centrifuge cups are recommended.

5. The supernatant, which contains the eluted antibody, is removed as quickly as possible. Test eluate by appropriate techniques.

## Procedure

### Preparation of Eluate

1. Break up a clotted specimen with applicator sticks or obtain 1–2 mL of free cells from an EDTA specimen. Manually wash the cells at least three times with large quantities of saline. If less than 1 mL of free cells is used, there will be insufficient eluate for testing.
2. Pack the cell mass and remove all of the last wash completely.
3. To one volume of red blood cells, add 1 volume of 6% bovine albumin and resuspend.
4. Constantly agitate the cell-albumin mixture in a 56° C waterbath for 7 minutes.
5. Preheat centrifuge holders by placing them in the 56° C waterbath.
6. Immediately centrifuge the cell-albumin mixture at 2000 rpm for 5 minutes.
7. Immediately remove the supernatant (eluate) and use it for testing. Do not remove any cells with the eluate, since they will reabsorb the antibody. This eluate is used in the same manner as serum.

Note: if antibodies other than Anti-A or Anti-B are suspected, identify the antibody using a reagent red blood cell panel with the eluate (see Identification of Antibodies).

### Testing of Eluate

1. Label four 10 × 75 mm test tubes: A, B, I, II.
2. Add 2 drops of eluate to each tube.
3. To each of labeled tubes, add 1 drop of 3% suspension of adult $A_1$ cells, B cells, and I, II.
4. Mix cells well and incubate at 37° C for 30 minutes.
5. Wash the contents of each tube three times with normal saline. Decant completely after the last wash.
6. Add 2 drops of antiglobulin sera to each tube.
7. Mix all tubes well and centrifuge at 3400 rpm for 15 seconds.
8. Gently resuspend the cells and examine each tube macroscopically and microscopically for agglutination. Record the results.
9. To each tube showing no agglutination after step 8, add 1 drop of Coombs control check cells.
10. Mix the tubes well and centrifuge for 15 seconds at 3400 rpm.
11. Gently resuspend the cells and examine each tube macroscopically for agglutination. If any of the tubes show no agglutination, the entire procedure is invalid and must be repeated.

## Reporting Results

Agglutination occurring when the eluate is tested against RBCs of appropriate phenotypes indicates that an antibody has been recovered from the original cells, subject to satisfactory control tests.

The absence of agglutination or of protein indicates that no antibody has been recovered from the cells.

## Procedure Notes

When cells are used to absorb antibody from serum, the lag periods between the adsorption, washing of the cells, and elution should be as short as possible. If the cells are allowed to remain in the serum after incubation, some of the adsorbed antibody may elute back into the original serum.

The strength of the AHG on a sample of the cells is an indication of the amount of antibody adsorbed on the cells. This will help determine the amount of fluid to be added to the cell mass for elution. If the AHG reaction is 3+ or 4+, the antibody can be eluted into a volume of fluid 1½ times the volume of the cells, and the reaction of the eluate will still be strong enough for definitive testing. If the AHG reaction is 2+, an equal volume of fluid and cell mass is used. If the AHG reaction is less than 2+, a smaller volume of fluid than the cell mass is indicated—thereby concentrating the antibody.

## Example

Results of eluate from Group A Cord Cells:

| Test Cells | Antiglobulin Test Results |
|---|---|
| A₁ | 3+ |
| B | 1+ |
| O | Neg |
| O | Neg |

Note: A weak reaction of the eluate with B cells indicates cross-reactivity of the antibody.

## Clinical Applications

Once an antibody has attached to red blood cells, either in vivo or in vitro, it can be recovered from those cells by a process called *elution*. The recovered antibody, in whatever fluid has been used to retrieve it, is called an *eluate*. Antibody elution is a valuable serologic tool and can be applied to:

1. Identification of antibodies from sera containing mixtures of antibodies.
2. Confirmation of antibody specificity.
3. Confirmation of the presence of weak antigens on red blood cell samples.
4. Identification of antibodies causing hemolytic disease of the newborn when the mother's serum is not available or verification of hemolytic disease of the newborn due to ABO incompatibility. In the case of severe hemolytic disease of the newborn (HDN), if the mother's serum is unavailable, the eluate should also be used to crossmatch blood for an exchange transfusion.
5. Identification of antibodies coating surviving incompatible donor red blood cells that have caused transfusion reactions.
6. Investigation of antibodies coating the red blood cells of patients with acquired hemolytic anemia.

## Limitations

Although heat elution is an easy and rapid procedure, it does not demonstrate good recovery of antibodies.

If washing is not adequate, the eluate will actually be a combination of free and eluted antibody. As many as a dozen or more washes may be necessary to remove free antibodies.

*Note:* The Landsteiner and Miller Heat Elution Technique is best suited for the investigation of ABO hemolytic disease of the newborn and the elution of IgM antibodies from red blood cells. It should not be routinely used for the investigation of immune red blood cell destruction by IgG auto or unexpected antibodies.

---

## TITLE: HEMOGLOBIN F DETERMINATION BY ACID ELUTION (KLEIHAUER-BETKE METHOD MODIFIED BY SHEPARD, WEATHERALL, AND CONLEY)

### Principle

After blood smears are fixed with ethyl alcohol, a citric acid-phosphate buffer solution removes (elutes) hemoglobin other than hemoglobin F from erythrocytes. The hemoglobin F (fetal hemoglobin)-containing erythrocytes are visibly identifiable upon microscopic examination when appropriately stained. Shortly after birth, the amount of hemoglobin F in humans decreases to low levels. Increased amounts of hemoglobin F are found in various hemoglobinopathies such as hereditary persistence of fetal hemoglobin, sickle cell anemia, and thalassemias.

### Specimen

Capillary blood or EDTA anticoagulated blood should be used. Smears made from fresh blood give the best results. Whole blood drawn into EDTA anticoagulant can be stored under refrigeration for no longer than 2 weeks. However, as soon as the blood smears are made, the test must be performed.

See Compatibility Testing procedure for full details of specimen collection.

Special Blood Banking Procedures **375**

## Reagents, Supplies, and Equipment

1. Ethyl alcohol, 80% (v/v)
2. Citric acid-phosphate buffer
   A. Stock Solutions
      (1) 0.2 M dibasic sodium phosphate ($Na_2HPO_4$). Weigh 2.84 g of dibasic sodium phosphate and transfer to 100 mL volumetric flask. Dilute to the 100 mL calibration mark with distilled water. Transfer to a dark brown bottle. Label the container with the reagent name and date. Refrigerate this stock solution.
      (2) 0.1 M citric acid. Weight 2.1 g of citric acid. Transfer to a 100 mL volumetric flask and dilute to the 100 mL calibration mark with distilled water. Transfer to a dark brown bottle. Label the container with the reagent name and date. Refrigerate this stock solution.
   B. Working Solution
      Before use, prepare the citric acid-phosphate buffer by mixing 13.3 mL of 0.2M dibasic sodium phosphate and 36.7 mL of 0.1M citric acid. A pH of 3.2 to 3.3 is critical; check with pH meter.
3. An aqueous solution of 0.1% erythrosin B. Weigh 0.2 g of erythrosin B and transfer to a 200 mL volumetric flask. Add approximately 170 mL of distilled water. Add two to three drops of glacial acetic acid. Dilute to the 200 mL calibration mark with distilled water. Mix and filter through #42 Whatman filter paper. Transfer to a labelled brown bottle. Store at room temperature and filter before use.
4. Mayer's hematoxylin. To prepare this solution, add 1 gram of hematoxylin (color index #75290) to an Erlenmeyer flask containing 500 mL of distilled water. Heat just to boiling on a hot plate and add another 500 mL of distilled water. Mix. Add 0.2 grams of sodium iodate. Mix. Add 50 grams of aluminum potassium sulfate (12 $H_2O$). Mix. Transfer to a large stoppered bottle and shake for 1 minute. Filter. Transfer to a brown bottle, label with reagent name and date. This solution should be stored at room temperature and keeps indefinitely.
5. 6 staining containers with covers and a timer.
6. Microscope, immersion oil, lens paper.

## Quality Control

Control tests using normal adult blood as well as blood from a neonate should be performed simultaneously with a patient specimen. The adult blood sample should have only a rare cell containing hemoglobin F, while the newborn infant sample should have a high percentage of acid resistant cells per microscopic field.

## Procedure

1. Make four thin blood smears from each specimen: patient, normal control, and neonatal control. Label.
2. Allow these smears to air-dry for 10 to 60 minutes.
3. Prepare the working citric acid-phosphate buffer solution. Transfer to a staining jar and cover. Incubate at 37° C for 30 minutes.
4. The solutions needed for steps 5 to 9 should be prepared and filtered (if needed) and dispensed into labelled containers before proceeding with the next step.
5. Place the dry slides into 80% ethyl alcohol for about 5 minutes. At the end of this time, gently rinse or dip the smears in distilled water and allow to air-dry.
6. After the smears are completely dry, place the slides in the prewarmed citric acid-phosphate buffer solution for 5 minutes. At the end of 1 minute, dip the slides up and down. Repeat again at 3 minutes.
7. After 5 minutes, remove the slides from the citric acid-phosphate buffer solution and rinse with distilled water. Air-dry.
8. After the smears are completely dry, stain in Mayer's hematoxylin for 3 minutes. Rinse with distilled water.
9. Place the slides in erythrosin B for 4 minutes. Rinse with distilled water and allow to air-dry.
10. Examine with (100×) oil immersion objective for hemoglobin F. Cells containing hemoglobin F stain a dark red-orange color depending upon the concentration of hemoglobin F. Normal adult erythrocytes appear as ghost cells. The neonatal blood sample should have many dense-appearing erythrocytes per field.

## Calculations

The percentage of hemoglobin F-containing cells can be determined by counting the number of dense-staining cells and the number of ghost cells per field. Using the high dry (43–44×) objective, count 500 ghost cells and record the number of dense hemoglobin F-containing cells seen during the count.

## Reporting Results

An adult specimen should have approximately the same number of dense hemoglobin F-containing cells as the normal adult blood. These cells should appear rarely. The results are expressed in percentage. Normal adults have less than 1% hemoglobin F-containing cells. Infant values are higher, with newborn infants having 70 to 90% hemoglobin F-containing cells.

## Procedure Notes

False positive results may be obtained if anticoagulated blood is allowed to stand overnight or if a patient has a very high percentage of reticulocytes. Reticulocytes may resist elution and give the appearance of cells containing hemoglobin F. To crosscheck high concentrations of hemoglobin F, a reticulocyte count can be performed.

In hemoglobinopathies such as sickle cell disease, the amount of hemoglobin F varies, producing inconsistent staining results. Cells containing small amounts of hemoglobin F stain lightly.

## Clinical Applications

Increased amounts of hemoglobin F are found in various hemoglobinopathies such as hereditary persistence of fetal hemoglobin, sickle cell anemia, and thalassemias. Refer to the Clinical Applications section of Hemoglobin F Determination by Alkaline Denaturation, this chapter, for additional special examples of disorders in which hemoglobin F is increased. Refer to Chapter 11, Hemolytic Disease of the Newborn, for a discussion of fetal-maternal hemorrhage and the significance of determining the extent of hemorrhage.

## Limitations

This procedure is a semiquantitative method. Hemoglobin electrophoresis can provide quantitative measurements of specific types of hemoglobin.

## TITLE: INDICATOR CELL ROSETTE TEST FOR FETOMATERNAL HEMORRHAGE

### Principle

This screening procedure detects fetal D positive cells in the circulation of a D negative postpartum woman. The test uses D positive indicator red blood cells to form easily identified rosettes around individual D+ fetal cells that may be present in the maternal circulation. The number of rosettes is roughly proportional to the number of D positive red blood cells present in the mixture. Because this procedure is considered only a screening test, specimens producing a positive result should be tested with a quantitative method, such as Kleihauer-Betke acid elution, to quantitate the number of fetal cells present.

### Specimen

No special preparation of the patient is required before specimen collection. She must be positively identified when the specimen is collected. The specimen must be labelled at the bedside and the label must include the patient's first and last name, the date when the specimen is collected, and the patient's hospital identification number. The time of collection and the phlebotomist's initials should be written on the required form.

Blood should be drawn by an aseptic technique and the specimen should be tested as soon as possible. Approxi-

mately 5 to 7 mL of blood should be collected in a red top (no anticoagulant) evacuated tube or lavender top (EDTA) evacuated tube. All specimens must be retained under refrigeration for 7 days.

### Reagents, Supplies and Equipment

Indicator red blood cells: 0.2 to 0.5% saline suspension of type O, $R_2R_2$ red blood cells (cDE/cDE). Either enzyme-treated or untreated red blood cells in an enhancing medium can be used.
Commercial anti-D antisera
Commercial antihuman globulin (AHG) reagent (broad-spectrum or IgG)
$10 \times 75$ mm or $12 \times 75$ mm disposable test tubes
Disposable pipettes, 4⅝" plastic or Pasteur
Test tube rack
Normal (0.9%) saline
37° C waterbath or heat block
High intensity lamp/optical magnifying lens
Centrifuge or cell washer

### Quality Control

Negative control: A 3 to 4% saline suspension of washed D-negative cells
Positive control: A 3 to 4% saline suspension of a mixture of D positive and D negative red blood cells. This mixture of 0.5% D positive cells can be prepared as follows:

1. Add 1 drop of a 3% saline suspension of washed D positive red blood cells to 15 drops of a 3% saline suspension of washed D negative red blood cells. Mix well.
2. Add 1 drop of the mixture prepared in step 1 to 9 drops of the 3% suspension of D negative cells. Mix well.

### Procedure

1. Prepare a 3 to 4% saline suspension of washed red blood cells from the patient's postpartum blood sample.
2. Label three $10 \times 75$ mm or $12 \times 75$ mm tubes: test, positive, and negative control.
3. Add 1 drop of anti-D antisera (or follow manufacturer's instructions) to each test tube.
4. Add 1 drop of maternal red blood cells, negative control cells, or positive control red blood cells to the respectively labeled tubes.
5. Incubate at 37° C for 15 to 30 minutes.
6. Wash the cell suspensions at least four times. Decant the saline completely after the last wash.
7. To the dry cell buttons, add 1 drop of indicator red blood cells to each tube and mix thoroughly to resuspend.
8. Centrifuge the tubes for 15 seconds at 3400 rpm.

9. Resuspend the cell button and examine the cell suspension microscopically at 100× magnification.
10. Examine at least 10 fields and count the number of cell rosettes in each field.

## Reporting Results

The absence of rosettes is a negative result. However, if enzyme-treated indicator red blood cells were used, a maximum of 1 rosette per 3 fields is considered a negative result. If the indicator red blood cells were treated with another type of enhancement media, a maximum of 6 rosettes per 5 fields constitutes a negative result.

If the number of rosettes exceeds the allowable maximums previously stated, the test is considered positive. In these cases, a quantitative test for the amount of fetal blood in the maternal circulation should be conducted.

## Procedure Notes

The presence of rosettes or agglutination in the negative control tube indicates inadequate washing after incubation. If washing is inadequate, enough residual anti-D antiserum is present to agglutinate the D positive indicator red blood cells.

## Limitations

Blood from a weak D (D^u) positive mother produces strongly positive results. It is important to establish that the mother is D and weak D (D^u) negative before performing the rosetting test. A massive fetal-maternal bleed may produce a rosetting pattern that is difficult to distinguish from weak D (D^u) blood.

## TITLE: PENICILLIN OR CEPHALOSPORIN ANTIBODY SCREENING

### Principle

Drug-coated red blood cells demonstrate agglutination if the serum or eluate from a patient's red cells contains an antibody to the drug. This procedure is helpful in identifying penicillin or cephalosporins as the cause of a positive direct antiglobulin test.

### Specimen

No special preparation of the patient is required before specimen collection. The patient must be positively identified when the specimen is collected. The specimen must be labelled at the bedside and must include the patient's first and last name, the date when the specimen is collected, and the patient's hospital identification number. The time of collection and the phlebotomist's initials should be written on the required form.

Blood should be drawn by an aseptic technique and the specimen tested as soon as possible. Approximately 5 to 7 mL of blood should be collected in a red top (no anticoagulant) evacuated tube.

### Reagents, Supplies, and Equipment

Drug-sensitized red cells, as follows:

*Penicillin-treated cells*

1. Prepare 1 mL of packed, well-washed, fresh red cells.
2. Add 15 mL of penicillin solution prepared by dissolving 0.6 g of penicillin in 15 mL of TMA-buffer (pH 10.0). Swirl occasionally.
3. Incubate at room temperature for 1 hour.
4. Wash cells 4 to 8 times in saline.
5. Resuspend in saline to a 3 to 4% suspension.

or

*Cephalothin-treated red cells*

1. Prepare 1 mL of packed, well-washed, fresh red cells.
2. Add 10 mL of Keflin solution prepared by dissolving 0.4 g of sodium cephalothin in 10 mL of TMA-buffer (pH 10.0). Swirl occasionally.
3. Incubate at 37° C for 1 hour.
4. Wash cells 4 to 8 times in saline.
5. Resuspend in saline to a 3 or 4% suspension.

2 to 4% suspension of group O washed red cells
Antihuman globulin antisera
10 × 75 mm or 12 × 75 mm disposable test tubes
Disposable pipettes, 4⅝" plastic or Pasteur
Test tube rack
Normal (0.9%) saline
37° C waterbath or heat block
High intensity lamp/optical magnifying lens
Centrifuge or cell washer

### Quality Control

Patient control and reagent control must be included in the test procedure.

### Procedure

1. Label four test tubes and add the following:

| Patient Test | Patient Control |
|---|---|
| 2 drops patient serum | 2 drops patient serum |
| 1 drop drug-coated red cells | 1 drop washed group O red cells |

| Control Test | Control Control |
|---|---|
| 2 drops positive control serum | 2 drops of positive control serum |
| 1 drop drug-coated red cells | 1 drop washed group O red cells |

2. Incubate all of the tubes at 37° C for 30 minutes.
3. Centrifuge, read and record results.
4. Wash all tubes 3 to 4 times with saline.
5. Add 2 drops of antiglobulin serum.
6. Mix, centrifuge for 10 to 15 seconds, read and record results.
7. Add 1 drop of Coombs' control red cells to each tube.
8. Mix, centrifuge for 10 to 15 seconds, read and record results. All tubes should be agglutinated after this step.

## Reporting Results

If the patient test is agglutinated in step 6, the patient has an antibody to the drug. For the patient results to be valid, the following reactions must also be observed:

Patient Control—No agglutination
Control Test—Agglutination
Control Control—No agglutination

## Procedure Notes

If the patient control exhibits agglutination, the patient may have an unexpected antibody. The identity of the antibody must be determined. After identification, red cells that lack the corresponding antigen should be coated with the drug and the procedure should be repeated.

If the control test demonstrates no agglutination, the cells are not adequately coated with drug.

If the control control exhibits agglutination, the control serum is contaminated. The procedure should be repeated with a new control specimen.

### Alternate Procedure

Prepare titrations of the patient's serum or an eluate using serial doubling dilution in saline of the patient serum or an eluate of the patient's red blood cells. Follow the previous procedure.

## Reporting Results

If the eluate demonstrates agglutination with the drug-coated red cells but fails to agglutinate uncoated red cells, the positive direct antiglobulin test has been caused by antibodies directed against the drug.

## Procedure Notes

Many normal sera have antibodies to penicillin or cephalothin-coated red cells that react at room temperature to a low titer. Individuals who have an antibody to the drug that is causing positive direct antiglobulin tests show reactivity to higher titers when tested with the indirect antiglobulin test. It is important to test the patient's serum to rule out a red cell unexpected antibody directed against the normal test cells.

## TITLE: TRANSFUSION REACTION PROTOCOL

### Principle

A sample standard protocol is established for the routine workup of transfusion reactions other than hives and urticaria. Refer to Chapter 12 for a complete discussion of transfusion reactions.

### Specimen

Approximately 5 to 7 mL of blood should be collected aseptically in a plain (no anticoagulant) evacuated tube and an additional specimen should be collected in an EDTA evacuated tube. Blood samples should be collected as soon as possible after notification of an adverse transfusion reaction. The blood samples must be examined as soon as possible. Hemolysis due to conditions such as traumatic venipuncture produces an inappropriate specimen.

The specimen must be labeled at the bedside and must include the patient's first and last name, the date and time when the specimen is collected, and the patient's hospital identification number. The phlebotomist's initials should be written in the required form.

### Reagents, Supplies, and Equipment

1. Antisera
   A. Direct blood grouping antisera: anti-A, anti-B, anti-A,B
   B. Rh typing antisera: anti-D, Rh control reagent
   C. Antiglobulin reagent polyspecific
2. Reagent red blood cells
   A. $A_1$ and B reagent red blood cells
   B. Coombs' control red blood cells
3. 10 × 75 mm disposable test tubes
4. Normal saline (0.9%).
5. Disposable pipettes, 4⅝"
6. Centrifuge
7. Cell washer (optional)
8. Magnifier
9. Transfusion Reaction Request Form

### Quality Control

Quality control steps should be implemented for each of the specific procedures. Refer to each specific procedure.

### Procedure

1. Symptoms: Hives, urticaria
   Response:
      A. The nurse in charge should notify the patient's physician for orders of treatment and should watch for more serious symptoms.

B. Transfusion need not be stopped unless symptoms worsen.

C. No lab workup is necessary unless the patient's physician requests it.

2. Symptoms: Chills, fever, pain (back, chest, local site of infusion), shortness of breath, hypotension, tachycardia, palpitations, hemorrhagic diathesis. Response on the floor:

A. The nurse should stop the transfusion immediately and notify the patient's physician and the blood bank.

B. A physician or nurse should evaluate the patient clinically for signs and symptoms of a severe reaction.

C. A clerical check of the patient's identification and the blood unit identification must be conducted at the patient's bedside.

D. The blood bag should be returned to the blood bank.

Response in the laboratory:

## Immediate Steps

1. Check the identification of the patient and the transfused unit of blood or component. Notify the medical director of the blood bank if any clerical or identification error exists. Check to see if any other patients are at risk.

2. Immediately obtain a post-transfusion blood specimen. Label appropriately as the *post-transfusion specimen.* Obtain the discontinued bag of blood, administration set, and any attached IV solutions. Request the collection of a urine sample from the patient as soon as possible. Intact red cells indicate hemorrhage into the urinary tract, not hemolysis. Test the urine specimen for the presence of free hemoglobin. If the urine specimen is not collected for several days, test for hemosiderin.

3. Examine the patient's post-transfusion specimens by:

A. Visually examining the patient's post-transfusion specimen for hemolysis. A pink color indicates that intravascular hemolysis has recently taken place. A sample obtained 4 to 10 hours after transfusion will have a yellow or brown color from increased bilirubin and other hemoglobin breakdown products.

B. Performing a direct antiglobulin test (DAT). If transfused incompatible cells (antibody or complement-coated) are not immediately destroyed, the direct AHG test will be positive with a mixed-field appearance.

If any of the above tests are positive or doubtful, perform the following laboratory procedures:

1. Perform ABO grouping and Rh typing of the pretransfusion, post-transfusion and blood from the bag or a segment attached to the unit.

2. Repeat the crossmatch with the pretransfusion and post-transfusion specimen.

3. Perform a direct antiglobulin test (DAT) on the pretransfusion specimen.

4. Repeat unexpected antibody screening tests on the pretransfusion and donor units as well as the post-transfusion specimen. If either the pretransfusion or donor unit has a previously unreported antibody, check for clerical errors in the pretransfusion testing. Perform a minor crossmatch using the patient's pretransfusion specimen if the donor unit has a previously unsuspected antibody.

5. If any of the unexpected antibody screening tests are positive, identify the antibody. Test the patient or donor erythrocytes for the corresponding antibody depending which serum contains the antibody.

## Additional Tests

If routine testing fails to provide information and immune hemolysis is suspected, the following tests may be helpful:

1. Antibody screening and compatibility tests with enhancement media or by increasing the ratio of serum to cells.

2. Perform DAT and alloantibody screening tests on several post-transfusion specimens collected from the patient at daily or frequent intervals.

3. Monitor the hemoglobin/hematocrit levels. In a nonbleeding patient, a unit of packed erythrocytes should produce an increase of 1 g/dL or packed cell volume (hematocrit) of 3%.

4. Genotype the erythrocytes of the patient's pretransfusion specimen and the donor cells. Examine the patient's postreaction specimen for the presence of cells bearing foreign antigens. If an antigen can be found that is present on the donor cells and absent on the patient's cells, its presence or absence in the post-transfusion sample indicates the degree to which the transfused cells have survived and remain in the circulation.

5. Test post-transfusion serum samples for the presence of unconjugated bilirubin.

6. Measure serum haptoglobin in pre- and post-transfusion patient specimens.

## Reporting Results

If a discrepancy occurs between the ABO grouping or Rh typing of the pretransfusion, post-transfusion, or donor unit, an error in patient identification, specimen labelling, donor unit identification or other clerical error is responsible. Notify the patient's physician and the medical director of the blood bank. Crosscheck all past patient records as well as the labelling of the blood product itself. The phlebotomist responsible for obtaining the blood specimen should be questioned *immediately* if the pretransfusion specimen does not agree with the post-transfusion specimen. Any other patient specimens drawn at approximately the same time should be rechecked, if the possibility of having another patient at risk exists.

An incompatible crossmatch with the pretransfusion specimen indicates that an error existed in the patient or donor specimen during pretransfusion testing. If the crossmatch is incompatible *only* with the post-transfusion specimen, an anamnestic reaction is suspect.

If only the DAT on the post-transfusion test is positive, the patient's erythrocytes have been coated with antibody or complement. Procedures for investigation of a positive DAT should be followed to determine the cause.

If the post-transfusion specimen has an antibody not present in the pretransfusion specimen, the cause may be an anamnestic reaction or passive administration of antibody in a transfusion component recently infused.

The presence of an unexpected antibody does not necessarily indicate that it is the cause of the reaction; the corresponding antigen must also be present.

A rising bilirubin may be detectable as early as 1 hour postreaction. Peak levels occur at 4 to 6 hours and disappear within 24 hours if bilirubin excretion is normal.

Visible hemoglobinemia develops only after haptoglobin depletion. Compare pretransfusion and post-transfusion values. A decline in haptoglobin is most useful in chronic hemolysis. If studies are performed several days after a hemolytic episode, normal levels may be restored because haptoglobin is an acute phase reactant that may regenerate rapidly after depletion.

## Other Tests

### Bacteremia

Carefully take specimens from the bag for cultures at 4° C, 20 to 24° C, and 35 to 37° C. Examine a smear of the blood stained with Gram stain or acridine orange (a DNA stain).

### Physical Damage

Examine the donor unit for physical damage (heat, cold storage/transport, or excessive heat from an in-line blood warmer) or chemical damage (drugs, hypotonic solutions). Discoloration (pink or red) of the donor unit can result from osmotic hemolysis caused by a hypotonic or dextrose solution entering the unit or present in the administration unit.

## TITLE: Rh IMMUNOGLOBULIN D PROTOCOL

### Principle

Refer to Chapter 11, Hemolytic Disease of the Newborn.

### Specimen

#### Maternal Specimen

No special preparation of the mother is required before specimen collection. She must be positively identified when the specimen is collected. The specimen must be labelled at the bedside and must include the patient's first and last name, the date the specimen is collected, and the patient's hospital identification number. The time of collection and the phlebotomist's initials should be written on the required form.

Blood should be drawn by an aseptic technique and the specimen should be tested as soon as possible. Approximately 5 to 7 mL of blood should be collected in a red top (no anticoagulant) or lavender top evacuated tube. All specimens must be retained under refrigeration for seven days.

#### Infant Specimen

Either a cord blood specimen collected in an EDTA or anticoagulated tube or a capillary blood specimen collected by the heelstick method can be used.

### Laboratory Criteria

The laboratory criteria for Rh IgG administration are as follows:

1. The mother is D and weak D ($D^u$) negative.
2. The mother's screening test for unexpected antibodies is negative for anti-D.
3. The infant is D or weak D ($D^u$) positive. In obstetric cases where the Rh cannot be determined, it must be assumed that this criterion has been met.
4. The direct antiglobulin test on cord cells or infant's cells, if available, is negative. If a positive DAT test result is obtained, an elution technique should be employed to establish that anti-D is not the coating antibody.

### Procedure Notes

Using an assay such as the Kleihauer-Betke test (in this chapter), the number of vials of Rh IgG can be determined. Calculation of the number of vials needed is presented in Chapter 11, Hemolytic Disease of the Newborn.

The criteria for the administration of antenatal Rh Immune Globulin omits the infant requirements because the Rh status of the fetus is unknown. A complete discussion of antenatal prophylaxis can be found in Chapter 10.

### Bibliography

Bauer, J.D.: Clinical Laboratory Methods (9th Ed.), St. Louis, C.V. Mosby Company, 1982, pp. 426–427.
Bowman, J.M. (Ed.): $Rh_o$ (D) Immune Globulin. Berkeley, CA, Cutter Biological, 1984.

Branh, D.R., Sy Siok Hian, A.L. and L.D. Petz. "A new elution procedure using chloroform, a nonflammable organic solvent," *Vox Sanguinis,* 42:46–53, 1982.

Burich, M.A., AuBuchon, J.P., and H.J. Anderson. "Antibody elution using citric acid," *Transfusion,* 26:116–117, 1986.

Cheng, M.S., and Lukomskyj, L.: Postpartum D$^u$-positive women and Rh immune globulin. Lab. Med., *17*(12):748–749, 1986.

Feng, C.S., Kirkley, K.C., Eicher, C.A., and DeJongh, D.S.: The Lui elution technique. Transfusion, *25*:433–434, 1985.

Gamma Biologicals, Inc., Houston, Texas: Reagent Red Blood Cells, package insert, January, 1986.

Hendry, E.B.: Osmolarity of human serum of chemical solution of biologic importance, Clin. Chem. *7*:156–164, 1961.

Henry, J.B. (Ed.): Clinical Diagnosis and Management by Laboratory Methods, 18th ed. Philadelphia, W.B. Saunders Co., p. 985, 1991.

Holland, P.V. Other Adverse Effects of Transfusion. In Clinical Practice of Blood Transfusion, Petz, L. W., and Swisher, S.N. (Ed.): NY, Churchill-Livingstone Inc., 1981, pp. 783–801.

Huestis, D., et al. Practical Blood Transfusion, 3rd Ed. Boston, Little, Brown and Co., 1982, pp. 106–107.

Huestis, D.W., Bove, J.R., and Case, J.: Practical Blood Transfusion. Boston, Little, Brown and Co., 1988, pp. 265–268.

Issitt, P.: Applied Blood Group Serology, 2nd Ed. Oxnard, CA, Spectra Biologics, 1975.

Mollison, P.L. Blood Transfusion in Clinical Medicine, 6th Ed. Oxford, Blackwell Scientific Publications, 1979, p. 556.

Morel, P.A., Bergren, M.O., and Frank, B.A.: A simple method for the detection of alloantibody in the presence of autoantibody, Transfusion, *18*:388, 1978.

Seiverd, C.E.: Hematology for Medical Technologists. Philadelphia, Lea & Febiger, 1972, p. 553.

Shepard, M.K., et al.: Semiquantitative estimation of the distribution of fetal hemoglobin in red cell populations. Bull. Johns Hopkins Hosp., *110*:293, 1962.

South, S.F., Rea, A.E., and Tregellas, W.M.: An evaluation of 11 red cell elution procedures. Transfusion, *26*(2):167–170, 1986.

Stec, N., Shirey, R.S., Smith, B., Kickler, T.S., and Ness, P.M.: The efficacy of performing red cell elution studies in the pretransfusion testing of patients with positive direct antiglobulin tests. Transfusion, *26*(3):225–226, 1986.

Walker, Richard H. (Ed.): AABB Technical Manual, 11th Ed. Bethesda, MD. American Association of Blood Banks, 1993, p. 642.

Walker, Richard H. (Ed.): AABB Technical Manual, 11th Ed. Bethesda, MD. American Association of Blood Banks, 1993, pp. 651–654.

Walker, Richard H. (Ed.): AABB Technical Manual, 11th Ed. Bethesda, MD. American Association of Blood Banks, 1993, pp. 661–664.

Walker, Richard H. (Ed.): AABB Technical Manual, 11th Ed. Bethesda, MD. American Association of Blood Banks, 1993, p. 665.

Walker, Richard H. (Ed.): AABB Technical Manual, 11th Ed. Bethesda, MD. American Association of Blood Banks, 1993, p. 668

Zonijewski, C.M.: Immunohematology, 2nd ed. NY, Appleton-Century-Crofts, 1972, p. 263.

# 16

# Transplantation

At the conclusion of the chapter, the reader should be able to:

- Describe briefly the history and scope of organ and tissue transplantation in terms of the number of donor organs and tissues harvested in a recent year.
- List the major limitations to liver transplantation.
- Describe the requirements of the Federal Required Request Law of 1986.
- Compare the different requirements for blood perfusion between organs and tissues.
- Name the four most commonly donated tissues and the most common type of donor.
- Describe storage conditions and the record keeping system, including retention of records, for tissues.
- Describe followup of complications, especially posttransplant HIV infection.
- Name the major areas of focus for transplantation donor testing procedures.
- Describe minimum procurement standards for potential donor evaluation.
- Name the two HLA antigens that should be identified to determine the best donor when HLA-selected blood components are sought for transfusion.

- State two general areas of laboratory monitoring posttransplantation.
- List three monitors for excess immunosuppression and three monitors for inadequate immunosuppression in transplant patients.
- Name two agents involved in the direct monitoring of immunosuppressive agent therapy.
- Name three biochemical markers of lymphocyte activation and describe the mode of action.
- Describe the selection process of bone marrow donors and explain issues related to donor consent.
- Briefly describe the process of collection and processing both bone marrow and peripheral blood progenitor cells.
- Explain laboratory testing, including quality control measures, as it relates to bone marrow and peripheral blood progenitor cell collection.

## INTRODUCTION

Transplantation can involve organs such as the kidneys, heart, and liver, or tissues such as the skin, bone, corneas, or bone marrow. Although the first tissue bank was established in 1949, there was minimal activity until 1974, and most banks were not organized until the 1980s. The American Association of Tissue Banks was formed in 1976 and has been responsible for the development of standards in the field.

Two pioneers in the field of transplantation shared the 1990 Nobel Prize for physiology and medicine. Joseph E. Murray transplanted the first human kidney from one individual to another on December 23, 1954. Donnall Thomas performed the first human bone-marrow transplant in 1956. In March 1963 Thomas Starzl performed the first liver transplant.

### Availability of Organs

The phenomenal growth in the number of transplants at approximately 260 centers is largely due to the development of improved immunosuppressant drugs. In 1990, about 15,000 organs were harvested from 4,500 donors. Organ procurement organizations and tissue banks also recovered tissues from an estimated 7,500 to 10,000 donors in the same year. These tissues were used in an estimated 250,000 to 300,000 allografts.

Organs and tissues are often in short supply and may not be available when needed. The time period between removal of an organ from a cadaveric donor (on life-support systems) and transplantation into the recipient is limited by initial deterioration in vivo within the moribund donor and by in vitro deterioration during the ischemic time of handling and transporting the isolated organ. For example, ischemia time for livers is beyond 24 hours and perhaps up to 48 hours. The major limitations to liver transplantation are matching of organ size and blood type. Occasionally, incompatible-blood-type organs are transplanted; segmental and living-related donor transplants have been performed recently.

### Requirements for Donation

The Federal Required Request law of 1986 requires hospitals that participate in Medicare and Medicaid reimbursement to establish guidelines for identifying potential donors, offering the choice of donation to legal next-of-kin, and notifying a procurement agency. Implementation of the Required Request protocols is one of the conditions of JCAHO accreditation.

The differing requirements for blood perfusion form the principal difference between organs and tissues. Solid organs, such as kidneys, heart, lungs, pancreas, and liver, require procurement from a "heart-beating donor." These organs are extremely susceptible to anoxia and will not function if necessary oxygenation is not maintained up to the time of procurement. Nonvascularized tissues, such as corneas, skin, bone, heart valves, and connective tissue, are much less sensitive to anoxia and do not require that the donor's heart be beating at the time of procurement. These tissues can be successfully removed for future use many hours after cessation of circulation.

Organs and tissues can be procured from the same donor. However, a patient who demonstrates oxygen deprivation, which occurs in conditions such as cardiac arrest, can only be a tissue donor.

### Commonly Donated Tissues

#### Bone

Bone is the most commonly transplanted tissue, because bone obtained from one donor can provide graft material for many recipients. Bones suitable for donation include the iliac crest, femur, patella, tibia, fibula, humerus, and rib. In addition, artificial bone or bone substitutes could provide alternative sources of bone.

Bone can be procured from either a living donor, as an autograft or allograft, or it can be obtained from a cadaver. Utilization of human allografts is presently preferred over metal reconstructive materials that have an increased risk of infection and loss of function over time. Human allografts remain the product of choice despite the continued development of substitutes. Bone growth factors, when available for routine use, will enhance allograft procedures and probably increase the number of procedures performed, as well as produce a higher probability of success.

Methods are needed to decrease bone graft failure due to immunologic rejection. The immune response to transplanted allogeneic marrow-free bone is usually cell-mediated, relatively mild, and manifested as a delayed hypersensitivity reaction. The components responsible for this reaction are not eliminated by irradiation, freezing, vacuum drying, or autoclaving. Short-term immunosuppression is currently being studied as a method to encourage graft incorporation.

Bone can be stored intact, cut into pieces, or broken up in small chips. Some bone products are stored frozen, while others are freeze dried.

## Corneas

Corneas are readily obtained, stored, and transplanted. Cornea donors are the most common type of donor; however, a nationwide shortage of transplantable corneas exists. A study conducted at Johns Hopkins Wilmer Eye Institute and other U.S. eye centers reports that ABO blood-group matching may be effective in reducing by 50% the risk of corneal graft failure from rejection.

## Skin

Skin is a commonly donated tissue. It can be procured and used within a few days as fresh skin, or cryopreserved and used many months later. Skin is commonly applied to burn patients as a temporary dressing.

At least one artificial skin product is available, but tissue bankers agree that there is no skin substitute that equals autologous or allograft skin. If human allografts are not available, artificial skin is used.

Artificial skin consists of two basic layers: epidermis (a synthetic material) and dermis (porcine collagen). Another product uses dermal cells (fibroblasts) and epidermal cells (keratinocytes) to fabricate a living skin equivalent. These cells supposedly do not trigger immune responses, and the grafts are therefore accepted as immunologically neutral implants. Another reported advantage of artificial skin is that the cells are genetically marked in order to track the continued viability of donor cells.

## Heart Valves

Heart valves have some advantages over mechanical valves because they last longer and do not require long-term anticoagulant therapy.

## Connective Tissue

Connective tissue can be procured from one donor and transplanted into several recipients. Dura mater, costal cartilage, fascia from various sites, and patellar tendons are examples of connective tissue that have been transplanted.

## TISSUE STORAGE, ISSUE, RECORDS, AND COMPLICATIONS

### Storage

Tissue storage should be centralized, with well-developed policies and procedures. Transportation and storage temperatures and conditions, and expiration dates and times, shall conform to the source facility's written directions for each tissue. Storage refrigerators and freezers shall have temperature monitoring, alarms, and emergency backup as required for blood and blood components.

Hospital practices regarding tissue storage varies greatly. Tissues tend to be stored in several locations, and proper records of tissue storage and recipient identification may not be kept. Tissue to be used as autografts are often stored without proper labeling or monitoring of storage conditions.

### Issue and Use

Tissues shall be prepared for use according to the source facility's written directions for each tissue. There shall be a unique numeric or alphanumeric identification for each tissue specimen. The recipient's chart shall document the type of tissue, the tissue identification number, and the quantity and date of use.

Records must permit tracing of any tissue from the donor (source facility) to all recipients or other final dispositions. Records must identify personnel who prepare or issue the tissue, the individual who accepts each tissue for use, and the dates of the activities. Although each facility is required to maintain specific records, and organ donation is nationally computerized, there is no central national registry for tissue. The Centers for Disease Control and Prevention (CDC) are about to publish formal guidelines for tracking organs and tissues from the time of donation until the post-convalescence period.

### Retention of Records

Records must be retained indefinitely to show the source facility, the original numeric or alphanumeric donor or lot identification, and the final disposition of each tissue. Records to be retained for a minimum of 5 years, or as required by applicable state and federal laws, include storage temperatures, control testing, and all superseded procedures, manuals, and publications described in the procedures manual and quality control.

### Complications

A system for investigating suspected tissue or donor infections, adverse effects, and disease transmission or other suspected complications of tissue use, and for promptly reporting such cases to the source facility, must be established and maintained. Requirements for recipient identification apply to tissue donors and recipients (patient notification–look back).

Posttransplant HIV reporting must include notification of positive HIV test results as soon as practical to any tissue bank and the director of any other transplant program that has received tissue or an organ from a positive donor. In addition, management of the investigation to determine whether the organ donor was infected with HIV must be conducted. Finally, a written report must be submitted to the United Network for Organ Sharing within 45 days. This report must outline the organizations and individuals who were notified, when the notification occurred, and the results of the investigation, including the HIV serology status of the organ recipients.

## CLINICAL LABORATORY TESTING

### Donor Testing

The objectives, concerns, and responsibilities of blood bankers are very similar to those of tissue bankers. Tests performed on both blood and tissue donors are basically the same. Testing procedures include:

1. Information needed before the transplant to determine if the organ should be used.
2. Information needed in the posttransplant management of the patient.

Protocols for pretesting of cadaveric candidate donors (Table 16-1) are primarily intended to rule out infectious diseases that may be transmitted by transplantation of the organ or with the donor blood perfusing the organ. In addition, the general condition of the organ or tissue is assessed. The transplant surgeon may request a frozen section to assess anoxic damage to the donor organ.

The proposed panel of tests for organ donors include: infectious disease markers such as hepatitis B surface antigen, antibodies to HIV-1, HIV-2, hepatitis C virus, and

hepatitis B core antigen. Other viruses that are tested for include: human T-cell lymphotropic virus (HTLV) type I, cytomegalovirus (CMV), Epstein-Barr virus (EBV), and parvovirus B19. The rapid plasma reagin and fluorescent treponemal antibody absorption tests for syphilis and the presence of *Toxoplasma gondii* are usually performed. In addition, the ABO group and Rh type are also tested.

If a donor has been hospitalized for 72 hours or longer, blood and urine cultures should be obtained. The only absolute contraindication to accepting organs from a candidate donor is the HIV status. A donor who is HIV positive must be excluded.

### Histocompatibility Antigens

#### General Characteristics

All vertebrates capable of acute rejection of foreign skin grafts possess a localized complex involving many genes that exert major control over the organism's immune reactions. Many nucleated cells possess cell-surface-protein antigens that are expressions of part of this complex and readily provoke an immune response if transferred into a genetically different (allogeneic) individual of the same species. Some of the expressed antigens are much more potent than others in provoking an immune response and are therefore called the *major histocompatibility complex (MHC)*.

In humans, the MHC is referred to as the human leukocyte antigen (HLA) system (see Chapter 3 for a basic discussion of the HLA system). The HLA system is the most complex immunogenetic system presently known in man; it is controlled by an MHC, or supergene, which includes several loci closely linked on the short arm of chromosome 6.

Class I includes the classic HLA-A, B, and C antigens. The three principal loci—A, B, and C, and their respective antigens—are numbered 1, 2, 3, and so on. The three specificities of class I are composed of a single heavy chain and a light chain, beta-2 microglobulin, which is controlled by a gene on chromosome 15. The Class II gene region antigens are encoded in the HLA-D region.

Multiple alleles occur at each locus and are followed by an arabic number (e.g., HLA-A1 or HLA-B27). Genes of class I, II, and III antigens at each locus are inherited as codominant alleles, and inheritance within families closely follows simple Mendelian-dominant characteristics.

The class I major transplantation antigens have been serologically defined. Class I and class II antigens can be found on body cells and in body fluids (Table 16-2). Class I and Class II molecules are surface membrane proteins. Class I molecules are transmembrane glycoproteins, but the Class II dimer molecule differs from Class I in that both dimers span the cell membrane. Class I and Class II gene products are biochemically distinct, although they

---

**Table 16-1. Minimum Procurement Standards[1]**

Potential donor evaluation should include:
- Verification of death
- Determination of conditions that may contraindicate donation. In addition to a confirmed HIV antibody seropositive status or indication of other infectious diseases, the presence of a malignant tumor or current sepsis are usual causes of exclusion
- Obtaining donor's history, reviewing medical chart, physical examination of donor, and recording of donor's vital signs. Potential donors who received human pituitary-derived growth hormone (HPDG) in the past or are positive for human T-lymphotropic virus type 1 (HTLV-1) are not suitable donors
- Laboratory testing

[1] United Network for Organ Sharing (UNOS). Lang, Heide, "Federally Mandated Program for Tracking Donor Tissue Advocated," *Advance for Medical Laboratory Professionals,* 5 (42) 10, October 18, 1993.

**Table 16-2. Expression of HLA Antigens on Surface Membranes**

| | |
|---|---|
| **Class I** | |
| Not expressed | Erythrocytes, corneal endothelium, villlus of trophoblast, exocrine pancreas, parotid acinar cells, and some duodenal Bruner's glands |
| Weakly expressed | Endocrine thyroid, parathyroid, pituitary, pancreatic islet cells, myocardial and skeletal muscle, gastric mucosa, and mature granulocytes |
| Variably expressed | Hepatocytes |
| Expressed | All other body cells |
| **Class II** | |
| Not expressed | Erythrocytes, all resting endocrine cells, hepatocytes and biliary epithelium, myocardial, skeletal, and smooth muscle cells, epithelial cells of the esophagus, stomach, Brunner's glands, colon, and rectum; parotid acinar and ductal epithelium; spermatozoa; bladder, prostate and ureter epithelium, neurons, platelets, mature granulocytes and resting T cells |
| Expressed | B cells, activated T cells and immature granulocytes, epithelium of the epiglottis, trachea, tonsils, and epididymis, renal glomeruli and tubules; dura, Langerhans cell, skin, dendritic cells, and epithelial cells of the deeper layers of the duodenum, ileum, and appendix |
| HLA-DR, expressed HLA-DQ, weakly expressed or absent | Monocytes, macrophages, and vascular endothelial cells |

From John Thompson, "The Human Leukocyte Antigen System," in *Internal Medicine*, 2nd ed. Jay H. Stein (ed.). Boston: Little, Brown, 1987, p. 1206.

appear to be distantly related through evolution. Class III gene products are incomplete, but these structures are defined by genes lying between or very near the HLA-B and -DR loci.

### The Role of MHC/HLA

The histocompatibility complex that encodes cell-surface antigens was first discovered in graft rejection experiments with mice. When the antigens were matched between donor and recipient, the ability of a graft to survive was remarkably improved. A comparable genetic system of alloantigens was subsequently identified in man. The presence of HLA was first recognized when multiply transfused patients experienced transfusion reactions despite proper crossmatching. It was discovered that these reactions resulted from leukocyte antibodies rather than antibodies directed against erythrocyte antigens. Similar antibodies were subsequently discovered in the sera of multiparous women.

The MHC gene products have an important role in clinical immunology. For example, transplants are rejected if performed against MHC barriers; thus, immunosuppressive therapy is required. These antigens are of extreme importance, second only to the ABO antigens in influencing the genetic basis of survival or rejection of transplanted organs.

Although HLA was originally identified by its role in transplant rejection, it is now recognized that the products of HLA genes play a crucial role in our immune system. T cells do not recognize antigens directly, but do so when the antigen is presented on the surface of an antigen-presenting cell, the macrophage. In addition to presentation of the antigen, the macrophage must present another molecule for this response to occur. This molecule is a cell-surface glycoprotein that is coded in each species by the MHC. T cells are able to interact with the histocompatibility molecules only if they are genetically identical (MHC restriction).

Both Class I and Class II antigens function as targets of T lymphocytes that regulate the immune response. Class I molecules regulate interaction between cytolytic T cells and target cells and class II molecules restrict the activity of regulatory T cells (helper, suppressor, and amplifier subsets). Hence, class II molecules regulate the interaction between helper T cells and antigen-presenting cells. Cytotoxic T cells directed against class I antigens are inhibited by T8 cells; cytotoxic T cells directed against class II antigens are inhibited by T4 cells. Many of the genes in both class I and class II gene families have no known functions.

Class III molecules bear no clear relations to class I and II molecules, aside from their genetic linkage (the presence of the gene in or near the MHC complex). Class III molecules are involved in immunologic phenomenon because they represent components of the complement pathway and tumor necrosis factor.

### HLA Applications

HLA matching is of value in organ transplantation as well as in the transplantation of bone marrow. In kidney allografts, the method of organ preservation, time elapsed between harvesting and transplanting, number of pretransplantation blood transfusions, recipient age, and primary cause for kidney failure are all important determinants of early transplant success or failure of kidney allograft. HLA compatibility, however, exerts the strongest influence on long-term kidney survival. The 1-year survival for kidneys transplanted from an HLA identical sibling approaches 95%. Approximately 50–65% of cadaver kidneys that are mismatched for all four HLA-A and B antigens function for 6 months but deteriorate thereafter with time. Only 15–25% of these mismatched cadaver kidneys remain functioning 4 years after transplantation.

It is obligatory to select HLA-identical donors for bone marrow transplantation to reduce the frequency of graft-versus-host disease (GVHD). However, a new method that depletes donor marrow T cells that are capable of recognizing foreign host antigens has markedly reduced the incidence of GVHD. HLA-matched platelets are useful to patients who are refractile to random donor platelets.

### Histocompatibility Testing

In addition to the previously outlined laboratory screening procedures that are performed pretransplantation, other testing—such as HLA testing—may be appropriate. In bone marrow transplantation, compatibility testing must include mixed leukocyte culture (MLC) testing. For renal transplantation, compatibility testing shall include a lymphocytotoxicity crossmatch. Protocol and procedures related to this phase of testing must follow the American Association of Blood Banks *Standards*.

### HLA Typing Antisera

*Documentation.* Documentation shall be available to ensure specificity of reagent antisera. Documentation should consist of prospective testing against a well-characterized cell panel, or retrospective analysis of the results of routine typing. The specificity of typing antisera obtained locally should be confirmed in at least one other laboratory. Serum, whether in bulk, aliquots, or loaded into typing trays, should be stored at −20° C or colder. If stored at warmer temperatures, there shall be documentation that reactivity is maintained.

*Control Sera.* Each typing or crossmatch tray shall include at least one complement-dependent positive control serum and at least one negative control serum (or serum from a pool known to lack cytotoxic antibody). Cell viability in the negative control well at the end of the incubation period shall be sufficient to permit accurate interpretation of the results. For most methods, viability should exceed 80%.

*Complement.* Each new batch of complement shall be tested to determine that it induces cytotoxicity in the presence of specific antibody, but is not cytotoxic in the absence of specific antibody. Control procedures should be established to ensure reactivity of stored complement.

### HLA Typing

The HLA terminology shall conform to World Health Organization (WHO) Committee on Nomenclature. Each HLA-A, -B, -C antigen should be defined either by at least two different monospecific sera, or by one monospecific and two multispecific sera, or by three multispecific sera. Each HLA-DR antigen should be defined either by at least five antisera or by three antisera that are operationally monospecific. In typing for a single antigen (e.g., HLA-B27) the procedure must include appropriate controls for cross-reactivity. A complement-dependent

lymphocytotoxic method or a method of demonstrated equivalence shall be used in cell testing.

### Compatibility Testing

Each specimen must be labeled in a manner to ensure positive identification of the individual from whom the sample was obtained. When HLA-selected blood components are sought for transfusion, donor and recipient HLA-A and -B antigens should be identified to determine the best donor. When living related persons are considered as transplantation donors, all available members of the immediate family should be typed to allow accurate haplotype assignment. For organ transplantation studies, donor and recipient shall be typed for ABO group, HLA-A, -B, and -DR antigens.

*Mixed Leukocyte Culture (MLC).* At the start of culture, viability of all cell suspensions should exceed 80%. Serum used in the culture medium must be shown to lack cytotoxic antibodies, be sterile, and support proliferative responses. Each MLC test must include an autologous control, as well as unrelated control responders and stimulators. For the latter, stimulator cell suspensions from three or more unrelated control individuals (preferably DR-mismatched or from two unrelated persons) and a pool of at least three or more unrelated persons must be used for each responder cell tested. The methods used for incubating and labeling shall be sufficient to discriminate positive from negative responses.

*Lymphocytotoxic Antibody Detection.* For this procedure, the panel used shall include cells representative of each commonly occurring recognized antigen and most working (w) specificities. When patients are awaiting renal transplantation, serum samples should be obtained at monthly intervals and tested for antibodies. If a potential renal transplant recipient has been transfused, pregnant, or had an allograft removed, a serum sample must be obtained for testing at least 14 days after the potentially immunizing event.

*Lymphocytotoxicity Crossmatching.* Crossmatches shall use methods to enhance sensitivity relative to routine microlymphocytotoxicity testing, such as incubation, washing, or augmentation with antiglobulin reagent. Crossmatches shall be done with the most reactive sample collected within 1 month of the time the testing is performed. If the recipient has had a sensitizing event or a Class I lymphocytotoxic panel reactivity greater than 15%, or if the history is uncertain or unavailable, the crossmatch should be done with a serum sample collected within 2 days of the transplant. If antibody testing indicates antibodies previously demonstrated are no longer present, the crossmatches may include available sera in which antibody showed its greatest reactivity. Each patient serum should be tested in both diluted and undiluted form. Serum samples used for crossmatches shall be retained in the frozen state for at least 3 months following transplantation.

**Table 16-3. Monitors for Excess Immunosuppression**

- Surveillance cultures for infections
- Total white blood cell count and differential count for indication of the response to infection
- Serologic examination for evidence of rise in titer to specific infectious agents, e.g., cytomegalovirus
- Measurement of cyclosporine (CsA) concentrations in blood
- Serum chemistry markers for organ injury

Records of tests including internal and external control tests must be retained, although they need not necessarily be immediately available. These records need to be stored for a minimum of 5 years, or as required by applicable laws.

## Monitoring Allogeneic Organ Transplantation

### Laboratory Monitors

The laboratory monitors in allogeneic organ transplantation include general indicators for excess immunosuppression (Table 16-3) that could lead to toxicity to other organs as well as opportunistic infection, and markers for inadequate immunosuppression (Table 16-4) that could lead to potential rejection of the transplanted organ. Patients who have received allogeneic organ transplants must have intense and continuous immunosuppressive therapy. However, patients who receive autologous transplantation of bone marrow can be at risk for similar sequelae, if they have ablation of their own bone marrow as part of the treatment of the primary disease—e.g., solid-tumor malignancy prior to reintroduction of marrow cells that have been harvested and processed.

### Direct Monitoring of Immunosuppressive Agent Therapy

***Cyclosporine (CsA) Monitoring.*** CsA is a potent inhibitor of T-cell lymphocyte function that was first derived from culture of a soil fungus. Since 1980, the number of liver transplants has increased dramatically following the introduction of cyclosporine as an immunosuppressant.

***FK-506.*** FK-506 is an experimental immunosuppressant that has been proposed to replace CsA for clinical use. Presumably, the toxic reactions from cyclosporine on

**Table 16-4. Monitors of Inadequate Immunosuppression**

- CsA concentration in blood
- Quantitation of lymphocyte subset populations, e.g., CD4 and CD8 lymphocyte absolute counts and ratios
- Organ biopsy for histologic evidence of rejection
- Serum chemistry markers for organ injury
- Urinalysis, especially in renal transplant

the kidneys, liver, and central nervous system may be less significant with FK-506 therapy.

### Biochemical Markers of Lymphocyte Activation

The goal of tracking biochemical markers is to quantitate lymphocyte-specific substances that theoretically are released during the initial part of an immune response before lymphocytes and other effectors of the immune system have the opportunity to cause organ damage. Early detection of rejection produces greater likelihood of reversing it with accelerated immunosuppression.

***Soluble Interleukin-2 Receptor and Lymphocyte Surface Markers.*** Lymphocytes are activated in vivo as part of an immune response either to infection or in the cell-mediated rejection of an allografted organ. Activation entails new synthesis of the interleuken-2 receptor (IL-2R) and its expression on the lymphocyte surface as a transmembrane protein. IL-2R on lymphocyte surfaces mediates the action of a lymphokine interleukin-2 (IL-2) when it binds IL-2. Lymphocyte activation and proliferation results in the synthesis of more IL-2R by lymphocytes.

***Beta-2($\beta$) Microglobulin.*** Beta-2 microglobulin ($\beta$2M) appears on the surface membrane of nucleated cells as the light chain of class I HLA molecules. It is naturally expressed and released with the membrane turnover accompanying cell division. Renal dysfunction has an impact on the clearance of $\beta$2M; therefore, it allows this substance to be used as a marker for success of renal transplantation.

***Neopterin.*** Neopterin appears to be produced by macrophages and lymphocytes during their activation and proliferation. Elevated levels have been observed in some malignancies (presumably due to the immune response to the tumor), autoimmune disorders, viral infection, and AIDS. Measurements in plasma and urine have been applied to renal transplant patients for the early detection of organ rejection. Another application may be the prediction of rejection episodes so severe that they will not respond to immunosuppression.

### Conventional Laboratory Tests

In the immediate postoperative period, transplant recipients require extensive monitoring of organ functions to assess whether the transplanted organ is viable and to determine the effect of surgery on the body as a whole. Common laboratory tests are arterial blood gases, basic chemistry panels, urinalysis, complete blood counts, and coagulation times.

## BONE MARROW AND PERIPHERAL BLOOD PROGENITOR CELLS

Bone marrow and peripheral blood progenitor cells contain lymphohematopoietic progenitor cells intended to provide temporary or permanent lymphohematopoietic engraftment in the recipient. In general, standards applying to blood components shall also apply to bone marrow and peripheral blood progenitor cells. Special consideration shall be given to maintaining the viability of the lymphohematopoietic progenitor cells contained in these preparations.

## Selection of Donors

If the blood bank or transfusion service is responsible for the selection of donors, donor selection procedures shall be in place that protect the safety of the donor and recipient. Prospective marrow donors shall be evaluated by history and physical examination for risks of anesthesia used in marrow harvesting.

For allogeneic marrow donors, review of donor health to determine suitability shall be performed before the recipient receives marrow ablative therapy and again when the donor is admitted for donation. For allogeneic bone marrow transplantation from an unrelated donor, the same rules apply as in donor selection for blood and blood components. Deviation from these requirements prescribed by the American Association of Blood Banks is permissible only with the documented approval of the donor's and recipient's physicians. Special circumstances related to allogeneic bone marrow transplantation from related donors may necessitate deviation from the AABB Standards. Approval for deviations must be documented.

For autologous donation of either bone marrow or hematopoietic progenitor cells, the criteria for selection are at the discretion of the patient's physician.

## Donor Consent

After the donor history, physical examination, and discussion with a physician familiar with the collection procedure, the donor's informed consent shall be documented. This should also include postphlebotomy advice and notification of test results.

## Collection and Processing

Collection and processing of bone marrow and peripheral blood progenitor cells should be done according to protocols defined in the facility's procedures manual. A written request from the recipient's physician must be available before collection and processing are initiated. Methods for collection and processing shall employ aseptic techniques and shall use methods known to result in acceptable progenitor cell viability. Lot numbers and expiration dates of reagents and disposables shall be recorded. Bone marrow and peripheral blood progenitor cells shall not receive gamma irradiation. In addition, personnel involved in collection and processing must be identified and their training shall be documented.

## Laboratory Testing

Allogeneic preparations are tested in the same way as donor blood. Autologous specimens are treated the same as autologous blood. Deviation from the requirements of the AABB Standards is permissible only with the documented approval of the donor's and the patient's physicians.

Required donor tests for infectious disease markers should be performed within 10 days prior to initiating the recipient preoperative regimen. For multiple blood or bone marrow collections from the same donor, the frequency of testing shall be the same as a cytopheresis donor dedicated to support of a specific patient. Testing must be performed prior to transfusion of the first apheresis component and at least every 10 days thereafter.

## Quality Control

Nucleated cell counts on each bone marrow or peripheral blood progenitor cell collection shall be performed according to procedures defined in the facility's procedures manual. The medical director is responsible for indicating the circumstances under which viability testing and progenitor cell content are to be determined and for ensuring that these protocols are followed. A representative sample of each bone marrow or peripheral blood progenitor cell harvest shall be tested for bacterial and fungal contamination after collection and processing. The medical director is responsible for review of the results.

Labeling of preparations must include information required in the labeling of blood or blood components and the name of the intended recipient. The label must list the storage temperature, expiration date, name of the preparing facility, and ABO group and Rh type of the contents.

## CHAPTER SUMMARY

### Introduction

Transplantation can involve organs such as the kidneys, heart, and liver or tissues such as the skin, bone, corneas, or bone marrow. The phenomenal growth in the number of transplants is largely due to the development of improved immunosuppressant drugs. The time period between removal of an organ from a cadaveric donor (on life support systems) and transplantation into the recipient is limited by initial deterioration in vivo within the moribund donor and by in vitro deterioration during the ischemic time of handling and transporting the isolated organ.

The Federal Required Request law of 1986 requires that hospitals that participate in Medicare and Medicaid reimbursement establish guidelines for identifying potential donors, offering the choice of donation to the legal next-of-kin, and notifying a procurement agency.

Bone is the most commonly transplanted tissue, because bone obtained from one donor can provide graft material for many recipients. Corneas are readily obtained, stored, and transplanted. Cornea donors are the most common type of donor.

### Tissue Storage, Issue, Records and Complications

At present, hospital practice regarding tissue storage varies greatly. Tissue storage can be improved, if storage is centralized and well-developed policies and procedures are followed. Records must be retained indefinitely to show the source facility, the original numeric or alphanumeric donor or lot identification, and the final disposition of each tissue.

### Clinical Laboratory Testing

Donor testing usually focuses on information needed to determine if an organ should be used, and information needed in posttransplant management of a patient. Tests performed on both blood and tissue donors are basically the same. Protocols for pretesting of cadaveric candidate donors are primarily intended to rule out infectious diseases that may be transmitted by transplantation of the organ or with the donor blood perfusing the organ.

The only absolute contraindication to accepting organs from a candidate donor relates to HIV status. A donor who is HIV positive must be excluded.

All vertebrates capable of acute rejection of foreign skin grafts possess a localized complex involving many genes that exerts major control over the organism's immune reactions. Many nucleated cells possess cell-surface-protein antigens that are part of this complex that readily provokes an immune response if transferred into a genetically different (allogeneic) individual of the same species.

In humans, the MHC is expressed as human leukocyte antigen (HLA).

HLA matching is of value in organ transplantation, as well as in the transplantation of bone marrow. In kidney allografts, the method of organ preservation, time elapsed between harvesting and transplanting, number of pretransplantation blood transfusions, recipient age, and primary cause for kidney failure are all important determinants of early transplant success or failure. HLA compatibility, however, exerts the strongest influence on long-term kidney survival.

The laboratory monitors in allogeneic organ transplantation include general indicators for excessive immunosuppression that could lead to toxicity to other organs as well as opportunistic infection, and markers for inadequate immunosuppression that could lead to potential rejection of the transplanted organ. Early detection of rejection produces a greater likelihood of reversing it with accelerated immunosuppression.

In the immediate postoperative period, transplant re-cipients require extensive monitoring of organ functions to assess whether the transplanted organ is viable and to determine the effect of surgery on the body as a whole. Common laboratory tests include arterial blood gases, basic chemistry panels, urinalysis, complete blood counts, and coagulation times.

### Bone Marrow and Peripheral Blood Progenitor Cells

Bone marrow and peripheral blood progenitor cells contain lymphohematopoietic progenitor cells intended to provide temporary or permanent lymphohematopoietic engraftment in the recipient. For allogeneic marrow donors, review of donor health to determine suitability shall be performed before the recipient receives marrow ablative therapy and again when the donor is admitted for donation.

---

## REVIEW QUESTIONS

1. Approximately _____ organs were harvested for transplantation in 1990.
   - **A.** 2500
   - **B.** 5000
   - **C.** 7500
   - **D.** 15000
2. The major limitation(s) to liver transplantation is (are):
   - **A.** Organ availability
   - **B.** Deterioration due to ischemia
   - **C.** Matching of organ size and blood type
   - **D.** Both A and B
3. The differing requirements for _____ form the principal difference between organs and tissues.
   - **A.** Oxygen
   - **B.** Blood perfusion
   - **C.** Compatibility testing
   - **D.** Both A and B
4. The most commonly transplanted tissue is:
   - **A.** Bone
   - **B.** Corneas
   - **C.** Skin
   - **D.** Heart valves
5. Reduction in corneal graft failure can be accomplished by:
   - **A.** Histocompatibility testing
   - **B.** ABO blood group matching
   - **C.** Depletion of lymphocytes
   - **D.** Use of artificial lens
6. Posttransplantation HIV reporting does *not* include:
   - **A.** Notification of positive HIV results to all involved medical directors and tissue banks
   - **B.** Management of the investigation to determine HIV status of donor
   - **C.** Submission of a written report within 24 hours
   - **D.** All of the above

7. Testing procedures related to transplantation focus on:
   A. Information needed to determine if an organ/tissue is suitable for transplantation
   B. Information needed for posttransplant management
   C. Laboratory assays related to the detection of infectious disease in a potential donor
   D. All of the above

8. Minimum Procurement Standards include:
   A. Exclusion of donors who are HIV positive
   B. Potential exclusion of a donor who has a malignant tumor
   C. Potential exclusion of a donor who currently suffers from sepsis
   D. All of the above

9. Which HLA antigen(s) is (are) of extreme importance in transplantation?
   A. A
   B. B
   C. A and B
   D. A and C

10. Monitoring a transplant patient for excess immunosuppression does not include:
    A. Total CD4 and CD8 count
    B. Surveillance cultures for infections
    C. Analysis of serum chemistry markers for organ injury
    D. Serologic examination for evidence of cytomegalovirus infection

11. Monitoring for inadequate immunosuppression in transplant patients does not include:
    A. CsA concentrations in the blood
    B. Total CD4 and CD8 count
    C. Organ biopsy for histologic evidence of rejection
    D. Surveillance cultures for infections

12. Biochemical markers are used to:
    A. Quantitate lymphocyte-specific substances before organ damage
    B. Prevent organ rejection
    C. Detect opportunistic infections
    D. Match compatible tissues

13. In the immediate posttransplantation period, laboratory tests that are commonly performed include:
    A. Arterial blood gases and basic chemistry panels
    B. Basic chemistry panels and urinalysis
    C. Complete blood count and coagulation studies
    D. All of the above

14. An overwhelming concern in the processing of lymphohematopoietic progenitor cells is:
    A. Maintaining cell viability
    B. Harvesting large quantities of cells
    C. The donor's age
    D. Processing with adequate gamma radiation

## Bibliography

Bennett, W.M., and Norman, D.J.: Action and toxicity of cyclosporine. Ann. Rev. Med., 37:215–224, 1986.

Bonnem, E.M.: Alpha interferon: Combinations with other antineoplastic modalities. Seminars in Oncology, XIV (2):48–60, Supp 2, 1987.

Collins, R.H., et al.: Donor-derived long-term multilineage hematopoiesis in a liver-transplant recipient. New Eng. J. Med., 328(11):762–765, 1993.

Comenzo, R.L., et al.: Anomalous ABO phenotype in a child after an ABO-incompatible liver transplantation. New Eng. J. Med., 326(13):867–870, 1992.

Cornea tissue matching proves unnecessary. Advance for Med. Lab. Professionals, November 2, 1992, p. 15.

Costello, R., and Duffaud, F.: Pretransplantation blood transfusion. New Eng. J. Med., 326(15):1027, 1992.

Curran, W.J.: Beyond the best interests of a child. New Eng. J. Med., 324(25):1818–1820, 1991.

Diagnostic and Therapeutic Technology Assessment (DATTA). Autologous bone marrow transplantation—reassessment. JAMA, 263(6):881–887, 1990.

Ellinger, P.J., and Crosson, J.T.: The role of the clinical lab in tissue banking. Med. Lab. Observer, 25(7):38–43, 1993.

Emery, R.W., and Lake, K.D.: Post-transplantation lymphoproliferative disorder and OKT 3. New Eng. J. Med., 324(20):1437–1442, 1991.

Fleischhauer, K., Kernan, N.A., O'Reilly, R.J., Dupont, B., and Yang, S.Y.: Bone marrow–allograft rejection by T lymphocytes recognizing a single amino acid difference in HLA-B44. New Eng. J. Med., 323(26):1818–1822, 1990.

Friend, S.H., Dryja, T.P., and Weinberg, R.A.: Oncogenes and tumor-suppressing genes. New Eng. J. Med., 318(10):618–623, 1988.

Good, R.A.: Mixed chimerism and immunologic tolerance. New Eng. J. Med., 328(11):801–802, 1993.

Goodrich, J.M., et al.: Early treatment with ganciclovir to prevent cytomegalovirus disease after allogeneic bone marrow transplantation. New Eng. J. Med., 325(23):1601–1607, 1991.

Graham, M.L., Simonis, T.B., and Davey, R.J.: Harvesting HLA antibodies from placentas. Lab. Med., 20(3):169–171, 1989.

Gribben, J.G., et al.: Immunologic purging of marrow assessed by PCR before autologous bone marrow transplantation for B-cell lymphoma. New Eng. J. Med., 325(22):1525–1533, 1991.

Kernan, N.A., et al.: Analysis of 462 transplantations from unrelated donors facilitated by the National Marrow Donor Program. New Eng. J. Med., 328(9):593–602, 1993.

Lang, H.K.: Federally mandated program for tracking of donor tissue advocated. Advance for Medical Laboratory Professionals, 5(42):10–11, 14, 1993.

Lazda, V.A., and Pollak, R.: Pretransplantation blood transfusion. New Eng. J. Med., 326(15):1027, 1992.

McPherson, R.A., and Markin, R.S.: Laboratory support for organ transplantation. Part I. Lab. Med., 22(4):243–252, 1991.

Markin, R.S., and McPherson, R.: Laboratory support for organ transplantation. Part II. Lab. Med., 22(5):319–324, 1991.

Ndimbie, O.K., and Riddle, P.B.: Serological assessment of the prospective organ donor. Lab. Med., 24(2):103–108, 1993.

Rao, K.V., Anderson, R., and Kasiske, B.L.: Value of liver biopsy in the evaluation and management of chronic liver disease in renal transplant recipients. Am. J. Med., 94:241–250, 1993.

Russell, P.S., Colvin, R.B., and Cosimi, A.B.: Monoclonal antibodies for the diagnosis and treatment of transplant rejection. Ann. Rev. Med., 37:63–79, 1986.

Simonds, R.J., et al.: Transmission of human immunodeficiency virus type 1 from a seronegative organ and tissue donor. New Eng. J. Med., *326*(11):726–732, 1992.

Solinger, A.M.: Organ transplantation and the immune response gene. *Symposium on Clinical Immunology I, Medical Clinics of North America, 69*(3):565–577, 1985.

Spiegel, R.J.: The alpha interferons: clinical overview. *Seminars in Oncology,* XIV(2):1–12, Supp 2, 1987.

Starzl, T.E.: Chimerism after liver transplantation for type IV glycogen storage disease and type 1 Gaucher's disease. New Eng. J. Med., *328*(11):745–749, 1993.

Starzl, T.E.: Chimerism after whole organ transplant. Guthrie J., *62*(2):49–53, 1993.

Starzl, T.E., et al.: Kidney transplantation under FK 506. JAMA, *264*(1):63–67, 1990.

Starzl, T.E.: Transplantation. JAMA, *263*(19):2686–2687, 1990.

Takemoto, S., et al.: Survival of nationally shared, HLA-matched kidney transplants from cadaveric donors. New Eng. J. Med., *327*(12):834–839, 1992.

Thompson, J.: The human leukocyte antigen system. In Internal Medicine, 2nd ed. Jay H. Stein (Ed.). Boston: Little, Brown, 1987, pp. 1205–1208.

Trigg, M.E.: Bone marrow transplantation for childhood diseases. Complements, *5*(1):2–5, 1985.

van Twuyver, E., et al.: Pretransplantation blood transfusion. New Eng. J. Med., *326*(15):1027–1028, 1992.

**17**

# Current Trends in Serologic Testing

At the conclusion of this chapter, the reader will be able to:

- Name the dates and locations of the beginning of microtechniques.
- Cite the two types of micromethods.
- List the applications of micromethods.
- Describe the advantages of microplate hemagglutination techniques.
- Explain the physical characteristics of microplates.
- Describe the principle of solid-phase assay.
- Compare the original method of automation in blood banking to the second-generation instruments.

**Chapter Outline**

Microplate Hemagglutination Techniques
The Gel Test
Solid-Phase Techniques
Automated Methods
    Original Approaches to Automation
        The Continuous-Flow Method
        The Hemagglutination Method
    Second-Generation Instrumentation
        Basic Considerations
        Examples of Instrumentation
        Galvanic Immunosensor Assay
Chapter Summary
Review Questions and Answers
Bibliography

Serologic testing in immunohematology has usually been performed by slide or test tube techniques, but increased emphasis on cost containment has stimulated interest in microtechniques as an alternative to conventional methods. Capillary tubes and microplates have been used in some laboratories for a long time. Capillary tube techniques have been used in the Rh Laboratory in Winnipeg since 1944 and microplates were invented in 1950 in Hungary by Takatsky. Microtesting for typing lymphocytes was introduced 20 years ago. This method has been adopted internationally and is basically the only method used for typing lymphocytes today.

The term *microtechnique* is deceptive because the amount of reagent is not as small as the quantities used in HLA testing. Micromethods for red cell antigen and antibody testing are either hemagglutination or solid phase adherence assays. These methods are still evolving, but are considered more economical than traditional methods because most methods require microliter quantities of reagent antisera or cells per test. These methods are also considered simpler to perform. Although the capillary tube technique has not yet been automated, the microplate method is the basis for several automated instruments.

Applications for micromethods include:

1. ABO grouping (forward and reverse)
2. Rh typing and Rh control
3. Unexpected antibody detection
4. Unexpected antibody identification
5. Antibody titration
6. Crossmatching
7. Reagent quality control

## MICROPLATE HEMAGGLUTINATION TECHNIQUES

In the 1960s, microplate technology was applied to blood banking. Subsequent modifications of the initial technique have succeeded in developing a reproducible and reliable test system without loss of reaction sensitivity. Use of microplates allows the performance of a large number of tests on a single plate, which eliminates time-consuming steps such as labelling test tubes. Although microplate testing was initially restricted to large-scale testing, the development of smaller microplates now allows smaller blood banks to use this technique.

The microplate is a compact plate of rigid or flexible plastic with multiple wells. The wells may be U-shaped or V-shaped or have a flat-bottom configuration. The U-shaped well has been the most commonly used in immunohematology. The volume capacity of each well is approximately 0.2 mL, which prevents spilling during mixing.

Samples and reagents are dispensed with small-bore Pasteur pipettes, recommended because they deliver 0.025

**395**

mL, which prevents splashing. After the specimens and reagents are added to the wells, they are mixed by gentle agitation of the plates. The microplate is then centrifuged for immediate reading. Countertop or floor model centrifuges are suitable if the are equipped with special rotors that can accommodate microplate centrifuge carriers and are capable of speeds between 400 and 2000 rpm. Smaller plates can be centrifuged in serologic centrifuges with an appropriate adapter.

After centrifugation, the cell buttons are resuspended by either gently tapping the microplate or using a flat-topped mechanical shaker. A shaker provides a more consistent and standard resuspension of the cells than manual tapping. After the cells are resuspended, the wells are examined with an optical aid or over a well-lighted surface. A positive reaction will settle in a diffuse, uneven button; negative reactions are manifested by a smooth, compact button (Fig. 17-1). Detection of weakly positive reactions is enhanced by allowing the red cells to settle.

It may be necessary to incubate the plates before centrifugation, depending on the type of test being performed. If a test requires a 37° C incubation, the plates are placed in a dry heat incubator or allowed to float in a waterbath. The wells must be covered during incubation to reduce evaporation of the specimen and reagents. An AHG test can be performed by washing the red cells manually with a dispenser designed to deliver a measured amount of saline to each well and centrifuging the plate between washings. After the last wash, AHG antiserum is added and the plate is recentrifuged. To read AHG reactions, the plate is placed at a 60 to 75-degree angle to allow the red

cells to stream. Positive reactions remain in an aggregated button or stream very slowly; negative reactions stream down the well in a smooth flow. A weakly positive reaction may be detected by gently resuspending the red cells and allowing them to resettle.

Although this technique is considered highly reliable, one problem with the microplates is that new microplates may have static charges. Static can cause adherence of cells and antisera to the sides of the microplate well and prevent the smooth settling of cells. This problem can, however, be avoided by pretreatment of the microplates.

## THE GEL TEST

The gel test employs the principle of controlled centrifugation of red blood cells (RBCs) through a suitable dextran acrylamide gel contained in a specifically devised microtube. The microtube consists of an upper reaction chamber and a barrel with a conical bottom. Centrifugation is an important step.

Gels may be used to perform the majority of applications in blood group serology. Three types of gel can be used: neutral gel, specific gels, and antiglobulin gels.

The gel test was introduced in 1988. It compares favorably to conventional techniques for ABO-Ch grouping, phenotyping, antibody detection and identification, crossmatching, and direct antiglobulin testing and titration in terms of safety, efficacy, and efficiency. A major feature of the gel test is that it addresses the issue of standardization while it incorporates sensitivity and efficiency; it also

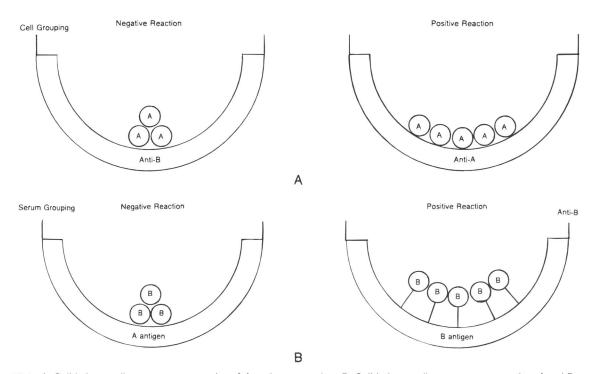

**Figure 17-1.** A, Solid-phase adherence assay results of A antigen grouping. B, Solid-phase adherence assay results of anti-B grouping.

is accessible to laboratories of all sizes and levels of expertise.

## SOLID-PHASE TECHNIQUES

Solid-phase adherence assays are a recent advancement in blood group serology to test erythrocytes for selected antigens, including weak antigen expression, subgroups A and B, and red cells classified by weak D (D^u) by conventional methods. These assays also test serum for erythrocyte antibodies, detect platelet antibodies, and perform compatibility and hepatitis testing. The sensitivity of solid-phase assays has been shown to be equivalent to or better than conventional agglutination methods.

For the past 90 years, the hemagglutination endpoint has remained the most widely used method in immunohematology to detect the interaction of erythrocyte antibodies and antigens. The major disadvantage of hemagglutination methods is the lack of an objective endpoint. Weakly positive reactions may be difficult to distinguish from negative reactions; therefore, test interpretation is subjective and relies on the technical ability and expertise of the technologist performing the test. By comparison, solid-phase assays have been designed to achieve endpoints that are more easily differentiated by manual or automated methods.

Solid-phase assays rely on adherence rather than hemagglutination for detection of antigen-antibody reactions. In 1976, it was demonstrated that monolayers of red cells could be immobilized on plastic tubes for the detection of antigen-antibody reactions. With this technique, either an antigen or an antibody is immobilized on a solid phase. Methods of immobilization are usually based on simple, passive adsorption of antibody or antigen onto the plastic surface. This phenomenon is believed to occur by hydrophobic bonding. Adsorption may be facilitated by pretreating the plates with chemicals such as glutaraldehyde before addition of antigen or antibody. Polystyrene microplates are the most commonly used, but polystyrene tubes and microplates or tubes made of polypropylene or polyvinyl plastics can also be used.

Erythrocyte antigen typing involves immobilization of specific antibodies such as anti-A or anti-D on the microplate wells. The red cells are enzyme-treated before testing to enhance antigen-antibody interaction. A dilute suspension of these treated red cells is prepared and added to the appropriate antibody-coated wells. Equipment used in solid-phase testing is the same as in microplate hemagglutination procedures. A centrifuge that can accommodate microplate centrifuge carriers and a 37° C dry heat incubator or waterbath are the minimum requirements. After addition of the appropriate reactants, the microplate is centrifuged and observed for a positive or negative reaction. A positive reaction is demonstrated by adherence of the red cells to the entire inner surface of the well; a nega-

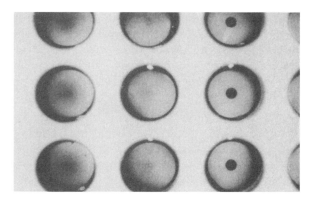

**Figure 17-2.** Buttons formed by nonagglutinated cells. Photograph courtesy of Olympus Corporation, Clinical Instruments Division, Lake Success, New York.

tive reaction is exhibited by nonadherence. Nonadhering red cells pellet into a discrete, compact button in the bottom of the well when centrifuged (Figure 17-2).

Solid-phase assays for antibody detection are more involved than antigen detection. One method is used for detection of IgM antibodies such as anti-A or anti-B and another for detection of IgG antibodies such as anti-D. The assay for anti-A or anti-B requires the immobilization of a red cell monolayer of A_1 or B red cells, or purified antigens on an immunologically active surface of the microplate well. Test serum is added to the appropriate wells, incubated, and decanted. Enzyme-treated A_1, B, or A_1B indicator red cells are added to each well and the microplate is centrifuged. Positive reactions are indicated by adherence of the indicator cells to either anti-A or anti-B that has been previously bound to the immobilized red cell monolayer. The reaction can be visualized as a "sandwich" of two layers of antigen linked together by antibody. Negative reactions are demonstrated by no adherence.

The assay for the detection of IgG alloantibodies also uses the immobilization of a red cell monolayer of red cells with a known selection of erythrocyte antigens. Test serum and a low ionic enhancement medium are added to each well. The mixture is incubated at 37° C and then washed with saline to remove free serum. Antiglobulin antiserum facilitates the linking of the antibody-coated indicator cells to the antibody bound to the red cell monolayer. The presence or absence of adherence is interpreted as a positive or negative result, respectively.

In addition to the adherence of erythrocytes, other indicators may be used to determine the reaction results. The results can be decided using a spectrophotometer designed for microplate reading. Adhering erythrocytes can be hemolyzed with distilled water and the resulting hemolysis can be read as a positive result. A chromogenic substrate may also be added for test interpretation. This type of substrate reacts with the hemoglobin peroxidase of the adhering erythrocytes to produce an interpretable color reaction.

The solid-phase antiglobulin test (SPAT) has been applied to crossmatching. This technique results in adherence of sensitized red cells to IgG-coated wells. Results can be read visually or automatically using a spectrophotometer designed for microplate readings. This application is considered to have more sensitivity than manual methods without loss of specificity.

## AUTOMATED METHODS

A major achievement in the past several decades has been the introduction of automation into the blood bank. Automated systems have the capabilities of positive sample identification; automatic dispensing of specimens and antisera; and interpretation, recording, and storing of results. One of the problems associated with early automated systems was the inability to detect weak antibody-antigen interactions.

### Original Approaches to Automation

#### The Continuous-Flow Method

In 1963, an adaptation of the continuous-flow method which was successfully implemented in clinical chemistry applications, was introduced to automate hemagglutination. Modifications of this basic technique have extended to applications such as special antigen typing, antibody screening, and antibody titration.

With the continuous-flow methodology, test specimens—erythrocytes, serum, or both—are aspirated, divided into aliquots, and routed through separate channels. Air bubbles are added to mechanically separate individual specimens and prevent liquid film formation on the mixing coils. The specimen mixes with appropriate reagents and agglutination occurs in a reaction coil. After mixing, a hypertonic salt solution is added to disperse clumps that are not bound by antibody. The mixture is sent through a settling coil to allow the resulting agglutinates to settle before passing over a T-fitting. As the mixture stream passes over the T-fitting, the agglutinates fall out of the sample stream.

Agglutination may be detected visually by examining deposits of agglutinates, which are removed at the T-fitting onto a strip of moving filter paper. If the stream is debubbled and infrared light-emitting diodes and sensors are positioned across the tubing, the optical density of the remaining liquid can be measured.

This type of instrumentation is limited to large blood processing centers because it is expensive and best suited for batch processing. A disadvantage of the system is that it is less effective than manual techniques in detecting all examples of clinically significant alloantibodies.

#### The Hemagglutination Method

Another system of automated hemagglutination is comparable to the manual tube method. Specimens and antisera are automatically dispensed into cuvettes. The mixtures are then incubated, centrifuged, and agitated. Agitation disperses all of the free erythrocytes into a homogeneous suspension and the clumps of agglutinated cells collect in the center of the cuvette. Agglutination is detected by comparing the optical density of the peripheral and central area of each cuvette.

A positive reaction is demonstrated by a reciprocal variation in the central and peripheral light intensities. The absence of variation in the optical density between the central and peripheral areas signifies a negative reaction. The instrument is interfaced to a computer, which interprets and prints the results.

This type of instrumentation is also limited to large blood processing centers because it is expensive and best suited for batch processing. A disadvantage of the system is that it is less effective than manual techniques in detecting all examples of clinically significant alloantibodies.

### Second-Generation Instrumentation

#### Basic Considerations

Newer systems that use microplate technology have been developed for large- and small-scale applications. Automated microplate systems may be used for routine blood grouping and antibody detection. These systems are considered more economical in terms of equipment costs than older systems. A disadvantage of the automated microplate systems, in general, is difficulty in detecting weak antigen-antibody reactions. In such cases, visual observation of the microplate and on-line manual editing require technologist interpretation of questionable reactions. The basic principle of automated systems is similar to manual microplate hemagglutination. The systems have incorporated densitometers to read microplate hemagglutination and interfaced them with computers that interpret and print or store the serologic results.

Specimens are dispensed to microplate wells either manually or automatically. The plate is processed by incubation, centrifugation, and gentle agitation. Free erythrocytes are resuspended and agglutinated cells remain in the center of the well. The optical density of each well is then read; the actual number of readings per well varies with the type of densitometer used. The readings are transferred through an interface to a computer for processing. Depending on the number of readings conducted, hemagglutination may be determined by either histogram analysis or a comparison of peripheral and central optical densities.

**Figure 17-3.** MicroBank system components. This system consists of the MicroBank™ reader (far right), which measures the optical density of red cell suspensions in U-bottom, 96-well microplates and processes the information by means of a resident computer and dedicated software. The reader microprocessor also accepts bar-coded tube and microplate information from the laser scanner. The reader houses one floppy disk drive for storage and transfer. The video terminal (far left) allows the operator to control and monitor the reader, scanner, and microprocessor operation. The dot matrix printer (rear) produces a hardcopy printout of serologic test results, quality control records, and administrative reports. The laser scanner (optional, second from right) reads bar-coded information from test tubes and microplates and transmits the information to the microprocessor for subsequent correlation of test sample numbers with blood group interpretations. The sample preparation device (optional, second from left) automatically prepares each test cell suspension and delivers the specimen and reagents to the appropriate microplate wells. Photograph courtesy of Dynatech Laboratories Inc., Chantilly, Virginia.

## Examples of Instrumentation

Two examples of second-generation instrumentation are the MicroBank™ Automated Blood Grouping System (Dynatech Laboratories, Inc., Chantilly, Virginia) and the Olympus PK 7100 (Olympus Corporation, Lake Success, New York).

The MicroBank system (Fig. 17-3) is designed to determine ABO grouping and Rh typing. A laser scanner identifies up to 8 bar code-labelled test tubes in the bar code-labelled microplate that is placed into a specially designed carrier (Fig. 17-4).

Specimens can be dispensed into the microplate by

**Figure 17-4.** Bar-coded tubes and plate in the scan position. Photograph courtesy of Dynatech Laboratories, Inc., Chantilly, Virginia.

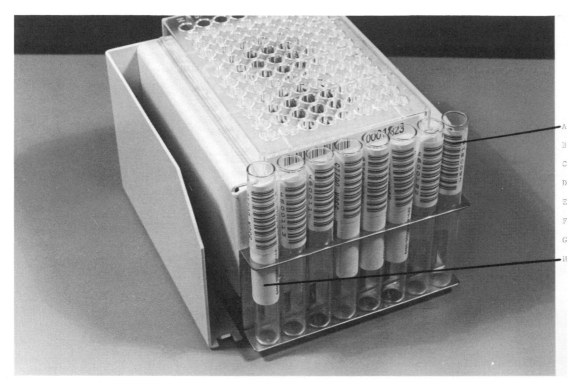

**Figure 17-5.** Test sample-microwell configuration. Photograph courtesy of Dynatech Laboratories, Inc., Chantilly, Virginia.

manual or semiautomated methods and maintain the pre-established test sample/microwell configuration (Fig. 17-5). Specimens and reagents are mixed in the wells of rigid U-bottom microplates. After centrifugation and resuspension of the test well mixtures, the microplate is placed on the reader platform. The microplate bar code is again scanned and multiple readings are made of each well (Fig. 17-6). The light absorbance of reactions is compared to preset threshold values for positive, negative, or questionable reactions. Specimens yielding negative results with

**Figure 17-6.** Laser scanner. Photograph courtesy of Dynatech Laboratories, Inc., Chantilly, Virginia.

**Figure 17-7.** Olympus system. Photograph courtesy of Olympus Corporation, Clinical Instruments Division, Lake Success, New York.

anti-D require further manual testing before the Rh type can be determined. Al results are stored on a floppy disk and/or transferred to a mainframe computer system.

The Olympus PK 7100 automated microplate-based, pretransfusion blood group system (Fig. 17-7) is a fully automated high-throughput instrument that performs forward and reverse ABO grouping and Rh typing. A bar code reader is standard for identification of patient specimens. Determination of ABO grouping is in saline without additives, but Rh typing includes treatment of the cells with bromelin using dual probes.

This system uses a unique terraced-well microplate (Fig. 17-8). The reaction wells have concentric rings cut into the walls, allowing agglutinated erythrocytes to settle evenly on the steps, or terraces, of the well. Nonagglutinated cells roll to the bottom of the well and form a tight concentric button, which will not dissociate or crumble

**Figure 17-8.** Olympus microwell construction. Photograph courtesy of Olympus Corporation, Clinical Instruments Division, Lake Success, New York.

due to automated handling.

Interpretation of reactions is made by comparing the optical densities at peripheral (P) and central (C) locations in each well, determining the P/C ratio, and comparing the results to the threshold levels of a known sample population. A built-in microcomputer records the results of each sample and controls the printout. Visual evaluation can be performed as the microplate enters the viewing station located on the top surface of the analyzer.

### Galvanic Immunosensor Assay

In an attempt to remove subjective interpretation and apply newer biotechnologies, biosensors have been used. A biosensor is a device that uses a biological-sensing, molecular-recognition element connected to a transducing or signal-gathering system that leads to the output of an electronic signal.

Using an immunosensor system, the first stage of cell sensitization can be detected within seconds of the combination of an antigen-antibody mixture. Commercially viable immunosensors will emerge eventually.

## CHAPTER SUMMARY

Microtechniques are becoming more popular because of an increased emphasis on cost containment. Micromethods for red cell antigen and antibody testing are hemagglutination or solid phase adherence assays. These methods are considered more economical than traditional methods. Applications of micromethods include ABO grouping, Rh typing and control, alloantibody detection and identification, antibody titration, crossmatching, and reagent quality control.

## Microplate Hemagglutination Techniques

Use of microplates allows performance of a large number of tests on a single plate, which eliminates time-consuming steps such as labelling test tubes. The microplate is a compact plate of rigid or flexible plastic with multiple wells. The U-shaped well has been the most commonly used in immunohematology. Although this technique is considered highly reliable, one problem with the microplates is that new microplates may have static charges that can cause adherence of cells and antisera to the sides of the microplate well and prevent smooth settling of cells. This can lead to erroneous results.

## Solid-Phase Techniques

Solid-phase assays rely on adherence rather than hemagglutination for detection of antigen-antibody reactions. With this technique, either an antigen or an antibody is immobilized on a solid phase. Erythrocyte antigen typing involves the immobilization of specific antibodies such as anti-A or anti-D on the microplate wells. Solid-phase assays for antibody detection are more involved than antigen detection. One method is used for the detection of IgM antibodies such as anti-A or anti-B and another for the detection of IgG antibodies such as anti-D. The solid-phase antiglobulin test (SPAT) has been applied to crossmatching. This technique results in adherence of sensitized red cells to IgG-coated wells. Results can be read visually or automatically using a spectrophotometer designed for microplate readings. This application is considered to have more sensitivity than manual methods without loss of specificity.

## The Gel Test

Gels may be used for serologic testing. This test method offers standardization of testing, incorporates sensitivity and efficiency, and is accessible to laboratories of all sizes and levels of expertise.

## Automated Methods

Automated systems have the capabilities of positive sample identification; automatic dispensing of specimens and antisera; and interpretation, recording, and storage of results. The first blood bank automated hemagglutination instrument was a modification of the continuous-flow method which had been successfully implemented in clinical chemistry. This type of instrumentation is limited to large blood processing centers because it is expensive and best suited for batch processing. A disadvantage of the system is that it is less effective than manual techniques in detecting all examples of clinically significant alloantibodies.

Another system of automated hemagglutination is comparable to the manual tube method. The instrument is interfaced to a computer, which interprets and prints the results. This type of instrumentation is also limited to large blood processing centers because it is expensive and best suited for batch processing.

Newer systems that use microplate technology have been developed for large- and small-scale applications. Automated microplate systems may be used for routine blood grouping and antibody detection. These systems are considered more economical in terms of equipment costs than older systems. A disadvantage of the automated microplate systems, in general, is difficulty in detecting weak antigen-antibody reactions. In such cases, visual observation of the microplate and on-line manual editing require technologist interpretation of questionable reactions. The basic principle of these systems is similar to manual microplate hemagglutination. The systems have incorporated densitometers to read microplate hemagglutination and interfaced them with computers that interpret and print or store the serologic results. Two examples of second-generation instrumentation are the MicroBank™ Automated Blood Grouping System and the Olympus PK 7100.

Immunosensors can detect the first stage of cell sensitization within seconds of the combination of an antigen-antibody mixture. This is a new and emerging technology.

---

## REVIEW QUESTIONS

1. Capillary tube microtechniques have been used in blood bank testing since:
   A. 1908
   B. 1924
   C. 1944
   D. 1963
   E. 1980
2. Micromethods can be used for:
   A. ABO grouping
   B. Rh Typing
   C. Alloantibody detection and identification
   D. Crossmatching
   E. All of the above
3. The advantage or advantages of the microplate technique is (are):
   A. Eliminates time-consuming steps
   B. Uses less specimen and reagents
   C. Uses less personnel time
   D. Is reliable
   E. All of the above
4. Solid phase assays rely on _____ for detection of antigen-antibody reactions.
   A. Hemagglutination
   B. Adherence
   C. Differential solubility rates
   D. Differences in optical density
   E. Competitive inhibition

**5.** The first automated systems in blood banking were adaptations of _____ methodology.
   **A.** Microplate hemagglutination
   **B.** Solid phase
   **C.** Continuous-flow
   **D.** Competitive inhibition
   **E.** Fluorescent

**6.** Most second-generation instrumentation is based on:
   **A.** Microplate hemagglutination
   **B.** Solid phase
   **C.** Continuous flow
   **D.** Competitive inhibition
   **E.** Fluorescence

## Bibliography

Alfano, J.A.: Solid-phase technology in the blood bank. Advance, 6(3):10–11, 1994.

Crawford, M.C.: A review of micromethods for blood bank laboratories. Lab. Med., 18(3):149–152, 1987.

Douglas, R., Schneider, J.V., Wilkie, D., and Harden, P.A.: A solid phase antiglobulin test. Transfusion, 27(4):378–383, 1987.

Friedman, L.I., Severns, M.L., Goodkofsky, I., and Holland, N.: The status of automation and data processing in the United States blood banking community. Transfusion, 26(6):514–518, 1986.

Gibbons, D.S., Kano, T., and Edelmann, M.: A terraced microplate system for automated ABO and Rh grouping. Am. Clin. Prod. Rev., 42–46, Nov. 1986.

Kohmann, T.F., Forey, J.E., Burch, J.W., and Au-Buchon, J.P.: Prelicensure evaluation of a microplate-based blood testing system. Transfusion, 26(6):550, 1986.

Kutt, S.M., Larison, P.J., and Lewis, C.A.: Evaluation of a microplate test system for blood banks. Am. Clin. Prod. Rev., 8–11, Jan., 1988.

Leong, S.W., and Terasaki, P.I.: Microtest for red cell typing. Transfusion, 25(2):149–151, 1985.

Malyska, H.M., and Weiland, D.: The gel test. Lab. Med., 25(2):81–85, 1994.

Moheng, M.C.: Blood Banking: State of the Art. In Pierce, S.R., and Wilson, J.K. (Eds.): Approaches to Serological Problems in the Hospital Transfusion Service. Arlington, VA, American Association of Blood Banks, 1985.

Moulds, J.J.: The galvanic immunosensor assay. Lab. Med., 25(2):86–89, 1994.

Peoples, J.C.A.: A retrospective survey of blood bank automation. Lab. Med., 16(12):763–765, 1985.

Rachel, J.M., Sinor, L.T., Beck, M.L., and Plapp, F.V.: A solid-phase antiglobulin test. Transfusion, 25(1):24–26, 1985.

Sinor, L.T., et al.: Solid-phase ABO grouping and Rh typing. Transfusion, 25(1):21–23, 1985.

Sosler, S.D.: Current trends in immunohematology and transfusion medicine. Lab. Med., 25(2):79–80, 1994.

Theuriere, M., Zelenski, K.R., Moore, V.K., and Logulo, A.C.: Automated detection of red cell antibodies in donor sera using an automated technology. Transfusion, 25(3):257–260, 1985.

Tomchick, C., Piccirilli, R., and Schmidt, A.P.: Evaluation of an automated microplate blood grouping system. Transfusion, 24(5):441, 1984.

# Appendix A

# The Foundations of Genetic Interactions

Genetics, the study of the transmission of inherited characteristics, is important in the study of antigen inheritance and inherited disorders. During the last 30 years a revolution has occurred in our understanding of genetics. More than 200 human genes have been cloned, and the chromosomal map location is known for more than 140 of these genes. Information is also rapidly emerging about alterations in genes for factors VIII and IX of the coagulation system.

Hereditary information resides in genes, which are present on chromosomes. The normal number of human chromosomes consists of 46 in each nucleated cell. Chromosomes are organized into 22 homologous autosomal pairs and one pair of sex chromosomes (XX or XY). Every normal individual has at least one X chromosome. Females are XX and males are XY.

In 1953, Watson and Crick described the double-helix model of DNA, in which genetic information is encoded into linear arrays in the form of the deoxyribonucleotide bases adenine (A), thymine (T), cytosine (C), and guanine (G). The two strands of DNA have antiparallel comple-

mentary sequences that pair by hydrogen bonding between the bases: thymine pairs with adenine and cytosine with guanine. The genetic code that stores hereditary information is stored as triplets of nucleotides, which encode for various amino acids (Figure A-1).

A *gene* is a segment of DNA that is arranged along the chromosome at a specific position called a *locus* (plural, *loci*). Genes at a specific locus that differ in their nucleotides sequence are called *alleles*. Thus, in each somatic cell, one member of a set of alleles is maternally derived and the other paternally derived. An individual who inherits identical alleles is *homozygous;* inheritance of nonidentical alleles is termed *heterozygous*. In some blood group systems, persons who are homozygous for a gene have more antigen on their red blood cells than individuals who are heterozygous. This may be referred to as a "double dose" or a "single dose" of antigen. Differences in the amount of antigen on the red blood cells can be detectable serologically. This variation in the strength of antigen reactivity is called *dosage effect*.

In addition, loci present on the same chromosome are

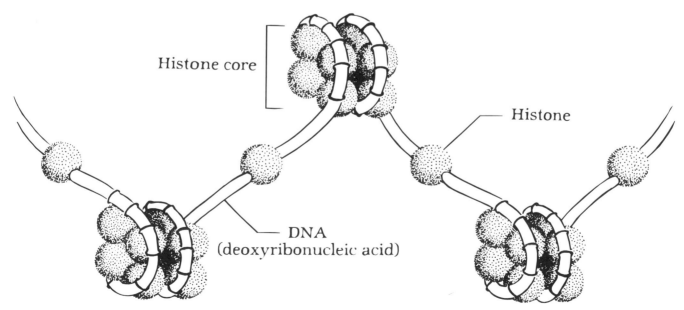

**Figure A-1.** A general model of the organization of DNA and histones.

**Table B-2. Genetic Markers Used in the Assessment of Parentage**

| A. Red Blood Cell Antigen Systems | Antigens |
|---|---|
| ABO | A, $A_1$, B |
| Rh | D, C, c, E, e |
| M, N, S | M, N, S, s |
| Kell | K, k, $K^{pa}$, $K^{pb}$ |
| Duffy | $Fy^a$, $Fy^b$ |
| Kidd | $JK^a$, $JK^b$ |

B. Red Blood Cell Enzymes
   Acid phosphatase
   Adenosine deaminase
   Adenylate kinase-1
   Carbonic anhydrase II
   Esterase-D
   Glucose-6-phosphate dehydrogenase (G-6-PD)
   Glyoxalase I
   Phosphoglucomutase-1
   Phosphoglucomutase-2
   6-phosphogluconic dehydrogenase (6PGD)

C. Serum Proteins
   Gm protein
   Complement (C3)
   Haptoglobin
   Transferrin

D. Human Leukocyte Antigens (HLA)
   HLA-A
   HLA-B
   HLA-C
   HLA-D
   HLA-DR

Deoxyribonucleic acid (DNA) analysis

relatively new technology has applicability in paternity testing. More than 30 DNA probes are currently available for investigating virtually any biologic parentage relationship.

To prepare DNA for study using a DNA probe, the DNA is cut into fragments using the restriction fragment length polymorphism (RFLP) test. DNA is removed from cells usually taken from blood samples and precisely cut apart at specific sequences using specialized restriction en-

**Table B-3. A Representative ABO Mating**

Female: Phenotype $A_1$, Genotype $A_1$/O
Male: Phenotype B, Genotype B/O

Female gametes: 50% $A_1$, 50% O
Male gametes: 50% B, 50% O

|  |  | Female gametes | |
|---|---|---|---|
|  |  | $A_1$ | O |
| Male gametes | B | $A_1$B | BO |
|  | O | AO | OO |

Probability of ABO groups of offspring:
Genotypes: 25% $A_1$/B; 25% B/O; 25% $A_1$/O; 25% O/O
Phenotypes: 25% $A_1$B; 25% B; 25% $A_1$; 25% O

## Example 1

| Mother | Alleged Father |
|---|---|
| A1 B8 C7/A2 B7 C2 | A11 B35 C4/A3 B14 C3 |

| Child |
|---|
| A2 B7 C2/A11 B35 C4 |

Summary: The mother contributed A2, B7, C2, therefore the biological father had to contribute A11, B35, and C4. The calculated probability that he is the actual father is based on HLA typing and the frequency of the obligatory genes in the random population.
Conclusion: Nonexclusion—a high probability of paternity.

## Example 2

| Mother | Alleged Father |
|---|---|
| A24 B13 C6/A30 B44 C5 | A25 B44 C3/A1 B55 C2 |

| Child |
|---|
| A30 B44 C5/A3 B7 C7 |

Summary: The mother contributed A30, B44, and C5 to the child. The biological father must have contributed A3, B7, C7. Because the alleged father in this case does not possess these markers, he is excluded.
Conclusion: Exclusion—no possibility of paternity.

**Figure B-1.** Examples of Exclusion and Nonexclusion in Parentage Assessment Using HLA Testing

zymes that act as biologic scissors. After electrophoresis (separation of proteins through the use of an electrical current), the bands of DNA fragments are transferred from the gel medium of the test onto a nylon membrane. The membrane is heated and gene probes labelled with a small amount of radioactive material are added. A gene probe is a small DNA segment manufactured in the laboratory and tagged with a radioactive marker. If the probe and the subject's DNA piece match, the probe displays the subject's polymorphic DNA position on the membrane by emitting radioactivity onto the film. This activity produces an x-ray–like picture, an *autoradiogram* of the DNA of the mother, the child, and the alleged father.

In the future, another method based on polymerase chain reaction (PCR) amplification may replace conventional DNA analysis. This technique, amplified fragment length polymorphism (AMPFLP), produces millions of copies of only the specific portion of the chromosome containing the fragment length polymorphism. This method is faster than traditional analysis, requires smaller blood samples, and works on aged blood samples. It is also less labor-intensive.

## DETERMINATION OF PATERNITY

In order to be able to determine exclusion or nonexclusion, the results of laboratory testing must be analyzed as to

**Table B-4. Examples of Exclusion Probabilities P for RBC antigens**

| Genetic Marker | Mean Probability of Exclusion of Nonfathers | |
|---|---|---|
| Red Cell Antigen | White | Black |
| ABO | 0.15 | 0.18 |
| Rh | 0.22 | 0.20 |
| MNSs | 0.31 | 0.15 |
| Kell | 0.04 | 0.01 |
| Duffy | 0.18 | 0.14 |
| Kidd | 0.19 | 0.16 |

the identity of the obligatory paternal genes. Obligatory paternal genes are those genes that the child must inherit from the biological father. The genetic systems currently in use have a cumulative power of exclusion (P) of greater than 95%. Little difficulty should be encountered in excluding an alleged father (Table B-4).

Two types of exclusion exist: first order and second order. A first-order exclusion is one in which the child has a gene that both the mother and alleged father lack. Second-order exclusions occur when the genes present in an alleged father are not represented in the child—that is, the paternal obligatory genes are not found in the alleged father but are present in the biological mother.

When an exclusion cannot be found, the results of the genetic testing are used to calculate the combined paternity index (PI) and/or cumulative probability of paternity (W). The PI is a ratio that compares the relative probability of paternity of the putative father to that of a random male for any given genetic system.

Illustration:

$$PI = X/Y$$

where  $X =$  the frequency with which the alleged father (af) passes on the obligatory gene, and

$Y =$  the frequency with which the random male (rm) passes on the obligatory gene.

The combined paternity index is achieved by multiplying the PI for each genetic system tested.

The probability of paternity (W) is the percent chance that the alleged father is the biological father based on the frequency of the genetic markers detected. The statistical formulas used for this calculation are predicted using Bayes Theorem, where a prior probability of 0.5 is assumed.

Illustration:

$$W = X/(X + Y)$$

Cumulative probability of paternity results from the multiplication of W for each genetic system tested.

**Bibliography**

Lang, H.K.: Improved paternity testing. Adv. Med. Lab. Prof., November 30, 1992, pp. 8, 9, 13.
Murphy. L.: Twintyping. Adv. Med. Lab. Prof., December 21, 1992, p. 12.
New PCR paternity test faster, more precise. Adv. Med. Lab. Prof., March 18, 1991.
Peck, S.: Parentage assessment and the technology available. Am. Clin. Lab., September, 1989, pp. 19–23.
Sebring, E.S., Polesky, H.F., and Schanfield, M.S.: Gm and Km allotypes in disputed parentage. A.J.C.P., 71(3):281–285, 1979.
Walker, R.H.: Technical Manual, 11th ed. Bethesda, MD. American Association of Blood Banks, 1993, pp. 289–290.

# Answers to Review Questions

## Chapter 1

1. C
2. C
3. C
4. D
5. A
6. E
7. B
8. B
9. D
10. D
11. D
12. A
13. D
14. A
15. A

## Chapter 2

1. D
2. C
3. E
4. D or B
5. B or D
6. A
7. E
8. A
9. C
10. D
11. B
12. A
13. C
14. B
15. C
16. D
17. D
18. D
19. C
20. C
21. D
22. C
23. A
24. C
25. E

26. A
27. C
28. B
29. D
30. B
31. D
32. A
33. C
34. B
35. A
36. D
37. C
38. A
39. D
40. B
41. A
42. C
43. D
44. A
45. C
46. A
47. A
48. D
49. D

## Chapter 3

1. D
2. A
3. D
4. D
5. B
6. C
7. A
8. A
9. B
10. B
11. A
12. D
13. C
14. A
15. D
16. D
17. E

18. A
19. B
20. C
21. C
22. A
23. B
24. A
25. D
26. A
27. B
28. D
29. D
30. C
31. A
32. D
33. B
34. B
35. D
36. E
37. C
38. A
39. D
40. B
41. D
42. D
43. A
44. D
45. D
46. A
47. B

## Chapter 4

1. B
2. B
3. D
4. A
5. C
6. B
7. A
8. D
9. C
10. B or C
11. A

| | | | | | | |
|---|---|---|---|---|---|---|
| **12.** | D | **68.** | C | **14.** | D | |
| **13.** | C | **69.** | A | **15.** | A | |
| **14.** | C | **70.** | D | **16.** | A | |
| **15.** | C | | | **17.** | A | |
| **16.** | D | **Chapter 5** | | **18.** | A | |
| **17.** | A | | | **19.** | B | |
| **18.** | B | **1.** | B | **20.** | B | |
| **19.** | C | **2.** | D | **21.** | C | |
| **20.** | D | **3.** | C | **22.** | B | |
| **21.** | C | **4.** | A | **23.** | B | |
| **22.** | A | **5.** | D | **24.** | A | |
| **23.** | B | **6.** | E | **25.** | D | |
| **24.** | A or D | **7.** | B | **26.** | D | |
| **25.** | A | **8.** | E | **27.** | C | |
| **26.** | D | **9.** | A | **28.** | D | |
| **27.** | D | **10.** | B | **29.** | D | |
| **28.** | C | **11.** | D | **30.** | B | |
| **29.** | D | **12.** | C | **31.** | D | |
| **30.** | E | **13.** | F | **32.** | A | |
| **31.** | C | **14.** | C | **33.** | D | |
| **32.** | E | **15.** | A | **34.** | A | |
| **33.** | D | **16.** | B | **35.** | B | |
| **34.** | A | **17.** | A | **36.** | E | |
| **35.** | D | **18.** | A | **37.** | A | |
| **36.** | A | **19.** | D | **38.** | C | |
| **37.** | B | **20.** | A | **39.** | C | |
| **38.** | C | **21.** | D | | | |
| **39.** | C | **22.** | B | **Chapter 7** | | |
| **40.** | D | **23.** | B | | | |
| **41.** | D | **24.** | D | **1.** | B | |
| **42.** | A | **25.** | A | **2.** | D | |
| **43.** | B | **26.** | C | **3.** | C | |
| **44.** | A | **27.** | D | **4.** | C | |
| **45.** | B | **28.** | B | **5.** | B | |
| **46.** | B | **29.** | A | **6.** | C | |
| **47.** | B | **30.** | B | **7.** | D | |
| **48.** | C | **31.** | B | **8.** | C | |
| **49.** | C | **32.** | B | **9.** | A | |
| **50.** | A | **33.** | A | **10.** | C | |
| **51.** | D | **34.** | A | **11.** | B | |
| **52.** | A | **35.** | D | **12.** | D | |
| **53.** | C | | | **13.** | B | |
| **54.** | A | **Chapter 6** | | **14.** | D | |
| **55.** | D | | | **15.** | A | |
| **56.** | B | **1.** | D | **16.** | C | |
| **57.** | A | **2.** | A | **17.** | E | |
| **58.** | B | **3.** | C | **18.** | A | |
| **59.** | B | **4.** | B | **19.** | A | |
| **60.** | A | **5.** | D | **20.** | B | |
| **61.** | A | **6.** | C | **21.** | B | |
| **62.** | A | **7.** | C | **22.** | B | |
| **63.** | B | **8.** | E | **23.** | A | |
| **64.** | C | **9.** | C | **24.** | D | |
| **65.** | D | **10.** | B | **25.** | C | |
| **66.** | A | **11.** | B | **26.** | D | |
| **67.** | B | **12.** | A | **27.** | C | |
| | | **13.** | B | | | |

28. D
29. D
30. D
31. B
32. B
33. D
34. A
35. B
36. E
37. C
38. B
39. A
40. B
41. D
42. A
43. B
44. D
45. D
46. A
47. C
48. D

## Chapter 9

1. B
2. E
3. A
4. C
5. C
6. D
7. D
8. D
9. A
10. B
11. D
12. A
13. C
14. B
15. E
16. C
17. C
18. D
19. C
20. B
21. D
22. C
23. D
24. A
25. D
26. D
27. C
28. D
29. B
30. B

## Chapter 10

1. A
2. E
3. B
4. D
5. D
6. D
7. A
8. B
9. D
10. C
11. B
12. D
13. C
14. C
15. B
16. D
17. A
18. B
19. D
20. D
21. D
22. D
23. D
24. B
25. B
26. D
27. D
28. C
29. D
30. A
31. D
32. B
33. C
34. C
35. B
36. B
37. B
38. D
39. D
40. C
41. C
42. D
43. D
44. C
45. D
46. A
47. C
48. B
49. D
50. D

## Chapter 11

1. B
2. B

3. D
4. D
5. B
6. C
7. C
8. D
9. D
10. D
11. C
12. D
13. A
14. C
15. C
16. A
17. A
18. C
19. B
20. B
21. D
22. C
23. D
24. B
25. A

## Chapter 12

1. D
2. C
3. B
4. A
5. D
6. C
7. D
8. A
9. D
10. B
11. D
12. A
13. D
14. A
15. D
16. D
17. D
18. D
19. C
20. D
21. C
22. A
23. B
24. D
25. D
26. B
27. C
28. D
29. C
30. C

| | | |
|---|---|---|
| **31.** D | **12.** D | **40.** C |
| **32.** D | **13.** B | **41.** D |
| **33.** C | **14.** A | |
| **34.** A | **15.** B | **Chapter 16** |
| **35.** E | **16.** B | |
| **36.** C | **17.** A | **1.** D |
| **37.** D | **18.** B | **2.** C |
| **38.** B | **19.** D | **3.** D |
| **39.** D | **20.** B | **4.** A |
| **40.** A | **21.** A | **5.** B |
| **41.** B | **22.** D | **6.** C |
| **42.** C | **23.** A | **7.** D |
| **43.** D | **24.** B | **8.** D |
| | **25.** D | **9.** C |
| **Chapter 13** | **26.** D | **10.** A |
| | **27.** C | **11.** D |
| **1.** B | **28.** D | **12.** A |
| **2.** D | **29.** D | **13.** D |
| **3.** B | **30.** B | **14.** A |
| **4.** D | **31.** D | |
| **5.** B | **32.** B | **Chapter 17** |
| **6.** D | **33.** D | |
| **7.** B | **34.** B | **1.** C |
| **8.** D | **35.** C | **2.** E |
| **9.** C | **36.** C | **3.** E |
| **10.** A | **37.** D | **4.** B |
| **11.** B | **38.** C | **5.** C |
| | **39.** D | **6.** A |

# Fundamentals of Immunohematology

# Glossary

**AABB.** American Association of Blood Banks

**AB cis gene.** A condition in which both the A and B genes seem to be inherited on a single chromosome.

**abruptio placentae.** The premature separation of a normally situated placenta.

**acquired immunodeficiency syndrome (AIDS).** An immune disorder affecting (T4) lymphocytes. This disorder is caused by the HTLV-III (human T cell leukemia virus) or LAV virus, also referred to as the human immunodeficiency virus (HIV).

**acriflavin.** The yellow dye used in some commercial anti-B reagents. This additive can produce false agglutination in some individuals but this is rare.

**acute.** Term for a condition of sudden and short duration.

**aerosol.** The introduction into the air of substances in droplet form.

**affinity.** The bond between a single antigenic determinant and an individual combining site.

**agammaglobulinemia.** The absence of plasma gamma globulin due to either congenital or acquired states.

**agglutination.** The clumping of particles that have antigens on their surface, such as erythrocytes, by antibody molecules that form bridges between the antigenic determinants.

**agglutinin.** The older term for an antibody.

**agglutinogen.** The older term for antigen.

**alleles.** Alternate forms of genes that code for traits of the same type; for example, the genes Fy$^a$ and Fy$^b$ are alleles.

**allergic reaction.** A reaction to soluble constituents in donor plasma.

**alloantibodies.** Immunoglobulins (antibodies) produced in response to exposure to foreign antigens of the same species.

**allogeneic.** Denotes genetically different individuals of the same species.

**amniocentesis.** The process of removing fluid from the amniotic sac for study, for example, chromosome analysis or biochemical studies.

**amorphic gene.** A gene that produces no detectable gene product, i.e., antigen.

**anamnestic antibody response.** An antibody "memory" response. This secondary response occurs on subsequent exposure to a previously encountered and recognized foreign antigen. An anamnestic response is characterized by rapid production of IgG antibodies.

**anaphylactic reaction.** A severe allergic reaction that can develop in IgA-deficient patients who have developed anti-IgA antibodies.

**anaphylactoid reaction.** A severe reaction to soluble constituents in donor plasma which produces edema.

**antenatal.** Before birth.

**antibodies.** Specific glycoproteins (immunoglobulins) produced in response to an antigenic challenge. Antibodies can be found in blood plasma and body fluids such as tears, saliva, and breast milk.

**antibody elution.** See eluate.

**antigen (antigenic, immunogenic).** A foreign substance that can elicit an immune (antibody) response.

**antigenicity.** The ability of an antigen to stimulate the immune response. The antigenicity of a substance may be influenced by the number of antigen receptor sites.

**antithetical antigens.** Two antigens controlled by a pair of allelic genes such as Kell (K) and Cellano (k).

**asymptomatic.** Exhibiting no symptoms of a disease or disorder.

**autocontrol.** A test consisting of the patient's erythrocytes and serum.

**autoimmune hemolytic anemia.** A condition of destruction of erythrocytes by self-produced antibodies.

**autologous donation.** Donation of blood for one's self. Autologous donation may take the form of predeposit or autotransfusion, for example, intraoperative autotransfusion, hemodilution, or postoperative autotransfusion.

**avidity.** The strength with which a multivalent antibody binds to a multivalent antigen.

**bilirubin.** A breakdown product of erythrocyte catabolism.

**blood substitutes.** Artificial substances that mimic the effect of a natural blood constituent, such as erythrocytes.

**Bombay phenotype.** The failure of an individual to express inherited A or B genes because of the lack of at least one H gene and the subsequent lack of the resulting H precursor substance.

**bursa equivalent.** Equal to the processing area, the bursa, in birds.

**carrier state.** The asymptomatic condition of harboring an infectious organism. This term may also refer to a heterozygous individual or the carrier of a recessive gene.

**chimeras.** Two-cell populations.

**chimerism.** A condition producing two cell populations in an individual.

**chorioamnionitis.** Inflammation of the membranes comprising the amniotic sac.

**chronic.** Term for condition of long duration.

**cis position.** Refers to the situation in which a gene on one chromosome of a homologous pair affects the actions of a related gene on the same chromosome.

**cold agglutinins.** Antibodies that react at room or colder temperatures.

**compatibility testing.** A term frequently used synonymously with the term crossmatch. Compatibility testing includes ABO and Rh grouping, screening of serum for alloantibodies, and crossmatching.

**complement.** A complex of plasma proteins.

**compound antigen.** The term used to express the idea that certain combinations of antigens demonstrate a combined effect, for example, the ce or f antigen.

**Coombs' test.** The older term for the antiglobulin test.

**critical incident.** A problem or any deviation from the standard operating procedures of the blood bank.

**Dane particle.** The intact, double-shelled hepatitis B virus.

**DAT.** Direct antiglobulin test.

**deglycerolized red blood cells.** See frozen blood.

**direct antiglobulin test (also called the direct antihuman globulin test.)** A test performed to detect the coating of erythrocytes with antibodies.

**disseminated intravascular coagulation (DIC).** Secondary fibrinolysis in which excessive clotting and fibrinolytic activity occur.

**dominant.** The gene that is expressed if present.

**dosage effect.** A variation in strength of agglutination between homozygous and heterozygous erythrocytes. The presence of a homozygous genotype can express itself with more antigen than the heterozygous genotype and can produce a stronger degree of agglutination.

**ectopic pregnancy.** The gestation of a fertilized egg outside the uterus, most commonly in a fallopian tube.

**edema.** Accumulation of fluid in the tissues that produces swelling.

**EDTA.** Tripotassium ethylenediamine tetra-acetate. This is a type of anticoagulant that removes calcium ($Ca^{++}$) through the process of chelation.

**eluate.** The product of deliberate manipulation of a red cell suspension to break an antigen-antibody complex (elu-

tion), with subsequent release of the antibody into the surrounding medium.

**endotoxemia.** A condition of having bacterial cell wall heat-stable toxins in the circulation. These toxins are pyrogenic and increase capillary permeability.

**epitope.** A specific segment of a molecule.

**Epstein-Barr virus (EBV).** A human herpes DNA virus that is the causative agent of infectious mononucleosis.

**erythrocytes.** The scientific term for red blood cells.

**erythropoiesis.** The process of producing red blood cells.

**etiology.** A synonym for cause (of a disease or disorder).

**exchange transfusion.** The replacement of an infant's coated erythrocytes with donor blood until a one or two total blood volume transfer is accomplished.

**extramedullary hematopoiesis.** Production of erythrocytes outside the bone marrow which can produce enlargement of the liver and spleen.

**extravascular hemolysis.** The phagocytizing and catabolizing of erythrocytes by the reticuloendothelial system, for example, the spleen.

**fab fragments.** The two antigen-binding fragments that result from the digestion of an antibody by proteolytic enzymes, e.g., papain.

**frozen blood.** A term used to refer to red blood cells that are coated with a substance such as glycerol, frozen to $-80°$ C, and deglycerolized when needed.

**genotype.** An individual's composite genetic inheritance of maternal and paternal genes. For example, A/O is one of the genotypes that a group O person may have.

**gestation.** The period of development and growth of the unborn in viviparous animals, including humans, from fertilization of the ovum to birth.

**glycosphingolipid.** A sphingolipid containing the sugar glucose or galactose. Sphingolipids are phospholipids containing sphingosine. Examples are ceramide and cerebroside.

**goodness of fit.** The complementary matching of antigenic determinants and the antigen-binding sites of corresponding antibodies that influences the strength of bonding between antigens and antibodies.

**graft-versus-host disease.** An intense and frequently fatal immunologic reaction of engrafted cells against the host caused by the infusion of immunocompetent lymphocytes into individuals with impaired immunity, such as organ transplantation patients.

**granulocyte.** A type of leukocytic white blood cell.

**haplotype.** The gene complex or genetic composition of an individual or population.

**hapten.** A very small molecule which can bind to a larger carrier molecule and behaves as an antigen.

**haptoglobin.** A plasma globulin which binds to hemoglobin alpha-beta dimers.

**hematoma.** A swollen area under the skin or membranes that results from blood collecting underneath. If this area is under the skin, a large bruised area results.

**hematopoietic tissues.** Blood-producing structures of the body, such as the liver, spleen, and bone marrow.

**hemochromatosis.** A condition of accumulation of iron in the tissues. This condition is likely to develop in chronically transfused patients.

**hemolysis.** The rupturing of a cell membrane, for example of an erythrocyte, with subsequent dumping of cytoplasmic contents.

**hemolytic disease of the newborn (previously called *Erythroblastosis fetalis*).** An immunologic incompatibility between mother and fetus that can produce severe or fatal consequences to the unborn or newborn infant due to destruction of erythrocytes and the accumulation of breakdown products.

**hemopexin.** A transport protein in the blood circulation.

**hemosiderin.** An insoluble storage form of iron.

**heterozygous.** The genetic state of having two dissimilar genes for the same trait.

**high protein solution.** A medium used in blood bank testing, for example, albumin.

**high titer-low avidity (HTLA) antibodies.** Antibodies with similar serologic characteristics that have a low antigen binding capacity and a high titration value, now referred to within the high-incidence group of antigens.

**histocompatibility (HLA) antigens.** Cell surface protein antigens found on blood and body cells, such as leukocytes and platelets, that readily provoke an immune response if transferred into a genetically different (allogeneic) individual of the same species.

**HIV.** See HTLV III.

**homozygous.** The genetic state of having two similar genes for the same trait, for example AA or cc.

**HTLV III.** Human T cell leukemia virus. A type of retrovirus that is also known as LAV or HIV.

**hypochromic or hypochromia.** A hematologic term used to describe erythrocytes that appear pale when examined microscopically.

**hypogammaglobulinemia.** A decreased gamma globulin fraction of plasma protein that can lead to errors in blood typing because of weak or missing antibodies.

**hypothermia.** A decrease in body temperature to below 30° C at the sino-atrial node of the heart that results in ventricular arrhythmias. The rapid infusion of large volumes of refrigerated blood can cause this condition.

**hypovolemic shock syndrome.** A physiologic condition, such as decreased blood pressure, resulting from the rapid loss of 15 to 20% or more of blood volume.

**icterus.** A synonym for jaundice or the yellow appearance of the skin and mucous membranes due to bilirubin (a product of red cell breakdown) accumulation.

**immunocompetent.** The term referring to lymphocytes that acquire thymus-dependent characteristics which allow them to function in an immune response.

**immunodominant sugar.** The carbohydrate residual that confers antigen specificity to a molecule.

**immunogenic.** See antigen.

**immunoglobulins.** A synonym for antibodies.

**immunohematology.** The study of blood-related antigens and antibodies as applied to situations such as blood transfusion and hemolytic disease of the newborn. Applications of immunohematology are related to blood transfusion.

**incompatibility.** Agglutination of antigen-bearing erythrocytes and their corresponding antibodies.

**intraperitoneal fetal transfusion (IPT).** The administration of blood to an unborn infant through the abdominal cavity.

**intrauterine.** Within the uterus.

**intravascular hemolysis.** The lysing of erythrocytes within the vessels of the circulatory system.

**intrinsic coagulation mechanism.** The initial stage of blood coagulation that can be activated by antigen-antibody complexes.

**in vitro.** Outside the body, for example, in the test tube.

**in vivo.** In a living organism.

**jaundice.** See icterus.

**kernicterus.** The deposition of increased bilirubin, a red cell breakdown product in lipid-rich nervous tissue such as the brain, which can produce mental retardation or death in the newborn. This condition can occur when circulating plasma bilirubin levels reach 20 mg/dL in a full-term infant and at lower levels in a premature infant.

**Kleinhauer-Betke test.** A procedure based on the differences in solubility between adult and fetal hemoglobin. The test is performed on a maternal blood specimen to detect fetal-maternal hemorrhage.

**latent infection.** Persistent infection characterized by periods of reactivation.

**LISS.** An antibody enhancement medium, low ionic strength salt solution.

**low incidence antigens.** Antigens that occur in very few individuals in a population.

**massive transfusion.** The administration of enough blood or components to constitute a complete volume replacement in 24 hours or less, for example, 8 to 10 or more units in an adult.

**microspherocytosis.** A hematologic term used to describe the microscopic appearance of smaller than normal, dense-appearing erythrocytes.

**monoclonal antibodies.** Purified immunoglobulins produced by cells that are cloned from a single fusion-type hybridoma cell.

**murine hybridomas.** A fusion product of malignant and normal cells which produces large quantities of monoclonal antibodies.

**neocytes.** Young red blood cells.

**neonatologist.** A physician specializing in the treatment of disorders of the newborn.

**nonsecretor.** The absence of water-soluble antigens in body fluids.

**oncogenic.** Associated with tumor formation.

**paroxysmal cold hemoglobinuria (PCH).** This form of destruction of erythrocytes is due to an IgG protein that reacts with the red blood cells in colder parts of the body and subsequently causes complement components to bind irreversibly to erythrocytes. It is commonly seen as an acute transient condition secondary to viral infection.

**paroxysmal nocturnal hemoglobinuria (PNH).** A disorder in which the patient's erythrocytes act as a complement activator. The activation of complement results in excessive lysis of the patient's erythrocytes.

**pathogenicity.** The disease-producing potential of a microorganism.

**phenotype.** The detectable or expressed characteristics of genes.

**phlebotomy.** The process of withdrawing blood from the circulatory system. The usual site for the phlebotomy procedure is a vein.

**phototherapy.** The use of ultraviolet light to accelerate the breakdown of bilirubin that has abnormally accumulated in the skin.

**plasma.** The straw-colored fluid in circulating or anticoagulated blood.

**polyagglutination.** Agglutination of erythrocytes by most normal human sera. Examples of polyagglutination include T and Tn activation as well as Cad polyagglutinability.

**postpartum.** After birth.

**post-transfusion viability.** The length of survival of blood cells after infusion into the human body, believed to be related to the structural and metabolic status of the cell membrane.

**potency.** Strength.

**potent.** To possess strength.

**prenatal.** Before birth.

**primary antibody response.** An immunologic (IgM antibody) response following a foreign antigen challenge.

**primiparous.** Term for a woman who has had at least one pregnancy that resulted in a live infant.

**proficiency testing.** Measure of accomplishment.

**properdin pathway.** The former term for the alternate pathway of complement activation.

**prophylaxis.** Prevention.

**prozone phenomenon.** A possible cause of false-negative antigen-antibody reactions due to an excessive amount of antibody.

**recessive.** Term used for a gene which is not expressed unless it is in the homozygous form.

**reticulocytosis.** A condition in which the number of cells in the normal developmental stage preceding the mature erythrocyte stage is increased.

**retrovirus.** A type of virus that carries a single, positive-stranded RNA and uses a special enzyme, reverse transcriptase, to convert viral RNA into DNA.

**Rh factor.** A blood group antigen, named for the Rhesus monkey, originally identified because an antibody agglu-tinated the erythrocytes of all rhesus monkeys and 85% of humans. The antibody was later discovered to be the Landsteiner-Wiener antibody, which is dissimilar from the Rh antibody; the antigen was actually the Landsteiner-Wiener antigen.

**Rh null.** The term used for the phenotype in which no Rh antigens are expressed.

**rouleaux.** Pseudoagglutination or the false clumping of erythrocytes when the cells are suspended in their own serum. This phenomenon resembles agglutination and is due to the presence of an abnormal protein in the serum, plasma expanders, such as dextran, or Wharton's jelly from cord blood samples.

**secretions.** Fluids such as tears, saliva, and semen that may contain water-soluble substances such as A, B, and/or H antigens.

**secretor.** The presence of water soluble antigens in body fluids.

**sepsis.** Microbial infection throughout the systemic circulation.

**serum.** The straw-colored fluid remaining when blood has clotted.

**specificity.** The complementary relationship between the binding sites of antibodies directed against determinants of a similar-type antigen.

**spherocytes.** Hematologic term to describe dense-appearing erythrocytes on microscopic examination.

**steric hindrance.** Mutual blocking of dissimilar antibodies with the same binding constant and directed against antigenic determinants located in close proximity to each other on a cell's surface.

**storage lesion.** The ATP-independent, irreversible loss of surface area of an erythrocyte stored in anticoagulant.

**subclinical infection.** An early or mild form of a disease without visible signs.

**surface of shear.** The outer edge of the ionic cloud surrounding a particle, for example erythrocytes, in an electrolyte solution.

**surrogate tests.** Tests that nonspecifically detect a condition or disorder. In hepatitis testing, the surrogate tests are the ALT and hepatitis B core antibody tests.

**symptom.** An indication of a disorder or disease or a variation in normal body function.

**therapeutic phlebotomy.** The process of removing venous blood as a treatment for a condition or disorder such as polycythemia vera.

**thrombocytopenia.** A decrease in the normal number of circulating platelets.

**titer.** The concentration or strength of an antibody expressed as the highest dilution of the serum that produces agglutination, for example 1:4, 1:8.

**transferase enzyme.** A type of enzyme that catalyzes the transfer of a monosaccharide molecule from a donor substrate to the precursor substance. This type of biochemical activity is related to the development of A, B, and H antigens.

**transplacental hemorrhage.** The entrance of fetal blood cells into the maternal circulation.

**transposition.** The situation of having a gene on one chromosome of a homologous pair affect the actions of a related gene on the other homolog.

**type and screen procedure.** This technique consists of performing an ABO and Rh typing and an indirect anti-globulin test.

**universal blood and body fluid precautions.** Specific regulations that conform to current state and Federal requirements. These precautions assume that *all* blood and body fluid specimens have the potential for transmitting disease.

**universal donor.** A misnomer often used for group O Rh negative blood.

**universal recipient.** A general term used to refer to a group AB patient.

**venous blood.** The circulating blood in the veins.

**WAIHA.** Warm autoimmune hemolytic anemia. This form of autoimmune anemia is associated with antibodies reactive at warm temperatures.

**weak D (D$^u$).** A phenotype of the Rh blood group system.

**weak D (D$^u$) rosette test.** A procedure that uses D positive indicator erythrocytes to form identifiable rosettes around individual D positive fetal cells that may be in the maternal circulation.

**zeta potential.** The difference in electrostatic potential between the net charge at the cell membrane and the charge at the surface of shear.

# Index

*Page numbers in italics refer to figures. Page numbers followed by the letter "t" refer to tables.*